# Restless Legs Syndrome

**NEUROLOGICAL DISEASE AND THERAPY**

1. Handbook of Parkinson's Disease, *edited by William C. Koller*
2. Medical Therapy of Acute Stroke, *edited by Mark Fisher*
3. Familial Alzheimer's Disease: Molecular Genetics and Clinical Perspectives, *edited by Gary D. Miner, Ralph W. Richter, John P. Blass, Jimmie L. Valentine, and Linda A. Winters-Miner*
4. Alzheimer's Disease: Treatment and Long-Term Management, *edited by Jeffrey L. Cummings and Bruce L. Miller*
5. Therapy of Parkinson's Disease, *edited by William C. Koller and George Paulson*
6. Handbook of Sleep Disorders, *edited by Michael J. Thorpy*
7. Epilepsy and Sudden Death, *edited by Claire M. Lathers and Paul L. Schraeder*
8. Handbook of Multiple Sclerosis, *edited by Stuart D. Cook*
9. Memory Disorders: Research and Clinical Practice, *edited by Takehiko Yanagihara and Ronald C. Petersen*
10. The Medical Treatment of Epilepsy, *edited by Stanley R. Resor, Jr., and Henn Kutt*
11. Cognitive Disorders: Pathophysiology and Treatment, *edited by Leon J. Thal, Walter H. Moos, and Elkan R. Gamzu*
12. Handbook of Amyotrophic Lateral Sclerosis, *edited by Richard Alan Smith*
13. Handbook of Parkinson's Disease: Second Edition, Revised and Expanded, *edited by William C. Koller*
14. Handbook of Pediatric Epilepsy, *edited by Jerome V. Murphy and Fereydoun Dehkharghani*
15. Handbook of Tourette's Syndrome and Related Tic and Behavioral Disorders, *edited by Roger Kurlan*
16. Handbook of Cerebellar Diseases, *edited by Richard Lechtenberg*
17. Handbook of Cerebrovascular Diseases, *edited by Harold P. Adams, Jr.*
18. Parkinsonian Syndromes, *edited by Matthew B. Stern and William C. Koller*
19. Handbook of Head and Spine Trauma, *edited by Jonathan Greenberg*
20. Brain Tumors: A Comprehensive Text, *edited by Robert A. Morantz and John W. Walsh*
21. Monoamine Oxidase Inhibitors in Neurological Diseases, *edited by Abraham Lieberman, C. Warren Olanow, Moussa B. H. Youdim, and Keith Tipton*
22. Handbook of Dementing Illnesses, *edited by John C. Morris*
23. Handbook of Myasthenia Gravis and Myasthenic Syndromes, *edited by Robert P. Lisak*
24. Handbook of Neurorehabilitation, *edited by David C. Good and James R. Couch, Jr.*
25. Therapy with Botulinum Toxin, *edited by Joseph Jankovic and Mark Hallett*
26. Principles of Neurotoxicology, *edited by Louis W. Chang*
27. Handbook of Neurovirology, *edited by Robert R. McKendall and William G. Stroop*
28. Handbook of Neuro-Urology, *edited by David N. Rushton*
29. Handbook of Neuroepidemiology, *edited by Philip B. Gorelick and Milton Alter*

30. Handbook of Tremor Disorders, *edited by Leslie J. Findley and William C. Koller*
31. Neuro-Ophthalmological Disorders: Diagnostic Work-Up and Management, *edited by Ronald J. Tusa and Steven A. Newman*
32. Handbook of Olfaction and Gustation, *edited by Richard L. Doty*
33. Handbook of Neurological Speech and Language Disorders, *edited by Howard S. Kirshner*
34. Therapy of Parkinson's Disease: Second Edition, Revised and Expanded, *edited by William C. Koller and George Paulson*
35. Evaluation and Management of Gait Disorders, *edited by Barney S. Spivack*
36. Handbook of Neurotoxicology, *edited by Louis W. Chang and Robert S. Dyer*
37. Neurological Complications of Cancer, *edited by Ronald G. Wiley*
38. Handbook of Autonomic Nervous System Dysfunction, *edited by Amos D. Korczyn*
39. Handbook of Dystonia, *edited by Joseph King Ching Tsui and Donald B. Calne*
40. Etiology of Parkinson's Disease, *edited by Jonas H. Ellenberg, William C. Koller and J. William Langston*
41. Practical Neurology of the Elderly, *edited by Jacob I. Sage and Margery H. Mark*
42. Handbook of Muscle Disease, *edited by Russell J. M. Lane*
43. Handbook of Multiple Sclerosis: Second Edition, Revised and Expanded, *edited by Stuart D. Cook*
44. Central Nervous System Infectious Diseases and Therapy, *edited by Karen L. Roos*
45. Subarachnoid Hemorrhage: Clinical Management, *edited by Takehiko Yanagihara, David G. Piepgras, and John L. D. Atkinson*
46. Neurology Practice Guidelines, *edited by Richard Lechtenberg and Henry S. Schutta*
47. Spinal Cord Diseases: Diagnosis and Treatment, *edited by Gordon L. Engler, Jonathan Cole, and W. Louis Merton*
48. Management of Acute Stroke, *edited by Ashfaq Shuaib and Larry B. Goldstein*
49. Sleep Disorders and Neurological Disease, *edited by Antonio Culebras*
50. Handbook of Ataxia Disorders, *edited by Thomas Klockgether*
51. The Autonomic Nervous System in Health and Disease, *David S. Goldstein*
52. Axonal Regeneration in the Central Nervous System, *edited by Nicholas A. Ingoglia and Marion Murray*
53. Handbook of Multiple Sclerosis: Third Edition, *edited by Stuart D. Cook*
54. Long-Term Effects of Stroke, *edited by Julien Bogousslavsky*
55. Handbook of the Autonomic Nervous System in Health and Disease, *edited by C. Liana Bolis, Julio Licinio, and Stefano Govoni*
56. Dopamine Receptors and Transporters: Function, Imaging, and Clinical Implication, Second Edition, *edited by Anita Sidhu, Marc Laruelle, and Philippe Vernier*
57. Handbook of Olfaction and Gustation: Second Edition, Revised and Expanded, *edited by Richard L. Doty*

58. Handbook of Stereotactic and Functional Neurosurgery, *edited by Michael Schulder*
59. Handbook of Parkinson's Disease: Third Edition, *edited by Rajesh Pahwa, Kelly E. Lyons, and William C. Koller*
60. Clinical Neurovirology, *edited by Avindra Nath and Joseph R. Berger*
61. Neuromuscular Junction Disorders: Diagnosis and Treatment, *Matthew N. Meriggioli, James F. Howard, Jr., and C. Michel Harper*
62. Drug-Induced Movement Disorders, *edited by Kapil D. Sethi*
63. Therapy of Parkinson's Disease: Third Edition, Revised and Expanded, *edited by Rajesh Pahwa, Kelly E. Lyons, and William C. Koller*
64. Epilepsy: Scientific Foundations of Clinical Practice, *edited by Jong M. Rho, Raman Sankar, and José E. Cavazos*
65. Handbook of Tourette's Syndrome and Related Tic and Behavioral Disorders: Second Edition, *edited by Roger Kurlan*
66. Handbook of Cerebrovascular Diseases: Second Edition, Revised and Expanded, *edited by Harold P. Adams, Jr.*
67. Emerging Neurological Infections, *edited by Christopher Power and Richard T. Johnson*
68. Treatment of Pediatric Neurologic Disorders, *edited by Harvey S. Singer, Eric H. Kossoff, Adam L. Hartman, and Thomas O. Crawford*
69. Synaptic Plasticity : Basic Mechanisms to Clinical Applications, *edited by Michel Baudry, Xiaoning Bi, and Steven S. Schreiber*
70. Handbook of Essential Tremor and Other Tremor Disorders, *edited by Kelly E. Lyons and Rajesh Pahwa*
71. Handbook of Peripheral Neuropathy, *edited by Mark B. Bromberg and A. Gordon Smith*
72. Carotid Artery Stenosis: Current and Emerging Treatments, *edited by Seemant Chaturvedi and Peter M. Rothwell*
73. Gait Disorders: Evaluation and Management, *edited by Jeffrey M. Hausdorff and Neil B. Alexander*
74. Surgical Management of Movement Disorders (HBK), *edited by Gordon H. Baltuch and Matthew B. Stern*
75. Neurogenetics: Scientific and Clinical Advances, *edited by David R. Lynch*
76. Epilepsy Surgery: Principles and Controversies, *edited by John W. Miller and Daniel L. Silbergeld*
77. Clinician's Guide To Sleep Disorders, *edited by Nathaniel F. Watson and Bradley Vaughn*
78. Amyotrophic Lateral Sclerosis, *edited by Hiroshi Mitsumoto, Serge Przedborski and Paul H. Gordon*
79. Duchenne Muscular Dystrophy: Advances in Therapeutics, *edited by Jeffrey S. Chamberlain and Thomas A. Rando*
80. Handbook of Multiple Sclerosis, Fourth Edition, *edited by Stuart D. Cook*

81. Brain Embolism, *edited by Louis R. Caplan and Warren J. Manning*
82. Handbook of Secondary Dementias, *edited by Roger Kurlan*
83. Parkinson's Disease: Genetics and Pathogenesis, *edited by Ted M. Dawson*
84. Migraine, *Russell Lane and Paul Davies*
85. Migraine and Other Headache Disorders, *edited by Richard B. Lipton and Marcelo Bigal*
86. Restless Legs Syndrome: Diagnosis and Treatment, *edited by William G. Ondo*
87. Handbook of Dementing Illnesses, Second Edition, *edited by John C. Morris, James E. Galvin, and David M. Holtzman*
88. Acute Stroke: Bench to Bedside, *edited by Anish Bhardwaj, Nabil J. Alkayed, Jeffrey R. Kirsch, and Richard J. Traystman*

# Restless Legs Syndrome

## Diagnosis and Treatment

edited by

William G. Ondo

*Baylor College of Medicine*
*Houston, Texas, U.S.A.*

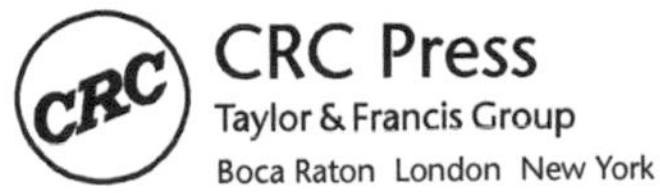

CRC Press
Taylor & Francis Group
Boca Raton London New York

CRC Press is an imprint of the
Taylor & Francis Group, an **informa** business

CRC Press
Taylor & Francis Group
6000 Broken Sound Parkway NW, Suite 300
Boca Raton, FL 33487-2742

First issued in paperback 2019



ISBN-13: 978-0-8493-3614-0 (hbk)
ISBN-13: 978-0-367-39021-1 (pbk)



A CIP record for this book is available from the British Library.

Library of Congress Cataloging-in-Publication Data available on application

**Visit the Taylor & Francis Web site at**
**http://www.taylorandfrancis.com**

**and the CRC Press Web site at**
**http://www.crcpress.com**

*I would like to dedicate this book to family, colleagues, and patients. My wife Vera and children, Carson and Sierra, provided perspective throughout the process. The authors, all leaders in the still collegial RLS research community, enthusiastically (well, usually enthusiastically) provided outstanding chapters, many of which have not been previously published. My patients with RLS initially stoked my interest in the condition and taught me almost everything I know about the disease, its consequences, and its management.*

# Preface

In 1996, I wrote my first paper as a movement disorder fellow. It was basically a clinical description of 54 restless legs syndrome patients with an emphasis on neuropathy. At the poster, I was approached by Art Walters, the leader of the fledgling International Restless Legs Study Group. Apparently, I was now a restless legs syndrome expert! I continued restless legs syndrome research in between the Parkinson's disease and dystonia cases that constituted the bulk of my clinic.

Ten years later, here I am editing a book on restless legs syndrome that contains thousands of references, almost all of which are more interesting and meaningful than my original paper. Most book prefaces discuss the rapid advances in their topic and the need for a current review, which constitutes the subsequent pages. However, few, if any, medical topics have evolved more rapidly than restless legs syndrome. Although restless legs syndrome was described centuries ago, most of the meaningful research concerning restless legs syndrome phenotype, epidemiology, pathophysiology, and treatment has occurred within the past decade. All objective measures of research interest, such as citation index numbers and governmental research funding, have increased dramatically during this period.

This book summarizes our current understanding of restless legs syndrome. The chapters cover all of the latest relevant restless legs syndrome science and pertinent related topics. The book is structured so that readers with focused interests can easily view specific sections and chapters. The book should be equally germane for the basic science researcher in restless legs syndrome, the clinical restless legs syndrome researcher, and the medical practitioner.

The book begins with a basic science section reviewing related background topics, such as sleep, circadian control, dopamine systems, and iron metabolism, and restless legs syndrome–specific chapters, including pathology, physiology, modeling, and genetics. Section II summarizes related clinical aspects, such as sleep deprivation and periodic limb movements; it includes restless legs syndrome–specific chapters on diagnosis and disease descriptions, epidemiology, and pediatric restless legs syndrome. Additional perspective is provided with a historic summary of restless legs syndrome and patient stories supplied by the director of the RLS Foundation , a patient organization. Section III consists of seven chapters that discuss individual diseases associated with restless legs syndrome. These include systemic iron deficiency, uremia, pregnancy, neuropathy, and Parkinson's disease.

Section IV concentrates on the rapidly expanding therapeutic options. After an overview, individual chapters focus on dopaminergics, opioids, iron, and other treatment-specific issues. Finally a "Future Directions" chapter summarizes where we are and where we are heading.

*William G. Ondo*

# Preface

# Contents

*Preface* .... *v*
*Contributors* .... *xvii*

***Section I: Basic Science***

**1. Overview of Sleep** ........................................ ***1***
*Allison V. Chan and Clete A. Kushida*
Introduction .... 1
Normal Sleep Architecture and Sleep Stages .... 1
Ontogeny of Sleep .... 3
Adequate Sleep .... 3
Sleep Deprivation .... 4
Phylogeny of Sleep .... 5
Physiological Determinants of Sleep .... 5
Biochemical Determinants of Sleep .... 8
Sleep Disorders Classification .... 8
Summary .... 10
References .... 10

**2. The Brain's Dopamine Systems and Their Relevance to Restless Legs Syndrome** ........................................ ***15***
*Alon A. Freeman and David B. Rye*
Synthesis and Metabolism of Dopamine .... 15
Physiological Effects of Dopamine (Cellular and Subcellular) .... 18
Functional Anatomy of Central Dopamine Systems .... 19
Circadian and Homeostatic Influences upon Central Dopamine Signaling .... 22
Summary: Dopamine in "State" Control and Its Relevance to Restless Legs Syndrome/Periodic Limb Movements .... 23
References .... 25

**3. Circadian Physiology** . . . . . . . . . . . . . . . . . . . . . . . . . . . . . . . *31*
*Mauro Manconi and Luigi Ferini-Strambi*
Introduction . . . . 31
Entrainment Effect of Light–Dark Alternation . . . . 31
Suprachiasmatic Nucleus . . . . 32
Melatonin . . . . 34
Circadian and Homeostatic Control of Sleep . . . . 37
Circadian Pattern of Restless Legs Syndrome/ Periodic Limb Movements . . . . 38
References . . . . 42

**4. Systemic Iron Regulation** . . . . . . . . . . . . . . . . . . . . . . . . . . . . . *49*
*John Beard*
Introduction . . . . 49
Regulation of Absorption . . . . 50
Control of Central Nervous System Iron . . . . 53
Iron Losses . . . . 54
References . . . . 58

**5. The Physiology of Restless Legs Syndrome** . . . . . . . . . . . . . . *61*
*Stephany Fulda and Thomas-Christian Wetter*
Introduction . . . . 61
Pathophysiology of Restless Legs Syndrome . . . . 63
What is the Role of Peripheral Neuropathy in Restless Legs Syndrome? . . . . 64
The Vascular Hypothesis—Exotic but Persisting? . . . . 65
The Spinal Cord . . . . 66
The Brain . . . . 68
Other Systems Relevant to Restless Legs Syndrome . . . . 72
Concluding Remarks . . . . 76
References . . . . 78

**6. Progress in the Animal Models of Restless Legs Syndrome** . . *89*
*Weidong Le, Hongru Zhao, and William G. Ondo*
Introduction . . . . 89
6-Hydroxydopamine–Lesioned Rat Model . . . . 89
6-OHDA–Lesioned and Iron-Deficient Mice . . . . 90
Dopamine D3 Receptor Knockout (D3KO) Mice Model . . . . 93
An Animal Model of Periodic Limb Movements of Sleep . . . . 95
Animal Models of Opioid Dopaminergic Interactions . . . . 97
References . . . . 97

**7. Pathology of Restless Legs Syndrome** .................... *101*
*James R. Connor and Xinsheng Wang*
Introduction .... 101
Neuropathological Evaluation .... 101
Iron Management Proteins .... 103
Proposed Consequences of Insufficient Iron in the Restless Legs Syndrome Substantia Nigra .... 105
Conclusion .... 106
References .... 107

**8. Genetics of Restless Legs Syndrome** .................... *111*
*Shaoqi Rao, Juliane Winkelmann, and Qing K. Wang*
Overview .... 111
Prevalence and Environmental Factors .... 111
Family History .... 112
Inheritance Models and Segregation Analysis .... 114
Familial Aggregation Analysis .... 114
Twin Studies .... 117
Linkage Studies .... 118
Genetic Association Studies .... 120
Conclusion and Outlook .... 121
References .... 121

***Section II: Clinical Diagnosis***

**9. Consequences of Sleep Deprivation** .................... *125*
*Li Ling Lim and Nancy Foldvary-Schaefer*
Introduction .... 125
Human Experimental Sleep Deprivation .... 126
Animal Sleep Deprivation Studies .... 132
Conclusions .... 133
References .... 133

**10. History of Restless Legs Syndrome** .................... *139*
*Wayne A. Hening*
Early Descriptions of Conditions Resembling Restless Legs Syndrome .... 139
The Work of Karl Ekbom .... 140
The Naming of Restless Legs .... 140
Nocturnal Myoclonus, Now Called Periodic Limb Movements .... 140
Early Therapeutic Trials of RLS .... 141

The RLS Foundation and the International RLS Study Group .... 141
Recent Development on Many Fronts .... 142
Summary Thoughts .... 143
References .... 144

**11. Restless Legs Syndrome: Diagnostic Criteria and Differential Diagnosis .............................. *147***
*Shahul Hameed and E. K. Tan*
Introduction .... 147
Diagnostic Criteria .... 147
Differential Diagnosis .... 153
Evaluation of the Restless Legs Syndrome Patient .... 155
Conclusions .... 156
References .... 156

**12. Occurrence of Restless Legs Syndrome ................ *159***
*Jan Ulfberg and Bjørn Bjorvatn*
Introduction .... 159
The Occurrence of Restless Legs Syndrome—Studies on Populations .... 160
Restless Legs Syndrome in Pregnancy .... 162
Restless Legs Syndrome and Parkinson's Disease .... 165
Restless Legs Syndrome in End-Stage Renal Disease .... 166
References .... 167

**13. Childhood-Onset Restless Legs Syndrome ............. *171***
*Suresh Kotagal and Michael H. Silber*
History .... 171
Clinical Features .... 171
Pathogenesis .... 172
Diagnosis .... 175
Treatment .... 175
Future Directions .... 177
References .... 177

**14. Periodic Limb Movements and Periodic Limb Movement Disorder .............................. *179***
*Margaret Park and Cynthia L. Comella*
Introduction .... 179
Epidemiology of Periodic Limb Movements Disorder .... 182
Associated Disease States .... 183
Pathophysiology .... 186

Imaging Studies . . . . 188
Treatment . . . . 189
References . . . . 191

**15. Restless Legs Syndrome Effects on Quality of Life . . . . . . . . . . . . . . . . . . . . . . . . . . . . . . . . . . *199***
*Richard P. Allen*
Introduction . . . . 199
Disease-Specific Quality of Life Evaluations of RLS . . . . 199
General Health-Related Quality of Life Evaluations . . . . 200
Treatment Benefits for Quality of Life . . . . 201
Summary . . . . 202
References . . . . 202

**16. Restless Legs Syndrome: Personal Perspectives . . . . . . . . . *205***
*Georgianna Bell*
The Faces of Restless Legs Syndrome . . . . 205
The RLS Foundation . . . . 205
Marlene's Story: "Good Physicians Make All the Difference" . . . . 206
Lynne's Story: "I Want to Live with Them, Not Them Live Around Me" . . . . 206
Clare's Story: "I Found a Way of Shutting It All Out" . . . . 207
Mike's Story: "Sleep Deprivation and Work Are an Incompatible Combination" . . . . 208
Sue's Story: "I Want Better for Them" . . . . 208
Jocelle's Story: "Never Give Up!" . . . . 209

***Section III: Secondary Restless Legs Syndrome***

**17. Iron Deficiency–Associated Restless Legs Syndrome . . . . . *211***
*William G. Ondo*
Introduction . . . . 211
Central Nervous System Iron Deficiency in RLS . . . . 211
Clinical Experience . . . . 213
Iron Deficiency and Other Associations of Restless Legs Syndrome . . . . 214
Iron Replacement . . . . 215
References . . . . 216

**18. Restless Legs Syndrome and Renal Failure** .............. *219*
*Kai Ming Chow and David Shu Cheong Hui*
Introduction .... 219
Epidemiology .... 219
Pathogenesis .... 221
Diagnosis .... 222
Treatment .... 224
Prognosis .... 225
Summary .... 226
References .... 226

**19. Restless Legs Syndrome and Neuropathy/Myelopathy** .............................. *229*
*Birgit Högl and Werner Poewe*
Introduction .... 229
Polyneuropathy, Radiculopathy, and Peripheral Nerve Lesions .... 229
Possible Interpretations of the Evidence .... 234
References .... 235

**20. Restless Legs Syndrome in Pregnancy** ................. *239*
*Luigi Ferini-Strambi and Mauro Manconi*
Introduction .... 239
Epidemiology .... 240
Clinical Course .... 241
Etiopathogenetic Hypotheses .... 242
Treatment .... 244
References .... 245

**21. Restless Legs Syndrome and Parkinson's Disease** .............................. *247*
*Vandana Dhawan and K. Ray Chaudhuri*
Background .... 247
Pathophysiology .... 247
Clinical Surveys .... 249
Conclusions .... 251
References .... 252

**22. Iatrogenic Restless Legs Syndrome** .................... *255*
*Changkook Yang and John W. Winkelman*
Introduction .... 255
Antidepressants .... 256

Antipsychotics .... 258
Histamine-Receptor Antagonists .... 260
Lithium .... 261
Antiepileptics .... 261
Smoking .... 261
Caffeine .... 262
Alcohol .... 262
Miscellaneous .... 262
Augmentation .... 263
Conclusion .... 263
References .... 264

**23. Other Restless Legs Syndrome Associations ............ *269***
*Irfan Lalani and William G. Ondo*
Introduction .... 269
Rheumatological Disorders .... 269
Ataxia .... 270
Tremor .... 271
Tourette's Syndrome .... 271
Multiple Sclerosis .... 272
Sleep Apnea .... 272
Miscellaneous Associations .... 273
Conclusion .... 273
References .... 273

***Section IV: Treatment of Restless Legs Syndrome***

**24. Treatment Overview ............................ *275***
*William G. Ondo*
Scales for Restless Legs Syndrome .... 275
Treatment Overview .... 278
References .... 280
Appendix A .... 282
Appendix B .... 284
Appendix C .... 285

**25. Dopaminergic Therapy for Restless Legs Syndrome ............................ *287***
*Philip M. Becker*
Introduction .... 287
Proposed Therapeutic Action .... 287
Pharmacology of Common Dopaminergic Agents .... 288

Investigational Dopamine Agonists . . . . 297
Augmentation Due to Dopaminergic Therapy . . . . 298
Conclusion . . . . 299
References . . . . 300

**26. Dopaminergic Augmentation** . . . . . . . . . . . . . . . . . . . . . . ***305***
*Diego García-Borreguero, Oscar Larrosa, Renata Egatz, Belen Cabrero, and Patrick Tröster*
Introduction . . . . 305
Clinical Description and Significance . . . . 305
Augmentation Under Dopaminergic Agents . . . . 307
Augmentation Under Nondopaminergic Agents . . . . 307
The Pathophysiology of Augmentation . . . . 307
Measurement of Augmentation . . . . 309
Differential Diagnosis of Augmentation . . . . 310
Treatment of Augmentation . . . . 312
References . . . . 312

**27. Opioids and the Restless Legs Syndrome: Treatment and Pathogenetic Considerations** . . . . . . . . . . . . . . . . . . . . ***315***
*Arthur S. Walters*
Introduction . . . . 315
Therapeutic Trials of Opioids in Restless Legs Syndrome/Periodic Limb Movements . . . . 315
Overall Therapeutic Recommendations . . . . 317
Role of the Endogenous Opiate System in the Pathogenesis of Restless Legs Syndrome/Periodic Limb Movements . . . . 318
Implications of the Receptor Blocking Studies . . . . 320
Other Evidence Supporting a Role of the Endogenous Opiate System in the Pathogenesis of Restless Legs Syndrome . . . . 320
References . . . . 322

**28. Iron Therapy in Restless Legs Syndrome** . . . . . . . . . . . . . . ***325***
*Charlene E. Gamaldo and Christopher J. Earley*
Introduction . . . . 325
Oral Iron Therapy . . . . 325
Intravenous Iron Therapy . . . . 328
Follow-up . . . . 332
References . . . . 332

**29. Other Therapies in Restless Legs Syndrome . . . . . . . . . . . . 335**
*Joohi Shahed and William G. Ondo*
Introduction . . . . 335
Antiepileptics . . . . 335
Clonidine . . . . 338
Benzodiazepines . . . . 338
Other Drugs . . . . 339
Nonpharmacologic Therapies . . . . 340
Conclusions . . . . 341
References . . . . 341

***Section V: Future Directions in Restless Legs Syndrome***

**30. Future Directions . . . . . . . . . . . . . . . . . . . . . . . . . . . . . . . . . 345**
*William G. Ondo*
Introduction . . . . 345
Diagnosis . . . . 345
Epidemiology . . . . 346
Disease Associations . . . . 347
Pathology . . . . 347
Treatment . . . . 348
Summary . . . . 349
References . . . . 349

*Index . . . . 351*

# Contributors

**Richard P. Allen** Department of Neurology, Johns Hopkins University, Baltimore, Maryland, U.S.A.

**John Beard** Department of Nutritional Sciences, Pennsylvania State University, University Park, Pennsylvania, U.S.A.

**Philip M. Becker** Department of Psychiatry, University of Texas Southwestern Medical Center at Dallas, Dallas, Texas, U.S.A.

**Georgianna Bell** Restless Legs Syndrome Foundation, Rochester, Minnesota, U.S.A.

**Bjørn Bjorvatn** Department of Public Health and Primary Health Care, University of Bergen, Bergen, Norway

**Belen Cabrero** Sleep Research Institute, Madrid, Spain

**Allison V. Chan** Stanford University Center of Excellence for Sleep Disorders, Stanford University, Stanford, California, U.S.A.

**K. Ray Chaudhuri** Regional Movement Disorders Unit, National Parkinson Foundation Centre of Excellence, Department of Neurology, King's College Hospital, Denmark Hill, and University Hospital Lewisham, and Guy's, King's, and St. Thomas' School of Biomedical Medicine, London, U.K.

**Kai Ming Chow** Department of Medicine and Therapeutics, Prince of Wales Hospital, Chinese University of Hong Kong, Shatin, New Territories, Hong Kong, P.R. China

**Cynthia L. Comella** Section on Movement Disorders, Department of Neurological Sciences, Rush University Medical Center, Chicago, Illinois, U.S.A.

**James R. Connor** Department of Neurosurgery, Pennsylvania State University College of Medicine, Milton S. Hershey Medical Center, Hershey, Pennsylvania, U.S.A.

**Vandana Dhawan** Regional Movement Disorders Unit, King's College Hospital, University Hospital Lewisham, London, U.K.

**Christopher J. Earley** Department of Neurology, Johns Hopkins School of Medicine, Baltimore, Maryland, U.S.A.

**Renata Egatz** Sleep Research Institute, Madrid, Spain

**Luigi Ferini-Strambi** Department of Neurology, Sleep Disorders Center, University Vita-Salute, IRCCS H San Raffaele, Milan, Italy

**Nancy Foldvary-Schaefer** Department of Neurology, Sleep Disorders Center, Cleveland Clinic Foundation, Cleveland, Ohio, U.S.A.

**Alon A. Freeman** Department of Neurology, Emory University, Atlanta, Georgia, U.S.A.

**Stephany Fulda** Max Planck Institute of Psychiatry, Munich, Germany

**Charlene E. Gamaldo** Department of Neurology, Johns Hopkins School of Medicine, Baltimore, Maryland, U.S.A.

**Diego García-Borreguero** Sleep Research Institute, Madrid, Spain

**Shahul Hameed** Department of Neurology, Singapore General Hospital, National Neuroscience Institute, Singapore, Republic of Singapore

**Wayne A. Hening** Department of Neurology, UMDNJ-RW Johnson Medical School, New Brunswick, New Jersey, U.S.A.

**Birgit Högl** Department of Neurology, Innsbruck Medical University, Innsbruck, Austria

**David Shu Cheong Hui** Department of Medicine and Therapeutics, Prince of Wales Hospital, Chinese University of Hong Kong, Shatin, New Territories, Hong Kong, P.R. China

**Suresh Kotagal** Department of Neurology and the Sleep Disorders Center, Mayo Clinic, Rochester, Minnesota, U.S.A.

**Clete A. Kushida** Stanford University Center of Excellence for Sleep Disorders, Stanford University, Stanford, California, U.S.A.

**Irfan Lalani** Section of Pain Management, Department of Anesthesiology, M.D. Anderson Cancer Center, Houston, Texas, U.S.A.

**Oscar Larrosa** Sleep Research Institute, Madrid, Spain

**Weidong Le** Department of Neurology, Baylor College of Medicine, Houston, Texas, U.S.A.

**Li Ling Lim** Department of Neurology, Sleep Disorders Unit, Singapore General Hospital, National Neuroscience Institute, Singapore, Republic of Singapore

**Mauro Manconi** Department of Neurology, Sleep Disorders Center, University Vita-Salute, IRCCS H San Raffaele, Milan, Italy

**William G. Ondo** Department of Neurology, Baylor College of Medicine, Houston, Texas, U.S.A.

**Margaret Park** Department of Behavioral Sciences, Sleep Disorders Service and Research Center, Rush University Medical Center, Chicago, Illinois, U.S.A.

**Werner Poewe** Department of Neurology, Innsbruck Medical University, Innsbruck, Austria

**Shaoqi Rao** Department of Molecular Cardiology, Lerner Research Institute, Centers for Cardiovascular Genetics and Molecular Genetics, The Cleveland Clinic Foundation, and Department of Molecular Medicine, Cleveland Clinic Lerner College of Medicine of Case Western Reserve University, Cleveland, Ohio, U.S.A.

**David B. Rye** Department of Neurology, Emory University, Atlanta, Georgia, U.S.A.

**Joohi Shahed** Department of Neurology, Baylor College of Medicine, Houston, Texas, U.S.A.

**Michael H. Silber** Department of Neurology and the Sleep Disorders Center, Mayo Clinic, Rochester, Minnesota, U.S.A.

**E. K. Tan** Department of Neurology, Singapore General Hospital, National Neuroscience Institute, Singapore, Republic of Singapore

**Patrick Tröster** Sleep Research Institute, Madrid, Spain

**Jan Ulfberg** Sleep Disorders Center, Avesta Hospital, Avesta, Sweden

**Arthur S. Walters** New Jersey Neuroscience Institute, Seton Hall University School of Graduate Medical Education, JFK Medical Center, Edison, New Jersey, U.S.A.

**Qing K. Wang** Department of Molecular Cardiology, Lerner Research Institute, Centers for Cardiovascular Genetics and Molecular Genetics, The Cleveland Clinic Foundation, and Department of Molecular Medicine, Cleveland Clinic Lerner College of Medicine of Case Western Reserve University, Cleveland, Ohio, U.S.A.

**Xinsheng Wang** Department of Neurosurgery, Pennsylvania State University College of Medicine, Milton S. Hershey Medical Center, Hershey, Pennsylvania, U.S.A.

**Thomas-Christian Wetter** Max Planck Institute of Psychiatry, Munich, Germany

**John W. Winkelman** Division of Sleep Medicine, Brigham and Women's Hospital, Harvard Medical School, Boston, Massachusetts, U.S.A.

**Juliane Winkelmann** Max Planck Institute of Psychiatry, RG Neurological Genetics, Institute of Human Genetics, Munich, Germany

**Changkook Yang** Sleep Disorders Clinic, Department of Psychiatry, Dong-A University College of Medicine, Busan, Korea

**Hongru Zhao** Department of Neurology, Baylor College of Medicine, Houston, Texas, U.S.A.

# 1 Overview of Sleep

**Allison V. Chan and Clete A. Kushida**
*Stanford University Center of Excellence for Sleep Disorders, Stanford University, Stanford, California, U.S.A.*

## INTRODUCTION

The field of sleep medicine remains a mystery because the precise biological function of sleep is still unclear. A significant portion of our existence is devoted to this experience; in fact, approximately one-third of human life is spent sleeping. Given that sleep deprivation leads to a rebound of sleep, it clearly has an important function. Whether the primary purpose of sleep is to provide thermoregulation, memory reinforcement, or body tissue restoration is unknown. But as this area of research continues to grow, we are provided a deeper and richer understanding of this complex process. In this chapter, we offer a brief overview of some of the fundamental aspects of sleep. Points of interest regarding sleep architecture and staging are reviewed, as well as sleep with age, the need for sleep, sleep deprivation, and the evolution of sleep. The intricate biochemical and physiological components of sleep are also detailed. Finally, the broad classification of sleep medicine disorders is categorized.

## NORMAL SLEEP ARCHITECTURE AND SLEEP STAGES

Sleep can be divided into two states: nonrapid eye movement (NREM) and rapid eye movement (REM) sleep. Each cycle of NREM and REM sleep lasts approximately 90 to 110 minutes, and about three to six cycles of NREM–REM sleep occur during a normal night of sleep (Fig. 1). Slow wave sleep (SWS), which will be discussed in more detail later, tends to dominate the first third of sleep, whereas REM sleep is most predominant in the last third of sleep. The first REM cycle is typically short; the final cycle of REM tends to be the longest. In terms of arousability, the deepest sleep occurs in the first third of the night, corresponding to SWS (NREM stages III and IV); an individual awakened during these stages of sleep is typically groggy and confused. If awakened during lighter stages of NREM sleep (stages I and II), there is the possibility that the individual may not be aware that he or she had fallen asleep. However, if one were awakened during REM sleep, a person may experience residual sleep paralysis or persistence of dreams intruding into the waking state because paralysis of voluntary muscles and dreams are normal components of REM sleep. Typical behavioral events that are observed following sleep onset, irrespective of type of sleep, include transient amnesia for the occurrence of sleep, fragmentary images, hypnic jerks, and automatic behavior.

An individual's sleep can be recorded via an overnight polysomnogram (PSG). Some of the most commonly measured variables include electroencephalography (EEG), electrooculography (EOG), electromyography (EMG), electrocardiography, respiration, oxygen saturation, snoring, and body position (Fig. 2). To score the various stages of sleep, an epoch of sleep, or a 30-second

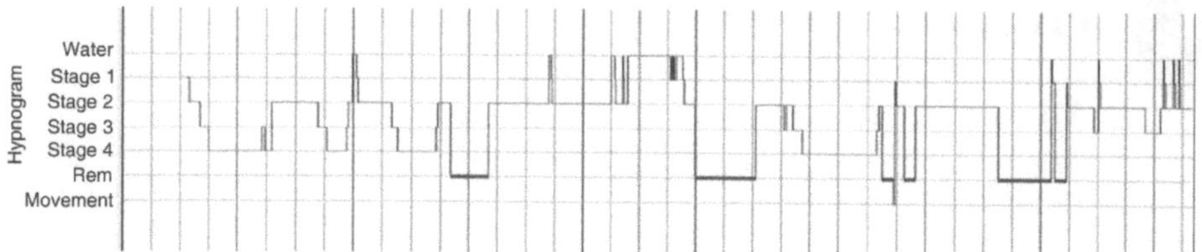


**FIGURE 1** Sleep hypnogram demonstrating typical shifting sleep stages during a single night.

polygraphic tracing at a speed of 10 mm/second, is evaluated according to defined criteria set forth in the international classification of sleep disorders (ICSD) (1).

In human adults, NREM sleep occupies 75% to 80% of the total sleep time. It is comprised of stages I through IV. Stage I sleep accounts for about 3% to 8% of the total sleep time. It is scored when an alpha rhythm (8–12 Hz) is present in less than half of the epoch. Theta (4–7 Hz) and beta frequencies (>13 Hz), slow rolling eye movements, and a slight decrease in electromyographic activity may be present in this stage of sleep. At the end of stage I, vertex waves lasting 50 to 200 msec can occur.

The largest portion of the total sleep time, about 45% to 55%, is spent in stage II sleep. Sleep spindles are present at this stage. These waveforms are generally 12 to

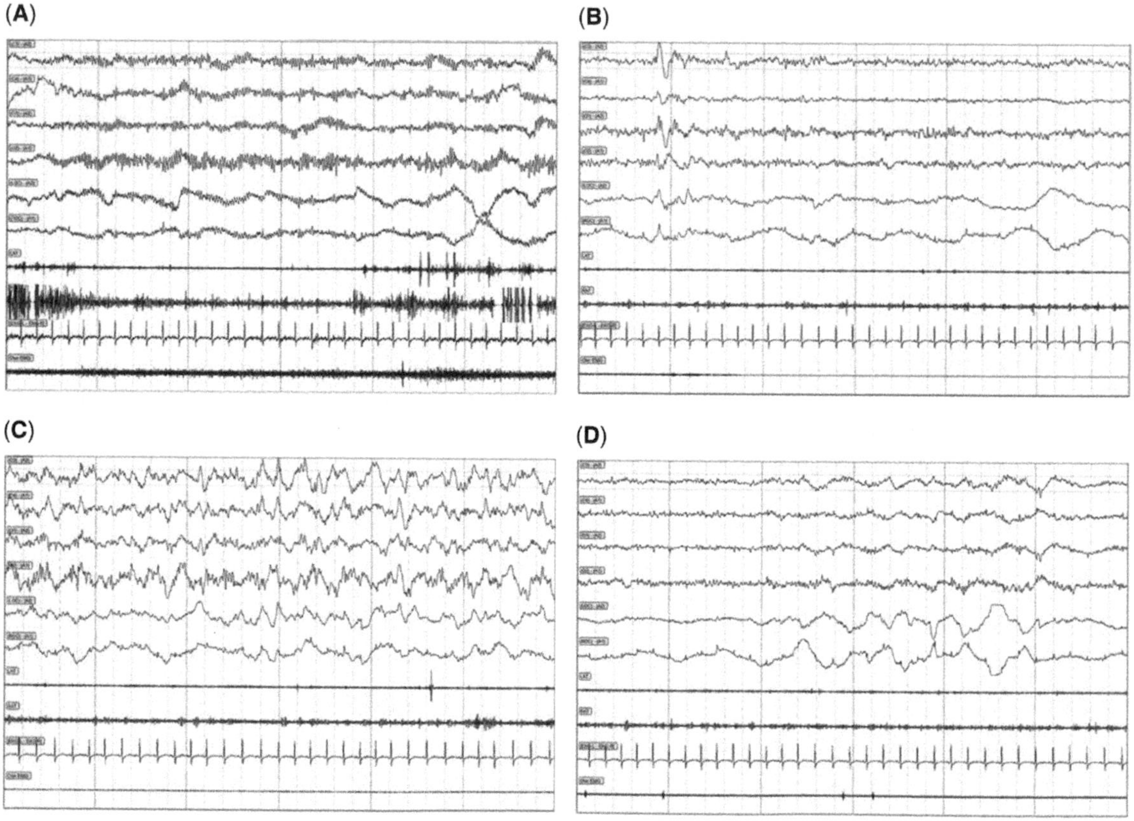

**FIGURE 2** (**A**) Wakefulness: desynchronized EEG, and very active chin EMG activity. One random eye blink. (**B**) Stage II: Alpha rhythm EEG with K complex and reduced but still active chin EMG. (**C**) Slow wave (delta) sleep: slow delta activity EEG and still active chin EMG. (**D**) REM: desynchronized EEG and no chin EMG activity. *Abbreviations*: EEG, electroencephalography; EMG, electromyography; REM, rapid eye movement.

14 Hz, with duration of about 0.5 seconds and have a "spindle-shaped" appearance. K complexes are waveforms with a negative wave followed by a positive wave; both waves last for greater than 0.5 seconds. Less than 20% of the epoch contains delta waves (0.5–4 Hz) in this stage of sleep.

SWS includes both stage III and stage IV sleep. Stage III is identified by the presence of delta waves (0.5–4 Hz) in 20% to 50% of the epoch. About 3% to 8% of the total sleep time is accounted for by this stage.

Stage IV sleep is characterized by the presence of delta waves in greater than 50% of the epoch and accounts for about 10% to 15% of the total sleep time. Body movements are registered as artifacts in PSG recordings at the end of SWS. In stages II through IV, eye movements are not present, and muscle tone is decreased from that seen in either wakefulness or stage I (2).

About 20% to 25% of total sleep time is spent in REM sleep. The first cycle of REM sleep occurs approximately 60 to 90 minutes after the onset of NREM sleep. A characteristic finding in REM sleep is the "saw tooth" appearance of theta waves on electroencephalographic tracings. Within REM sleep, tonic and phasic stages occur. The hallmarks of tonic REM sleep include hypotonia or atonia of major muscle groups, desynchronization of the EEG, and depression of monosynaptic and polysynaptic reflexes. Phasic REM sleep is characterized by tongue movements, REMs in all directions, phasic swings in blood pressure and heart rate, irregular respiration, spontaneous middle ear muscle activity, and myoclonic twitching of chin and limb muscles (3–6).

## ONTOGENY OF SLEEP

With age, sleep requirements change. Newborns can spend greater than 16 hours per day sleeping; approximately 50% of their total sleep time is composed of REM sleep. In fact, when newborns first fall asleep, they immediately enter REM sleep, also known as active sleep. Restless movements of the facial muscles, arms, and legs occur during active sleep; it can be difficult to distinguish wakefulness from REM sleep on PSG. There is a gradual change from the infant's multiphasic sleep to the adult's monophasic pattern (7–9). REM sleep begins to decrease during the first few months of a newborn's existence. By about three months of age, infants sleep a total of about 10 hours a day, sleep through the night, and take two or more naps during the day. At this time, the newborn's EEG begins to adopt an adult sleep pattern with the appearance of spindles (10); by six months, K complexes are present (11). Children who are one year of age tend to have a NREM–REM cycle with a duration of 45 to 50 minutes. By five years of age, children have a major nocturnal sleep period and may take one nap during the day. Between the ages of 5 and 10 years, the NREM–REM cycle lengthens to—60 to 70 minutes. Adult REM cycles lasting 90 to 110 minutes and REM percentages that decreased to 20% to 25% are seen in children by the age of about 10 years. Through puberty and adulthood, individuals maintain the major nocturnal period without a nap, although this may be somewhat culturally dependent. Older adults frequently complain of poor sleep. Their sleep is marked by an attenuation of delta waves, frequent nocturnal awakenings, and early morning awakenings. However, both their total amount of REM sleep as well as total sleep time do not actually decrease (12).

## ADEQUATE SLEEP

Irrespective of one's cultural or environmental differences, the average adult requires about 7.5 to 8 hours of sleep (9,13,14). A study of college students demonstrated that about 1.1% of this population sleeps for less than 5.5 hours/night, and about 3.2% sleeps more than 9.5 hours/night (15). An epidemiological study conducted by Kripke et al. demonstrated that people who sleep less than four hours/night or more than nine hours/night were at a higher risk than those sleeping seven to eight hours/night of death due to cancer, stroke, or coronary artery disease (16). There have been no other psychological factors or personality traits to distinguish "short" or "long" sleepers from average sleepers.

Excess sleep appears to be related with decreased sleep efficiency and can be followed by exhaustion and irritability. Although long sleepers spend more time asleep, they have been found to have relatively decreased amounts of stages III and IV sleep and an increased amount of stage II sleep (17).

## SLEEP DEPRIVATION

Numerous jobs today require their employees to maintain irregular sleep–wake schedules and alternating shifts. Physicians, nurses, and other health care providers to police officers, firefighters, truck drivers, and others may be essentially sleep deprived on a chronic basis (18,19). Compared with a study of about 2000 Americans between 1910 and 1911, a study of 311 Americans in recent times showed that we are sleeping about 1.5 hours less (18). Despite the possible sampling error, it is unlikely that Americans have become more resilient and need less sleep. It seems more plausible that we are simply deprived of sleep, perhaps due to the presence of televisions and radios, increased environmental light, and increased numbers of individuals involved in shift work (20,21). While it has been demonstrated that 5% to 36% of the Western population is excessively sleepy (22), others maintain that individuals are actually choosing to sleep less and are not chronically sleep deprived (23).

Studies of total, partial, and selective sleep deprivation (e.g., loss of REM sleep vs. stage IV sleep) have been performed to determine the consequences of sleeplessness (24–33). There is clear evidence of sleepiness, worsened reaction time, and impairment of concentration, performance, attention, and vigilance. Periods of microsleep may be related to the performance impairment seen in sleep deprivation. The term "microsleep" refers to a transient physiologic sleep (an EEG pattern change from that seen in wakefulness to that of NREM stage I sleep for a duration of 3–14 seconds). It may or may not be associated with slow rolling eye movements and behavioral sleep, including head sagging/nodding or eyelid heaviness/drooping. There does not appear to be a permanent loss of memory or other major central nervous system changes associated with sleep deprivation (20,21).

Sleep deprivation is the most common cause of excessive daytime somnolence (EDS) (Chapter 9 for a detailed discussion). An epidemiological study by Partinen demonstrated that chronic partial sleep deprivation caused 33% of young adults to suffer from EDS; middle-aged adults attributed their EDS to sleep disorders in 7% of the cases and to shift work in 2% (22). The danger to the individual suffering from EDS, and to the population as a whole, cannot be overstated. International consequences from EDS due to sleep deprivation include the Three Mile Island nuclear accident, the Chernobyl nuclear plant disaster, the Challenger explosion, and the Exxon Valdez oil spill (34). The recently estimated cost of sleep-related accidents in the United States is between approximately 2 and 56 billion dollars (35,36).

Two types of sleepiness are hypothesized to exist: physiologic and subjective (37). Physiologic sleepiness refers to the body's need for sleep and depends on the sleep factor and the circadian phase. The sleep factor involves the prior period of wakefulness and sleep debt; the longer the period of preceding wakefulness, the greater the tendency to sleep. Additional sleep satisfies but does not equal this sleep debt in terms of exact hours. Extra SWS is needed for restoration in a sleep-deprived person. The circadian factor describes the body's proclivity for sleep, which is greatest between 3:00 to 5:00 A.M. Sleep-deprived people may be helped by scheduling 20- to 30-minute long naps. If sleep deprivation is anticipated, a prophylactic nap may be helpful (37).

Subjective sleepiness pertains to one's perception of sleepiness. Many different types of external factors can affect subjective sleepiness, including caffeine consumption, the presence of bright light or loud noise, or being engaged in stimulating activities. Sleepiness tends to peak in humans between 2:00 and 6:00 A.M. and 2:00 and 6:00 P.M.; the majority of sleep-related catastrophes appear to occur between these time periods (38).

## PHYLOGENY OF SLEEP

There have been studies to determine if other mammals experience sleep stages like humans (39–43). Mammalian and human EEG recordings share many similarities. The EEG, EMG, and EOG can be used in animals to distinguish between their NREM and REM sleep. It has been suggested that features of NREM and REM sleep are combined into a single sleep state in the echidna, which are egg-laying mammals (44).

Mammals can also be short or long sleepers, much like humans. Although small and large animals have many similarities in terms of their sleep lengths and lengths of their sleep cycles, small animals have a higher metabolic rate, shorter life span, and increased relative sleep time compared to large animals with decreased metabolic rates (45). Larger animals have a longer REM–NREM cycle than smaller animals.

Dolphins, porpoises, and pilot whales demonstrate episodes of unihemispheric sleep (46). During sleep, one half of a dolphin's brain demonstrates the characteristic EEG findings consistent with sleep, while the other half demonstrates EEG findings of wakefulness (47). The dolphin's sleep period persists for about 30 to 60 minutes. At the end of this period, each hemisphere changes to the opposite function.

Sleep and wakefulness are present in vertebrates as well as invertebrates (48). Specifically, insects, worms, and scorpions display the behavioral criteria of sleep (49). Over the course of 24 hours, fundamental rest-activity cycles are present in many animals. Although the REM–NREM cycles of birds are quite brief, EEG and behavioral data indicate that birds do experience sleep (50). Whether or not reptiles, from which birds are considered to have evolved, truly experience REM sleep is still questioned (48). Another area that remains unclear is if NREM and REM sleep evolved independently in birds and mammals.

## PHYSIOLOGICAL DETERMINANTS OF SLEEP

NREM sleep is associated with altered transmission at the level of the thalamus. In this way, incoming messages are inhibited, and the cortex is deprived of signals from the outside world. One of the major oscillations present during this stage is

(A)

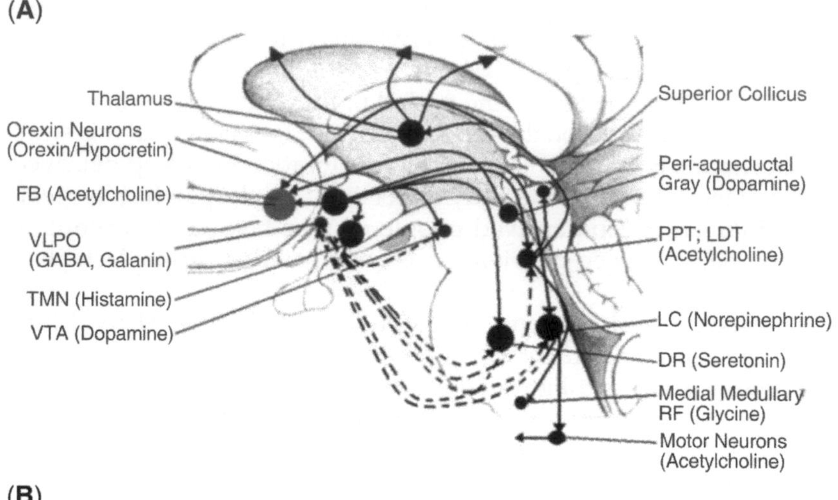


(B)

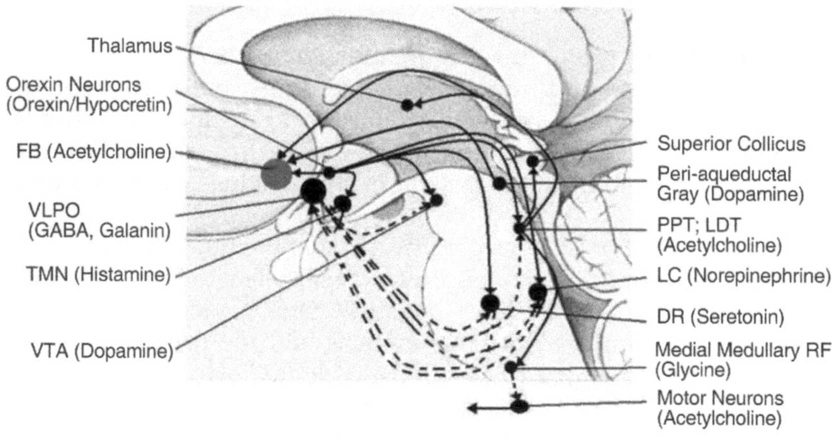


(C)

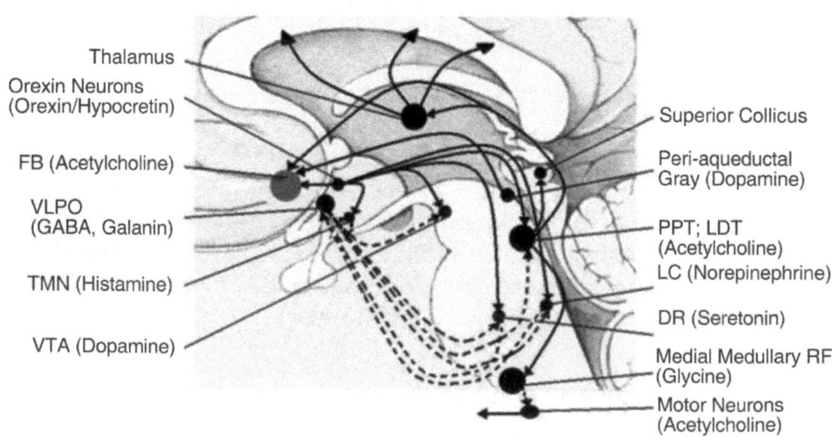


**FIGURE 3** (*Caption on facing page*)

spindles. Thalamic reticular neurons generate this particular waveform and impose rhythmic inhibitory sequences onto thalamocortical neurons. Corticothalamic projections govern the widespread synchronization of this rhythm.

Two other major oscillations that characterize NREM sleep include two different types of delta activity (51,52). Generated in thalamocortical neurons, the first type of oscillation is "clock-like" waves with a frequency of 1 to 4 Hz. The second type of oscillation also has a frequency of 1 to 4 Hz; however, they are cortical waves that persist despite extensive thalamectomy. But the slow (less than 1 Hz) oscillation generated intracortically is the hallmark of NREM sleep. This intracortical oscillator has the ability to coalesce the different rhythms by grouping the thalamically generated spindles as well as the delta oscillations generated in the thalamus and cortex (53,54).

REM sleep generation is critically related to the pontomesencephalic region, as transection studies have demonstrated (55). When the mesopontine region is connected to rostral structures, REM sleep phenomena such as desynchronized EEG and ponto-geniculo-occipital (PGO) spikes are seen in the forebrain; when this region is continuous with the medulla and the spinal cord, the REM sleep phenomenon of skeletal muscle atonia can be seen.

The cholinergic "REM-on" nuclei, including the laterodorsal tegmental (LDT) nuclei and the pedunculopontine (PPT) nuclei, are found within the pontomesencephalic area (Fig. 3). The LDT and PPT nuclei project through the thalamus to the cortex, producing the EEG desynchronization of REM sleep. PGO spikes are a precursor to the REMs of REM sleep. They are formed in the cholinergic mesopontine nuclei and propagate rostrally through the lateral geniculate and other thalamic nuclei to the occipital cortex (56). LDT and PPT nuclei project caudally via the ventral medulla to the alpha motor neurons in the spinal cord, where skeletal muscle tone is inhibited during REM sleep by the release of glycine (57). As NREM sleep transitions to REM sleep, tonic inhibition of REM-generating cholinergic pontomesencephalic nuclei by brainstem serotoninergic and adrenergic

---

**FIGURE 3** (*Facing page*) (**A**) During wakefulness, the hypocretin system is activated. It stimulates the FB acetylcholine system, the TMN histamine neurons, the VT dopaminergic neurons, and the reticular activating system: LC norepinephrine neurons, DR serotonin neurons, and PPN and LDT acetylcholine neurons. The activated PPN/LDT tracks ascend to "open" the thalamic pathways, which causes EEG desynchronization. The LC descends to the motor neurons to activate them. The other nuclei (FB, TMN, VT, DR, LC) ascend to activate the cortex. The DR, LC TMN inhibit the VLPO nucleus. (**B**) During NREM sleep the VLPO in the preoptic area is active and sends GABA and galanin to inhibit the DR, LC, TMN, as well as the FB and VT. Therefore, the VLPO and DR/LC/TMN are reciprocally inhibitory and create a sleep–wake flip-flop circuit that has many inputs (light, circadian rhythm, melatonin, adenosine build-up) but is ultimately mediated by the hypocretin system, which is much less active during sleep. During NREM sleep the DR and LC still have some activity. (**C**) During REM sleep, the VLPO firing is at its highest and DR, LC, TMN firing almost disappears. This combination disinhibits (activates) a specific "REM on" acetylcholine center within the PPN/LDT. FB acetylcholine also increases. The REM center ascends to the thalamus causing the EEG asynchrony (similar to wakefulness). They also descend to stimulate neurons in the medial medulla (not specifically named) that send inhibitory glycine axons to the alpha motor neurons in the spinal cord, thus inhibiting them and causing the atonia. The absence of LC activity also reduces motor tone during REM. (——) indicates excitatory fibers and (----) indicates inhibitory fibers. *Abbreviations*: GABA, gamma-aminobutyric acid; VLPO, ventrolateral preoptic area; TMN, tuberomammillary nucleus; VTA, ventral tegmental area; LC, locus coeruleus; PPT, pedunculopontine nucleus; LDT, laterodorsal tegmental nucleus; DR, dorsal raphe; FB, forebrain; PPN, pedunculopontine; RF, reticular formation; EEG, electroencephalography.

nuclei decreases, thereby allowing the development of PGO spikes and muscle atonia (58). The cholinergic REM-on nuclei of the PPT and LDT slowly activate the monoaminergic "REM-off" nuclei of the dorsal raphe and locus ceruleus, which, in turn, inhibit REM-on nuclei.

## BIOCHEMICAL DETERMINANTS OF SLEEP

The major neurotransmitter pathways that regulate the wakefulness system are the ascending reticular activating systems (ARAS). Projecting to the thalamus, hypothalamus, and basal forebrain, the ARAS includes cholinergic, noradrenergic, dopaminergic, and histaminergic neurons. Within the laterodorsal and PPT tegmental nuclei at the pontomesencephalic junction, cholinergic neurons project to the thalamus, posterior hypothalamus, and basal forebrain region. These cholinergic neurons fire at their highest rates during wakefulness and also during REM sleep, but they decrease their rates of firing at the onset of NREM sleep. Through both nicotinic and muscarinic receptors, acetylcholine depolarizes and excites the thalamocortical projecting neurons, promoting tonic firing. Cholinergic receptor antagonists inhibit cortical activation. The role of dopamine is uncertain, but pharmacologic, biochemical, and physiologic studies suggest dopamine helps maintain wakefulness. The $D_1$, and possibly the $D_2$ receptors, may modulate this activity. Nevertheless, marked alterations in dopaminergic signaling have not been observed as a function of the sleep/wake cycle. Norepinephrine-containing locus ceruleus neurons show their highest firing rates during wakefulness, reduced firing during NREM and almost no activity during REM sleep. Although the noradrenergic system promotes wakefulness, the role of various noradrenergic receptor subtypes in maintaining sleep vs. wakefulness needs to be clarified. Pharmacologic studies suggest that posterior hypothalamic histaminergic neurons help maintain wakefulness and, possibly, vigilance. Glutamate and aspartate, the excitatory amino acids, are present in many neurons projecting to the cerebral cortex, forebrain, and brainstem; they are maximally released during wakefulness. Glutamate or aspartate-containing neurons are intermingled within the ARAS. Prolonged cortical activation is produced by glutamate agonists. Many peptides and hormones, including corticotrophin-releasing factor, thyrotropin-releasing factor, vasoactive intestinal polypeptide, thyroid-stimulating hormone, epinephrine, and adrenocorticotrophic hormone, may also participate in wakefulness (59).

Hypocretin is secreted by neurons in the lateral hypothalamus. These neurons project widely to the brainstem and forebrain areas, densely innervating monoaminergic and cholinergic cells. They promote wakefulness and inhibit REM sleep. Increased levels of hypocretin during active waking and in REM sleep compared to quiet waking and slow-wave sleep suggest a role for hypocretin in the central programming of motor activity (60). Hypocretin projections to the nucleus pontis oralis may play a role in the generation of active REM sleep and muscle atonia (61). In patients with the sleep disorder narcolepsy with cataplexy, hypocretin levels from the cerebrospinal fluid have been shown to be low compared to healthy controls and those with other sleep disorders (62).

## SLEEP DISORDERS CLASSIFICATION

The Association of Sleep Disorders Centers initially classified sleep–wake disorders into four categories, including disorders of initiating and maintaining sleep;

disorders of excessive somnolence; disorders of sleep–wake schedule; and dysfunctions associated with sleep, sleep stages, or partial arousals. In 1990, the ICSD described a system, which was slightly revised in 1997, that divided the 84 sleep disorders into four classes: dyssomnias, parasomnias, sleep disorders associated with medical or psychiatric disorders, and proposed sleep disorders.

The latest ICSD was published in 2005 (63). ICSD-2 divides sleep disorders into eight categories: insomnias; sleep-related breathing disorders; hypersomnias of central origin not due to a circadian rhythm sleep disorder, sleep-related breathing disorder, or other cause of disturbed nocturnal sleep; circadian rhythm sleep disorders; parasomnias; sleep-related movement disorders; isolated symptoms, apparently normal variants, and unresolved issues; and other sleep disorders. Some divisions were based according to a common complaint, others on etiology, and still others on the organ system from which the disorder arose.

Insomnias are further subdivided into 11 categories. An adjustment (acute) insomnia is due to an identifiable stressor and has a duration of a few days to a few weeks; once the patient adjusts to or experiences resolution of the inciting stressor, the insomnia resolves. Psychophysiological insomnia is characterized by learned sleep-preventing associations and heightened arousal with decreased functioning during wakefulness. Paradoxical insomnia occurs without either objective sleep disturbance or the level of daytime impairment expected with the degree of reported sleep deficits. Idiopathic insomnia is a chronic problem with insomnia that had an insidious onset appreciated during infancy or childhood. The fifth category of insomnia includes those cases due to an underlying mental disorder. The next category, inadequate sleep hygiene, is produced from an individual's activities, which increase arousal and are inconsistent with sleep organization. Behavioral insomnia of childhood includes both the sleep-association type and the limit-setting type. Insomnia due to a drug or substance includes a suppression or disruption of sleep from a prescribed medicine, recreational drug, alcohol, caffeine, food, or environmental toxin. Insomnia due to a medical condition can entail difficulty with either initiation or maintenance of sleep or be interpreted as poor quality sleep. Insomnia that is not due to substance use or a known physiologic condition (nonorganic insomnia, not otherwise specified) is suspected to be due to an underlying mental disorder, psychological factors, or sleep-disruptive practices. The final category of insomnia, physiologic (organic) insomnia, unspecified, includes those cases thought to be related to an underlying medical disorder, physiological state, or substance use.

Sleep-related breathing disorders include central sleep apnea syndromes (including primary in adults or children as well as those related to Cheyne Stokes, high-altitude, medical conditions, or drugs), obstructive sleep apnea syndromes, sleep-related hypoventilation/hypoxemic syndromes (related to alveolar hypoventilation or a medical condition), and other sleep-related breathing disorders. Hypersomnias of central origin include narcolepsy, recurrent hypersomnia (as in Kleine–Levin syndrome or as related to menses), idiopathic hypersomnia (with or without a long sleep time), behaviorally induced insufficient sleep syndrome, or hypersomnia due to a medical condition, drug, or nonorganic or physiological (organic) factors.

Circadian rhythm disorders are caused by disruption of sleep–wake schedule changes and share an underlying chronophysiological basis. The primary feature of delayed sleep phase syndrome, advanced sleep phases syndrome, and non-24-hour sleep–wake syndrome is that the patient's sleep pattern does not match their desired (or socially acceptable) sleep pattern. The irregular sleep–wake pattern is characterized by intermittent sleep episodes. Time-zone (jet lag) syndrome is familiar to most of us who have crossed multiple time zones. Shift work sleep disorder occurs when the work hours of the employee impose an abnormal shift in their sleep–wake cycle.

Parasomnias usually associated with REM sleep share a common pathophysiological mechanism related to REM sleep. Unlike sleep terrors, sleepwalking, and confusional arousals, which are all associated with SWS, nightmares are REM sleep phenomena. Sleep paralysis is its own entity but can occur in narcoleptics. REM sleep-related sinus arrest is quite rare. REM sleep behavior disorder (RBD) is more common and can manifest in association with other disorders. Acute cases of RBD have toxic, metabolic etiologies, particularly withdrawal from ethanol (64). Chronic cases can be due to neurological disorders [e.g., Parkinson's disease and other neurodegenerative disorders (65), subarachnoid hemorrhage (66), pontine neoplasm (67), or narcolepsy (68)] or may be idiopathic (66). Other types of parasomnias include sleep-related dissociative disorders, sleep enuresis, sleep-related groaning, exploding head syndrome, sleep-related hallucinations, and sleep-related eating disorder.

Sleep-related movement disorders include restless legs syndrome, periodic limb movement disorder, leg cramps, bruxism, and rhythmic movement disorder. These conditions are characterized by relatively simple, usually stereotyped, movements.

Sleep disorders within the isolated symptoms category include long sleeping, short sleeping, snoring, sleeptalking, sleep starts (hypnic jerks), benign sleep myoclonus of infancy, hypnangogic foot tremor and alternating leg muscle activation during sleep, propriospinal myoclonus at sleep onset, and excessive fragmentary myoclonus. Sleep disorders that cannot be classified elsewhere are assigned to the final category, other sleep disorders. These include physiological (organic) sleep disorders and environmental sleep disorders.

## SUMMARY

The field of sleep medicine is still poorly understood. Undoubtedly, further investigation is warranted given that the consequences of various sleep disorders are potentially far-reaching, with life-threatening consequences to the individual, community, and the global environment. Understanding sleep medicine begins with a basic appreciation for the interpretation of the overnight PSG; this chapter provides the fundamental aspects of sleep staging and scoring. Because sleep is not a static process, we reviewed how sleep in humans changes with age. Much of what we are able to perceive about sleep has been derived from the work on many different types of animals; therefore, sleep in other species is described. The highly relevant topic of sleep deprivation has also been briefly explored in this chapter. Finally, a brief overview of the classification of sleep disorders is provided. It is our hope that the reader will be inspired to delve further into the fascinating and challenging world of sleep.

## REFERENCES

1. Diagnostic Classification Steering Committee. International Classification of Sleep Disorders: diagnostic and coding manual. Rochester, MN: American Sleep Disorders Association, 1990.

2. Rechtschaffen A, Kales A, eds. A Manual of Standardized Terminology, Techniques and Scoring System for Sleep Stages of Human Subjects. Los Angeles, CA: Brain Information Service/Brain Research Institute, UCLA, 1968:1–12.
3. Baust W, Holzbach E, Zechlin O. Phasic changes in heart rate and respiration correlated with PGO-spike activity during REM sleep. Pflugers Arch 1972; 331(2):113–123.
4. Orem J. Neuronal mechanisms of respiration in REM sleep. Sleep 1980; 3(3–4): 251–267.
5. Oksenberg A, Gordon C, Arons E, et al. Phasic activities of rapid eye movement sleep in vegetative state patients. Sleep 2001; 24(6):703–706.
6. Chokroverty S. Phasic tongue movements in human rapid-eye movement in sleep. Neurology 1980; 30(6):665–668.
7. Williams RL, Karacan I, Hursch CJ. Electroencephalography (EEG) of Human Sleep: Clinical Applications. New York, NY: John Wiley and Sons, 1974.
8. Anders TF. Maturation of Sleep Patterns in the Newborn Infant. In: Weitzman ED, ed. Advances in Sleep Research. New York, NY: Spectrum, 1975:43.
9. Riter S. Sleep wars: research and opinion. Pediatr Clin North Am 2004; 51(1):1–13.
10. Metcalf DR. EEG sleep spindle ontogenesis. Neuropadiatrie 1970; 1(4):428–433.
11. Metcalf DR, Mondale J, Burler FK. Ontogenesis of spontaneous K complexes. Psychophysiology 1971; 8(3):340–347.
12. Kales A, Kales JD. Sleep disorders. Recent findings in the diagnosis and treatment of disturbed sleep. N Engl J Med 1974; 290(9):487–499.
13. Kleitman N. Phylogenetic, ontogenetic, and environmental determinants in the evolution of sleep-wakefulness cycles. Research Publications–Association for Research in Nervous & Mental Disease 1967; 45:30–38.
14. White RM Jr. The Lengths of Sleep. Washington, D.C.: America Psychological Association, 1975.
15. Webb WB, Friel J. Sleep stage and personality characteristics of "natural" long and short sleepers. Science 1971; 171(971):587–588.
16. Kripke DF, Simons RN, Garfinkel L, et al. Short and long sleep and sleeping pills. Is increased mortality associated? Arch Gen Psychiatry 1979; 36(1):103–116.
17. Benoit O, Foret J, Bouard G. The time course of slow wave sleep and REM sleep in habitual long and short sleepers: effect of prior wakefulness. Hum Neurobiol 1983; 2(2):91–96.
18. Webb WB, Agnew HW. Are we chronically sleep-deprived? Bull Psychonomic Soc 1975; 6:47–48.
19. Bonnet MH, Arand DL. We are chronically sleep-deprived. Sleep 1995; 18(10): 908–911.
20. Kushida C. Sleep Deprivation: Basic Science, Physiology, and Behavior. New York, NY: Marcel Dekker, 2005:1–506.
21. Kushida C. Sleep Deprivation: Clinical Issues, Pharmacology, and Sleep Loss Effects. New York, NY: Marcel Dekker, 2005:1–572.
22. Partinen M. Epidemiology of Sleep Disorders. In: Kryger MH, Roth T, Dement WC, eds. Principles and Practice of Sleep Medicine. 2nd ed. Philadelphia, PA: Saunders, 1994:437.
23. Harrison Y, Horne JA. Should we be taking more sleep? Sleep 1995; 18(10):901–907.
24. Rechtschaffen A, Gilliland MA, Bergmann BM, et al. Physiological correlates of prolonged sleep deprivation in rats. Science 1983; 221(4606):182–184.
25. Clemes SR, Dement WC. Effect of REM sleep deprivation on psychological functioning. J Nerv Ment Dis 1967; 144(6):485–491.
26. Johnson LC, MacLeod WL. Sleep and awake behavior during gradual sleep reduction. Percept Mot Skills 1973; 36(1):87–97.
27. Carskadon MA, Dement WC. Effects of total sleep loss on sleep tendency. Percept Mot Skills 1979; 48(2):495–506.
28. Carskadon MA, Dement WC. Cumulative effects of sleep restriction on daytime sleepiness. Psychophysiololgy 1981; 18(2):107–113.
29. Webb WB, Agnew HW Jr. The effects of a chronic limitation of sleep length. Psychophysiology 1974; 11(3):265–274.

30. Freidmann JK, Globus G, Huntley A, et al. Performance and mood during and after gradual sleep reduction. Psychophysiology 1977; 14(3):245–250.
31. Carskadon MA, Dement WC. Sleep loss in elderly volunteers. Sleep 1985; 8(3): 207–221.
32. Kales A, Tan TL, Kollar EJ, et al. Sleep patterns following 205 hours of sleep deprivation. Psychosom Med 1970; 32(2):189–200.
33. Agnew HW Jr, Webb WB, Williams RL. Comparison of stage 4 and 1-REM sleep deprivation. Percept Mot Skills 1967; 24(3):851–858.
34. National Commission on Sleep Disorders. Wake up America. Washington, D.C.: US Government Printing Office, 1993.
35. Leger D. The cost of sleep related accidents: a report for the National Commission on Sleep Disorders Research. Sleep 1994; 17(1):84–93.
36. Webb WB. The cost of sleep-related accidents: a reanalysis. Sleep 1995; 18(4):276–280.
37. Dinges DF, Broughton RJ. Sleep and Alertness: Chronobiological, Behavioral, and Medical Aspects of Napping. New York, NY: Raven, 1989.
38. Mitler MM, Carskadon MA, Czeisler CA, et al. Catastrophes, sleep and public policy: consensus report. Sleep 1988; 11(1):100–109.
39. Borbely A. Secrets of Sleep. New York, NY: Basic Books, 1984.
40. Zepelin H. Mammalian sleep. In: Kryger MH, Roth T, Dement WC, eds. Principles and Practice of Sleep Medicine. Philadelphia, PA: Saunders, 1994:69.
41. Tauber ES. Phylogeny of Sleep. In: Weitzman ED, ed. Advances in Sleep Research. Vol. I. Flushing, NY: Spectrum, 1974:133.
42. Tobler I, Horne J. Phylogenetic Approaches to the Functions of Sleep. In: Koella WP, ed. Sleep 1982. Basel: S Karger, 1983:126.
43. Tobler I. Evolution of the sleep process: a phylogenetic approach. In: Borbely AA, Valatx JL, eds. Sleep Mechanisms: Experimental Brain Research. Heidelberg: Springer, 1984; 8(Suppl):227.
44. Siegel JM, Manger PR, Nienhuis R, Fahringer HM, Pettigrew JD. The echidna Tachyglossus aculeatus combines REM and NREM aspects in a single sleep state: implications for the evolution of sleep. J Neurosci 1996; 16(10):3500–3506.
45. Zepelin H, Rechtschaffen A. Mammalian sleep, longevity and energy metabolism. Brain Behav Evol 1974; 10(6):425–470.
46. Tobler I. Is sleep fundamentally different between mammalian species? Behav Brain Res 1995; 69(1–2):35–41.
47. Mukhametov LM, Supin AY, Polyakova IG. Interhemispheric asymmetry of the electroencephalographic sleep patterns in dolphins. Brain Res 1977; 134(3):581–584.
48. Hartse KM. Sleep in Insects and Nonmammalian Vertebrates. In: Kryger MH, Roth T, Dement WC, eds. Principles and Practice of Sleep Medicine. 2nd ed. Philadelphia, PA: Saunders, 1994:95.
49. Flannigan WF Jr. Behavioral States and Electroencephalogram of Reptiles. In: Chase MH, ed. The Sleeping Brain: Perspectives in Brain Sciences. Los Angeles, CA: UCLA Brain Information Service/Brain Research Institute, 1972:14.
50. Amlaner CJ Jr, Ball NJ. Avian Sleep. In: Kryger MH, Roth T, Dement WC, eds. Principles and Practice of Sleep Medicine. 2nd ed. Philadelphia, PA: Saunders, 1994:81.
51. Steriade M, Nunez A, Amzica F. A novel slow (<1 Hz) oscillation of neocortical neurons in vivo: depolarizing and hyperpolarizing components. J Neurosci 1993; 13(8):3252–3265.
52. Steriade M, Contreras D, Curro Dossi R, et al. The slow (<1 Hz) oscillation in reticular thalamic and thalamocortical neurons: scenario of sleep rhythm generation in interacting thalamic and neocortical networks. J Neurosci 1993; 13(8):3284–3299.
53. Steriade M, Amzica F. Coalescence of sleep rhythms and their chronology in corticothalamic networks. Sleep Res Online 1998; 1(1):1–10.
54. Amzica F, Steriade M. Electrophysiological correlates of sleep delta waves. Electroencephalogr Clin Neurophysiol 1998; 107(2):69–83.
55. Siegel JM. Brainstem Mechanisms Generating REM sleep. In: Kryger MH, Roth T, Dement WC, eds. Principles and Practice of Sleep Medicine. Philadelphia: W.B. Saunders, 2000:112–133.

56. Steriade M, Pare D, Datta S, et al. Different cellular types in mesopontine cholinergic nuclei related to ponto-geniculo-occipital waves. J Neurosci 1990; 10(8):2560–2579.
57. Holmes CJ, Jones BE. Importance of cholinergic, GABAergic, serotonergic and other neurons in the medial medullary reticular formation for sleep-wake states studied by cytotoxic lesions in the cat. Neuroscience 1994; 62(4):1179–1200.
58. Aston-Jones G, Bloom FE. Activity of norepinephrine-containing locus coeruleus neurons in behaving rats anticipates fluctuations in the sleep-waking cycle. J Neurosci 1981; 1(8):876–886.
59. Estabrooke IV, McCarthy MT, Ko E, et al. Fos expression in orexin neurons varies with behavioral state. J Neurosci 2001; 21(5):1656–1662.
60. Kiyashchenko LI, Mileykovskiy BY, Maidment N, et al. Release of hypocretin (orexin) in during wake and sleep states. J Neurosci 2002; 22(13):5282–5286.
61. Xi MC, Fung SJ, Yamuy J, et al. Induction of active (REM) sleep and motor inhibition by hypocretin in the nucleus pontis oralis of the cat. J Neurophysiol 2002; 87(6):2880–2888.
62. Mignot E, Lammers GJ, Ripley B, et al. The role of cerebrospinal fluid hypocretin measurement in the diagnosis of narcolepsy and other hypersomnias. Arch Neurol 2002; 59(10):1553–1562.
63. The International Classification of Sleep Disorders. Westchester, IL: American Academy of Sleep Medicine, 2005.
64. Gross MM, Goodenough D, Tobin M, et al. Sleep disturbances and hallucinations in the acute alcoholic psychoses. J Nerv Ment Dis 1966; 142(6):493–514.
65. Schenck CH, Bundlie SR, Mahowald MW. Delayed emergence of a parkinsonian disorder in 38% of 29 older men initially diagnosed with idiopathic rapid eye movement sleep behavior disorder. Neurology 1996; 46(6):388–393.
66. Schenck CH, Bundlie SR, Ettinger MG, et al. Chronic behavioral disorders of human REM sleep: a new category of parasomnia. Sleep 1986; 9(2):293–308.
67. De Barros-Ferreira M, Chodkiewicz JP, Lairy GC, et al. Disorganized relations of tonic and phasic events of REM sleep in a case of brain-stem tumour. Electroencephalogr Neurophysiol 1975; 38(2):203–207.
68. Schenck CH, Mahowald MW. Motor dyscontrol in narcolepsy: rapid-eye-movement (REM) sleep without atonia and REM sleep behavior disorder. Ann Neurol 1992; 32(1):3–10.

# 2 The Brain's Dopamine Systems and Their Relevance to Restless Legs Syndrome

**Alon A. Freeman and David B. Rye**

*Department of Neurology, Emory University, Atlanta, Georgia, U.S.A.*

## SYNTHESIS AND METABOLISM OF DOPAMINE

The family of catecholamines includes norepinephrine, epinephrine, and dopamine; of which dopamine is the most abundant in the central nervous system. It was not until the 1950s that dopamine was recognized as a critical neurotransmitter, and not simply an intermediate in the single biosynthetic pathway it shares with norepinephrine and epinephrine. In the first and rate-limiting step of the pathway, L-tyrosine is hydroxylated via the enzyme tyrosine hydroxylase (TH) to form L-dihydroxyphenylalanine (-DOPA) (1). Removal of a carboxyl group from L-DOPA by DOPA decarboxylase then produces dopamine. In subsequent steps, dopamine can then be further converted to norepinephrine and then to epinephrine by dopamine β-hydroxylase and phenylethanolamine-*N*-methyltrasferase, respectively (Fig. 1).

Activation of TH is the rate-limiting step in the production of dopamine and it is under strict regulatory control by a variety of factors, including inhibitory feedback by the catecholamine products (e.g., dopamine). In order to convert tyrosine to L-DOPA, TH requires the binding of iron to the catalytic domain at the C-terminal. Catalytic activity of TH also requires (6R) -(l-erythro-1′, 2′-dihydroxypropyl) -2-amino-4-hydroxu-5,6,7,8-tetrahydropteridine (6R-tetrahydrobiopterin; 6RBPH4, more commonly known as tetrahydrobiopterin (BH4), a naturally occurring pteridine cofactor, to reduce the iron to the ferrous form ($Fe^{2+}$). This allows the binding of the substrates (e.g., L-tyrosine and molecular oxygen) to the C-terminal (2). Following a catalytic cycle, the molecular oxygen can oxidize a fraction of the iron to the ferric form, thus increasing the binding affinity for dopamine and L-DOPA. When either L-DOPA or dopamine is bound to the regulatory domain of the N-terminus, the complex is inactivated by preventing the binding of $BH_4$. Biosynthesis of L-DOPA, and consequently dopamine, can be restored by phosphorylation of the TH enzyme at serine 40 by cyclic adenosine monophosphate (cAMP) -dependent protein kinase (PKA) phosphorylation, thus decreasing the binding affinity for dopamine 300-fold and increasing the binding affinity for the pteridine cofactor (3,4). Meanwhile, endogenous levels of $BH_4$ are regulated by guanosine triphosphate (GTP) cyclohydrolase activity, as its synthesis is downstream of the rate-limiting GTP enzyme (5). Mutations in the GTP cyclohydrolase I gene contribute to hereditary L-DOPA–responsive dystonia (6), which manifests a dopamine-responsive circadian distribution of symptoms with greater penetrance in women, sharing these two features in common with restless legs syndrome (RLS) (7,8).

Following the release of dopamine, the primary mode of removal from the synapse is reuptake into the presynaptic neuron via the dopamine transporter

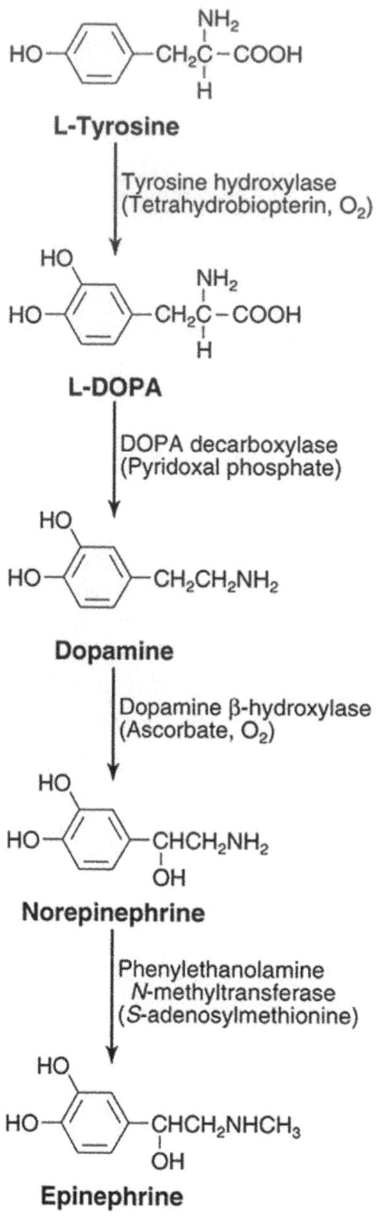

**L-Tyrosine**

Tyrosine hydroxylase
(Tetrahydrobiopterin, $O_2$)

**L-DOPA**

DOPA decarboxylase
(Pyridoxal phosphate)

**Dopamine**

Dopamine β-hydroxylase
(Ascorbate, $O_2$)

**Norepinephrine**

Phenylethanolamine
*N*-methyltransferase
(*S*-adenosylmethionine)

**Epinephrine**

**FIGURE 1** Metabolic pathway leading to the production of dopamine. *Abbreviation*: DOPA, dihydroxyphenylalanine.

(DAT) (Fig. 2). DAT is dependent upon the energy created by the $Na^+/K^+$ pump and is a member of the $Na^+/Cl^-$-dependent plasma membrane transporter family, as are the norepinephrine and γ-aminobutyric acid (GABA) transporters. Imaging studies utilizing compounds with highly specific affinity for DAT (i.e., 3β-(4-iodo-phenyl) tropane-2-carboxylate (B-CIT) permit visualization of the integrity of the DA system.

Once returned to the presynaptic terminal, dopamine is repackaged in synaptic vesicles via the vesicular monoamine transporter-2 (VMAT-2) or metabolized to dihydroxyphenylacetic acid (DOPAC) by monoamine oxidase (MAO). Two alternative pathways are available for dopamine catabolism in the synapse,

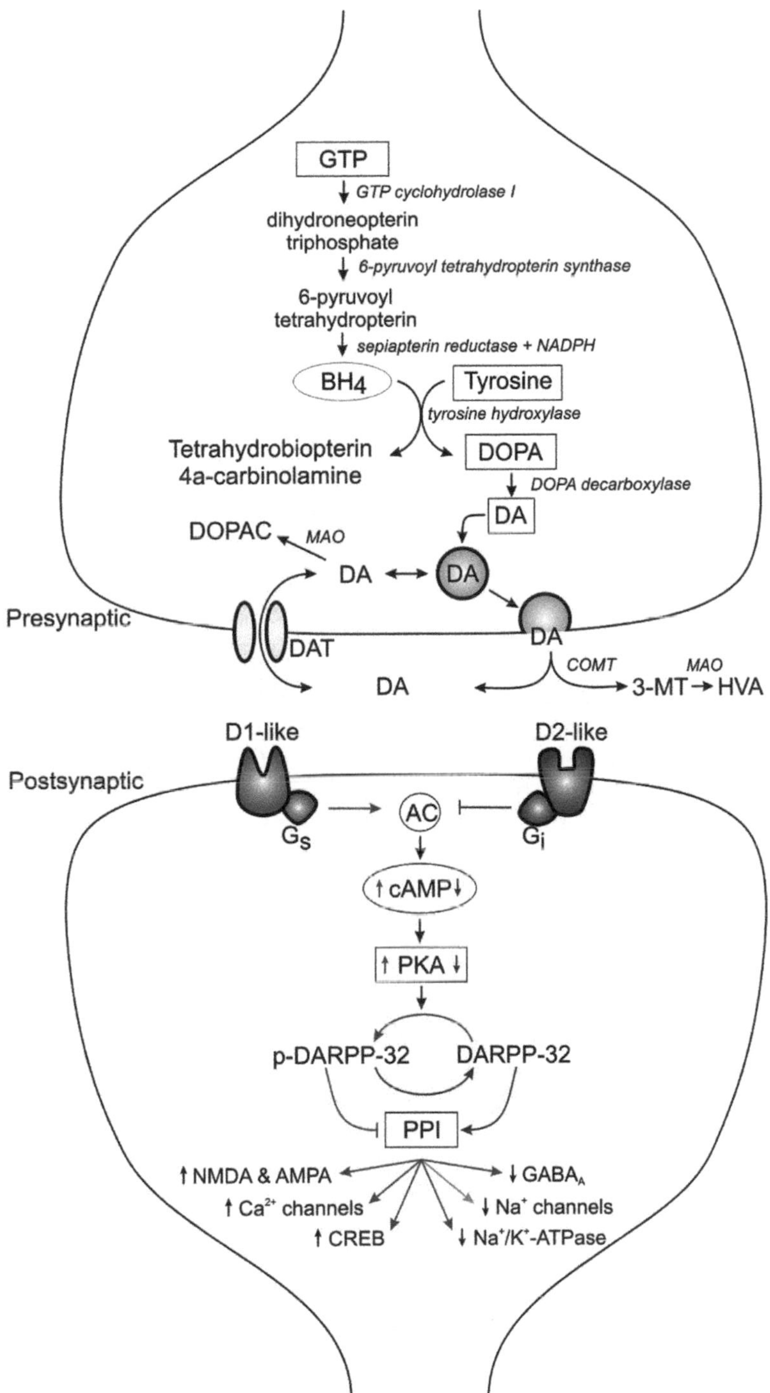


**FIGURE 2** Overview of dopamine: presynaptic, synaptic, and postsynaptic. *Abbreviations*: DOPA, dihydroxyphenylalanine; GTP, guanosine triphosphate; DAT, dopamine transporter; 3-MT, 3-methoxytyramine; HVA, homovanillic acid; cAMP, cyclic adenosine monophosphate; GABA, $\gamma$-aminobutyric acid; PKA, protein kinase; PP1, protein phosphatase-1; MAO, monoamine oxidase; COMT, catechol-O-methyltransferase.

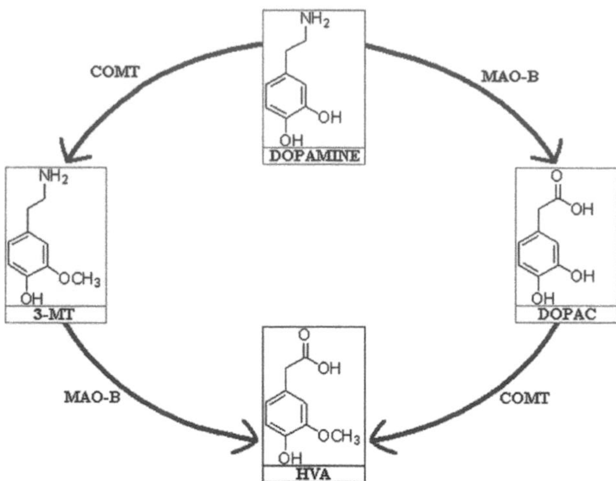


**FIGURE 3** Enzymatic metabolism of dopamine. *Abbreviations*: DOPAC, 3,4-dihydroxyphenyl acetic acid; 3-MT, 3-methoxytyramine; HVA, homovanillic acid; MAO-B, monoamine oxidase-B; COMT, catechol-O-methyltransferase.

depending on whether the first step is catalyzed by MAO or by catechol-O-methyltransferase (COMT). Thus, dopamine can be either deaminated to 3,4-DOPAC or methylated to 3-methoxytyramine (3-MT). In turn, deamination of 3-MT and methylation of DOPAC lead to homovanillic acid (HVA) (Fig. 3). In humans, cerebrospinal fluid levels of HVA have been used as a proxy for levels of dopaminergic activity within the brain. The fidelity of this measure as a true marker of dopaminergic function is not clear.

## PHYSIOLOGICAL EFFECTS OF DOPAMINE (CELLULAR AND SUBCELLULAR)

The physiological effects of the dopaminergic system are best operationalized as "neuromodulatory." Rather than eliciting excitatory (EPSPs) or inhibitory postsynaptic potentials (IPSPs) in a manner similar to glutamate and GABA, dopamine allows the gating of inputs via alteration of membrane properties and specific ion conductances (9). This enhanced or decreased response to other inputs affects the intensity, duration, and timing of output commensurate with environmental and homeostatic demands (10–12). Dopamine's multivariate control is provided through five subtypes of seven transmembrane domain G-protein–coupled receptors (D1–D5), which based upon similarities in pharmacology, biochemistry, and amino acid homology are divided into two classes: $D_1$-like-(D1, D5) and $D_{2\text{-like}}$ (D2, D3, D4) (13). D3 demonstrates the highest affinity for endogenous dopamine followed, in decreasing order of affinity, by D4, D2, D5, and D1 (14,15). Furthermore, each receptor subtype has unique patterns of localization throughout the brain that increases the array of dopamine's behavioral effects.

$D_{1\text{-like}}$ receptors activate the $G_s$ transduction pathway, stimulating the production of adenylyl cyclase that increases the formation of cAMP and ultimately increases the activity of cAMP-dependent PKA. PKA activates DARPP-32 (dopamine and cyclic adenosine 3,5-monophosphate-regulated phosphoprotein,

32 kDa) via phosphorylation, permitting phospho-DARPP-32 to then inhibit protein phosphatase-1 (PP-1). The downstream effect of decreased PP-1 activity is an increase in the phosphorylation states of assorted downstream effector proteins regulating neurotransmitter receptors and voltage-gated ion channels. Ultimately, this results in increased activity of glutamate receptors *N*-methyl-L-aspartate (NMDA) and α-amino-5-hydroxy-3-methyl-4-isoxazole propionic acid (AMPA), $Ca^{2+}$ channels (L-, N-, and P-types), and cAMP response element binding protein (CREB), as well as decreased activity of $GABA_A$ receptors, $Na^+$ channels, and $Na^+/K^+$-ATPase (16). Alternatively, $D_{2\text{-like}}$ receptors stimulate the $G_i$ transduction pathway, which is negatively coupled to the production of adenylyl cyclase. Activation of $D_{2\text{-like}}$ receptors also leads to an increase in intracellular calcium concentrations. These two pathways can act independently, through decreased PKA and increased calcineurin, respectively, to return phospho-DARPP-32 to the inactive DARPP-32. Additionally, calcineurin activity can be stimulated by the increase in intracellular calcium concentrations caused by glutamatergic activation of NMDA receptors. Other mechanisms of action mediated by $D_{2\text{-like}}$ receptors include increasing $K^+$ conductance and inhibiting $Ca^{2+}$ entry via voltage-gated $Ca^{2+}$ channels.

Both $D_{1\text{-like}}$ and $D_{2\text{-like}}$ receptors are found postsynaptically, exerting their effect on nondopaminergic cells targeted by dopaminergic projections. $D_{2\text{-like}}$ receptors can also be localized presynaptically on the dendrites, soma, and presynaptic terminals of dopaminergic cells. The presynaptic localization of these autoreceptors enables them to provide an inhibitory feedback mechanism. The regulation in the somatodendritic region includes modulation of the firing rate of the dopaminergic cell, and in the nerve terminal autoreceptors control the synthesis and release of dopamine. In addition, dopamine appears to act on receptors present on endothelial cells lining the brain's microvasculature promoting vasoconstriction (17). While the exact mechanisms for the regulation of dopamine synthesis and for dopamine release remain to be elucidated, evidence does exist that these are distinct mechanisms (18). For example, in the prefrontal and cingulated cortices, activation of autoreceptors regulates the release, but not the synthesis of dopamine (18). Very low dose effects of dopaminomimetics are mediated by autoreceptor activation, as opposed to postsynaptic receptors, due to their 10-fold higher affinity for dopamine.

## FUNCTIONAL ANATOMY OF CENTRAL DOPAMINE SYSTEMS

It has now been some 40 years since a group of Swedish scientists first described the nigrostriatal, mesocorticolimbic, and tuberoinfundibular dopamine neurons as giving rise to the three most conspicuous and behaviorally relevant dopamine circuits in the brain (19). Using histofluoresence and subsequently immunohistochemical identification of TH (20,21), 16 unique monoaminergic cell groups were identified and given designations A1–A16. Dopamine has been identified as the major transmitter in a portion of A2 in the dorsal motor vagal complex and in groups A8–A16 (22). There is generally marked conversation in the cellular and receptor distributions and major pathways across species with limited exceptions (23). Operationally, these groups can be characterized as long projection vs. local circuit neurons with unique functions (Table 1).

The nigrostriatal pathway originates in the midbrain, from catecholamine cell groups A8 and A9, and projects to the caudate nucleus and putamen (collectively,

**TABLE 1** Major Dopaminergic Modulatory Systems of the Brain

| Origin | | 1° projections | Function |
|---|---|---|---|
| *Long projecting systems* | | | |
| A8 | Midbrain—retrorubral field | Forebrain | (?) |
| A9 | Midbrain—substantia nigra | Caudate/putamen | Motor behaviors |
| A10 | Midbrain—ventral tegmental area | Nucleus accumbens<br>"Limbic" cortical and subcortical structures | Reward<br>Motivation<br>Arousal<br>Appetite |
| A11 | Subparafascicular thalamus | Spinal cord | Sensorimotor<br><br>Autonomic modulation |
| *Local circuits* | | | |
| A12 | Arcuate/periventricular | Median eminence/ infundibular stalk | Modulate hormone release (See text) |
| | Hypothalamus | Intermediate and neural lobes of the hypophysis | |
| A13 | Medial zona incerta | Local; anterior hypothalamus<br>MPO | ? |
| A14 | Periventricular hypothalamus | Local; anterior hypothalamus<br>MPO | ? |
| A15 | Olfactory tubercle | Local | Increase dynamic range for odor detection (24) |
| A16 | Olfactory bulb<br>Periglomerular cells | | |
| A17 | Retina inner nuclear layer Amacrine cells | | Light adaptation—contrast sensitivity (25) |

*Note*: See text for further description or individual references.
*Abbreviation*: MPO, medial preoptic area.
*Source*: From Refs. 21, 26.

often referred to as the dorsal striatum). This pathway is traditionally taught to modulate voluntary (waking) movement and its destruction or degeneration, as seen in Parkinson's disease (PD), results in impairments in the planning, initiation, and execution of movement and motor engrams (26–29). Heuristic models of this major dopaminergic circuit focus themselves upon dopamine's indirect actions (i.e., via the dorsal striatum) upon the internal segment of the globus pallidus and substantia nigra pars reticulata, and a series of parallel, segregated striato-pallidal-thalamocortical recurrent loops centered upon functionally distinct cortical regions (30,31) (Fig. 4). The anatomy of the input and output connections of the A8–A9 neurons and associated behaviors are most often considered in isolation with the basal ganglia nuclei and the thalamus. Moreover, wakefulness has been the "default" medium through which the behavioral correlates of dopamine dysfunction are thought to play out in this major pathway. It is less well established or understood what relevance this dopaminergic system might have to modulation of normal and pathological wake/sleep states such as RLS/periodic limb movements (PLMS) in sleep (32,33).

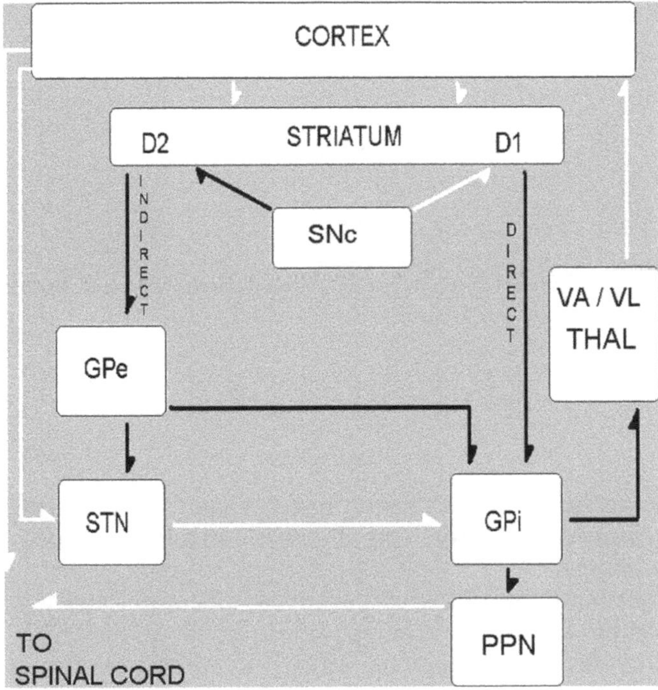


**FIGURE 4** Simplified schematic of basal ganglia circuitry. *Abbreviations*: $SN_c$, substantia nigra pars compacta; $GP_e$, globus pallidus external; VA, ventral anterior; VL, ventral lateral; THAL, thalaine; STN, subthalamic nucleus; GPi, globus pallidus internal; PPN, pedunculopotine nucleus; TO, to spinal cord.

The mesocorticolimbic pathway arises from the midbrain catecholamine cell group A10, within the ventral tegmental area (VTA), and targets the ventral striatum (nucleus accumbens), subcortical limbic nuclei (such as the septum and amygdala), the hippocampus, and prefrontal cortex (34). Activation of this pathway is known to modulate various cognitive/emotive functions including reward, the psychomotor effects associated with drugs of abuse, and working memory (35–37). Disruption of this pathway is thought to modify schizophrenia, attention deficit hyperactivity disorder, Tourette's syndrome, and major depression. Together, the nigrostriatal and mesocorticolimbic systems account for nearly 80% of the brain's dopamine content.

The third major circuit, the tuberoinfundibular and tuberohypophyseal pathways, originates in the hypothalamic arcuate/periarcuate nuclei and periventricular hypothalamus (catecholamine cell groups A12 and A14, respectively). Activation of the A12 cluster modulates the release of numerous hormones in very complex ways; i.e., often in opposing ways at the cellular vs. presynaptic level. Dopamine in the tuberoinfundibular system/anterior pituitary tonically inhibits release of prolactin, and luteinizing and thyroid stimulating hormones, and promotes growth hormone release, primarily via effects on releasing hormones (38–42). The effects of dopamine upon the tuberohypophyseal system include generally inhibitory modulation of vasopressin release and facilitation of oxytocin release (21).

The little-studied A11 catecholamine cell group in the subparafascicular thalamus is the largest source of spinal DA (43–46), although the A14 cell group does send minor projections into the spinal chord, and even the A10 group projects into the cord in some species. Within the spinal cord, these A11 axons target the intermediolateral column housing preganglionic sympathetic neurons, dorsal horn regions related to afferent nerve processing, interneurons (e.g., Renshaw cells), and

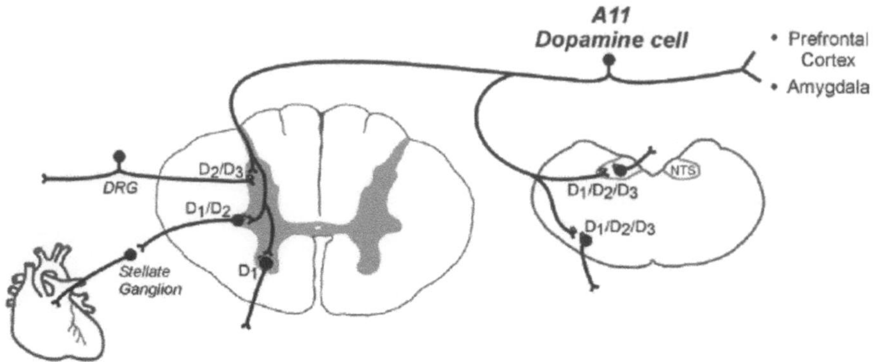


**FIGURE 5** Schematic of A11 dopaminergic pathways.

somatic motoneurons (45), where they likely dampen spinal nociceptive processing and sympathetic outflow, and enhance motor output predominantly via $D_{2\text{-like}}$ receptor mechanisms (Fig. 5) (47,48).

The axons of major projecting brain dopamine systems have a proclivity to collateralize extensively, i.e., individual axons branch, and innervate two or more physically, and perhaps functionally, unique regions (49–51). In addition to innervating the striatum and frontal cortex, for example, A8-A9-A10 neurons also target the thalamus (principally the midline, intralaminar, and reticular nuclei that modulate thalamocortical excitability), the extended amygdala, the noradrenergic locus coeruleus, and the serotonergic raphe system. Axons of individual A11 cells branch extensively to all spinal cord levels along their course in the dorsolateral funiculi, as well as to the prefrontal cortex, amygdala, and nucleus of the solitary tract (52). These arrangements are ideally suited to coordinate behaviors affected by disparate brain areas (e.g., environmental stimuli, cardiorespiratory homeostasis, and sleep/wake state) and bear remarkable semblance to other nuclei traditionally thought of as influencing the organism's arousal state (i.e., comprising the Ascending Reticular Activating System).

## CIRCADIAN AND HOMEOSTATIC INFLUENCES UPON CENTRAL DOPAMINE SIGNALING

It has long been appreciated that there are ultradian rhythms in content, turnover, release, and behavioral responses of many of the brain's dopamine systems outlined above. While we are far from a complete understanding, it is relatively safe to posit that dopamine signaling is under circadian influences that manifest as a peak in activity during the active period and a nadir in the major inactive period (i.e., sleep). This rhythmicity is retained in cultures containing hypothalamic dopamine neurons that are in close proximity to the principal circadian pacemaker (i.e., the suprachiasmatic nucleus), and less evident or absent in cultures containing forebrain or midbrain dopamine neurons (53). Circadian influences upon brain dopamine systems are conveyed in part via melatonin because pinealectomy dampens rhythms in striatal dopamine content (54). There is also increasing evidence of molecular control of dopaminergic transmission by genes involved in the circadian clock (55). Mice expressing an inactive protein of the circadian-associated gene *Clock*, for example, exhibit increased expression and phosphorylation of TH and increased activity in A10 neurons and associated behaviors (55). The first studies to look at circadian variations in human brain monoamine content were those undertaken by Carlsson and colleagues on the hypothalamus in postmortem tissue (56). Hypothalamic dopamine content probably peaks in midday and then drops continuously through the evening reaching its nadir in early morning. It crescendos markedly after 4 to 6 A.M. in people. The greatest variations in dopamine content in the nocturnally active mouse occur within the hypothalamus (57), peaking at midnight then dropping significantly by 4 a.m. At least in part, this appears attributable to diurnal modulation in the expression of TH, which nadirs several hours prior to the major wake period and peaks in the middle of the subjective day coincident with levels of extracellular dopamine, DOPAC and HVA, and motor activity (58–63). Expression of DAT also exhibits a diurnal rhythm that appears to lead these other rhythms in dopamine transmission, at least in the striatum (63). It remains unclear whether these rhythms are mirrored by changes in striatal receptor density (60,64), and whether they might be more pronounced in limbic (65) or motor (66) subcircuits.

Some of the brain's dopamine systems also appear to be under homeostatic influences and this has been most studied in the nigrostriatal pathway. Amongst the brain's dopamine systems, plasticity of the nigrostriatal pathway attending increased drives to sleep appears unique. Hypothalamic dopamine receptors, for example, are unaffected by sleep deprivation (67). Dopamine and its metabolites, as opposed to other monoamines, are increased in the striatum of rapid eye movement (REM)-sleep–deprived rats (68–73). There is disagreement, on the other hand, concerning the precise receptor and regional changes that occur. Some investigators argue for no changes in the absolute receptor number (70,74), while others describe increases in $D_{2\text{-like}}$ receptor binding (75–77). Still others argue for a $D_{1\text{-like}}$ receptor–mediated increase in adenylate cyclase within mesocortical limbic pathways whose reversal with $D_{1\text{-like}}$, as opposed to $D_{2\text{-like}}$ antagonists, facilitates rebound sleep (78–80).

## SUMMARY: DOPAMINE IN "STATE" CONTROL AND ITS RELEVANCE TO RESTLESS LEGS SYNDROME/PERIODIC LIMB MOVEMENTS

Pharmacologic agents that alter neural dopaminergic signaling are some of the most prescribed and effective agents for treating sleepiness and sleep disorders such as RLS/PLMs. While this clinical experience argues that dopamine signaling is integral to the regulation of arousal state, a complete understanding is only beginning to emerge from recent scientific inquiries (32,33,81). To summarize very briefly, differential binding affinities and localizations of the various dopamine receptor subtypes likely account for the biphasic effects that dopaminomimetics have on behavioral state. Low doses promote sleep, including REM sleep that can be antagonized by nonsedating doses of neuroleptics, suggesting a presynaptic $D_{2\text{-like}}$ inhibitory mechanism on terminals or somata of dopaminergic VTA or substantia nigra pars compacta neurons. Higher doses of nonspecific dopaminergic agonists increase locomotor activity, enhance wakefulness, and suppress SWS and REM sleep likely via $D_{1\text{-like}}$ postsynaptic receptors.

A central dopamine hypothesis (viz., a hypofunctioning) to RLS derives from the exquisite sensitivity of most patients to improve with even low doses

**TABLE 2** Dopaminergic Drugs Used to Treat Restless Legs Syndrome Are High-Affinity $D_3$ Receptor Agonists

| Drug | Receptor type affinities[a] |
|---|---|
| Dopamine | High, with $D_{3,4} >> D_{1,2,5}$ |
| Pergolide | High, with $D_3 > D_2 > D_4 >> D_{1,5}$ |
| Pramipexole | High, with $D_3 > D_4 > D_2 >> D_{1,5}$ |
| Cabergoline | High, with $D_3 \sim D_2 > D_5 > D_4 > D_1$ |
| Ropinirole | Very high, with $D_3 >> D_{2,4} >> D_{1,5}$ |
| Rotigotine | High, with $D_3 > D_2 >> D_1$ |

[a]Data obtained from PDSP drug database comparison: http://pdsp.cwru.edu/

*Note*: The table shows the relative affinity of currently used dopaminergics and for comparison, the relative affinity of dopamine for the individual molecularly defined receptors.

of dopaminomimetics (Table 2). This hypothesis endures despite the lack of any compelling biological evidence of dopaminergic dysfunction in RLS patients. Genetic association studies do not point to RLS susceptibility residing in variants of proteins involved in dopamine's synthesis or signaling (82) [see, however (83)]. Cerebrospinal fluid analyses of dopamine and its major metabolites have also been unrevealing (84,85). Imaging studies of the most conspicuous of brain dopamine pathways, the nigrostriatal system, have yielded inconsistent data that have been unable to differentiate between a post- vs. presynaptic dysfunction, or a relative excess vs. deficiency in the availability of synaptic dopamine (86). Decreased fluoro-dopa uptake (87,88) and D2 receptor binding (87,89,90) have been described by some investigators, yet these changes are small, occur in the face of normal DAT binding (90,91), and are not substantiated by another study (92). Difficult to reconcile with a significant presynaptic dysfunction in nigrostriatal terminals underlying the expression of RLS is the clinical experience that RLS (as well as PLMs) occur more, rather than less frequently, in PD in which greater than 80% of midbrain dopaminergic neurons have been lost (93–95). These findings can be reconciled if a dysfunction of dopamine signaling postsynaptically, rather than presynaptically, underlies RLS. Dysfunction of the synapse itself is also possible. Alternatively, this collective data may point to the primary pathophysiology residing in hypofunctioning of the little studied A11 dopaminergic diencephalospinal pathways (*vide supra*) that, despite their small size, exert potent modulatory actions upon spinal networks principally via $D_{2\text{-like}}$ receptors (including the $D_3$ receptor subtype) (47,96–98). One preliminary lesion study of this pathway suggests that interruption of this sole source of spinal dopamine may induce an RLS-like phenotype (99) (Chapter 6). Additional behavioral analysis and specifics concerning the synaptic, cellular, and network mechanisms involved are beginning to emerge. Dopamine and $D_{2\text{-like}}$ agonists, for example, depress the monosynaptic reflex amplitude in the mouse spinal cord in vitro, and that at low but physiological levels of dopamine this modulation is mediated by $D_3$ receptors (i.e., it is absent in functional $D_3$ receptor knockout animals) (98). Mice lacking a functional $D_3$ receptor also exhibit a reversal of their circadian profile of TH in spinal sympathetic neurons (100), and behaviorally are motorically hyperactive and manifest increased wakefulness across the rest–activity cycle (101). Given circadian nadirs of dopamine function discussed above, behavioral effects of any natural or disease-related (e.g., in RLS) reductions in this dopamine circuit would therefore favor an increase in spinal cord nociceptive inputs, reflexes, sympathetic drive, and potentially a phenotype resembling RLS.

## ACKNOWLEDGMENTS

This work was supported by USPHS-NS43374 (DBR) and MH064312 (AF) and the RLS Foundation. We thank Drs. Stefan Clemens and Shawn Hochman for their thoughtful insights and discussions.

## REFERENCES

1. Nagatsu T, Levitt M, Udenfriend S. Tyrosine hydroxylase the initial step in norepinephrine synthesis. J Biol Chem 1964; 239:2910–2917.
2. Nakashima A, Mori K, Suzuki T, et al. Dopamine inhibition of human tyrosine hydroxylase type I is controlled by the specific portion in the N-terminus of the enzyme. J Neurochem 1999; 72:2145–2153.
3. Ramsey A, Fitzpatrick P. Effects of phosphorylation of serine 40 of tyrosine hydroxylase on binding of catecholamines: evidence for a novel regulatory mechanism. Biochemistry 1998; 37:8980–8986.
4. Ramsey A, Hillas P, Fitzpatrick P. Characterization of the active site iron in tyrosine hydroxylase redox states of the iron. J Biol Chem 1996; 271:24395–24400.
5. Nagatsu I. Tyrosine hydroxylase: human isoforms, structure and regulation in physiology and pathology. Essays Biochem 1995; 30:15–35.
6. Bandmann O, Valente E, Holmans P, et al. Dopa-responsive dystonia: a clinical and molecular genetic study. Ann Neurol 1998; 44:649–656.
7. Nygaard T, Marsden C, Duvoisin R. Dopa-responsive dystonia. Adv Neurol 1988; 50:377–384.
8. Nygaard T. Dopa-responsive dystonia. Delineation of the clinical syndrome and clues to pathogenesis. Adv Neurol 1993; 1993:577–585.
9. Nicola S, Surmeier J, Malenka R. Dopaminergic modulation of neuronal excitability in the striatum and nucleus accumbens. Ann Rev Neurosci 2000; 23:185–215.
10. Barbeau H, Rossignol S. Initiation and modulation of the locomotor pattern in the adult chronic spinal cat by noradrenergic, serotonergic and dopaminergic drugs. Brain Res 1991; 546(2):250–260.
11. Kiehn O, Kjaerulff O. Spatiotemporal characteristics of 5-HT and dopamine-induced rhythmic hindlimb activity in the in vitro neonatal rat. J Neurophysio 1996; 75(4):1472–1482.
12. Katz P. Neurons, networks, and motor behavior. Neuron 1996; 16:245–253.
13. Missale C, Nash SR, Robinson SW, Jaber M, Caron MG. Dopamine receptors: from structure to function. Physiol Rev 1998; 78(1):189–225.
14. Sautel F, Griffon N, Levesque D, Pilon C, Schwartz J, Sokoloff P. A functional test identifies dopamine agonists selective for D3 versus D2 receptors. Neuroreport 1995; 6:329–332.
15. Sokoloff P, Andrieux M, Besancon R, et al. Pharmacology of human dopamine D3 receptor expressed in a mammalian cell line: comparison with D2 receptor. Eur J Pharmacol 1992; 225:331–337.
16. Greengard P, Allen P, Nairn A. Beyond the dopamine receptor: the DARPP-32/protein phosphatase-1 cascade. Neuron 1999; 23:435–447.
17. Krimer LS, Muly EC III, Williams GV, Goldman-Rakic PS. Dopaminergic regulation of cerebral cortical microcirculation. Nat Neurosci 1998; 1(4):286–289.
18. Cooper J, Bloom F, Roth R. The Biochemical Basis of Neuropharmacology. 8th ed. New York: Oxford University Press, 2002.
19. Dahlstrom A, Fuxe K. Evidence for the existence of monoamine-containing neurones in the central nervous system. I. Demonstration of monoamines in the cell bodies of brain stem neurones. Acta Physiol Scand 1964; 232(suppl):1–55.
20. Hokfelt T, Martensson R, Bjorklund A, Kleinau S, Goldstein M. Distributional maps of tyrosine-hydroxylase-immunoreactive neurons in the rat brain. In: Bjorklund A, Hokfelt T, eds. Handbook of Chemical Neuroanatomy. New York: Elsevier, 1984:277–379.
21. The Dopaminergic System. New York: Springer Verlag, 1985.

22. Lindvall O, Bjorklund A. Neuroanatomy of central dopamine pathways: review of recent progress. In: al. MKe, ed. Advances in Dopamine Research. Oxford and New York: Pergamon Press, 1982:297–311.
23. Smeets W, Gonzalez A. Catecholamine systems in the brain of vertebrates: new perspectives through a comparative approach. Brain Res Brain Res Rev 2000; 33:308–379.
24. Ennis M, Zhou F, Ciombor K, et al. Dopamine D2 receptor-mediated presynaptic inhibition of olfactory nerve terminals. J Neurophysiol 2001; 86:2986–2997.
25. Witkovsky P. Dopamine and retinal function. Doc Ophthalmol 2004; 108:17–40.
26. Kandel ER, Schwartz JH, Jessell TM. Principles of Neural Science. 4th ed. New York: McGraw-Hill, 2000.
27. Grillner S, Hellgren J, Menard A, Saitoh K, Wikstrom M. Mechanisms for selection of basic motor programs–roles for the striatum and pallidum. Trends Neurosci 2005; 28:364–370.
28. Albin R, Young A, Penney J. The functional anatomy of basal ganglia disorders. Trends Neurosci 1989; 12:366–375.
29. DeLong MR. Primate models of movement disorders of basal ganglia origin. Trends Neurosci 1990; 13:281–285.
30. Alexander GE, Crutcher MD, DeLong MR. Basal ganglia-thalamocortical circuits: parallel substrates for motor, oculomotor, "prefrontal" and "limbic" functions. Prog Brain Res 1990; 85:119–146.
31. Alexander G. Anatomy of the basal ganglia and related motor structures. In: Watts R, Koller W, eds. Movement Disorders: Neurologic Principles and Practice. New York: McGraw-Hill, 1997:73–86.
32. Rye D. Parkinson's disease and RLS: the dopaminergic bridge. Sleep Med 2004; 5: 317–328.
33. Rye D. The two faces of Eve: dopamine's modulation of wakefulness and sleep. Neurology 2004; 63(suppl 3):S2–S7.
34. Williams SM, Goldman-Rakic PS. Widespread origin of the primate mesofrontal dopamine system. Cereb Cortex 1998; 8(4):321–345.
35. Tzschentke T, Schmidt W. Functional relationship among medial prefrontal cortex, nucleus accumbens, and ventral tegmental area in locomotion and reward. Crit Rev Neurobiol 2000; 14:131–142.
36. Fibiger H, Phillips A. Reward, motivation, cognition: psychobiology of mesotelencephalic dopamine systems. In: Handbook of Physiology. Vol. 4. Intrinsic regulatory systems of the brain. Bethesda: American Physiology Society 1986:647–675.
37. Goldman-Rakic PS. Cellular basis of working memory. Neuron 1995; 14(3):477–485.
38. Krulich L. Central neurotransmitters and the secretion of prolactin, GH, LH and TSH. Ann Rev Physiol 1979; 41:603–615.
39. Behrends J, Prank K, Dogu E, Brabant G. Central nervous system control of thyrotropin secretion during sleep and wakefulness. Horm Res 1998; 49:173–177.
40. Martin J. Neural regulation of growth hormone secretion. Med Clin North Am 1978; 62:327–336.
41. Benker G, Jaspers C, Hausler G, Reinwein D. Control of prolactin secretion. Klin Wochenschr 1990; 68:1157–1167.
42. Muller E. Nervous control of growth hormone secretion. Neuroendocrinology 1973; 11:338–369.
43. Bjorklund A, Skagerberg G. Evidence for a major spinal cord projection from the diencephalic A11 dopamine cell group in the rat using transmitter-specific fluorescent retrograde tracing. Brain Res 1979; 177(1):170–175.
44. Hokfelt T, Phillipson O, Goldstein M. Evidence for a dopaminergic pathway in the rat descending from the A11 cell group to the spinal cord. Acta Physiol Scand 1979; 107(4):393–395.
45. Skagerberg G, Bjorklund A, Lindvall O, Schmidt RH. Origin and termination of the diencephalo-spinal dopamine system in the rat. Brain Res Bull 1982; 9(1–6):237–244.
46. Skagerberg G, Lindvall O. Organization of diencephalic dopamine neurones projecting to the spinal cord in the rat. Brain Res 1985; 342(2):340–351.

47. Fleetwood-Walker S, Hope P, Mitchell R. Antinociceptive actions of descending dopaminergic tracts on cat and rat dorsal horn somatosensory neurones. J. Physiol (Lond) 1988; 399:335–348.
48. Gladwell S, Coote J. Inhibitory and indirect excitatory effects of dopamine on sympathetic preganglionic neurones in the neonate rat spinal cord in vitro. Brain Res 1999; 818:397–407.
49. Sanchez-Gonzalez M, Garcia-Cabezas M, Rico B, Cavada C. The primate thalamus is a key target for brain dopamine. J Neurosci 2005; 25:6076–6083.
50. Freeman A, Ciliax B, Bakay R, et al. Nigrostriatal collaterals to thalamus degenerate in parkinsonian animal models. Ann Neurol 2001; 50:321–329.
51. Gaspar P, Stepniewska I, Kaas JH. Topography and collateralization of the dopaminergic projections to motor and lateral prefrontal cortex in owl monkeys. J Comp Neurol 1992; 325(1):1–21.
52. Takada M. Widespread dopaminergic projections of the subparafascicular thalamic nucleus in the rat. Brain Res Bull 1993; 32:301–309.
53. Abe M, Herzog ED, Yamazaki S, et al. Circadian rhythms in isolated brain regions. J Neurosci 2002; 22(1):350–356.
54. Khaldy H, Leon J, Escames G, Bikjdaouene L, Garcia JJ, Acuna-Castroviejo D. Circadian rhythms of dopamine and dihydroxyphenyl acetic acid in the mouse striatum: effects of pinealectomy and of melatonin treatment. Neuroendocrinology 2002; 75(3):201–208.
55. McClung C, Sidiropoulou K, Vitaterna M, et al. Regulation of dopaminergic transmission and cocaine reward by the Clock gene. Proc Natl Acad Sci USA 2005; 102:9377–9381.
56. Carlsson A, Svennerholm L, Winblad B. Seasonal and circadian monoamine variations in human brain examined post mortem. Acta Pyschiatr Scan Suppl 1980; 280: 275–285.
57. Matsumoto M, Kimura K, Fujisawa A, et al. Diurnal variations in monoamine contents in discrete brain regions of the mongolian gerbil (Meriones unguiculatus). J Neurochem 1981; 37:792–794.
58. McGeer E, McGeer P. Some characteristics of brain tyrosine hydroxylase. In: Mandel A, ed. New Concepts in Neurotransmitter Regulation. New York: Plenum Press, 1973: 53–68.
59. Simon ML, George R. Diurnal variations in plasma corticosterone and growth hormone as correlated with regional variations in norepinephrine, dopamine and serotonin content of rat brain. Neuroendocrinology 1975; 17(2):125–138.
60. Bruinink A, Lichtensteiger W, Schlumpf M. Ontogeny of diurnal rhythms of central dopamine, serotonin and spirodecanone binding sites and of motor activity in the rat. Life Sci 1983; 33(1):31–38.
61. Smith AD, Olson RJ, Justice JB Jr. Quantitative microdialysis of dopamine in the striatum: effect of circadian variation. J Neurosci Methods 1992; 44(1):33–41.
62. Schade R, Vick K, Sohr R, et al. Correlative circadian rhythms of cholecystokinin and dopamine content in nucleus accumbens and striatum of rat brain. Behav Brain Res 1993; 59(1–2):211–214.
63. Whittaker J, Morcol T, Patrickson J. Circadian plasticity in dopaminergic parameters in the rat substantia nigra. Soc Neurosci Abstr 1997; 23(80.2):190.
64. Watanabe S, Seeman P. D2 dopamine receptor density in rat striatum over 24 hours: lack of detectable changes. Biol Psychiatry 1984; 19(8):1249–1253.
65. O'Neill RD, Fillenz M. Simultaneous monitoring of dopamine release in rat frontal cortex, nucleus accumbens and striatum: effect of drugs, circadian changes and correlations with motor activity. Neuroscience 1985; 16(1):49–55.
66. Paulson PE, Robinson TE. Relationship between circadian changes in spontaneous motor activity and dorsal versus ventral striatal dopamine neurotransmission assessed with on-line microdialysis. Behav Neurosci 1994; 108(3):624–635.
67. Lal S, Thavundayil J, Nair NP, et al. Effect of sleep deprivation on dopamine receptor function in normal subjects. J Neural Transm 1981; 50(1):39–45.

68. Ghosh PK, Hrdina PD, Ling GM. Effects of REMS deprivation on striatal dopamine and acetylcholine in rats. Pharmacol Biochem Behav 1976; 4(4):401–405.
69. Tufik S, Lindsey CJ, Carlini EA. Does REM sleep deprivation induce a supersensitivity of dopaminergic receptors in the rat brain?. Pharmacology 1978; 16(2):98–105.
70. Farber J, Miller JD, Crawford KA, McMillen BA. Dopamine metabolism and receptor sensitivity in rat brain after REM sleep deprivation. Pharmacol Biochem Behav 1983; 18(4):509–513.
71. Asakura W, Matsumoto K, Ohta H, Watanabe H. REM sleep deprivation decreases apomorphine-induced stimulation of locomotor activity but not stereotyped behavior in mice. Gen Pharmacol 1992; 23:337–341.
72. Farooqui SM, Brock JW, Zhou J. Changes in monoamines and their metabolite concentrations in REM sleep-deprived rat forebrain nuclei. Pharmacol Biochem Behav 1996; 54(2):385–391.
73. Lara-Lemus A, Drucker-Colin R, Mendez-Franco J, Palomero-Rivero M, Perez de la Mora M. Biochemical effects induced by REM sleep deprivation in naive and in D-amphetamine treated rats. Neurobiology 1998; 6(1):13–22.
74. Hamdi A, Brock J, Ross K, Prasad C. Effects of rapid eye movement sleep deprivation on the properties of striatal dopaminergic system. Pharmacol Biochem Behav 1993; 46:863–866.
75. Zwicker A, Calil H. The effects of REM sleep deprivation on striatal dopamine receptor sites. Pharmacol Biochem Behav 1986; 24:809–812.
76. Nunes G Jr, Tufik S, Nobrega N. Autoradiographic analysis of D1 and D2 dopaminergic receptors in rat brain after paradoxical sleep deprivation. Brain Res Bull 1994; 34(5):453–456.
77. Brock JW, Hamdi A, Ross K, Payne S, Prasad C. REM sleep deprivation alters dopamine D2 receptor binding in the rat frontal cortex. Pharmacol Biochem Behav 1995; 52(1):43–48.
78. Fadda P, Martellotta MC, De Montis MG, Gessa GL, Fratta W. Dopamine D1 and opioid receptor binding changes in the limbic system of sleep deprived rats. Neurochem Int 1992; 20(suppl):153S–156S.
79. Fadda P, Martellotta MC, Gessa GL, Fratta W. Dopamine and opioids interactions in sleep deprivation. Prog Neuropsychopharmacol Biol Psychiatry 1993; 17(2):269–278.
80. Durán-Vázquez A, Drucker-Colín R. Differential role of dopamine receptors on motor asymmetries of nigro-stratal lesioned animals that are REM sleep deprived. Brain Res 1997; 744:171–174.
81. Rye DB, Jankovic J. Emerging views of dopamine in modulating sleep/wake state from an unlikely source: PD. Neurology 2002; 58(3):341–346.
82. Desautels A, Turecki G, Montplaisir J, et al. Dopaminergic neurotransmission and restless legs syndrome: a genetic association analysis. Neurology 2001; 57:1304–1306.
83. Desautels A, Turecki G, Montplaisir J, et al. Evidence for a genetic association between monoamine oxidase A and restless legs syndrome. Neurology 2002; 59:215–219.
84. Earley C, Hyland K, Allen R. CSF dopamine, serotonin, and biopterin metabolites in patients with restless legs syndrome. Mov Disord 2001; 16:144–149.
85. Stiasny-Kolster K, Moller J, Zschocke J, et al. Normal dopaminergic and serotonergic metabolites in cerebrospinal fluid and blood of restless legs syndrome patients. Mov Disord 2004; 19:192–196.
86. Wetter T, Eisensehr I, Trenkwalder C. Functional neuroimaging studies in restless legs syndrome. Sleep Med 2004; 5:401–406.
87. Turjanski N, Lees A, Brooks D. Striatal dopaminergic function in restless legs syndrome. Neurology 1999; 52:932–937.
88. Routtinen H, Partinen M, Hublin C, Bergman J, Haaparanta M, Solin O, et al. An FDOPA PET study in patients with periodic limb movement disorders and restless legs syndrome. Neurology 2000; 54:502–504.
89. Staedt J, Stoppe G, Kogler A, et al. Nocturnal myoclonus syndrome (periodic movements in sleep) related to central dopamine D2-receptor alteration. Eur Arch Psychiatr Clin Neurosci 1995; 245:8–10.

90. Michaud M, Soucy J, Chabli A, Lavigne G, Montplaisir J. SPECT imaging of striatal pre- and postsynaptic dopaminergic status in restless legs syndrome with periodic leg movements in sleep. J Neurol 2002; 249:164–170.
91. Linke R, Eisensehr I, Wetter T, et al. Presynaptic dopaminergic function in patients with restless legs syndrome: are there common features with early Parkinson's disease? Mov Disord 2004; 19:1158–1162.
92. Eisensehr I, Wetter TC, Linke R, et al. Normal IPT and IBZM SPECT in drug-naive and levodopa-treated idiopathic restless legs syndrome. Neurology 2001; 57:1307–1309.
93. Bliwise D, Rye D, Dihenia B, et al. Periodic leg movements in elderly patients with Parkinsonism. Sleep 1998; 21(suppl):196.
94. Wetter T, Collado-Seidel V, Pollmacher T, Yassouridis A, Trenkwalder C. Sleep and periodic leg movement patterns in drug-free patients with Parkinson's disease and multiple system atrophy. Sleep 2000; 23(3):361–367.
95. Ondo WG, Vuong KV, Khan H, Atassi F, Kwak C, Jankovic J. Daytime sleepiness and other sleep disorders in Parkinson's disease. Neurology 2001; 57:1392–1396.
96. Garraway S, Hochman S. Modulatory actions of serotonin, norepinephrine, dopamine, and acetylcholine in spinal cord deep dorsal horn neurons. J Neurophysiol 2001; 86:2183–2194.
97. Barriere G, Mellen N, Cazalets J. Neuromodulation of the locomotor network by dopamine in the isolated spinal cord of the newborn rat. J Neurophysiol 2004; 19:1325–1335.
98. Clemens S, Hochman S. Conversion of the modulatory actions of dopamine on spinal reflexes from depression to facilitation in D3 receptor knock-out mice. J Neurosci 2004; 24:11337–11345.
99. Ondo WG, He Y, Rajasekaran S, Le WD. Clinical correlates of 6-hydroxydopamine injections into A11 dopaminergic neurons in rats: a possible model for restless legs syndrome. Mov Disord 2000; 15(1):154–158.
100. Clemens S, Sawchuk M, Hochman S. Reversal of the circadian expression of tyrosine-hydroxylase but not nitric oxide synthase levels in the spinal cord of D3 receptor knockout mice. Neurosci 2005; 133:353–357.
101. Hue G, Decker M, Solomon I, Rye D. Increased wakefulness and hyper-responsivity to novel environments in mice lacking functional dopamine D3 receptors. In: Society for Neuroscience, 2003.

# 3 Circadian Physiology

**Mauro Manconi and Luigi Ferini-Strambi**

*Department of Neurology, Sleep Disorders Center, University Vita-Salute, IRCCS H San Raffaele, Milan, Italy*

## INTRODUCTION

Some biological phenomena occur once in a lifetime, whereas others occur repeatedly. Repeated events that occur over regular intervals become cyclic phenomena. One cycle is represented by the necessary route of that phenomenon to repeat itself. The duration of a cycle is defined as a period. The biological cyclic phenomena with a period of 24 hours are termed "circadian" (from latin "circa diem" meaning about one day), those with a period shorter than 24 hours, for instance, the respiratory or the heart beat rhythms, are called "ultradian," and those with a period longer than circadian, such as the menstrual cycle, are called "infradian." The rhythmic oscillations of most of these phenomena are under the control of both endogenous and exogenous factors. The former usually correspond to specialized cells that exhibit the property of autodepolarization, called "pacemakers." The second are represented by all the external factors able to influence or overcome the pacemaker's rhythm. In animals, the main endogenous clock is constituted by the suprachiasmatic nucleus (SCN) (1), while the dark–light alternation, due to the axial earth rotation, represents the most important external environment (2). Body core temperature, sleep, motor activity, and melatonin (MLT) secretion are typical examples of physiological circadian phenomena. Hypnic headache, paroxysmal nocturnal hemoglobinuria, and restless legs syndrome (RLS) are only a few of many pathological conditions that, for different reasons, follow a circadian rhythm of expression. Chronobiology is a young science that studies the basis of physiological and pathological circadian phenomena. The most common method used by this scientific branch to measure the burden of each exogenous or endogenous factor in driving a specific circadian cycle is to eliminate or strengthen the considered factor, keeping constant all the others, and then detect the consequences on the circadian system. If this operation causes a period shift on the given rhythm, it means that the factor has a role in deciding the circadian oscillation of the system. During the last decades, the application of this study's paradigm under standard laboratory conditions has noticeably improved the knowledge around the pathophysiology of the circadian phenomena.

## ENTRAINMENT EFFECT OF LIGHT–DARK ALTERNATION

It is no coincidence that the internal biological clock of most living things, from single-cell prokaryotes to humans, has a periodicity of approximately 24 hours. Obviously, evolution selected the species with a behavioral rhythm more or less synchronous to the rotation of the earth. Among all potential environmental factors on circadian rhythms, light was the first, and remains the most studied.

In about the middle of the 20th century it was demonstrated that the artificial administration of light stimulus on biological systems was able to induce a phase shift on circadian rhythm (3). The direction and the intensity of the shift changed according to when the stimulus was provided within the 24-hour day. The mathematical relationship between the time of light administration and the shift in the circadian system is graphically synthesized by the so-called phase-response curve (PRC) (4). The PRC shows that when the light stimulus is presented during the early subjective night it provokes a phase-delay shift, while the same stimulus presented in the late subjective night advances the circadian rhythm. The light effect during the subjective day is markedly reduced in some animals and, even abolished in others, during a time of the day known as the "dead zone" (5). Dark stimulus during the day usually has no effect. Until recently, several studies demonstrated that the experimental exposure to bright light induces phase shift on the majority of circadian biological phenomena, such as sleep, body temperature, MLT, and cortisol secretion (6–9).

According to the theory of the dose–response curve (DRC), the magnitude of the phase shift also depends, with nonlinear behavior, on the intrinsic characteristics of the light, such as the duration of exposure (10), the intensity of stimulus (11), and the spectral composition in terms of wavelength (12).

The majority of understanding regarding the mechanisms of light effect on animals remains unclear. The retina is a necessary target for light entrainment. Because PRC and DRC are also preserved in postchiasmatic blind people without conscious light perception, and even in different sightless experimental animals, it is likely that the photoreception apparatus accountable for these responses is distinct from that one responsible for the sensorial visual function (13–15). From these specialized cone photoreceptors the signal activates a pool of ganglion cells that project by the retinohypothalamic tract (RHT) to the SCN, and by the geniculohypothalamic tract (GHT) to the intergeniculate leaflet (IGL) of the thalamus (16). The RHT consists of monosynaptic glutamatergic neurons whose postsynaptic effect is mediated by *N*-methyl-d-aspartate (NMDA) and α-amino-5-hydroxy-3-methyl-4-isoxazole propionic acid receptors coupled with cyclic adenosine monophosphate (cAMP). Intracellular increases of calcium and cAMP in SCN cells results in a phosphorylation of nuclear DNA-binding proteins that regulate the transcription of specific genes. Reciprocal nervous connections between SCN and IGL nuclei have been demonstrated. Experimental lesions of RHT or GHT affect the light entrainment on circadian rhythm (17).

Although the strongest, light is not the only exogenous entrainment. Especially in human beings, food intake, locomotor activity, knowledge of the clock time, or different social cues, such as bedtime and work schedule, can reset the biological rhythms.

## SUPRACHIASMATIC NUCLEUS

The existence of an endogenous pacemaker has been strengthened by more recent experiments conducted on humans and animals in free-running conditions. One study protocol showed that the main circadian rhythms (temperature, sleep, and hormone secretion) also persist in experimental isolation from all the exogenous entrainments, including light (18). Under constant external environmental conditions, the persistent biological rhythm of the majority of living beings has a period not exactly of 24 hours, but of around 25 hours (about a day). In the early 1970s, the finding that a bilateral lesion of a small part of the hypothalamus of rodents led to a disruption of the circadian biological fluctuations represented the first step in identifying the location of the endogenous pacemaker in the SCN (19,20). When the SCN cells are isolated in vitro or in vivo they maintain a rhythm of firing and secretion of approximately 24 hours; this demonstrates that these cells owe the intrinsic fundamental capacity of autodepolarization to a neurophysiologic mechanism that should reside, and can be generated, within the same neurons (21). Transplantation of SCN tissue into the diencephalon of SCN-lesioned animals restores circadian oscillations, with a rhythm that reflects the specific characteristics of the donor and not of the recipient (22). The physiology of SCN can be simplified into three main functions: autodepolarization, a response to external input stimuli as light, and a faculty to influence circadian rhythms by output signals (23,24). Even though most of the underlying cellular mechanisms supporting the SCN autodepolarization are still unsolved, the discovery of clock (*circadian locomotor output cycles kaput*) genes represented an important step toward understanding the problem. The term clock genes identifies a family of loci involved in circadian physiology, which exhibit a clear circadian rhythm of transcription, or a transcriptional response, to entrainment inputs (24). Period (*Per*), Cryptochrome (*Cry*), and *Rev-Erbα* are typical examples of clock genes.

Mammals' SCN consists in a bilateral symmetric group of about 20,000 neurons, located in the anterior part of the hypothalamus (25). Cells of the SCN have differing phenotype, innervation, functions, and gene expression. In rodents, the dorsal medial shell part of SCN produces vasopressin (VP), and receives little afferent neurons from the retina. The ventrolateral part of the SCN receives more consistent innervations from the retina, and is composed of three different kinds of cells containing: vasoactive intestinal peptide (VIP), calbinding and substance P (SP), and gastrin-releasing peptide (GRP). The shell part of the SCN has a self-sustained rhythm ascribed to a circadian autoregulatory transcriptional–translation loop involving clock gene expression (26–29). In these cells, the dimerization of two nuclear proteins CLOCK and BMAL allows their binding to the promoter region of *Per*, *Cry*, and *Rev-Erbα* genes, activating their transcription. As the respective *Per* and *Cry* proteins accumulate in the cytoplasm, they dimerize and move into the nucleus to exert an inhibitory effect on the CLOCK and BMAL, resulting in an inhibition of their own transcription and closing of a negative feedback cycle. The SCN shell neurons converse with the targets by γ-amino butyric acid (GABA) and VP secretion (24).

Although the core part of the SCN does not express an autonomous circadian rhythm, it shows a strong expression of *Per* genes in response to light stimulus, and it seems to be essential for an harmonic synchronization of the different parts of the SCN (30). Light stimulus, through the retina and RHT, induces glutamate (GLU) and SP release in the SCN core (31,32). GLU binding with NMDA is followed by an increase of influx calcium, which activates protein kinases that phosphorylate the c-AMP-response-element-binding protein (CREB) (33). Phosphorylated CREB binds the promoter regions of *Per-1* and *Per-2*, inducing their transcription. By VIP, GRP, and SP, the SCN core neurons communicate to the SCN shell cells where *Per* transcription occurs with a constant delay with respect to the external stimulus and the *Per* transcription in the SCN core (34).

While the two main RHT and GHT afferent nervous pathways to the SCN are well-defined, the efferent projections from SCN are less well-known, especially in humans. Efferent neurons to the paraventricular nucleus (PVN), ventromedialis nucleus, subparaventricular zone (SPZ) of the hypothalamus, and SCN itself have been demonstrated (35). The SPZ could be differentiated into a ventral and in a dorsal part. Lesional experiments showed that the ventral SPZ is a relay region mainly involved in the circadian control of sleep–wake and locomotor activity, while the dorsal SPZ principally regulates temperature body rhythm. The SCN could also drive circadian rhythm via diffusible substance, in agreement with the evidence that driving function is preserved in SCN cell transplantation (35,36). Therefore, local nuclei could be affected without direct traditional axonal connections. Because in vivo monitoring of the SCN is almost impossible, body core temperature and MLT secretion are generally used as phase markers of SCN activity, given that their oscillation periods closely resemble that of the hypothalamic pacemaker.

When free-running experiments are extended for a long time, some vegetative functions, such as body temperature, cortisol secretion, and REM sleep, desynchronized from the behavioral functions such as motor activity or food and drink intake, which continue to follow the SCN rhythm. This phenomenon, described as "internal desynchronization," suggested the existence of other different endogenous clocks, and a strong dependence of behavioral input to the SCN rhythm. The existence of these different endogenous pacemakers and this possible hierarchical relationship with the SCN is still debated (37).

## MELATONIN

Before its molecular structure and its multiple roles were deciphered, melatonin (MLT) was merely a mysterious substance produced by the pineal gland (PG). It became an object of interest because of its control of skin coloration on amphibians. In 1917, McCord and Allen, applying extract of bovine PG to frog skin, produced a skin lightening (38). This extract was later (1958) identified to be *N*-acetyl-5-methoxytryptamine, and named by their discoverers Lerner et al. as MLT because of its effect on amphibian skin (39). A few years before, Bargman had suggested that the secretion of this substance was regulated by the light (40). Simultaneously, Kitay and Altschule demonstrated the influence of MLT in regulating the animal seasonal reproductive function (41,42). Implications of MLT in circadian and seasonal reproduction control, and stimulation on amphibian's skin melanophores, represent the main roles of this hormone, whereas its involvement in regulation of immune system, gut, retina, and antioxidant and antiaging function are likely but still not well-established (42).

### Synthesis and Catabolism

Even though the retina and gastrointestinal tract contribute to MLT synthesis, vertebrate PG is the most important tissue of secretion (43). The anabolism pathway of MLT begins with the drawing of tryptophan from the bloodstream and its conversion into 5-hydroxy-tryptophan in pineal mitochondria by tryptophan hydroxylase (44). After translocation into the cytosol, the molecule is decarboxylated to serotonin (5-HT) (45). Among the five different indoleamines that are created from 5-HT, MLT exerts the main physiological role. 5-HT is acetylated into *N*-acetyl-serotonin by arylalkylamine-*N*-acetyl-transferase (NAT), and finally methylated into MLT by hydroxyndole-*O*-methyltransferase (HIOMT) (46,47). The mRNA expression, protein, and enzymatic activity of both NAT and HIOMT are almost undetectable during the day and increase significantly (more than 100-fold for NAT) during the night (48,49). The nocturnal peak even persists in constant darkness, and it is strongly suppressed by light exposition (50). NAT (chromosome 17q25) and HIOMT (chromosome X) genes transcription are regulated by clock proteins, which seem to be critical for the circadian rhythmic expression of the respective enzymes (51,52). NAT is considered the rate-limiting enzyme for MLT synthesis, while HIOMT represents the majority of cytosolic proteins of pinealocytes (48). Although monoamine oxidase (MAO) enzymes do not participate directly in the MLT synthesis, they are detectable in pinealocytes (MAO B) and in nervous terminals to PG (MAO A), where their activity follows a circadian rhythm with the highest value during the day (53).

Because MLT has a short half-life (20–40 minutes), its plasma concentration mainly depends on its rate of production. MLT is degraded via cytochrome 450 in the liver and then sulfanated in the kidney and eliminated as 6-sulfatoxy-MLT in the urine (54).

## Input to Pineal Gland and Sites of Action of Melatonin

The foremost neuronal input to PG consists of a multisynaptic pathway named the retinohypotalamic–pineal tract. The first step of this pathway is represented by the previously mentioned RHT, which comes from the retina and ends in the ventrolateral SCN (55,56). The endogenous pacemaker (SCN) projects inhibitory and excitatory neurons to the PVN mediated by GABA and VIP/VP, respectively (57). The PVN projects to the intermediolateral neurons of the first three cervical spinal levels via oxytocin and VP, where the injection of these two neurotransmitters to this spinal area decreases MLT plasma concentrations (58). From there, cholinergic excitatory neurons reach the superior cervical ganglion that projects sympathetic innervation to the PG (59). Besides norepinephrine, these nerve endings contain dopamine, serotonin, VIP, and neuropeptide Y (NPY). Other neuronal input to the PG originated from: the thalamic IGL via NPY, the PVN via VP and oxytocin, the lateral hypothalamus via hypocretin, and the habenular nucleus via SP (60). Non-neuronal input to epiphysis is represented by several hormones and substances, including delta-sleep–inducing peptide and luteinizing-releasing hormone; they may exert control by endocrine, paracrine, and autocrine effects (Fig. 1) (61).

Although MLT reaches several non-nervous tissues such as the gut, ovaries, blood vessels, and others, the highest concentration of MLT receptors is documented in the brain (62). Three categories of MLT receptors (MLT-R) have been demonstrated. MLT-$R_1$ is a G-protein-coupled receptor mostly expressed in brain with the highest concentration in the pars tuberalis of the adenohypophysis and in the SCN (63). MLT-$R_2$ are widespread in the retina and the brain, while MLT-$R_3$ is a low-affinity receptor identifiable with quinone reductase 2 (63,64). In SCN, MLT-$R_1$ seems to mediate an inhibitory electrical effect of hyperpolarization, while the MLT-$R_2$ could be involved in the shift-phase mechanism (42).

## Melatonin as a Circadian Hormone

In all mammals MLT has a circadian expression; it is secreted during the dark phase and inhibited by light. Thus, in diurnal animals, the MLT peak occurs during sleep. While the dependence of MLT by light/dark alternation through the SCN is well-accepted, it still remains unclear which effects MLT exerts on the SCN and on circadian phenomena in general. Furthermore, the effects of MLT on circadian

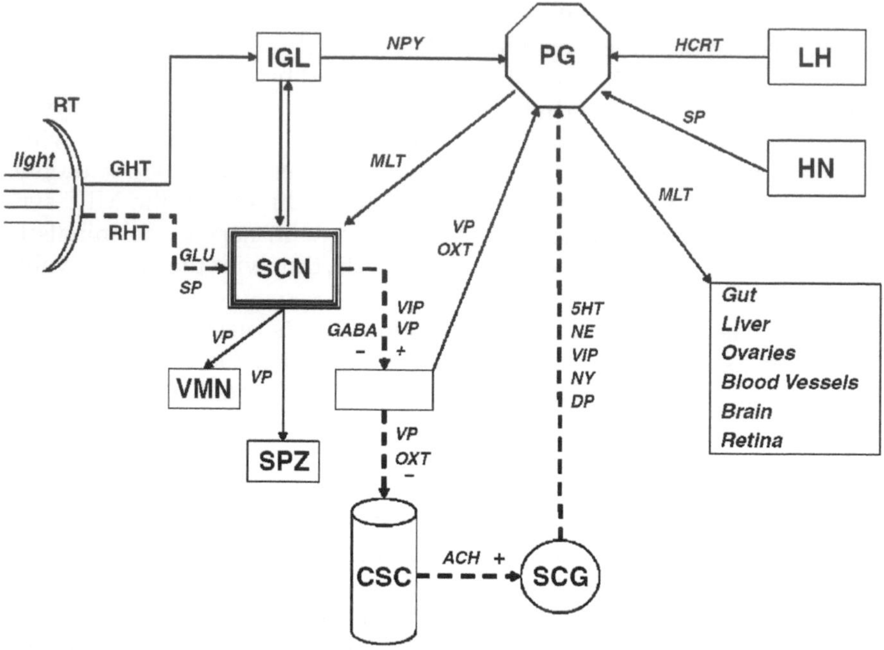


**FIGURE 1** Schematic organization of nervous network for circadian control. Light exerts its entrainment on SCN by the RHT. The nervous terminal of this pathway contains GLU and SP. Thanks to its autodepolarization property, the SCN represents the endogenous pacemaker. VIP, VP, and GABA are the main neurotrasmitters for the SCN efferents to VMN, SPZ, and PVN. SCN is also connected by a reciprocal innervation to IGL. SNC acts on PG through the multisynaptic retinohypothalamic–pineal pathway, which is represented in the figure by sketched line. Other inputs to PG are from IGL, LH, and HN. PG produces MLT, which reaches its targets via paracrine and endocrine secretion. MLT receptors are located in several neuronal and extraneuronal tissues. *Abbreviations:* RT, retina; GHT, geniculohypothalamic tract; IGL, intergeniculate leaflet; RHT, retino-hypothalamic tract; SCN, suprachiasmatic nucleus; VMN, ventromedialis nucleus; SPZ, subparaventricular zone; PVN, paraventricular nucleus; CSC, cervical spinal cord; SCG, superior cervical ganglia; PG, pineal gland; LH, lateral hypothalamus; HN, habenular nucleus; GLU, glutamate; VP, vasopressin; VIP, vasointestinal peptide; OXT, oxytocin; ACH, acetylcoline; 5-HT, 5-hydroxy-triptamine; NE, norepinephrine; DP, dopamine; NY, neuropeptide Y; SP, substance P; MLT, melatonin; HCRT, hypocretin.

rhythm varied widely across different animal species. In some avian species, pinealectomy almost abolishes the circadian organization of body temperature, locomotor activity, or feeding (65). In rats, pinealectomy failed to alter rest–motor circadian pattern. Pinealectomy experiments may be affected by numerous methodological limits: in many species the PG is not the only MLT source, results could depend on the level and timing of light exposure, and the PG could influence circadian rhythms by other non-MLT substances. In constant dark free-running conditions, high doses of exogenous MLT could entrain circadian rhythms (66). In vitro, MLT advances the circadian phase on SCN cells only if administrated during permissive time windows (67). In humans, the hypnotic effect of exogenous MLT is still debated, while the chronobiologic capability in shifting the circadian phase is more accepted. The current point of view considers MLT as a rapidly delivered mediator, used primarily by the SCN, to inform the various MLT target tissues of the circadian timing. In other words, MLT may represent a time-giver hormone with a synchronization role on the activities of different structures. MLT is like a biological reporter who keeps the organism informed on the external (light for first) and internal entrainment, giving them a better adaptation to the daily and seasonal variations. Nevertheless, MLT-agonist drugs have proven to be effective sedative hypnotics.

## CIRCADIAN AND HOMEOSTATIC CONTROL OF SLEEP

Sleep, as feeding and locomotor activity, strictly follows a circadian expression (68,69). In humans, sleep occurs during dark, together with high levels of circulating MLT and low values of body temperature (70). Circadian organization of sleep depends on the internal SCN drive and external factors mainly represented by light. Exogenous entrainments exert a so-called masking effect on endogenous rhythm, so sleep timing is the natural consequence of a harmonic fight between geophysical and internal pacemaker influences. Light exposure during dark phase stimulates wakefulness, locomotor activity, and increases body temperature, while light suppression during the day does the opposite (23). The light entrainment is mostly mediated by the already described RHT pathway through the SCN. In constant dark/light free-running conditions, sleep rhythm maintains a cyclic organization that prolongs to 25.5 hours. The acute free-running results seem, therefore, to assign a prominent role to SCN compared to light. The chronic effect of long free-running condition appears to produce a further extension of the sleep/wake cycle that, in some experiments, may reach duration up to 40 hours (71). A few authors reported that in this extreme condition the body temperature could maintain its 25 hours cycle, yielding to the above-mentioned desynchronization state (37,72). The respective independence of sleep from the endogenous pacemaker is simulated by the experimental lesion of the SCN. In mammals, the consequences of this procedure severely disrupt circadian sleep organization (25). The manner by which the SCN, through its efferent branches, exerts its control on sleep centers, remains elusive. The SCN projects by different neurotransmitters to several brain regions (73,74). Because the experiments of midbrain transection do not affect circadian expression of sleep, it is supposed that SCN regulation is mediated by direct influences on supratentorial structures. Possible sites of action of SCN could be represented by the ventral preoptic area and by the histaminergic neurons of the posterior hypothalamus. The last region projects diffusely to several brain areas involved in the arousal control of the cortex (75–77). Cholinergic forebrain and midbrain areas are also considered. On the other side, a humoral control of sleep by SCN is strongly supported by the fact that transplantation of SCN cells in animals previously lesioned in the SCN restores this circadian sleep rhythm without needing direct neuronal connections (22).

Although very disorganized, sleep is also possible after SCN lesion. Moreover, long free-running protocol may show a desynchronization between SCN and sleep rhythm. These results suggest the existence of another control mechanism for sleep occurrence. This mechanism could be in part identified in the homeostatic process. In mammals, the EEG delta power of NREM sleep is proportional to the duration of prior wakefulness (78). Sleep propensity increases in a nonlinear way during the day and decreases during the night. Sleep deprivation induces sleep pressure, which allows falling asleep during a circadian period that is usually not permissive to sleep. In humans, sleep deprivation of greater than 18 hours is sufficiently high to overcome endogenous circadian drive (79). An accumulation of specific substances in cerebral spinal fluid during wakefulness, and their removal during sleep, could stand for the base of homeostatic process. Adenosine, GABA, dopamine, prostaglandins, and other neuropeptides could be implicated in the homeostatic control of sleep (80–84).

Both circadian and homeostatic processes modulate the sleep propensity by acting on the so-called "sleep gate." The opening level of the "sleep gate" depends on the combination of circadian and homeostatic pressure. In humans, sleep usually occurs about 2 hours before MLT peak and 4 hours before temperature body nadir, and continues for about 2 hours after temperature nadir and 5 to 6 hours after MLT peak (85,86).

In mammals, a rest/activity circadian expression is demonstrable after the last gestational period of the fetus (87). Maternal SCN activity, in concert with the external light/dark influence and by using circulating MLT, could exert an entrainment effect in synchronizing the fetal SCN activity. The homeostatic control of sleep seems to develop itself around the first weeks of life (88).

## CIRCADIAN PATTERN OF RESTLESS LEGS SYNDROME/PERIODIC LIMB MOVEMENTS

RLS symptoms are "worst during the evening and/or night hours." Although the circadian physiology of RLS had not been yet scientifically demonstrated when the above statement was first made, it had already appeared as the fourth decisive item in the (1995) diagnostic criteria for RLS (89). This is because the daily rhythm of RLS has always been one of the most solid and undisputed empiric feature of RLS. The oldest dated RLS description, made by Willis in 1683, already underlined the temporal relationship between symptoms and sleep/bed, with these words: "when being a *Bed* they betake themselves to sleep, presently in the Arms and Legs, Leapings and Contractions of the Tendons, and so great a Restlessness and Tossings of their Members ensue, that the diseased are no more able to sleep, than if they were in a Place of the greatest Torture" (90). Later, this link was confirmed by Ekbom, who stated that: "The patients cannot sleep, but are forced to lie and move their legs and continually change their position, to sit on the edge of the bed and kick, or walk about on the floor" (91). In both reports, the evening worsening of RLS was correlated with the words sleep and bed, as sleepiness and rest could have some causal relationship with the symptoms (90,91). Even though unanimously recognized and estimated as an essential feature, only in the last decade did very few experimental protocols focus on the circadian aspect of RLS (92–98). Probing deep into this topic essentially means to collect data regarding three fundamental issues: RLS circadian pattern observation, temporal description of its trend, and assessment of eventual causal relationships of RLS with external and internal circadian phenomena. While the first issue is nearly assessed, the second needs a better definition, and the third is almost unexplored.

### Definition of RLS and PLMs Circadianity

Unfortunately, there are no biological markers for objectively assessing the daily RLS course. The only objective measure available for this topic may be represented by the periodic limb movements (PLM) index. Therefore, in order to obtain reliable and comparable data, investigators first of all should decide which parameter to observe, and then to monitor its trend by the same standard methods and in the same standard environmental conditions. Sensory RLS symptoms could be assessed only through the patient, by repetitive subjective evaluation. The conventional RLS scale of severity is not suitable for this purpose because it is validated to measure the symptoms' intensity of the previous 30 days before its compilation (99). Existing studies were forced to use the visual analogical scale to quantify symptoms at different day times (93,94,96). During sleep, symptoms could be evaluated only by waking patients up at regular intervals or by using a sleep deprivation protocol. A continuous video recording of patient movements or the more reliable assessment of PLM are generally used to quantify the motor component. The number of PLM during sleep (PLMS) per standard time intervals of the night is an easy and solid index of RLS course. Moreover, it has recently been demonstrated that there is a fairly good correlation between RLS symptoms' severity and PLMS index (100). During the day, and in general during wakefulness, the PLMS index could be substituted by the index of PLM during wakefulness by applying the suggested immobilization test (SIT) more times per day (101).

The earliest investigation performed by using the aforementioned methods goes back to 1995, when Montplaisir et al. demonstrated a significant increase of RLS symptoms and PLM from morning to evening (92). Later, a few investigations delineated a better symptom course by assessing at a higher frequency and by evaluating multiple features (93,94,96). Hening et al., acquiring sensory and PLM data every three hours in nine subjects, described the circadian pattern, finding a peak of severity of both factors between midnight and 4:00 A.M., and a nadir between 9:00 A.M. and 1.00 P.M. (93). The same results were obtained by Trenkwalder et al., who confirmed the close link between symptoms and PLM trend (94). Using a higher frequency of detection (every 2 hours), Michaud et al. established that the symptoms and PLM peaked around 3:00 A.M. and nadired around 9:00 A.M. Although these are the only studies available at this time, their results appear to be quite homogeneous. PLMS index progressively decreases during night. Because the percentage of PLMS correlated to arousal seems to remain stable through the sleep cycles of the night, it has been assumed that PLMS course could not be directly dependent on the arousal threshold and sleep propensity (102). The trend of both the sensory and the motor components imitate the course of body temperature (93,94,96). PLM and sensory symptoms increase during the descending phase of the temperature curve, with a peak around the temperature nadir, and improve together with temperature arising. Body temperature follows a normal course in RLS patients, suggesting a regular function of circadian endogenous pacemaker (Fig. 2).

## Entrainment Effect of Motor Activity and Sleep

The second and the third standard diagnostic criteria state that RLS symptoms "begin or worsen during rest or inactivity, and are partially or totally relieved by movement" (99). Experiments using SIT demonstrated that this assumption is valid also for PLM which, as with the sensation discomfort, increase linearly with rest (100). Such evidences suggested that the evening and night worsening of RLS severity was due to a generic and physiological decrease of locomotor activity during the late part of the day. To verify this hypothesis, it is necessary to observe the symptoms while eliminating the influence of the motor variable. Since the forcing of rest for a long period is indeed impractical, a constant routine protocol has been

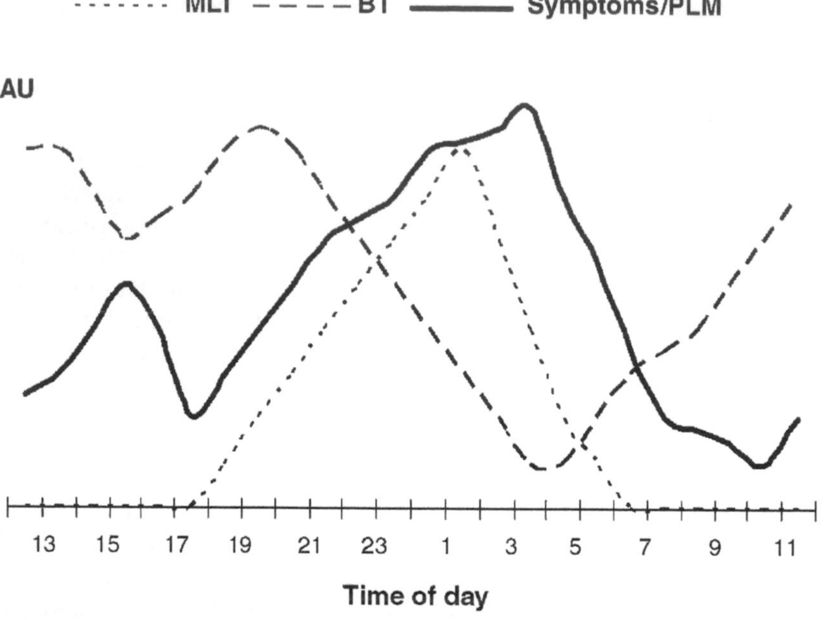


**FIGURE 2** Circadian course of RLS symptoms and PLM. *Abbreviations*: AU, arbitrary unit; MLT, melatonin; BT, body temperature; RLS, restless legs syndrome; PLM, periodic limb movements.

usually adopted for this purpose. This approach failed to affect the circadian trend of RLS intensity (93,94,96). Almost the same considerations can be done regarding the influence of sleep pressure. Actually, in according with the homeostatic sleep process, RLS symptoms worsened concurrently with the increase of sleepiness and decrease of vigilance, and improved progressively with reduction in delta power and resumption of arousal system during the night. Is the sleep process determinant for the RLS circadiancy? Applying the sleep deprivation protocol, Hening et al. and Trenkwalder et al. tried to answer this question (93,94). They assessed sensory symptoms and PLM course in nine and eight RLS patients, respectively, for 3 nights and 3 days in constant routine conditions. Patients underwent 2 days of physiological sleep/wake alternation, followed by a night and successive day of sleep deprivation. In both investigations, although a mild worsening of symptoms was noticed during the third day compared to the two previous days, the circadian trend of RLS was not overcome by the sleep deprivation, and the usual morning improvement and the evening worsening was confirmed (93,94). In other words, despite the fact that sleepiness and rest may modulate RLS symptoms, their suppression did not affect RLS circadian expression, which is probably regulated by an unknown independent circadian factor. In conclusion, the distinction between rest/motor activity and circadian influences, operating by the diagnostic criteria, seems to be appropriate because it is motivated by experimental evidences that suggest an autonomous effect of each factor on RLS (103).

### Role of Dopamine and Melatonin in RLS Circadian Expression

Some evidence supports the idea that dopamine hypofunctioning plays an important role in RLS pathogenesis: symptoms improve by dopaminergic drugs and worsen with antidopaminergic drugs. PLM and RLS are often noticed in patients affected by Parkinson's disease. Motor hyperexcitability in animal models has been induced by lesions of the hypothalamic dopaminergic neurons that project to spinal centers. Iron deficiency (iron is a key coenzyme in the dopamine anabolism) is a strong risk factor for RLS and data from a few single-photon emission computed tomography (SPECT) and positron emission tomography (PET) analysis showed modest dopamine abnormality in basal ganglia of RLS patients (104).

Dopamine is very widespread in the brain, and its modulation effect on locomotor and motor activity is well-known. The main dopaminergic encephalic nuclei are represented by the substantia nigra (nigrostriatal system) and by the midbrain ventral tegmental area (mesocorticolimbic system). However, a conspicuous group of dopamine-producing cells is also documented in the hypothalamus, in particular the posterior (A11), arcuate (A12), dorsocaudalis (A13), and periventricular (A14) areas (105). Among the other functions, hypothalamic dopamine exerts an inhibitory action on pituitary prolactin (PRL) secretion and a descending control on the dorsal horn spinal neurons, which are likely relevant in modulating pain afferents (106). The interest around dopamine as a possible key neurotransmitter in RLS pathogenesis became more relevant after the discovery of several links between dopamine and circadian physiology. Central nervous system dopamine concentration follows a circadian trend with higher levels during the subjective day, especially at the beginning of the day, together with high locomotor activity and low levels of MLT (107). Tyrosine hydroxylase (TH), the rate-limiting enzyme in dopamine synthesis, shows also a circadian trend in brain cells (108). In D3 receptor knockout mice, the circadian trend of TH is disrupted (109). Moreover, a circadian course has been demonstrated for the cellular surface expression of D2 and D3 receptors, possibly under Clock gene transcription control (109). A possible explanation of the circadian dopamine oscillation could be represented by SCN influences on dopaminergic neurons. The SCN projects directly to the A11 hypothalamic area (105,110,111). Furthermore, lesion of the SCN results in a disruption of dopamine circadian rhythm. Because the dopamine rhythm does not restore after a reimplantation of SCN cells, it is likely that efferent SCN control on dopamine centers is neuronal and not humorally mediated (112). In patients affected by idiopathic RLS, PRL and growth hormone show an exaggerated response to L-Dopa administration only during nighttime. This enhanced response could be a consequence of a D2/D3 receptor's upregulation (95).

Circadian expression of dopamine could also be explained by its significant interactions with MLT (113). D1 and D2 dopamine receptors are demonstrated in PG cells (113). In some mammals, D1 agonist binding enhances NAT activity, increasing MLT level, while a D2 activation inhibited NAT activity, decreasing MLT level. Both functions are mediated by an opposite regulation of intracellular cAMP and CREB (114). Dopamine receptors are also confirmed on dopamine-productive cells of retina. In these photoreceptors, MLT synthesis is strongly inhibited by light and dopamine (115–117). On the opposite side, MLT inhibits dopamine release in several nervous system areas such as the hippocampus and brainstem, but also the hypothalamus and retina (113). Antidopaminergic activities of MLT are also well-documented in basal ganglia, where they can modulate motor activity. In patients with Parkinson's disease, MLT, likely because of its action on dopamine, could worsen motor symptoms, but also could improve tardive dyskinesia (118–120). In idiopathic RLS, symptoms peak together with temperature and vigilance nadir, but follow about 2 hours MLT zenith (96).

Taken together, the above data suggest that the circadian expression of RLS could be the consequence of a nightly decrease in dopamine level as a direct result of interaction with MLT, and indirectly through more complex interactions with SCN activity, without excluding a possible modulation activity exerted by sleep propensity and light influence. Further research is needed to support this suggestive hypothesis, especially regarding the potential modulation of RLS symptoms by exogenous MLT administration.

## ACKNOWLEDGMENT

The book edited by Fred W. Turek and Phyllis C. Zee (1), as well as the article reviewed by Valerie Simonneaux and Christophe Ribelayga (42) have been two precious sources in writing this chapter. The authors also thank Chadron Rose for intellectual suggestions and English revision.

## REFERENCES

1. Zee PC, Turek FW. Introduction to sleep and circadian rhythms. In: Turek FW, Zee PC, eds. Lung Biology in Health and Disease, Vol.133. New York: Basel, 1999:1–17.
2. Aschoff J, Fatranska M, Giedke H, et al. Human circadian rhythms in continuous darkness: entrainment by social cues. Science 1971; 171(967):213–215.
3. Hastings JW, Sweeney BM. A persistent diurnal rhythm of luminiscence in Gonyaulax polyedra. Bio Bull 1959; 115:440–458.
4. Winfee AT. The geometry of biological time. New York: Springler-Verlag, 1980.
5. Pohl H. Characteristics and variability in entrainment of circadian rhythms to light in diurnal rodents. In: Structure and Physiology. Berlin: Springler-Verlag, 1982:339–346.
6. Dijk DJ, Beersma DG, Daan S, et al. Bright morning light advances the human circadian system without affecting NREM sleep homeostasis. Am J Physiol 1989; 256(1 Pt 2): R106–R111.
7. Lewy AJ, Sack RL, Miller LS, et al. Antidepressant and circadian phase-shifting effects of light. Science 1987 16; 235(4786):352–354.
8. Dijk DJ, Visscher CA, Bloem GM, et al. Reduction of human sleep duration after bright light exposure in the morning. Neurosci Lett 1987; 73(2):181–186.
9. Czeisler CA, Allan JS, Strogatz SH, et al. Bright light resets the human circadian pacemaker independent of the timing of the sleep-wake cycle. Science 1986; 233(4764):667–671.
10. Johnson CH, Hastings JW. Circadian phototransduction: phase resetting and frequency of the circadian clock of Gonyaulax cells in red light. J Biol Rhythms 1989; 4(4):417–437.
11. Nelson DE, Takahashi JS. Sensitivity and integration in a visual pathway for circadian entrainment in the hamster (Mesocricetus auratus). J Physiol 1991; 439:115–145.
12. DeCoursey PJ, Buggy J. Circadian rhythmicity after neural transplant to hamster third ventricle: specificity of suprachiasmatic nuclei. Brain Res 1989; 500(1–2):263–275.
13. Vuillez P, Herbin M, Cooper HM, et al. Photic induction of Fos immunoreactivity in the suprachiasmatic nuclei of the blind mole rat (Spalax ehrenbergi). Brain Res 1994; 654(1):81–84.
14. Foster RG, Provencio I, Hudson D, et al. Circadian photoreception in the retinally degenerate mouse (rd/rd). J Comp Physiol 1991; 169(1):39–50.
15. Meijer JH, Groos GA, Rusak B. Luminance coding in a circadian pacemaker: the suprachiasmatic nucleus of the rat and the hamster. Brain Res 1986; 382(1):109–118.
16. Card JP, Whealy ME, Robbins AK, et al. Two alpha–herpesvirus strains are transported differentially in the rodent visual system. Neuron 1991; 6(6):957–969.
17. Harrington ME. The ventral lateral geniculate nucleus and the intergeniculate leaflet: interrelated structures in the visual and circadian systems. Neurosci Biobehav Rev 1997; 21(5):705–727.

18. Dijk DJ, Czeisler CA. Contribution of the circadian pacemaker and the sleep homeostat to sleep propensity, sleep structure, electroencephalographic slow waves, and sleep spindle activity in humans. J Neurosci 1995; 15(5 Pt 1):3526–3538.
19. Stephan FK, Zucker I. Circadian rhythms in drinking behavior and locomotor activity of rats are eliminated by hypothalamic lesions. Proc Natl Acad Sci U S A 1972; 69(6): 1583–1586.
20. Ibuka N, Kawamura H. Loss of circadian rhythm in sleep-wakefulness cycle in the rat by suprachiasmatic nucleus lesions. Brain Res 1975; 96(1):76–81.
21. Welsh DK, Logothetis DE, Meister M, et al. Individual neurons dissociated from rat suprachiasmatic nucleus express independently phased circadian firing rhythms. Neuron 1995; 14(4):697–706.
22. Ralph MR, Foster RG, Davis FC, et al. Transplanted suprachiasmatic nucleus determines circadian period. Science 1990; 247(4945):975–978.
23. Saper CB, Lu J, Chou TC, et al. The hypothalamic integrator for circadian rhythms. Trends Neurosci 2005; 28(3):152–157.
24. Antle MC, Silver R. Orchestrating time: arrangements of the brain circadian clock. Trends Neurosci 2005; 28(3):145–151.
25. Weaver DR. The suprachiasmatic nucleus: a 25-year retrospective. J Biol Rhythms 1998; 13(2):100–112.
26. Mai JK, Kedziora O, Teckhaus D, et al. Evidence for subdivisions in the human suprachiasmatic nucleus. J Comp Neurol 1991; 305:508–525.
27. Card JP, Moore RY. The suprachiasmatic nucleus of the golden hamster: immunohistochemical analysis of cell fiber distribution. Neuroscience 1984; 13:415–443.
28. Moore RY, Speh JC, Leak RK. Suprachiasmatic nucleus organization. Cell Tissue Res 2002; 309:89–98.
29. Abrahamson EE and Moore RY. Suprachiasmatic nucleus in the mouse: retinal innervation, intrinsic organization and efferent projections. Brain Res 2001; 916:172–191.
30. Meijer JH, Rusak B, Ganshirt G. The relation between light-induced discharge in the suprachiasmatic nucleus and phase shifts of hamster circadian rhythms. Brain Res 1992; 598:257–263.
31. Bryant DN, LeSauter J, Silver R, et al. Retinal innervation of calbindin-D28K cells in the hamster suprachiasmatic nucleus: ultrastructural characterization. J Biol Rhythms 2000; 15:103–111.
32. Tanaka M, Hayashi S, Tamada Y, et al. Direct retinal projections to GRP neurons in the suprachiasmatic nucleus of the rat. Neuroreport 1997; 8(9–10):22187–22191.
33. Yan L, Silver R. Differential induction and localization of mPer1 mPer2 during advancing delaying phase shifts . Eur J Neurosci 2002; 16:1531–1540.
34. Yan L and Silver R. Resetting the brain clock: time course and localization of mPER1 and mPER2 protein expression in suprachiasmatic nuclei during phase shifts. Eur J Neurosci 2004; 19:1105–1109.
35. Dai J, Swaab DF, Buijs RM. Distribution of vasopressin and vasoactive intestinal polypeptide (VIP) fibers in the human hypothalamus with special emphasis on suprachiasmatic nucleus efferent projections. J Comp Neurol 1997; 383(4):397–414.
36. Roenneberg T, Morse D. Two circadian oscillators in one cell. Nature 1993; 362: 362–364.
37. Erkert HG. Internal desynchronization of the circadian activity and feeding rhythm in an owl monkey (Aotus lemurinus griseimembra): a case study. Chronobiol Int 2000; 17(2):147–153.
38. McCord CP and Allen FB. Evidence associating pineal gland function with alterations in pigmentation. J Exp Zool 1917; 23:207–224.
39. Lerner AB, Takahashi Y, Lee TH, et al. Isolation of melatonin, the pineal gland factor that lightens melanocytes. J Am Chem Soc 1958; 80:2587.
40. Iuvone PM, Tosini G, Pozdeyev N, et al. Circadian clocks, clock networks, arylalkylamine N-acetyltransferase, and melatonin in the retina. Prog Retin Eye Res 2005; 24(4):433–456.
41. Miller AL. Epidemiology, etiology, and natural treatment of seasonal affective disorder. Altern Med Rev 2005; 10(1):5–13.

42. Simonneaux V, Ribelayga C. Generation of the melatonin endocrine message in mammals: a review of the complex regulation of melatonin synthesis by norepinephrine, peptides, and other pineal transmitters. Pharmacol Rev 2003; 55(2):325–395.
43. Arendt J. Melatonin and the Mammalian Pineal Gland. London: Chapman and Hall, 1995.
44. Lovenberg W, Jequier E, Sjoerdsma A. Tryptophan hydroxylation: measurement in pineal gland, brain stem and carcinoid tumor. Science (Washington D.C.) 1967; 155: 217–219.
45. Lovenberg W, Weissbach H, Undenfriend S. Aromatic L-amino acid decarboxylase. J Biol Chem 1962; 237:89–92.
46. Weissbach H, Redfield BG, Axelrod J. Biosynthesis of melatonin: enzymatic conversion of serotonin to N-acetyl-serotonin. Biochem Biophys Acta 1960; 43:352–353.
47. Axelrod J, Weissbach H. Enzymatic O-methylation of N-acetylserotonin to melatonin. Science (Washington D.C.) 1960; 131:1312.
48. Miguez JM, Simonneaux V, Pévet P. Role of intracellular and extracellular serotonin in the regulation of melatonin production in rat pinealocytes. J Pineal Res 1997; 23: 63–71.
49. Ribelayga C, Pévet P, Simonneaux V. Adrenergic and peptidergic regulations of hydroxyindole-O-methyltransferase in rat pineal gland. Brain Res 1997; 777:247–250.
50. Ribelayga C, Gauer F, Pévet P, et al. Photoneural regulation of rat pineal hydroxyindole-O-methyltransferase (HIOMT) messenger ribonucleic acid expression: an analysis of its complex relationship with HIOMT activity. Endocrinology 1999; 140: 1375–1384.
51. Coon SL, Mazuruk K, Bernard M, et al. The human serotonin N-acetyltransferase (EC 2.3.1.87) gene (AANAT): structure, chromosomal localization and tissue expression. Genomics 1996; 34:76–84.
52. Weber M, Lauterburg T, Tobler I, et al. Circadian patterns of neurotransmitter related gene expression in motor regions of the rat brain. Neurosci Lett 2004; 358(1):17–20.
53. Yang HYT, Goridis C, Neff NH. Properties of monoamine oxydases in sympathetic nerve and pineal gland. J Neurochem 1972; 19:1241–1250.
54. Waldhauser F, Waldhauser M, Lieberman HR, et al. Bioavailability of oral melatonin in humans. Neuroendocrinology 1984; 39(4):307–313.
55. Moore RY, Klein DC. Visual pathways and the central neural control of a circadian rhythm in pineal serotonin N-acetyltransferase activity. Brain Res 1974; 71:17–33.
56. Klein DC, Moore RY. Pineal N-acetyltransferase and hydroxyindole-O-methyltransferase: control by the retinohypothalamic tract and the suprachiasmatic nucleus. Brain Res 1979; 174:245–262.
57. Lucas RJ, Freedman MS, Munoz M, et al. Regulation of the mammalian pineal by non-rod, non-cone ocular photoreceptors. Science (Washington D.C.)1999; 284:423–425.
58. Gilbey MP, Coote JH, Fleetwood-Walker S, et al. The influence of the paraventriculo-spinal pathway and oxytocin and vasopressin on sympathetic preganglionic neurons. Brain Res 1982; 251:283–290.
59. Strack AM, Sawyer WB, Marubio LM, et al. Spinal origin of sympathetic preganglionic neurons in the rat. Brain Res 1988; 455:187–191.
60. Card JP, Moore RY. Ventral lateral geniculate nucleus efferents to the rat suprachiasmatic nucleus exhibit avian pancreatic polypeptide-like immunoreactivity. J Comp Neurol 1982; 206:390–396.
61. Graf MV, Kastin AJ. Delta-sleep inducing peptide: a review. Neurosci Behav Rev 1984; 8:83–93.
62. Weaver DR, Rivkees SA, Carlson LL, et al. Localization of melatonin receptors in mammalian brain. In: Klein DC, Moore RY, and Reppert SM, eds. The Suprachiasmatic Nucleus, The Mind's Clock. New York: Oxford University Press, 1991:289–308.
63. Nosjean O, Ferro M, Coge F, et al. Identification of the melatonin-binding site $MT_3$ as the quinone reductase 2. J Biol Chem 2000; 275:31311–31317.
64. Reppert SM, Godson C, Mahle CD, et al. Molecular characterization of a second melatonin receptor expressed in human retina and brain: the $Mel_{1b}$ melatonin receptor. Proc Natl Acad Sci USA 1995; 92:8734–8738.

65. Gwinner E, Hau M, Heigl S. Melatonin: generation and modulation of avian circadian rhythms. Brain Res Bull 1997; 44(4):439–444.
66. Slotten HA, Pitrosky B, Pevet P. Influence of the mode of daily melatonin administration on entrainment of rat circadian rhythms. J Biol Rhythms 1999; 14(5):347–353.
67. Prosser RA. Melatonin inhibits in vitro serotonergic phase shifts of the suprachiasmatic circadian clock. Brain Res 1999; 818(2):408–413.
68. Rogers NL, Dorrian J, Dinges DF. Sleep, waking and neurobehavioral performance. Front Biosci 2003; 8:s1056–s1067.
69. Stanley N. Actigraphy in human psychopharmacology: a review. Hum Psychopharmacol 2003; 18(1):39–49.
70. Kunz D, Herrmann WM. Sleep-wake cycle, sleep-related disturbances, and sleep disorders: a chronobiological approach. Compr Psychiatry 2000; 41(2 suppl 1):104–115.
71. Ferraro JS, Sulzman FM. The effects of feedback lighting on the circadian drinking rhythm in the diurnal new world primate Saimiri sciureus. Am J Primatol 1988; 15(2): 143–155.
72. Copinschi G, Van Reeth O, Van Cauter E. Biologic rhythms. Effect of aging on the desynchronization of endogenous rhythmicity and environmental conditions. Presse Med 1999; 28(17):942–946.
73. Watts AG, Swanson LW, Sanchez-Watts G. Efferent projections of the suprachiasmatic nucleus: I. Studies using anterograde transport of Phaseolus vulgaris leucoagglutinin in the rat. J Comp Neurol 1987; 258(2):204–229.
74. Watts AG, Swanson LW. Efferent projections of the suprachiasmatic nucleus: II Studies using retrograde transport of fluorescent dyes and simultaneous peptide immunohistochemistry in the rat. J Comp Neurol 1987; 258(2):230–252.
75. Hashimoto S, Kohsaka M, Nakamura K, et al. Midday exposure to bright light changes the circadian organization of plasma melatonin rhythm in humans. Neurosci Lett 1997; 221(2–3):89–92.
76. Malinowski JR, Laval-Martin DL, Edmunds LN Jr. Circadian oscillators, cell cycles, and singularities: light perturbations of the free-running rhythm of cell division in Euglena. J Comp Physiol 1985; 155(2):257–267.
77. Daan S, Damassa D, Pittendrigh CS, et al. An effect of castration and testosterone replacement on a circadian pacemaker in mice (Mus musculus). Proc Natl Acad Sci USA 1975; 72(9):3744–3747.
78. Trachsel L, Tobler I, Borbely AA. Sleep regulation in rats: effects of sleep deprivation, light, and circadian phase. Am J Physiol 1986; 251(6 Pt 2):R1037–R1044.
79. Webb WB, Agnew HW Jr. Stage 4 sleep: influence of time course variables. Science 1971; 174(16):1354–1356.
80. Benington JH, Kodali SK, Heller HC. Stimulation of A1 adenosine receptors mimics the electroencephalographic effects of sleep deprivation. Brain Res 1995; 692(1–2):79–85.
81. Gaillard JM. Neurochemical regulation of the states of alertness. Ann Clin Res 1985; 17:175–184.
82. Hayaishi O. Prostaglandin D2 and sleep. Adv Prostaglandin Thromboxane Leukot Res 1989; 19:26–33.
83. Hayaishi O. Sleep-wake regulation by prostaglandins D2 and E2. J Biol Chem 1988; 263(29):14593–14596.
84. Inoue S. Sleep and sleep substances. Brain Dev 1986; 8(4):469–473.
85. Wyatt JK, Ritz-De Cecco A, Czeisler CA, et al. Circadian temperature and melatonin rhythms, sleep, and neurobehavioral function in humans living on a 20-h day. Am J Physiol 1999; 277(4 Pt 2):R1152–R1163.
86. Shochat T, Luboshitzky R, Lavie P. Nocturnal melatonin onset is phase locked to the primary sleep gate. Am J Physiol 1997; 273(1 Pt 2):R364–R370.
87. Corner MA. Sleep and the beginnings of behavior in the animal kingdom—studies of ultradian motility cycles in early life. Prog Neurobiol 1977; 8(4):279–295.
88. Schechtman VL, Harper RK, Harper RM. Distribution of slow-wave EEG activity across the night in developing infants. Sleep 1994; 17(4):316–322.
89. Walters AS. Toward a better definition of the restless legs syndrome. The International Restless Legs Syndrome Study Group. Mov Disord 1995; 10(5):634–642.

90. Willis T. The London practice of Physik. In: Basse T, Crooke W., eds. 1st ed. London, 1685:404.
91. Ekbom K. Restless legs syndrome. Neurology 1960; 10:868–873.
92. Montplaisir J, Boucher S, Gosselin A, et al. The restless legs syndrome: evening vs morning restlessness. Sleep Res 1995; 24:302.
93. Hening WA, Walters AS, Wagner M, et al. Circadian rhythm of motor restlessness and sensory symptoms in the idiopathic restless legs syndrome. Sleep 1999; 22(7):901–912.
94. Trenkwalder C, Hening WA, Walters AS, et al. Circadian rhythm of periodic limb movements and sensory symptoms of restless legs syndrome. Mov Disord 1999; 14(1):102–110.
95. Garcia-Borreguero D, Larrosa O, Granizo JJ, et al. Circadian variation in neuroendocrine response to L-dopa in patients with restless legs syndrome. Sleep 2004; 27(4):669–673.
96. Michaud M, Dumont M, Selmaoui B, et al. Circadian rhythm of restless legs syndrome: relationship with biological markers. Ann Neurol 2004; 55(3):372–380.
97. Garcia-Borreguero D, Larrosa O, de la Llave Y. Circadian aspects in the pathophysiology of the restless legs syndrome. Sleep Med 2002; 3(suppl):S17–S21.
98. Tribl GG, Waldhauser F, Sycha T, et al. Urinary 6-hydroxy-melatonin-sulfate excretion and circadian rhythm in patients with restless legs syndrome. J Pineal Res 2003; 35(4):295–296.
99. Allen RP, Picchietti D, Hening WA, et al. Restless legs syndrome: diagnostic criteria, special considerations, and epidemiology. A report from the restless legs syndrome diagnosis and epidemiology workshop at the National Institutes of Health. Sleep Med 2003; 4(2):101–119.
100. Birinyi PV, Allen RP, Lesage S, et al. Investigation into the correlation between sensation and leg movement in restless legs syndrome (p NA). Mov Dis 2005; 20(9):1097–1103.
101. Montplaisir J, Boucher S, Nicolas A, et al. Immobilization tests and periodic leg movements in sleep for the diagnosis of restless leg syndrome. Mov Disord 1998; 13(2): 324–329.
102. Sforza E, Jouny C, Ibanez V. Time course of arousal response during periodic leg movements in patients with periodic leg movements and restless legs syndrome. Clin Neurophysiol 2003; 114(6):1116–1124.
103. Trenkwalder C, Paulus W. Why do restless legs occur at rest?—pathophysiology of neuronal structures in RLS. Neurophysiology of RLS (part 2). Clin Neurophysiol 2004; 115(9):1975–1988.
104. Stiasny-Kolster K, Trenkwalder C, Fogel W, et al. Restless legs syndrome—new insights into clinical characteristics, pathophysiology, and treatment options. J Neurol 2004; 1(suppl 6):VI/39–43.
105. Kitahama K, Ikemoto K, Jouvet A, et al. Aromatic L-amino acid decarboxylase- and tyrosine hydroxylase-immunohistochemistry in the adult human hypothalamus. J Chem Neuroanat 1998; 16(1):43–55.
106. Ondo WG, He Y, Rajasekaran S, Le WD. Clinical correlates of 6-hydroxydopamine injections into A11 dopaminergic neurons in rats: a possible model for restless legs syndrome. Mov Disord 2000; 15(1):154–158.
107. Carlsson A, Svennerholm L, Winblad B. Seasonal and circadian monoamine variations in human brains examined post mortem. Acta Psychiatr Scand Suppl 1980; 280:75–85.
108. Sawchuk MA, Clemens S, Hochman S. Tyrosine-hydroxylase levels in spinal sympathetic regions Circadian variation and greatly reduced staining in D3 knockout mice. Proc San Diego Soc Neurosci 2004; 546:15.
109. Clemens S, Sawchuk MA, Hochman S. Reversal of the circadian expression of tyrosine-hydroxylase but not nitricoxide synthase levels in the spinal cord of dopamine D(3) receptor knockout mice. Neuroscience 2005; 133(2):353–357.
110. van den Pol AN, Herbst RS, Powell JF. Tyrosine hydroxylase-immunoreactive neurons of the hypothalamus: a light and electron microscopic study. Neuroscience 1984; 13(4):1117–1156.
111. Reuss S. Components and connections of the circadian timing system in mammals. Cell Tissue Res 1996; 285:353–378.

112. Arutiunian AV, Kerkeshko GO, Stepanov MG, et al. Disruption of circadian rhythms of biogenic amines in rat hypothalamus upon administration of 1,2-dimethylhydrazine. Vopr Onkol 2001; 47(5):608–615.
113. Zisapel N. Melatonin-dopamine interactions: from basic neurochemistry to a clinical setting. Cell Mol Neurobiol 2001; 21(6):605–616.
114. Santanavanich C, Ebadi M, Govitrapong P. Dopamine receptor activation in bovine pinealocyte via a cAMP-dependent transcription pathway. J Pineal Res 2005; 38(3):170–175.
115. Rosiak J, Zawilska JB. Near-ultraviolet light perceived by the retina generates the signal suppressing melatonin synthesis in the chick pineal gland-an involvement of NMDA glutamate receptors. Neurosci Lett 2005; 379(3):214–217.
116. Wiechmann AF, Udin SB, Summers Rada JA. Localization of Mel1b melatonin receptor-like immunoreactivity in ocular tissues of Xenopus laevis. Exp Eye Res 2004; 79(4):585–594.
117. Zawilska JB, Berezinska M, Rosiak J, et al. Suppression of melatonin biosynthesis in the chicken pineal gland by retinally perceived light–involvement of D1-dopamine receptors. J Pineal Res 2004; 36(2):80–86.
118. Bordet R, Devos D, Brique S, et al. Study of circadian melatonin secretion pattern at different stages of Parkinson's disease. Clin Neuropharmacol 2003; 26(2):65–72.
119. Willis GL, Armstrong SM. A therapeutic role for melatonin antagonism in experimental models of Parkinson's disease. Physiol Behav 1999; 66(5):785–795.
120. Mayo JC, Sainz RM, Uria H, et al. Melatonin prevents apoptosis induced by 6-hydroxydopamine in neuronal cells: implications for Parkinson's disease. J Pineal Res 1998; 24(3):179–192.

# 4 Systemic Iron Regulation

**John Beard**

*Department of Nutritional Sciences, Pennsylvania State University, University Park, Pennsylvania, U.S.A.*

## INTRODUCTION

Iron is one of the essential micronutrients, and, as such, is required for growth, development, and normal cellular functioning. In contrast to some other micronutrients such as water-soluble vitamins, there is a significant danger of toxicity if excessive amounts of iron accumulate in the body. A finely tuned feedback control system functions to limit this excessive accumulation by limiting absorption of iron. This chapter will discuss systemic iron homeostasis, as well as specific brain metabolism.

### Common and Scientific Name

Iron is element number 26 in the periodic table and has an atomic weight of 55.85. It is the fourth most abundant element and the second most abundant metal in the earth's crust. In simple aqueous solutions, iron exists in two principal oxidation states: ferrous ($Fe^{2+}$) and ferric ($Fe^{3+}$). The two forms of iron in solution are interchanged by the addition or subtraction of an electron. Many common reducing agents (e.g., ascorbic acid) will convert ferric iron to ferrous iron, while simple exposure to oxygen in solution will convert ferrous back to ferric iron. The amount of "free" iron within cells or in the fluid spaces of the body is quite low because iron can easily participate in redox reactions, which underlie the inherent toxicity of excess free iron within cells. This well-known Haber–Weiss–Fenton reaction is illustrated below

$$Fe^{2+} + O^2 \Rightarrow Fe^{3+} + O^{2^-}$$

$$2O^{2^-} + 2H^+ \Rightarrow H^2O^2 + O^2$$

$$Fe^{2+} + H^2O^2 \Rightarrow OH \cdot + \cdot OH^- + Fe^{3+}$$

The hydroxyl radical, OH·, is capable of attacking most proteins, nucleic acids, and carbohydrates, and in initiating lipid peroxidation reactions (1). The vast majority of iron within cells of plants and animals is (i) stored within large complex proteins such as hemosiderin or ferritin, (ii) contained as an essential component with proteins and enzymes and is critical for their functioning, or (iii) contained in proteins of iron transport that move iron from one cellular organelle to another, or move iron from one cell to another cell or between organs [transferrin (Tf) is an example of this iron protein complex].

### Dietary Forms of Iron

Iron occurs in two fundamental forms in the human diet: heme and nonheme iron (2). Heme iron refers to all forms of iron from plant and animal sources, in which the iron molecule is tightly bound within the porphyrin ring structure as is found in both myoglobin and hemoglobin. Nonheme iron refers to all other forms of iron. Contaminant iron that is derived from dust and soil iron is relatively unavailable to the absorptive cells, but may constitute a significant amount of iron intake in developing countries. There is substantial information that demonstrates that nearly all nonheme dietary iron mixes in a luminal "pool" of iron in the upper gastrointestinal (GI) tract because of acidification in the stomach and then exposure to pancreatic and GI enzymes. Inorganic iron is solubilized and ionized by gastric acid juice, reduced to the ferrous form, and kept soluble in the upper GI tract by chelation to compounds such as citrate and ascorbic acid. The type and amount of other materials, such as ascorbic acid, that can chelate iron to keep it in solution, also determine the amount of nonheme iron in a soluble luminal pool. The number of "inhibitors" of nonheme iron absorption is substantial with phytate, polyphenols, and tannins leading the list. These inhibitors typically bind either ferric or ferrous iron in a tight complex in the lumen of the gut and make it unavailable for the absorptive proteins. Thus, a diet that contains a large amount of unrefined grains, nondigestible fibers, etc. results in poor iron bioavailability. In contrast, a diet that is highly refined contains little roughage, and substantial portions of meat will have a greater iron bioavailability regardless of other factors. The American diet typically contains about 50% of its iron intake from grain products in which the iron concentration is between 0.1 and 0.4 mg/serving. Some fortified cereals, however, may contain as much as 24 mg of iron in a single serving. Heme iron is more highly bioavailable than nonheme iron and its bioavailability is less affected by other components of the diet than is the nonheme iron. Heme iron represents only about 10% of total dietary iron intake in many western countries.

## REGULATION OF ABSORPTION

There are two fundamental regulators or determinants of the amount of iron absorbed in humans. The first is the total amount and form of iron compounds ingested (discussed above) and the second is the iron status of the individual (3). Thus, individuals with a high iron status will absorb proportionally less of any amount of iron consumed than will an iron-deficient individual and individuals with a lower iron status will absorb more of any dietary intake. This process of selective absorption is the fundamental mechanism whereby humans regulate iron balance (4). While the details of the regulation are still not yet entirely clear, major discoveries in the last decade have added substantially to our understanding. At supraphysiological levels (as in high-dose iron supplementation), iron can apparently move across the gut by paracellular diffusion following a concentration gradient. At more physiological concentrations, as would be expected with the consumption of food, iron uptake is mediated by a series of receptors and binding proteins, which distinguish heme and nonheme iron.

### Heme Iron Absorption

Heme iron is soluble in an alkaline environment; hence, no binding proteins are necessary for its luminal absorption. Specific transporters exist for heme on the surface of enterocytes and efforts are being made to characterize this heme transporter (5,6). After binding to its receptor, the heme molecule is then internalized and acted upon by heme oxygenase (HOX1) to release the iron to the soluble cytoplasmic pool (7). HOX1 is not induced by oral administration of hemoglobin (a source of heme) but is induced by iron deficiency, suggesting some form of feedback regulation from the iron stores "signal" (7). The distribution in the intestine is identical to the areas of maximal heme iron absorption and is far more efficient at absorption than in the nonheme iron pathway (8). In a typical American diet, it is reasonable to expect that overall dietary nonheme iron is absorbed at approximately 5% to 10% efficiency, whereas heme iron is nearly 40% efficient.

### Nonheme Iron Absorption

Divalent metal transporter (DMT) is a transmembrane protein that resides on the luminal membrane and has a strong preference for divalent metals. It exists in several isoforms (DMT1 and DMT2) (2,9). The nonheme iron in the lumen of the gut has variable solubility, depending on the various amounts of ferric and ferrous iron and the amount of iron-binding compounds. The rapid conversion of ferric to ferrous iron is accomplished by a membrane-bound member of the cytochrome P450 family, *Dcytb*, which is in sufficient abundance as to not be limiting to the transport capacity of DMT1, and internalization via vesicle endocytosis. The internalized vesicle undergoes further modification and acidification with resulting release of iron into the cytoplasmic space. This iron is then free to be transported to the basolateral membrane for export by some yet undescribed, intracellular iron-binding protein(s), or it can be incorporated into ferritin (10). A candidate for this Tf-like protein may be mobilferrin, a 56 kDa cytosolic protein isolated from rat and human duodenal mucosa, which can bind iron ($K_d = 9 \times 10^{-5}$ M) (11). It is a homologue of calreticulin, a protein that plays a role in the assembly and transport of major histocompatability complex class 1 molecules and can bind calcium, copper, and zinc (12).

Given the frequent observation of increased efficiency of iron absorption in individuals with low iron stores and decreased absorption with high iron stores, it has long been predicted that some sort of plasma-born signal communicates to enterocytes as part of this homeostatic control loop (13). This signal compound could tell the basolateral membrane to export iron (or not), or signal internal iron-binding proteins to preferentially move iron to ferritin within the enterocyte, or somehow communicate with the luminal membrane to change the amount of iron imported into the cell. It is now clear that the signal is the newly described protein, hepcidin (14). This protein was first identified as a small peptide with antimicrobial activity. Mice that lacked the hepcidin gene accumulate toxic amounts of iron in liver while overexpressing mice developed iron deficiency (15). The amount of hepcidin in the plasma is proportional to the amount of liver iron stores.

After GI absorption, the intraerythrocyte regulation of iron flux is an evolving story given the identification of new iron importers, exporters, and their regulation by cytoplasmic iron concentrations. The amount of ferritin that is synthesized by the enterocyte is under the regulation of the mRNA-binding protein, interferon gamma iron response protein (IRP), which binds with high affinity at an iron response element (IRE) located in the 5′-untranslated end of the ferritin mRNA (10,16). There is also a similar set of IREs on the 3′ end of the mRNA for TfR and DMT-1 that allows for a reciprocal regulation of iron storage and iron uptake. This IRE–IRP system of regulation, however, is also susceptible to oxidative stress because nitric oxide may alter the affinity of this regulator of protein translation (8,17,18). The amount of IRP1 is, in turn, dependent on the cytosolic free iron concentration. In the presence of cytosolic iron, IRP1 becomes cytoplasmic aconitase with the iron in a 4 Fe–4 sulfur complex. In the absence of iron, IRP1 (now a 3 Fe–4 S complex) binds to the IREs of various iron proteins to regulate the translation of mRNA transcripts. IRP2, a second isoform, appears to primarily be an oxygen sensor, which is also sensitive to cytosolic free iron and has somewhat different binding affinities to IREs than does IRP1 (10). Lower duodenal levels of ferritin mRNA found in iron-deficient subjects and higher duodenal levels of ferritin mRNA found in secondary iron overload support the role of mucosal ferritin as a major regulator of iron absorption (19). Thus, enterocyte ferritin is the mucosal "iron sink" and can serve as a means of limiting iron absorption because the enterocytes are sloughed off the tip of the microvillus in 3 to 4 days. IRP2 is produced and metabolism in a distinctly different fashion than the aconitase-related IRP1 appears to be quite sensitive to oxygen partial pressure. At the physiological pO2 of most cells, IRP2 is the predominant regulator of IRE binding (20). Hypoxia increases iron absorption (21) independently of erythropoiesis (22). Increased plasma iron turnover, which occurs not only in erythropoiesis but also in disorders of ineffective erythropoiesis such as thalassemia, hemolytic anemias, and sideroblastic anemias, is associated with increased iron absorption (23). Thus, it is now reasonable to assume that the IRPs are the principal iron sensors in the enterocyte and determine the fate of iron movement for export or storage in ferritin (20). Consistent with this hypothesis is the fact that the concentrations of mucosal cell ferritin mRNA and ferritin protein in patients with familial hemochromatosis are lower than those of patients with secondary iron overload (13,19,24).

### Basolateral Membrane Iron Export

As previously alluded, hepcidin has been identified as the putative plasma regulator of iron absorption. It is a small 25 amino acid protein secreted by hepatocytes in amounts proportional to iron stores (14). This secreted protein appears to have two primary targets: the macrophage and the basolateral membrane of the enterocyte. In the macrophage, they regulate the release of iron from ferritin stores into the plasma pool. Hepcidin binds to another transmembrane protein, ferroportin, with a resulting internalization and destruction (25). Hepcidin appears to be released from liver in response to both iron accumulation and cytokines released during inflammation. This newly described iron exporter also contains IRE (like ferritin, and DMT1, TfR) and interacts, in some undefined fashion, with the hemochromatosis factor (HFE) protein on the abluminal enterocyte surface. Mutant forms of this protein are associated with very severe iron overload (14).

### Plasma Transport

The ferroportin protein releases ferrous iron into the plasma pool where association with hephastin and ceruloplasmin act in a redox couple to form ferric iron for high-efficiency binding to Tf. This taxicab for iron is produced in a number of cells, but the liver is the primary donor to the plasma pool. The rate of production of Tf is affected by the iron status of the individual via transcriptional regulation (3). Individuals with depleted iron stores and a plasma Fe concentration less than 40 to 60 μg/dL will increase Tf production and increase the plasma Tf concentration by nearly 100%. The two binding sites on Tf are nearly identical in binding affinity for iron ($K_d = 10^{-22}$ M). In vivo Tf is normally 25% to 50% saturated with iron, but in iron deficiency it can be less than 5% saturated in the extreme (1). One of the criteria for establishing iron deficiency is for the

Tf saturation (ratio of serum Fe/total iron-binding capacity) to be less than 15% (4). At this level of saturation, there is insufficient delivery of iron to bone marrow to maintain normal rates of erythropoiesis. Thus, under normal physiological circumstances, the iron-binding capacity of plasma is always in excess of iron concentration. The rate and location of the uptake of iron from the plasma pool are proportional to the number of Tf receptors expressed on plasma membranes (3). The normal concentration of iron in the human body is between 30 and 40 mg/kg, but nearly 85% of the nonstorage iron is found in the erythroid mass (red blood cells). The iron storage concentration in the body varies from 0 to 15 mg/kg depending on the sex and iron status of the individual. The liver contains greater than 60% of the storage pool of iron with the metal sequestered inside a 24-subunit protein, ferritin. The core of this ferritin molecule can contain up to 4000 atoms of iron as ferric-hydrite. The amount of ferritin produced is determined by the IRP–IRE interaction previously described in the enterocyte. The remaining 40% of stored iron is found in muscle tissues and cells of the reticuloendothelial system (4). Normally, 95% of the stored iron in liver tissue is found in hepatocytes as ferritin. Hemosiderin constitutes the remaining 5% and is found predominately in Kupffer cell lysosomal remnants. However, during iron overload, the mass of hemosiderin in the liver accumulates at 10 times the rate of ferritin (26).

Because the bone marrow has by far the greatest daily demand for iron that is where greater than 80% of the plasma iron ends up on a daily basis. It is estimated that nearly 20 mg of Fe/d goes to the bone marrow erthryoblasts for insertion into the porphyrin ring structure to form hemoglobin. As the plasma pool of iron is frequently less than 4 mg of iron, it is easy to compute that the half-life of an iron molecule in plasma is quite short. The other contributors to the plasma pool of iron apart from the GI are macrophages, other RE cells, and hepatocytes. Iron turnover is primarily mediated by destruction of senescent erythrocytes by the reticuloendothelial system (27). Erythrocytes, which contain about 80% of the body's functional iron, have a mean functional lifetime of 120 days in humans. At the end of their functional lifetime, they are recognized as senescent by changes in the structure of their membranes and are catabolized at extravascular sites by Kupffer cells and spleen macrophages. After phagocytosis, the globin chains of hemoglobin are denatured, which releases bound heme. Intracellular unbound heme is ultimately degraded by HOX1, which liberates iron. About 85% of the iron derived from hemoglobin degradation is re-released to the body in the form of iron bound to Tf or ferritin. Each day 0.66% of the body's total iron content is recycled in this manner (28). Smaller contributions are made to plasma iron turnover by the degradation of myoglobin and iron-containing enzymes. As noted previously, macrophage release of iron is affected by hepcidin, which is altering the export of iron to the plasma pool (25).

## CONTROL OF CENTRAL NERVOUS SYSTEM IRON

The brain has specific requirements that demand exacting control of iron (29,30). Not only is iron required for the usual metabolic needs, such as adenosine triphosphate formation and ribonucleotide synthesis, but within the brain iron also subserves myelin formation, synaptic regulation, and neurotransmission. Furthermore, iron distribution is highly heterogeneous and is highest in the cerebellum and midbrain. This distribution, however, is not apparent at birth and tends to increase over time. In humans this is not seen until adolescence.

A large number of diseases are associated with excessive central nervous system (CNS) iron. In some diseases, such as neuroferritinopathy, aceruloplasminemia, Freiderich's ataxia, and Hallervordan-Spatz (aka, neuronodegeneration with brain iron accumulation 1), the iron accumulation is culpable, resulting in direct neurotoxicity. Other diseases, such as Parkinson's disease, Alzheimer's disease, tardive dyskinesia, and multiple sclerosis, demonstrate excessive iron deposits, but the exact relationship between this and the disease process is not known. Restless legs syndrome (discussed in detail in Chapter 7) demonstrates reduced CNS iron.

The mechanisms that regulate iron flow into the brain are not well understood. Like most substances, iron must transverse the blood–brain barrier, mediated by endothelial cells surrounding the microvasculature. It may then enter directly into the brain or through the ependymal cells that line the ventricles.

Cerebral spinal fluid levels of ferritin are less than 10% of those in the serum. Tf levels are also lower and are probably fully saturated with iron. The brain also makes endogenous Tf in the choroid plexus and the oligodendrocytes. The endothelial cells contain high levels of Tf receptors. They also contain DMT-1, melanotransferrin (aka p97, a homologue of Tf), metal transport protein-1 (MTP-1), and HFE. These appear to be fairly evenly distributed throughout the microvasculature. In rats, the endothelial cells contain high levels of ferritin, suggesting that they possess abundant iron stores. Regulation of these iron transport proteins is only rudimentarily understood. Systemic iron deficiency does not seem to affect iron transport protein levels in the endothelial cells. Brain deficiency, seen in Belgrade rats, does result in upregulation of TfR and DMT-1, but not ferritin or Tf.

## IRON LOSSES

The low solubility of iron at physiologic pH precludes urinary excretion as a major mechanism of maintaining iron homeostasis. Thus, in contrast to most other trace minerals whose homeostasis in maintained by excretion, the primary mechanism of maintaining whole body iron homeostasis is to regulate the amount of iron absorbed so that it approximates iron losses. Iron losses can vary considerably with the gender of the individual. In male humans, total iron losses from the body have been calculated to be 1 mg/day. For premenopausal female humans, this loss is slightly higher. The predominant route of loss is from the GI tract and amounts to 0.6 mg/day in adult males (28). Fecal iron losses derive from shed enterocytes, extravasated red blood cells, and biliary heme breakdown products, which are poorly absorbed. Urogenital and integumental iron losses have been estimated to be greater than 0.1 mg/day and 0.3 mg/day, respectively, in adult males (27). Menstrual iron loss, estimated from an average blood loss of 33 mL/month, equals 1.5 mg/day, but may range as high as 2.1 mg/day (31). Oral contraceptives reduce this loss and intrauterine devices increase it (32,33).

Pregnancy is associated with losses approximating 1 g, which consists of basal loss of 230 mg iron, increased maternal red cell mass of 450 mg iron, fetal needs of 270–300 mg iron, and placenta, decidua, and amniotic fluid iron content of 50–90 mg. All maternal iron stores are called upon to provide Fe for these needs. Women at partum are often iron deficient and sometimes also quite anemic. Because iron need and distribution are different while pregnant, assessment of iron status can be difficult in this population.

A number of clinical and pathological conditions are attended by variable amounts of blood loss. These include hemorrhage, hookworm infestation, peptic gastric or anastomotic ulceration, ulcerative colitis, colonic neoplasia, cow's milk feeding to infants, aspirin, nonsteroidal anti-inflammatory drugs or corticosteroid administration, and hereditary hemorrhagic telangiectasia [see (4) for review]. In addition to these conditions, a significant amount of iron (210–240 mg/unit) can be lost with regular blood donation.

## Iron Overload

Iron overload diseases have received much attention in the last decade, especially in the last 5 years, with the discovery of the gene associated with hereditary hemochromatosis, HFE. One in 200 to 400 individuals of Anglo-Saxon ancestry is affected by an autosomal recessive gene mutation that results in the iron overload disease called hereditary hemochromatosis (3). The gene mutation of the HFE gene in position C282Y accounts for the vast majority of the cases of hemochromatosis in individuals with Celtic origins. Various other mutations have also been described and, in most cases, the mutations are associated with a failure of the HFE protein to be able to bind effectively with the β-2 microglobular protein and the TfR1 protein at the plasma membrane. The failure of the association to occur is related to the lack of control of iron flux across the enterocyte. Hereditary hemochromatosis is thus characterized by a failure to control iron absorption in the enterocyte with a resulting accumulation of iron in iron storage pools, primarily in cells of the reticuloendothelial system. Without treatment, clinical signs of iron toxicity occur in homozygous individuals in the fourth decade of life, or earlier, at which time their total body iron content is more than 20 g. Lack of treatment by chelation and phlebotomy results in cirrhosis of the liver, heptocellular carcinoma, myocardial pathology, and damage to the pancreatic function (34). This accumulation of iron in the liver and the accompanying hepatic fibrosis and cirrhosis appear to be causal in nature. The evidence for iron accumulation in heterozygous individuals is less clear and the role of dietary iron bioavailability in body iron accumulation in these individuals is still being debated (35). At the time, it appears prudent for known heterozygous individuals to limit their consumption of iron supplements.

Other forms of iron overload due to chronic excessively high iron intakes have been reported, but these intakes of approximately 200–1200 mg of Fe per day for long periods are unusual. Bantu siderosis in Africa is an additional example of iron toxicity due to excessively high iron intakes for prolonged periods of time (4). Home brewing of beer in large iron pots was associated with an intake of iron in excess of 50–100 mg of Fe per day with a resulting iron overload disease. There is some evidence as well, that there is a genetic component to this disease (36).

Transfusional iron overload may result from the accumulation of iron after senescent transfused red cells are metabolized in the reticuloendothelial system. Because each unit of blood contains approximately 225 mg of Fe, there is a real danger of hepatic iron overload with repeated transfusions. Individuals with disorders in erythropoiesis who receive transfusions have the additional iron burden of excessive iron absorption. That is, iron accumulation in the RES occurs due to both high rates of red cell turnover and high rates of iron absorption.

## Treatment of Iron Deficiency

In 2001, the United States Food and Nutrition Board of the National Academy of Sciences released the current evaluation of recommended intakes and upper limits of safe intakes (35). That committee had the perspective that functional consequences of iron deficiency occurred only when there were depleted iron stores and there was insufficient delivery of iron to the essential iron pools in all tissues. The erythroid mass has the largest essential iron pool in the form of hemoglobin; bone marrow uptake is responsible for greater than 70% of the plasma iron turnover on a daily basis.

In the evaluation of assessment of iron status, the review panel utilized the following indicators: (i) serum or plasma ferritin as an indicator of iron storage pool size, (ii) plasma-soluble Tf receptor as an indicator of adequacy of iron delivery to rapidly growing cells, (iii) plasma or serum Tf saturation as an indicator of iron transport, and (iv) hemoglobin concentration, hematocrit, or red cell counts as an indication of the existence of anemia. It should be noted that free iron is highly variable and should not be used in isolate to assess iron status. The need to utilize all of these indicators is well-justified, given the impact that acute and chronic infections have on the evaluation of iron status (37). The soluble form of the transferrin receptor (sTfR) is the cleaved portion of the protein that floats around in the plasma. The amount of the cleaved protein in plasma is proportional to the cellular "iron status" because the more iron deficient a cell becomes, the greater is the expression of this protein. This is a relatively new test for iron status but, unlike ferritin, is not sensitive to inflammation, so there is great promise that it will prove to be a valuable indicator in complicated clinical and nutritional diagnosis. The suggested levels of intake represent the required intakes to ensure adequate nutrition in 95% to 97.5% of the population and are an overestimation of the level needed for most people in any given group. Individuals who do not routinely consume the suggested level of iron from foods should be encouraged to supplement their diets with iron compounds.

Iron deficiency has traditionally been separated into iron deficiency anemia and tissue iron deficiency, also referred to as "depleted iron stores." Iron deficiency anemia is diagnosed as a low serum Tf saturation (less than 15%), a low serum ferritin concentration (<12 μg/L), and an elevated soluble TfR (>6 mg/dL) in the setting of microcytic anemia. However, anemia reflects a late stage of iron depletion with earlier stages often evidenced by low serum ferritin and slightly elevated TfR levels. Because both serum ferritin and serum iron concentrations are acute phase reactants to inflammatory cytokines, the presence of inflammation must be considered in a diagnosis of iron deficiency. After the diagnosis of true iron deficiency, restoration of an iron-replete state can be achieved by administering 125–250 mg of ferrous sulfate orally per day. This dose of the salt will deliver 39–72 mg of highly bioavailable iron per day. There is some evidence that doses greater than 250 mg ferrous sulfate convey additional benefits and it is still common practice in severe anemia of pregnancy to administer this dose twice per day. This, however, results in a high prevalence of complaints of GI distress, constipation, and blackened stools. Thus, compliance with these high doses drops considerably from prescribed amounts. Once the iron deficiency is resolved, daily intake of iron based at recommended dietary allowance levels should be maintained.

## Approaches to Preventative Iron Supplementation

One of the great concerns regarding iron deficiency anemia is the adequacy of iron intake during periods of high iron losses. This has led to a reevaluation of the concept of "daily iron supplements" (38,39). At issue is the relative effectiveness of daily therapeutic doses of iron compared to the administration of lower "preventative intermittent iron" doses. The concept is this: because the GI enterocyte will

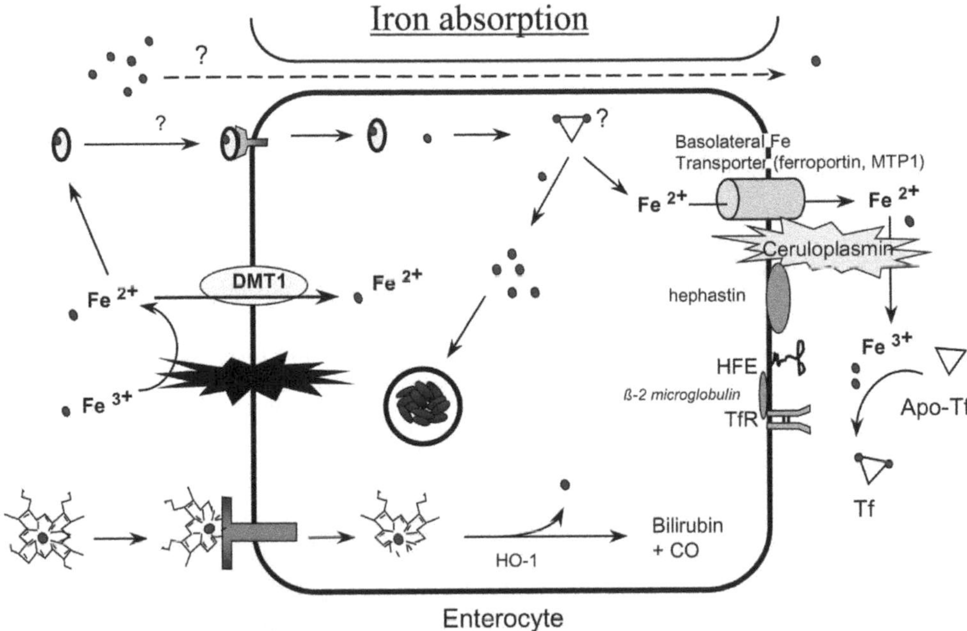


**FIGURE 1** Putative mechanism for the absorption of iron in enterocytes of the upper gastrointestinal tract in humans. On the left side of the diagram is a putative heme iron transporter, the DMT-1, DMT–mediated uptake coupled to a ferroxidase, and a poorly described nonheme iron transporter independent of DMT1. Soluble intracellular iron can be inserted into ferritin (center of the cell) or exported through the metal transport protein-1 shuttle system located in close proximity to copper containing hepastin or ceruloplasmin. The hemochromatosis gene product, HFE, is likely to exert its influence at this site of iron export from the absorptive cell. *Abbreviations*: DMT, divalent metal transporter; HFE, hemochromatosis factor; MTP, metal transport protein; TfR, transferrin receptor; Tf, transferrin.

"reset" its set point for iron absorption every 3 to 4 days because a new crop of crypt cells migrates up to the tip of the villus, the large doses of iron given on days 2 and 3 are wasted and may in fact result in oxidative damage and mucosal injury. To test this hypothesis, a number of studies in developing countries have compared the efficacy of daily doses compared to an intermittent dose in correcting iron deficiency anemia in adolescents, reproductive age women, pregnant women, and children. The daily dosage approach had a faster response, but with lower compliance, than did the intermittent oral iron dose. The end result in terms of correcting the anemia was similar in nearly all studies, with the exception of pregnancy, where daily iron therapy clearly provided a greater benefit (40). Cleary, blood loss from the body is the single largest cause of increased or altered iron requirements. Bleeding ulcers, lesions, and leaking inflammatory states in the gut will all be associated with a decreased iron status due to increased rates of blood and iron loss.

Doses of iron as low as 180 mg may be lethal in adults if the iron is in a highly bioavailable form (41). High acute intakes of iron may be associated with necrotizing gastritis and enteritis, pallor, lassitude, and frequent diarrhea. The rapid rise in the plasma iron concentration within 60 minutes to levels in excess of 500 μg/dL is common and is likely related to the pathology. Rapid treatment with iron chelators, like desferrioxamine, will rapidly decrease plasma iron concentration, and gastric lavage has improved recovery rates.

A number of iron compounds exist in the market place that can effectively and safely supplement dietary iron to bring individuals back into iron balance. There is risk, however, that overzealous use of supplements can lead to GI distress and in some individuals with genetic mutations, toxic iron overload and even death. New understanding of the genetic causality of iron overload syndromes will provide greater avenues for preventing accidental iron overload in the near future.

## REFERENCES


1. Gutteridge JM, Halliwell B. Free radicals and antioxidants in the year 2000. A historical look to the future. Ann NY Acad Sci 2000; 899:136–147.
2. Hurrell R. Improvement of trace element status through food fortification: technological, biological and health aspects. Bibl Nutr Dieta 1998; 54:40–57.
3. Aisen P, Enns C, Wessling-Resnick M. Chemistry and biology of eukaryotic iron metabolism. Int J Biochem Cell Biol 2001; 33:940–959.
4. Bothwell TH, Charlton RW, Cook JD, Finch CA. Iron metabolism in man. Oxford: Blackwell Scientific Publications, 1979.
5. Conrad M, Burton B, Williams H, Foy A. Human absorption of hemoglobin-iron. Gastroenterology 1967; 53:5–10.
6. Grasbeck R, Majuri I, Kouvonen I, Tenhun R. Spectral and other studies on the intestinal haem receptor of the pig. Biochem Biophys Acta 1982; 700:137–147.
7. Raffin SB, Woo CH, Roost KT, Price DC, Schmid R. Intestinal absorption of hemoglobin heme iron cleavage by mucosal heme oxygenase. J Clin Invest 1974; 54:1344.
8. Rouault T, Klausner R. Regulation of iron metabolism in eukaryotes. Curr Top Cell Regul 1997; 35:1–19.
9. Gunshin H, Mackeasie B, Berger UV, et al. Cloning and characterization of a mammalian proton-coupled metal-ion transporter. Nature 1997; 388:472.
10. Eisenstein RS. Iron regulatory proteins and the molecular control of mammalian iron metabolism. Annu Rev Nutr 2000; 20:627–662.
11. Conrad ME, Umbreit JN, Peterson RDA, Moore EG, Harper KP. Function of integrin in duodenal mucosal uptake of iron. Blood 1993; 81:517–521.
12. Conrad ME, Umbreit JN, Moore EG. Rat duodenal iron-binding protein mobilferrin is a homologue of calreticulin. Gastroenterology 1993; 104:1700–1704.
13. Lee P, Gelbart T, West C, Halloran C, Beutler E. Seeking candidate mutations that affect iron homeostasis. Blood Cells Molecules Dis 2002; 29:471–487.
14. Nicolas G, Bennoun M, Devaux I, et al. Lack of hepcidin gene expression and severe tissue iron overload in upstream stimulatory factor 2 knockout mice. Proc Natl Acad Sci USA 2001; 98:8780–8785.
15. Nicolas G, Bennoun M, Porteu A, et al. Severe iron deficiency anemia in transgenic mice expressing liver hepcidin. Proc Natl Acad Sci USA 2002; 98:994596–994601.
16. Owen D, Kuhn LC. Noncoding 3′ sequences of the transferrin receptor gene are required for mRNA regulation by iron. EMBO J 1987; 6(5):1287–1293.
17. Rouault TA. Post-transcriptional regulation of human iron metabolism by iron regulatory proteins. Blood Cells Mol Dis 2002; 29(3):309–314.
18. Hentze MW, Kuhn LC. Molecular control of vertebrate iron metabolism: mRNA-based regulatory circuits operated by iron, nitric oxide, and oxidative stress. Proc Natl Acad Sci USA 1996; 93(16):8175–8182.
19. Pietrangelo A, Rocchi E, Casalgrandi G, et al. Regulation of transferrin, transferrin receptor, and ferritin genes in human duodenum. Gastroenterology 1992; 102: 802–809.
20. Meyron-Holtz EG, Ghosh MC, Rouault RA. Mammalian tissue oxygen levels modulate iron-regulatory protein activities in vivo. Science 2004; 306(5704):2087–2090.
21. Mendel GA. Studies on iron absorption. I: The relationship between the rate of erythropoiesis, hypoxia and iron absorption. Blood 1961; 18:727–736.

22. Raja KB, Simpson RJ, Pippard MJ, Peters TJ. In vivo studies on the relationship between intestinal iron ($Fe^{3+}$) absorption, hypoxia, and erythropoiesis in the mouse. Br J Haematol 1988; 68:373–384.
23. Weintraub LR, Conrad ME, Crosby WH. The significance of iron turnover in the control of iron absorption. Blood 1964; 24:19–24.
24. Fracanzani AL, Fargion S, Romano R, et al. Immunohistochemical evidence for a lack of ferritin in duodenal absorptive epithelial cells in idiopathic hemochromatosis. Gastroenterology 1989; 96:1071–1078.
25. Nemeth E, Tuttle MS, Powelson J, et al. Hepcidin regulates cellular iron efflux by binding to ferroportin and inducing its internalization. Science 2004; 306(5704): 2090–2093.
26. Selden C, Owen JMP, Hopkins JMP, Peters TJ. Studies on the concentration and intracellular localization of iron proteins in liver biopsy specimens from patients with iron overload with special reference to their role in lysosomal disruption. Br J Haematol 1980; 44:593–603.
27. Finch CA, Deubelbliss K, Cook JD, et al. Ferrokinetics in man. Medicine 1970; 49:17–53.
28. Green R, Charlton R, Seftel H, Bothwell TH, Mayet F. Body iron excretion in man: a collaborative study. Am J Med 1968; 45:336–353.
29. Burdo JR, Connor JR. Brain iron uptake and homeostatic mechanisms: an overview. Biometals 2003; 16(1):63–75.
30. Burdo JR, Simpson IA, Menzies S, Beard J, Connor JR. Regulation of the profile of iron-management proteins in brain microvasculature. J Cereb Blood Flow Metab 2004; 24(1):67–74.
31. Cole SK, Billewicz WZ, Thomson AM. Sources of variation in menstrual blood loss. J Obstet Gynaecol Br Comm 1971; 78:933–939.
32. Frassinelli-Gunderson EP, Margen S, Brown JR. Iron stores in users of oral contraceptive agents. Am J Clin Nutr 1985; 41:703–712.
33. Kivijarvi A, Timonen H, Rajamaki A, Gronroos M. Iron deficiency in women using modern copper intrauterine devices. Obstet Gynecol 1986; 67:95–98.
34. Bothwell TH, MacPhail PA. Hereditary hemochromatosis: etiologic, pathologic, and clinical aspects. Semin Hematol 1998; 35:55–71.
35. National Academy of Science-Institute of Medicine Panel on Micronutrients, Dietary Reference Intakes for Vitamin A, Vitamin K, Arsenic, Boron, chromium, Copper, Iodine, Iron, Manganese, Molybdenum, Nickel, Silicon, Vanadium, and Zinc. National Academy Press, Washington, D.C., 2001.
36. Gordeuk VR, Caleffi A, Corradini E, et al. Iron overload in Africans and African-Americans and a common mutation in the SCL40A1 (ferroportin 1) gene. Blood Cells Mol Dis 2003; 31(3):299–304.
37. Schuman K. Safety aspects of Iron in food. Annals Nutr Metab 2001; 45:91–101.
38. Beard JL. Weekly iron intervention: the case for intermittent iron supplementation. Am J Clin Nutr 1998; 68(2):209–212.
39. Hallberg L. Combating iron deficiency: daily administration of iron is far superior to weekly administration. Am J Clin Nutr 1998; 68(2):213–217.
40. Beaton GH, McCabe GP. Efficacy of Intermittent Iron Supplementation in the control of Iron Deficiency Anemia in Developing Countries: An Analysis of Experience. Ottawa: Micronutrients Initiative Report, 1999.
41. Ellenhorn MJ, Barceloux DG, eds. Iron. Medical Toxicology. New York: Elsevier, 1988:1023–1030.

# 5 The Physiology of Restless Legs Syndrome

**Stephany Fulda and Thomas-Christian Wetter**
*Max Planck Institute of Psychiatry, Munich, Germany*

## INTRODUCTION

The most prominent symptom of the restless legs syndrome (RLS) is an unpleasant sensation in the legs, and occasionally in the arms, that the patients describe as crawling, creeping, extremely unpleasant, and sometimes painful. In addition, motor symptoms such as periodic leg movements (PLM) during sleep (PLMS) and wakefulness (PLMW), as well as nonperiodic involuntary leg movements, are present in a majority of patients. The present chapter is organized along the anatomical structures that may be involved in the origin of these sensory and motor symptoms summarizing neurophysiologic, neuroendocrinologic, and brain-imaging studies. To that end, we will first review research pertaining to peripheral factors in RLS (see Section "The Periphery"), and then in more detail the involvement of the spinal cord (see Section "The Spinal Cord") and the brain (see Section "The Brain") including subcortical (see Section "Brainstem") and cortical structures (see Section "Cortex").

Typically, the sensory and motor symptoms of RLS occur at specific times during the 24-hour day, mostly in the evening and at night. Thus, the quest is open for factors that at least covary with these times; neuroendocrine factors may be the prime candidates. Because these factors do not map precisely on single anatomical regions, we have added an overview of specific systems implicated in RLS pathophysiology. Because other chapters in this book are devoted to central nervous system (CNS) dopaminergic systems (Chapter 2), the role of iron (Chapter 4), and circadian physiology (Chapter 3), we will only touch briefly on these issues, but review the opiate system (see Section "Asthenia Crurum Dolorosa—Pain and the Opiate System in RLS") and neuroendocrine factors (see Sections "Melatonin, Sexual Steroid Hormones," Serotorin and "Other Neuroendocrine Factors") in more detail.

Research into the pathophysiology of RLS matches the complexity of this disorder with the use of several different methods. Although many studies describe isolated pathological findings not replicated or extended, and rarely relating to each other, there are some basic problems that are central to this research: The question whether the origin of RLS lies within the CNS or in the periphery has been disputed for a long time. Both sides of the *central vs. peripheral* debate contribute diverse evidence. One of the arguments is that peripheral nerve damage such as peripheral neuropathy constitutes a recognized secondary form of RLS. The frequency of RLS patients with subclinical nerve damage without clinical signs of neuropathy arises as research methods to diagnose peripheral nerve damage become more sophisticated (1). On the other hand, the dramatic relief of RLS symptoms achieved with a dopamine agonist cannot be reversed by a peripherally acting dopamine antagonist (e.g., domperidone) pointing to a central process (2).

Another intriguing debate evolves around the question whether there is a *structural vs. functional* abnormality underlying RLS. The question is fundamental to research strategies and becomes especially apparent in the evaluation of brain-imaging studies that have failed to reveal consistent abnormalities (see Section "Basal Ganglia"). From a structural point of view it should make no difference at which time point measurements [e.g., positron-emission tomography (PET) and single photon emission-computed tomography (SPECT)] are performed; however, from a functional regulatory standpoint, measurements should be performed at the time of the strongest symptom expression; i.e., in the evening or at night. This question might not boil down to exactly those two opposites—fixed vs. time dependent—but may also involve the possibility that a time-dependent measurement might unmask a structural deficit.

A further controversial issue is the association between RLS and PLMS (3,4). While some authors regard PLMS and PLMW as the motor side of RLS, and sensations and the urge to move as the sensory side of RLS, there is some evidence supporting dissociation between both symptoms. At least 80% of RLS patients have PLMS (5–7); however, PLMS are also a frequent finding in noncomplaining subjects, especially in the elderly (8–10). Therefore, PLMS is a sensitive but not specific marker of RLS. Because of this one-sided incomplete overlap, closely related but not identical mechanisms are expected to contribute to both disorders. In addition, both syndromes respond to dopaminergic and opioidergic treatment. On a group level, the frequency of PLM correlates with the severity of RLS (11). However, the analysis of individual time courses of leg movements and dysesthesia suggests that their occurrence is partly independent (12) and governed by different time-related factors (13). Interestingly, brain-imaging studies may point to more distinct findings in patient groups selected with respect to PLMS rather than RLS (14).

An important question concerns the interpretation of research results in terms of pathogenic factors. There are recognized secondary forms of RLS such as iron deficiency, pregnancy, end-stage renal disease (ESRD), and neuropathy. While iron treatment in the case of iron deficiency (15,16), delivery in the case of pregnancy (17,18), and kidney transplantation in the case of ESRD (19,20) have all been shown to ameliorate RLS, the case is more difficult for neuropathy, which tends to be a chronic disease that is mostly treated symptomatically. However, only some of the patients affected by these disorders will exhibit RLS, making it highly probable that there has to be a predisposing factor or vulnerability (a necessary but not sufficient factor) to develop RLS. An opposite argument may also apply: there might be protective factors against developing RLS even in cases with a high load of risk factors; however, this question has not received any interest so far. Furthermore, findings may only be coincidental epiphenomena of a more general process such as aging. Especially in the case of chronic and frequent disorders such as diabetes or hypertension, a large overlap between the two conditions would be expected by chance alone. It must be distinguished whether a factor is a trigger for RLS or a factor maintaining RLS once it has occurred. Furthermore, it must be kept in mind that RLS is a chronic condition and thus findings may be the expression of a long-term adaptation or compensation process if not a consequence of a given treatment for RLS. Any factor relevant to the pathogenesis of RLS must explain a whole range of findings; i.e., the heterogeneous disease course with frequent and long periods of complete remission at least in the beginning of the disorder, the pronounced circadian variation of symptoms, and the provocation of symptoms at rest. It seems likely that such a complex pattern might only emerge by the interaction between several factors, most likely only in persons with a possible genetically determined vulnerability and in the presence of a specific set of triggering and symptom-maintaining factors.

## PATHOPHYSIOLOGY OF RESTLESS LEGS SYNDROME

Pathogenic factors in the physiology of RLS have been looked for in the periphery, spinal mechanisms, and subcortical and cortical brain structures. Some of the structures are more implicated in the sensory or motor symptoms of RLS. The present review is grouped along these broad categories and will review in each section the evidence pertaining to RLS sensory symptoms and leg movements during sleep and wakefulness.

This review will begin with a short overview of studies that have employed neurophysiological examination techniques, such as sensory-evoked potentials (SEP) or motor-evoked potentials (MEP) using transcranial magnetic stimulation (TMS) that evaluate the complete somatosensory or motor pathway. Although these methods might be supplemented with more specific examination designs that allow for a localization of abnormal findings, ultimately abnormal results may in principle be located anywhere between the basic sensory receptors/motor units and the cortex.

SEP have been evaluated in RLS patients only in one study (21) that found normal results in all subjects. Active and resting motor thresholds elicited with TMS of the motor cortex in idiopathic RLS patients were normal for muscles of the hand (M. abductor digiti minimi and M. abductor pollicis brevis) (22–25), foot (M. abductor halllucis) (25), and leg (M. tibialis anterior) (22,24). One study (23) found a higher active motor threshold both in the morning and in the evening for the tibialis anterior muscle, but not for the hand muscles when comparing RLS to healthy controls. Another TMS study recently did show a reduced cortical silent period that normalized after dopaminergic therapy (24a). The above studies also failed to reveal any abnormalities in MEP parameters, such as recruitment pattern, amplitudes, or latencies (24–26). In addition, two studies that have employed detailed movement analysis found no differences between RLS patients and controls in various movement components (27,28).

Quantitative sensory testing employing temperature perception has been performed in three studies (29–31). In a small study of eight patients with RLS, five showed an increased cold and seven an increased warm perception threshold, but all patients also showed evidence of peripheral axonal neuropathy (29). On a group level, another study (30) showed that idiopathic RLS patients had a decreased cold perception threshold when compared to a control group, while warm and heat pain thresholds did not differ. In the same study, 32% of RLS patients, but also 10% of the control subjects, showed at least one pathological threshold value. A third study (31) found that cold and heat pain thresholds were normal in all patients, but reported abnormal temperature limens (difference between cold and heat pain thresholds) in 72% of 22 secondary RLS subjects and 55% of 20 idiopathic RLS subjects when compared to age-related normal values.

Overall, evaluations of the entire somatosensory and motor pathways give no over indications of abnormalities in the motor system, but some distinctive findings related to temperature perception in the somatosensory system. Whether this is a consequence of abnormal sensory input or abnormalities of sensory processing will be discussed in the following sections.

### The Periphery

Because sensory symptoms are primarily located in the legs, it makes sense to look there for a potential disturbing stimulus or process that gives rise to these sensations. There are two main approaches that have investigated the periphery; i.e., a peripheral nerve etiology and a vascular etiology with peripheral circulatory disturbances.

## WHAT IS THE ROLE OF PERIPHERAL NEUROPATHY IN RESTLESS LEGS SYNDROME?

Peripheral neuropathy is an assumed cause of secondary RLS and reviewed in detail in Chapter 19. It is thought that at the basic perceptual level sensory stimuli are distorted, possibly leading to a hypersensitization of the sensory pathway that may induce a *circulus vitiosus* maintaining restless legs symptoms. Peripheral neuropathy can be evoked by a broad range of medical diseases, toxins, and drugs. The overall prevalence is about 2% to 4%, and in persons older than 55 years rises to about 8% of the population (32). In unselected groups of RLS patients, the prevalence of neuropathy or abnormal electrophysiological results ranged from 10% (33,34) to 30% (1,35). These abnormal results may be more frequent in sporadic vs. familial RLS (36) and in those with older age at onset of RLS (1) and mostly point to an axonal type of neuropathy (29,33,37).

In a study of 154 consecutive patients with neuropathy, the prevalence of RLS was only 5.2% (38). However, all other studies with patients suffering from neuropathy of various origins such as cryoglubolinemia (39–41), Charcot–Marie–Tooth neuropathy (41,42), small sensory fiber neuropathy (43), or other neuropathies (41,44) have found prevalence rates of roughly 30% in these samples. Of special interest are two observations pertaining to the temporal relationship between the occurrence of RLS and neuropathy. Salvi et al. (45) could show that in four of five members of a family with familial amyloid polyneuropathy, RLS actually started before any clinical signs of neuropathy could be detected. Iannaccone et al. (46) corroborate this finding by their own observation of 31 patients with RLS and neuropathy of various origins where RLS was heralding neuropathy in 94% of the patients. Furthermore, during a two-year follow-up period, RLS disappeared in 16 patients who complained of a worsening of neuropathy. Thus, subtle changes at peripheral nerves and nerve endings—undetectable by routine examination—might serve as abnormal sensory input to trigger and maintain RLS symptoms.

By definition, results from clinical examinations including electromyography (EMG) and nerve conduction velocity studies are inconspicuous in idiopathic RLS. In addition, compound motor action potentials, F-responses (24), peripheral silent periods elicited by TMS (22,24,47), or the quantitative nociceptor axon reflex (31) were normal in subjects with idiopathic RLS (22,24,31) and RLS secondary to iron deficiency (47). Nerve conduction studies in persons with periodic limb movement disorder (PLMD) also yielded normal results (48), but in one study of elderly volunteers the occurrence of PLMS was related rather unsystematically to sensory and motor latencies or velocities (49). Electrophysiological routine evaluations do not evaluate the small sensory fibers for which muscle biopsy or quantitative sensory testing (see above) is more suited. Nerve and muscle biopsy studies (1,29,37,50) in RLS patients have detected evidence of an axonal involvement (29,37) and abnormalities of small sensory fibers (1) and nerve endings (29,50), although this might not be specific to RLS (50).

Overall, although a greater percentage of RLS patients than previously expected may show subtle abnormalities when examined using electrophysiological or other sophisticated techniques, it is also obvious that these abnormalities are not a necessary precondition for the development of RLS. And although the prevalence of RLS in patients with neuropathy may be higher than expected in the general population, the majority of patients even with severe neuropathy will not develop RLS. Whether neuropathy is a sufficient cause in selected patients to trigger or maintain RLS is still open to debate.

## THE VASCULAR HYPOTHESIS—EXOTIC BUT PERSISTING?

Ekbom decidedly favored a vascular pathogenesis of RLS predominantly based on the good therapeutic results obtained by the use of two vasodilatative agents (carbachol and tolazoline) in 23 out of 29 patients (51). Ekbom also noted that RLS patients often reported cold feet, which pointed to a certain degree of circulatory insufficiency. In addition, Ekbom described the resemblance of RLS to acroparesthesia of the hands (intermittent paresthesias mostly at night), which was then thought to be a vasomotor disorder. At the same time and independently from Ekbom, Allison also reported that *"the disagreeable sensation stops at once when 1/100 g of nitroglycerin is chewed, suggesting that the cause is vascular"* [in Ref. (51), p.14].

This, of course, is reminiscent of the clonidine treatment that has been found to be effective in two double-blind studies in idiopathic (52) and uremic RLS (53). The response rates in 70% (52) to 80% (53) of the patients even correspond roughly to the rate of improvement (80%) reported by Ekbom (51). Surprisingly, there is one large open-label study (54) that reported that 98% (111/113) of patients searching treatment for varicose veins and suffering from concomitant RLS reported a complete or near complete relief of RLS symptoms after a few sessions with sclerotherapy, and in approximately 70% of patients this relief lasted for 2 years. Even more recently, a 35-day treatment with enhanced counterpulsation (55) and the wearing of a low-pressure device on the legs (56) ameliorated RLS in individual patients. The actual pressure sensation, however, could account for this independent of any vascular effect. Circumstantial evidence could also be evoked by the link between smoking and RLS in the general population that has been reported in some (57–59) though by no means all studies (60–62). However, in two large studies with 1566 primary care patients in the United Kingdom (63) and 2404 subjects in the United States (64), the presence of RLS symptoms was unrelated to venous reflux or venous obstruction determined by duplex ultrasonography.

Reduced peripheral blood circulation has also been discussed as the cause of PLMS. Ancoli-Israel et al. (65) reported that about a third of elderly subjects with significant PLMS complained about cold feet, and in a case study thermal biofeedback training reduced the PLMS index dramatically in a single patient. In a small case series (66), treatment with the alpha-receptor blocker phenoxybenzamine was initiated in six PLMD patients (one subject with RLS). Follow-up polysomnograms of four patients revealed a reduction of PLMS in three of them. However, for the single RLS subject, the treatment had no positive impact on restless legs symptoms. The authors regarded the subjective complaints of cold feet and observed decreased peripheral pulses as the consequence of an overactive sympathetic nervous system (SNS) possibly mediated by norepinephrine. Arguments in favor of this include that the SNS has a normal 20- to 40-second periodicity (67) that matches that of PLM nicely. However, clonidine—an alpha-adrenergic–stimulating agent that inhibits norepinephrine activity at presynaptic neurons—ameliorated RLS symptoms but failed to reduce PLM (52).

Like peripheral neuropathy, vascular disturbances can be caused by a multitude of common factors, but they also have wide-ranging consequences including peripheral nerve damage. Although the vascular hypothesis has not received much scientific interest in recent years, it persists and cannot be ruled out completely. Similar to peripheral neuropathy there might be patients—although probably much fewer—in whom a disturbance of vascular circulation may trigger or maintain restless legs symptoms.

### RLS and Amputation

It would be a strong argument against a purely peripheral origin of RLS if RLS symptoms exist in an amputated leg. Ekbom (68) described a patient with preexisting RLS whose right lower leg had to be amputated due to diabetic gangrene, and who no longer experienced RLS symptoms in the amputated leg. Similarly, Hedén (69) reported a patient with childhood amputation of right leg who developed RLS in adulthood with symptoms being restricted to the intact leg. At the same time, however, Nordlander (70) described a patient who experienced phantom sensations in the amputated leg that were relieved when moving the stump. Very recently, there were two further independent case reports (71,72) on subjects with amputation of both lower legs who developed RLS in these amputated limbs, being responsive to dopamine agonists in both cases.

## THE SPINAL CORD

Involvement of the spinal cord in the pathophysiology of RLS is suggested by the fact that sensory and motor symptoms are bilateral and segmentally localized in the legs in most cases. Possibly, either a sensory signal from the periphery to the sensory cortex is affected at the level of the spinal cord or the abnormal input itself is generated at that level. The two major lines linking RLS and PLMS to the spinal cord are observations of both phenomena in association with spinal cord pathological processes and research findings pertaining to segmental reflexes such as the flexor reflex or the H-reflex.

### RLS Associated with Spinal Cord Lesions

There are numerous case reports describing the onset of RLS in close temporal association with spinal pathologies such as lumbosacral radiculopathy (73), borrelia-induced myelitis (74), transverse myelitis (75), vascular injury of the spinal cord (76), multiple sclerosis (77), traumatic lesions (77), cervical spondylotic myelopathy (77), or syringomyelia (77). After spinal anesthesia, 8.7% of 161 patients developed transient new onset RLS (78). Many subjects in these reports responded to dopaminergic treatment (74,75,77,79), while in one subject (76) relief was obtained by a combination of tilidin and zolpidem.

The autosomal-dominant spinocerebellar ataxias (SCA) are a heterogeneous group of neurodegenerative disorders, and the subtypes SCA-3 (80), SCA-2 and -3 (81), and SCA-1, -2, and -3 (82) have been linked to an increased prevalence of RLS. Although spinal processes—among a range of diverse subcortical structures—have been implicated in SCA, the authors focused on a possible genetic contribution to RLS.

The evidence for a spinal origin of the sensory symptoms of RLS is less robust. Given the high prevalence of RLS, the scarcity of the case reports does not argue convincingly in favor of a spinal generator of sensory RLS symptoms. Even in "pure" spinal pathologies such as syringomyelia or syringobulbia, where

62% of unselected patients showed PLM, none of them had symptoms of RLS (83). However, spinal pathologies may serve as a trigger for restless legs symptoms.

## PLMS Associated with Spinal Cord Lesions

In animals, complex motor performance such as walking behavior can still be performed in the case of a complete spinal transection, arguing in favor of complex motor pattern generators in the spinal cord (84). Also, in animals with spinal cord lesions PLM emerged during sleep (85). Spinal pathologies that have been associated with PLMS include syringomyelia (78,83) and syringobulbia (83), lumbrosacral radiculopathy (73), traumatic injuries (86), and other lesions (87). Even in completely paraplegic patients PLMS have been observed (86,88,89), strongly suggesting a spinal origin of PLMS. Interestingly, the known lower occurrence of PLMS during rapid eye movement (REM) sleep is maintained in patients with spinal pathologies and only abolished in patients with complete spinal cord transsections (86,88). Watanabe et al. (90) reported a well-documented case of an 86-year-old male who exhibited PLM during midthoracic epidural anesthesia. Careful observation in the hospital did not reveal any PLMS, and, furthermore, the PLM could be repeatedly induced by spinal anesthesia. These observations suggest that PLM might be generated in the spinal cord and sleep may unmask a possible generator by diminishing inhibitory supraspinal influences.

## Reflexes and the Spinal Cord

PLM have been thought to be highly stereotyped movements, possibly resembling the Babinski sign (91) or the flexor reflex (92) and could thus be the consequence of a transitory loss of supraspinal inhibitory influences on descending motor pathway function. Another line of research has explored segmentally localized reflexes in RLS patients, especially the H-reflex, in search for a spinal hyperexcitability.

PLMS have been likened to the Babinski sign (91,93), which in healthy persons is absent during wakefulness and REM sleep, but can be elicited during non-REM (NREM) sleep (94). More recently, it has been shown that the elicited flexor reflex and especially its late components are disinhibited in idiopathic RLS patients compared to controls during sleep and wakefulness (92), which has been confirmed in uremic patients (95). Both studies corroborate earlier findings (96) that the flexor reflex failed to show habituation and was followed by long-latency components.

Interestingly, in a case study, an injection with apomorphine abolished both the PLMS and the flexor reflex in a subject with severe PLM after dopamine withdrawal (97). There is evolving evidence, however, that PLMS are not stereotyped movements that follow a regular spinal recruitment pattern, not even in the same patient (21,98). The EMG recruitment pattern of involuntary limb movements during wakefulness might exhibit a slightly higher intraindividual stability as reported by Trenkwalder et al. (99).

As early as 1974, Martinelli and Coccagna (96) reported that three of their five RLS patients and a subject with PLMD showed an impaired excitability curve of the H-reflex with strong indications for reduced inhibition. In addition, these findings were even more pronounced in the evening. An indication for a disinhibition of the H-reflex was also found in two of six subjects with PLMD (48), while two independent studies found no abnormalities in idiopathic RLS (100) and RLS related to iron deficiency (47). In a recent study including nine subjects with PLMD

(PLMS-index >25)—of whom eight also had RLS—standard parameters of the H-reflex did not differ between PLMD/RLS subjects and controls. However, elicitation of the H-reflex during vibration showed significantly larger amplitudes in PLMD/RLS subjects, and the H-reflex recovery curve for paired stimuli was suggestive of a distinct disinhibition.

Together with the results of a disinhibition of the flexor reflex in RLS patients (92), there is evidence of a spinal hyperexcitability, which is currently more robust for PLMD. Circumstantially, spinal cord disinhibition from supraspinal dopaminergic systems remains an intriguing hypothesis, despite little human data to support it (92a). Animal models destroying dopaminergic spinal projections result in increased motor activity (92b). Whether this phenomenon is specifically located at the spinal cord level or reflects a loss of supraspinal inhibitory influences has not yet been resolved.

## THE BRAIN

There is no evidence of systematic structural abnormalities of the brain in RLS subjects as shown by magnetic resonance imaging (MRI) (21,92,100) or autopsy (101,102). Brain glucose metabolism as revealed by a PET study was normal in six RLS subjects (103). Central motor conduction times did not differ between RLS (23) or PLMD patients (104) and controls, nor between persons with syringomyelia and PLMS vs. those without PLMS (83). Olfactory functioning, disturbed in Parkinson's disease, was normal in RLS (105).

### Brainstem

Hypotheses specifically involving the brainstem in sensory symptoms of RLS are sparse. However, a significant role has been proposed in a recent comprehensive review (106) for the inferior olive and the red nucleus as centers of sensory–motor integration crucial for RLS. It must be noted that RLS symptoms depend not only on physical rest but also on decreased arousal levels. Patients report decreased symptom intensities in situations that are mentally alerting. This central arousal level is regulated in the brainstem. Also, the rostromedial medulla has been suggested to play a role in sensory–motor disorders including RLS (107).

In the first and to date only functional MRI (fMRI) study in patients with RLS (108) no activations were found in the pons, the mesencephalon, or the red nucleus at times of sensory discomfort. PLMW, however, did activate these structures, implicating the brainstem in the generation of RLS motor symptoms. In contrast to the substantia nigra and putamen, imaging of brain iron content in the pons and the red nucleus did not show any differences between RLS subjects and controls (109). The smaller size of these structures may have contributed to this. The same MRI methodology applied in two patients with hemochromatosis and RLS found an iron content below the range of a control group in the red nucleus, the substantia nigra, and the pallidum, but not in the putamen or caudate (110).

Brainstem reflexes have been investigated in the search for increased excitability. While two studies have reported a hyperexcitability of the blink reflex in patients with PLMD (48,111), no abnormalities were found in RLS subjects (47,100). Normal results were also obtained for the temporalis inhibitory reflex in RLS subjects (100) and brainstem auditory-evoked responses in PLMD patients (112). Coleman proposed that PLMS are controlled by a pacemaker at the reticular level that may be disinhibited in subjects with PLMD (113). In addition, two cases of new onset of PLM after a pontine lesions were reported, both responded to dopaminergic agents (114). There is now a consolidated body of evidence that PLMS are heralded and accompanied by systematic autonomic changes of the heart rate (115–117), which most likely reflects an increase in sympathetic activity (118). In the ongoing debate whether cortical arousals and PLM both originate from a single source, the brainstem is the candidate structure.

### Basal Ganglia/Striatum

Imaging of brain iron content in patients with RLS (109) revealed a decreased iron content in the substantia nigra and the putamen, but not in the caudate nucleus or the globus pallidus.

Most imaging studies have investigated dopamine metabolism in the basal ganglia and specifically in the striatum. Imaging of presynaptic dopamine transporter protein (DAT) in the basal ganglia during the daytime with $^{123}$I-IPT SPECT (119,120) or $^{123}$I-β-CIT-SPECT (28,121) consistently revealed no differences between drug-naive (119–121) or pretreated RLS patients (28,119,120) and matched control subjects. F-dopa uptake ($^{18}$F-fluorodopamine PET) in the caudate or putamen did not differ from that of controls in a small study with only four RLS subjects (103), while another study including nine RLS subjects reported a subtle but statistically significant reduction of F-dopa uptake in the caudate and putamen. Specifically, uptake values that were more than two standard deviations below that of the control group were seen in the caudate in two patients and in the putamen in five RLS patients (103). A mildly reduced dopamine uptake has also been found in another study (122) with 13 RLS subjects, although dopamine uptake was in the normal range for all patients.

The same study (122) also employed $^{11}$C-raclopride PET to explore postsynaptic dopamine binding and found a reduction in both the putamen and the caudate in RLS patients. Another $^{11}$C-raclopride study also showed increased receptor availability in the striatum, but also the anterior cingulated cortex and the thalamus (122a). This was similar in the morning and evening. In addition, postsynaptic D2 binding capacities using $^{123}$I-IBZM-SPECT have been explored by four independent research groups (14,119–121,123,124). The groups in Munich and Vienna did not find any difference in basal ganglia dopamine binding between drug-naive or pretreated RLS patients and age- and gender-matched controls (119,120,124). In contrast, the Montreal group scanned dopamine agonist-naive RLS patients in the late afternoon (16:30–21:30 hours) and found that striatal binding was significantly reduced in RLS subjects vs. healthy controls. Previous studies by Staedt et al. from Göttingen (14,123) including a mixed group of PLMD and RLS patients found a distinct lower dopamine binding in the basal ganglia compared to controls that were 16 years younger on average.

Comparison across studies is hampered by the use of different methodologies to compute the dopamine binding capacity. Overall, there is little indication that on a group level RLS patients have significantly and systematically decreased pre- or postsynaptic D2-binding capacities during the daytime. Post synaptic binding seems to be more abnormal than dopamine binding or dopamine transport imaging. Another interpretation of this, not mentioned in any of the actual reports, is that there are normal dopamine levels but the endogenous dopamine can not reach the receptor. This is consistent with some recent work hypothesizing synaptic abnormalities in RLS (Chapter 7). Importantly, imaging in the evening or at night, at the time of expression of RLS symptoms, might reveal more robust abnormalities of striatal dopamine metabolism. Additionally, higher resolution scanners should also be able to examine other smaller dopaminergic areas outside the striatum.

### Cerebellum

In the above-discussed fMRI study (108), the cerebellum was activated during sensory discomfort in RLS patients, although to a lesser extent than in association with PLMW. MRI measurement of brain iron did not reveal any differences between five RLS subjects and five matched controls with regard to the iron content of the dentate nucleus (109).

### Thalamus

The thalamus is the ultimate relay station and sensory gate for all incoming information to the sensory cortex. There are six different imaging studies that have explored the role of the thalamus in RLS. Unsurprisingly, the fMRI study (108) showed that the thalamus was activated bilaterally during sensory discomfort and sensory discomfort with PLMW in all seven patients with RLS. The activation of the thalamus did not differ between both conditions, suggesting that the sensory discomfort is the main cause of the activation. In a case study of familial painful RLS in a father and a daughter (125), increasing pain brought on by increasing durations of immobilization correlated with increased cerebral blood flow in the thalamus and anterior cingulate, while blood flow in the caudate was reduced. However, cerebral blood flow was expressed in relation to blood flow of the cerebellum—thought of as an uninvolved region—which in light of the findings of Bucher et al. (108) (activation of the cerebellum at times with sensory discomfort) must be questioned. A recent study by von Spiczak et al. (126) studied opioid receptor availability with [$^{11}$C]diprenophine PET. The authors found no difference in ligand binding between 15 idiopathic RLS and 12 age-matched controls. However, a higher International Restless Legs Syndrome Severity Scale score (127) correlated with lower bilateral medial thalamus opioid receptor availability among other structures. Allen et al. (128) employed $^{1}$H MR spectroscopy of the thalamus in 32 idiopathic RLS patients and 13 matched controls. Preliminary results showed a reduction of creatine and subsequently an increased *N*-acetyl aspartate (NAA)/creatine ratio. Choline and NAA did not differ between patients and controls. In RLS patients, the thalamic creatine levels correlated with tetrahydrobiopterin obtained from a nighttime lumbar cerebrospinal fluid (CSF) sample. The same authors also measured the brain iron content in patients with RLS and found no difference in the thalamus when compared to a matched control group (109). Etgen et al. (129) employed voxel-based morphometry in two independent samples of 28 and 23 idiopathic-medicated RLS patients and age- and gender-matched controls and found a significant bilateral increase in gray matter in the dorsal part of the thalamus suggesting the pulvinar. Finally, Ondo et al. did not observe any improvement in RLS when a deep brain stimulator was placed into the ventral intermedial nucleus of the thalamus for subjects with concurrent essential tremor (129a).

To summarize, the findings demonstrate a wealth of different approaches to the thalamus and point to its role for the sensory symptoms of RLS. However, on the basis of these studies it remains unclear whether the involvement of the thalamus in RLS represents a normal processing, a normal processing with increased or distorted input, or an abnormal mode of processing.

## Cortex

In the cortex, somatosensory stimuli are ultimately processed and voluntary movement activity is mediated. As mentioned above, SEP were basically normal in RLS patients (21), however, the sensory cortex has not otherwise received any systematic attention. There is only one study exploring cortical activity in RLS patients during a three-minute vigilance EEG (130). In comparison to control subjects, RLS patients showed an increased delta and fast alpha power, while slow alpha was decreased. The clinical significance of these findings is unclear, but the authors (130) suggested that these findings resemble those observed in depressive patients.

Other lines of research predominantly focused on the role of the motor cortex in RLS with two conceptually different approaches: the first involves the question of whether involuntary movements during wakefulness or PLMS are preceded by systematic cortical activity; the second line focuses on (motor) cortical inhibition and facilitation, which has been explored with TMS.

### *Leg Movements and Cortical Involvement*

EEG analysis showed consistently that PLMS (21,131,132) and involuntary leg movements during wakefulness (133) are not preceded by a Bereitschaftspotential, thus making a cortical origin of the movements unlikely. In a recent small study (134), event-related desynchronization in the beta-band preceded both voluntary and involuntary leg movements in RLS subjects, although with different premovement latencies. Although this is no indication of a voluntary and/or conscious activity, it suggests that there might be some cortical activity of the preparatory type.

A solid body of evidence now shows that PLMS are heralded by systematic changes in cortical and autonomic activity. In the case of visual polysomnogram scoring, signs of arousals precede PLMS in roughly half of the cases (135). Even in the absence of visually identified microarousals, PLMS are systematically preceded by an increase in delta activity (115,116,136) at least in NREM sleep (115). The faster frequencies also increase during the leg movements (115,116,132,137). A comprehensive framework to reconcile these findings with PLM and associated autonomic variations (see Section "Brainstem") is offered by the concept of the cyclic alternating pattern (CAP) (138). The vast majority of PLMS occurred during CAP and within CAP during phase A (139). Indeed, it has been proposed that CAP acts as a phasing mechanism that entrains the motor pattern of PLM to the dominant 20- to 40-second periodicity (139,140).

### *Cortical Inhibition and Facilitation*

TMS has been widely used as a noninvasive technique to explore the integrity and excitability of the motor system (141,142). One of its measures, the cortical silent period (CSP), is most likely generated at the motor cortical level resulting from intracortical inhibition with only the very first part ($<50$ msec) attributable to spinal mechanisms (143). Six studies comparing CSP of RLS patients to that of healthy controls have yielded mixed results (24a,23–26) with studies finding no difference between CSP of the hand (M. abductor digiti minimi) (24,25), foot (M. abductor hallucis) (25), or leg (M. tibialis anterior) (24) in the morning (24) or late afternoon (25). Two other studies reported significantly shorter CSP for the hand (22,26) and the leg (24a). Preliminary evidence from a small study in four RLS patients with painful neuropathy also showed a shortened CSP for the leg but not the hand in these patients (144). The most extensive exploration of CSP to date has been performed by Stiasny-Kolster et al. (23) who measured CSP of the hand and leg in the evening (20:00 hours) and morning (08:00 hours) in patients and controls as well as in patients after a single evening dose of 200/50 levodopa/benserazide. They found a significantly shorter CSP for the tibialis anterior in the evening and a trend for a shorter CSP in the morning, which was not observed for the hand muscle. After levodopa treatment CSP was prolonged in the leg but not the arm and only in the evening.

Paired pulse TMS is another nonstandard TMS technique that demonstrates changes in cortical excitability that cannot be measured using other techniques (145). All three studies comparing intracortical inhibition at short interstimulus intervals (ISIs) found a reduced inhibition in RLS patients compared to controls for hand (24–26), foot (25), and leg areas (24) of the motor cortex. Increased facilitation at long ISIs was observed in one (24) of two studies (24,25). Accordingly, another study reported that RLS subjects did not differ from controls in EEG activity before a voluntary brisk hand movement, but showed an increased postmovement event-related synchronization in the fast beta range suggesting a reduced inhibition (146).

In summary, there is a strong indication of a decreased intracortical inhibition in RLS subjects. The origin, consequences, and meaning of this finding have not been elucidated so far. Possible causes could be simply the long-standing increased peripheral input (147,148); it is, however, of special interest that experimental studies in healthy subjects have shown that the cerebellum may be involved in intracortical inhibition (149,150).

## OTHER SYSTEMS RELEVANT TO RESTLESS LEGS SYNDROME

Although neuroanatomy is a logical starting point into the physiology of RLS, other structures, in particular neurotransmitter and neuroendocrine systems, do not map precisely onto single structures and might be more suited to explain the multifactorial nature of RLS symptoms. Two major systems are reviewed in detail elsewhere, the dopaminergic pathways and the iron metabolism will only be discussed briefly here.

### The Dopaminergic System

Some involvement of a dopaminergic system in the pathophysiology of RLS is undisputed. The strongest argument is based on the rapid and dramatic improvement of RLS with dopaminergic agents (151,152). As reviewed above, brain-imaging studies of the dopaminergic system in the basal ganglia have not revealed consistent abnormalities (see Section "Basal Ganglia"). Another way to explore the integrity of the dopamine system is by measuring neuroendocrine responses to challenges with dopaminergic agonists or dopamine-blocking substances. For example, metoclopramide (a dopamine blocker) normally causes an increase in both prolactin and human growth hormone (hGH). Basic 24-hour time courses of prolactin and growth hormone do not differ between RLS subjects and controls (153). Furthermore, challenges with a dopamine antagonist in the early afternoon revealed a normal response in RLS subjects (154). Neuroendocrine response to a levodopa challenge was more pronounced during the night vs. the morning in both RLS subjects and controls, but both the decrease in prolactin and the increase in hGH were especially pronounced in RLS subjects at night. This might suggest a hypersensitivity of postsynaptic dopamine receptors at night in the RLS population (155).

The measurement of metabolites of the dopamine synthesis and degradation in CSF is another way to explore this system. High levels of free dopamine, homovanillic acid (HVA), free norepinephrine, and 3-methoxy-4-hydroxyphenylethyleneglycol have been found in the morning CSF of a single patient with severe, familial, early-onset RLS (156). A subsequent systematic study in RLS subjects in the evening found normal dopaminergic metabolites in the CSF and blood (157). In an earlier study (158) with morning CSF samples, HVA and neopterin did not differ between RLS subjects and age-matched controls, but biopterin was increased in RLS subjects. Serendipitously, one study found lower dopamine, 3, 4-dihydroxyphenylacetic acid and HVA nocturnal urinary excretion levels in four subjects with a PLMS index of >5 in a placebo night (159). Earley et al. also looked for circadian changes in CSF dopamine metabolites (159a). Compared to controls, they found larger changes (A.M. vs. P.M.) in tetrahydrobiopterin (BH4), HVA:5HIAA ratio, and 3-OMD for RLS patients. All three metabolites were higher at 10 A.M. compared to 10 P.M. sample. Therefore RLS patients seem to have a greater diurnal variation than controls. In summary, the response to dopaminergic agents is probably one of the most closely associated features of RLS. Finding a marker for an altered dopamine system in RLS has proven to be more difficult, and it seems likely that the dopamine system is predominantly involved in the circadian expression of restless legs symptoms.

## Brain Iron Metabolism

There is strong evidence confirming the role of iron in RLS [reviewed in (160,161)]. First, systemic iron insufficiency is associated with secondary RLS, possibly also including ESRD and pregnancy. Second, studies using CSF measurements, MRI, or autopsy material to determine the brain iron status in RLS subjects indicate low brain iron content in RLS (101,109,162). Most interestingly, iron is a cofactor of tyrosine hydroxylase, the rate-limiting enzyme for the dopamine synthesis. Thus, iron is needed for dopamine synthesis and in case of deficiency may impair the normal production of dopamine. Oral iron supplementation may improve RLS in patients with low ferritin (16) but not in those with normal ferritin levels (163). However, in subjects with normal iron stores only 1% to 2% of the orally given iron is absorbed and oral supplementation is often poorly tolerated due to gastroenterologic side effects. Intravenously administered iron does not exhibit this limitation. Successful treatment of RLS with intravenous (IV) iron has already been reported more than half a century ago (15). A recent open-label study showed that 6 out of 10 patients experienced a complete remission of RLS symptoms for 3 to 36 months after only a single IV iron treatment (164). Importantly, the same study (164) reported that the treatment did actually increase brain iron concentrations based on imaging results. However, in the weeks following IV iron treatment serum ferritin levels showed an unexpectedly rapid linear decrease. Iron and the dopamine–iron connection in the brain is one of the most promising avenues of research into the pathophysiology of RLS.

## Asthenia Crurum Dolorosa—Pain and the Opiate System in RLS

In a 1945 monograph, Ekbom (51) distinguished two forms of RLS: *asthenia crurum paraesthetica*, the now classical description of RLS with paresthesia and *asthenia crurum dolorosa*, the painful form of RLS. Ekbom found the painful forms not as simple to diagnose and more difficult to treat but thought of them as "*probably only variants of the same basic disease (P 61).*" While current definitions (165) do not include a painful component of RLS sensory symptoms, they recognize that painful sensations can be part of RLS. Indeed, in two independent studies the percentage of RLS patients that described their symptoms as painful ranged from 56% (166) to 85% (33).

There is an increased prevalence of RLS symptoms in patients with frequent and diffuse body pain (167) such as that seen in fibromyalgia (168–170) or rheumatoid arthritis (171,172). Also, 34% of patients with intractable headaches had RLS (173), and these subjects were especially vulnerable to develop drug-induced akathisia during the treatment with IV dopamine receptor–blocking agents. On the other hand, in a population study working-aged men and women with RLS were more likely to report morning or daytime headaches (174,175). This, however, was not the case when comparing blood donors with and without RLS in another larger-scaled study by the same authors (176). However, in a study including 218 RLS patients, roughly 15% were taking pain medications (177), and in another study with 243 patients from a single psychiatric practice the occurrence of RLS was related to the intake of nonopioid analgesics (178), leading the authors to speculate that central sensitization by nonopioid analgesic overuse might play a role in RLS (179).

An increase in pain sensitivity; i.e., static mechanical hyperalgesia, was shown in one study in RLS patients (180). Interestingly, this increased pain sensitivity was significantly reduced after long-term (one year) but not short-term levodopa treatment. However, pain sensitivity is also associated with poor sleep and depression (181) and slow wave sleep deprivation (182), all factors present to a certain degree in RLS. The above-mentioned study (see Section "Thalamus") with [$^{11}$C]diprenorphine PET (126) found no difference of opioid binding between RLS subjects and controls, but within the group of RLS subjects opioid receptor binding correlated with RLS severity and questionnaire-based pain scores. The most convincing evidence supporting involvement of the opiate system, of course, is based on the effectiveness of opioidergic treatment in RLS (183–185), (Chapter 27). Challenges of the opiate system in RLS patients (186) showed that administration of naloxone to opiate-treated patients reactivates RLS symptoms, while it has no consistent effect in subjects treated with dopaminergic agents. According to a case report (187), administration of a dopamine receptor blocker to an opiate-treated RLS patient also reactivated RLS symptoms. The challenge of untreated RLS patients with naloxone seems to have no effect on RLS symptoms (154,188,189). Furthermore, untreated RLS patients showed a normal hormonal response (increases in hGH, cortisol, and adrenocorticotropic hormone) following naloxone challenge (154).

Overall, RLS responds to opioidergic agents and is associated with painful medical conditions. Similar to the dopamine system, a specific biomarker for an altered endogenous opiate system in RLS has not been identified.

## Serotonin

There is a relatively higher psychiatric comorbidity in subjects with RLS; furthermore, RLS might be more prevalent in psychiatric patients. Systematic studies have linked RLS to depression (190), anxiety disorders (130,191,192), and attention-deficit hyperactivity disorder (193). A high proportion of RLS subjects are treated with antidepressant medications (177), and in a large survey study selective serotonin reuptake inhibitors (SSRIs) but not tricyclic antidepressants were associated with a higher risk for RLS (59). Metabolites of serotonin in CSF evening (157) did not differ between RLS patients and (age-matched) controls. Serotonin metabolites taken in the morning did not show any absolute differences compared to a control group; however, when these were normalized for differences in age, the serotonin metabolite 5-hydroxyindoleacetic acid was lower in RLS subjects (158). SSRIs can provoke or aggravate symptoms of RLS (194,195); however, the opposite has also been reported (196). Recent systematic evidence also showed that patients taking SSRI had significantly more PLMS than controls without SSRI medication (197).

## Melatonin

RLS symptoms occur at specific times during the 24-hour day, preferentially in the evening and at night. The circadian rhythm (independent from sleep–wake behavior) has been associated with both the sensory and the motor symptoms of this disorder (198–200). The relationship between the duration of rest and the occurrence of symptoms also showed a circadian variation (201). A prime marker of circadian rhythm, the core body temperature, did not show any abnormalities in RLS subjects (198–200,202).

Melatonin is a "chronobioticum," a substance that adjusts the timing of biological rhythms. A rather summative measure of daytime (07:00–22:00 hours) and nighttime (22:00–07:00 hours) urinary 6-OH-melatonin-sulfate excretion did not differ between RLS subjects and controls (203). Melatonin also had a normal circadian rhythm in a 28-hour modified constant routine study, but there was a shorter nocturnal melatonin secretion in RLS patients and a strong cross-correlation with melatonin levels preceding both sensory symptoms and PLM by 2 hours (200). In an uncontrolled, open-label study, daily intake of melatonin reduced PLM in nine patients with PLMD but without RLS (204). Interestingly, 21 days of levodopa treatment in RLS subjects advanced dim light melatonin onset, in particular in a subgroup of patients with augmentation (205). These studies suggest a role of melatonin in RLS. So far, it has not been clear if melatonin is merely a marker of an altered circadian system in RLS patients or more directly involved in the pathophysiology of RLS, possibly by exerting an inhibitory effect on dopamine secretion as has been shown for some areas of the mammalian CNS (206).

## Sexual Steroid Hormones

Several epidemiological studies have shown a higher prevalence of RLS in women than in men (59,62,207). Elderly women seem to be particularly affected (207), which points to the postmenopausal hormonal status as a possible cause. Prospective (208,209), concurrent (210,211), or retrospective assessment (18) of RLS occurrence during pregnancy consistently indicates that approximately 25% of females will experience RLS symptoms, with the highest prevalence during the last trimester (see Chapter 20). In many females, RLS symptoms during pregnancy are mild and infrequent (18,208,210) and disappear shortly after delivery (18,208–210). Hormonal changes during pregnancy predominantly manifest by increases in plasma estrogen, progesterone, and prolactin. A recent study (212) that followed pregnant women with and without RLS from the 35th week of gestation to approximately 12 weeks postpartum has found markedly elevated estradiol levels in pregnant women with RLS during late-term pregnancy but not after delivery.

In addition, a population study (57) has shown that the prevalence of RLS was related to the number of pregnancies.

In light of these findings, hormone replacement therapy (HRT) would be expected to worsen RLS symptomatology but evidence for this is scarce. In one study (62), the percentage of elderly women with RLS who took estrogens was higher than that of those without RLS, but numbers were low and the difference was not statistically significant. Another study (213) has examined the incidence of PLMS during estrogen replacement therapy for up to 7 months and found no effect of HRT on PLMS and PLMS-associated arousals. This was corroborated by another treatment study (214) with an estrogen or an estrogen–progesterone combination.

Female hormones are candidate measures to explain prevalence differences between men and women and the high incidence of RLS during pregnancy. The available evidence, however, is sparse and only tentatively identifies estrogens as a possible factor. It may be possible that only very high levels of steroid hormones, as they are found in pregnancy, play a role in RLS.

#### Other Neuroendocrine Factors

To date, three studies (215–217) have measured *hypocretin* in patients with RLS. While one (215) has found increased evening CSF hypocretin-1 levels in RLS patients and particularly in those with early onset of RLS, this finding has not been replicated by two other reports measuring both evening (217) and daytime (216) levels of hypocretin.

Close temporal associations between *hypothyroidism* and the occurrence of RLS has been reported for single patients (218,219). In large-scale studies of the general population and in a primary care setting, RLS patients demonstrated a higher prevalence of thyroid disorders (57,177), though other studies found no difference in hypothyroidism (220), intake of thyroid medication (62), or thyroid-stimulating hormone levels (57,60). Furthermore, the prevalence of RLS in patients with thyroid disorders was not increased (221).

In a general population study, *parathyroid hormone* levels did not differ between subjects with and without RLS (60). In uremic patients with RLS a reduced parathyroid hormone level has been reported (222) but was not confirmed in several other studies (223–225). Abnormal calcium levels were not seen (222).

## CONCLUDING REMARKS

The most sought question in RLS pathophysiology today is the "common final pathway" of restless legs symptoms and the exact nature of the processes at the time of their expression. The fMRI study identified activation of the thalamus and cerebellum during times of sensory symptoms and additional activations of the brainstem at times of motor symptoms during wakefulness as a correlate of sensory/motor symptoms. This study, however, has never been replicated. The temporal nature of these symptoms makes it unlikely that "stable" traits can explain them sufficiently and more studies exploring circadian time-related processes are clearly needed.

The available evidence shows that RLS subjects differ from healthy controls at specific times during the 24-hour day. All studies that have assessed diverse functions at various times during the day and night have revealed differences in most functions and point to contrasts between patients and controls only at times of RLS symptom expression in many instances. This makes it more difficult to interpret negative findings, because most of them have been performed during the day and it is thus unclear whether there truly are no differences or whether differences will only become apparent at a later time of the day.

For PLMS there is strong evidence of a (sleep) state-dependent increased excitability or loss of inhibitory influences at various levels of the motor pathway including the motor cortex and other supraspinal structures. It seems that the spinal cord provides everything necessary to generate and maintain a rhythmic motor activity of the lower limbs. During sleep, inhibitory influences on spinal processes are dampened—as evidenced by the elicitation of the Babinski reflex during NREM sleep in healthy subjects—and it might only be a small step to further reduce these influences below a critical level. Spinal pathological processes but also disorders of subcortical structures at the level of the brainstem or basal ganglia are especially likely to give rise to PLMS. While the rhythmicity can be generated within the spinal cord, the temporal association with other physiological processes point to the brainstem—at the level of the reticular substance—as "coordinating" center in the case of an intact spinal cord. Given the high prevalence of PLM in the general population, increasing with age, and the systematic coupling with the CAP A phase during sleep, it could also be argued that PLM are physiological events occurring during all forms of unstable sleep—but maybe only in persons with a certain but by no means rare predisposition. This, in turn, would mean that the disturbed sleep in RLS provokes the PLM rather than vice versa. The extrapolation of these concepts to PLMW or even involuntary leg movements is questionable.

The corresponding sensory side of RLS is less well-understood. While it seems that peripheral processes are able to trigger RLS in selected subjects, the preponderance of evidence points to abnormalities in sensory processing rather than sensory input. An as yet concealed process possibly involving hypersensitization is prompted by another process yet to be defined that is closely bound to the circadian system and for which melatonin could be a prime candidate. However, iron metabolism and dopamine also show characteristic variations over the 24-hour day, with evidence suggesting that the amplitude of these variations is larger in RLS subjects. Most likely an interaction between diverse factors such as iron and dopamine act in concert to produce restless legs symptoms.

A wealth of independent studies ranging from large-scale population-based epidemiological studies to carefully described single case reports has been accumulated. Thus, the important question arises how to interpret the research results in terms of pathogenic factors. As discussed in the introduction, a given factor might be a factor triggering RLS, or maintaining RLS, or might be simply an epiphenomenon of RLS, an associated risk factor or even a consequence of RLS. A factor may be related to the occurrence of RLS or the circadian expression of RLS symptoms. Ultimately, these questions have to be determined empirically. In epidemiological research, it is accepted that causal risk factors for the occurrence of a disorder precede this outcome in a temporal dimension (226). Thus, several conditions have been associated with RLS; however, for many of them it is unknown how they relate to the onset and course of RLS. This applies to the association of RLS with peripheral neuropathy, but also the many pathophysiological findings such as impaired temperature perception, increased pain thresholds, reduced intracortical inhibition, an increased spinal hyperexcitability, decreased brain iron content, or possible thalamic structural or metabolic alterations. On the other hand, ESRD, pregnancy, and spinal lesions are conditions that precede the occurrence of RLS, although this is better documented for the first two conditions. RLS is a disorder with many faces and prospective studies are needed to determine what is a symptom, a consequence, or a causally operating factor of this disorder.

## REFERENCES


1. Polydefkis M, Allen RP, Hauer P, et al. Subclinical sensory neuropathy in late-onset restless legs syndrome. Neurology 2000; 55:1115–1121.
2. Wetter TC, Stiasny K, Winkelmann J, et al. A randomized controlled study of pergolide in patients with restless legs syndrome. Neurology 1999; 52:944–950.
3. Montplaisir J, Michaud M, Denesle R, et al. Periodic leg movements are not more prevalent in insomnia or hypersomnia but are specifically associated with sleep disorders involving a dopaminergic impairment. Sleep Med 2000; 1:163–167.
4. Silber MH. Commentary on controversies in sleep medicine. Montplaisir et al. Periodic leg movements are not more prevalent in insomnia or hypersomnia but are specifically associated with sleep disorders involving a dopaminergic mechanism. Sleep Med 2001; 2:367–369.
5. Michaud M, Paquet J, Lavigne G, et al. Sleep laboratory diagnosis of restless legs syndrome. Eur Neurol 2002; 48:108–113.
6. Montplaisir J, Boucher S, Poirier G, et al. Clinical, polysomnographic, and genetic characteristics of restless legs syndrome: a study of 133 patients diagnosed with new standard criteria. Mov Disord 1997; 12:61–65.
7. Montplaisir J, Boucher S, Nicolas A, et al. Immobilization tests and periodic leg movements in sleep for the diagnosis of restless legs syndrome. Mov Disord 1998; 13:324–329.
8. Bixler EO, Kales A, Vela-Bueno A, et al. Nocturnal myoclonus and nocturnal myoclonic activity in the normal population. Res Commun Chem Pathol Pharmacol 1982; 36:129–140.
9. Ancoli-Israel S, Kripke DF, Klauber MR, et al. Periodic limb movements in sleep in community-dwelling elderly. Sleep 1991; 14(6):496–500.
10. Wetter TC, Collado-Seidel V, Pollmächer T, et al. Sleep and periodic leg movement patterns in drug-free patients with Parkinson's disease and multiple system atrophy. Sleep 2000; 23(3):361–367.
11. Garcia-Borreguero D, Larrosa O, de la Llave Y, et al. Correlation between rating scales and sleep laboratory measurements in restless legs syndrome. Sleep Med 2004; 5: 561–565.
12. Pelletier G, Lorrain D, Montplaisir J. Sensory and motor components of the restless legs syndrome. Neurology 1992; 42:1663–1666.
13. Birinyi PV, Allen RP, Lesage S, et al. Investigation into the correlation between sensation and leg movements in restless legs syndrome. Mov Disord 2005; 20: 1097–1103.
14. Staedt J, Stoppe G, Kogler A, et al. Nocturnal myoclonus syndrome (periodic movements in sleep) related to central dopamine D2-receptor alteration. Eur Arch Psychiatry Clin Neurosci 1995; 245:8–10.
15. Nordlander NB. Therapy in restless legs. Acta Med Scand 1953; 145:453–457.
16. O'Keeffe ST, Gavin K, Lavan JN. Iron status and restless legs syndrome in the elderly. Age Ageing 1994; 23:200–203.
17. Ekbom K. Akroparestesier och restless legs under graviditet. Sven Lakartidn 1960; 57:2597–2603.
18. Manconi M, Govoni V, De Vito A, et al. Restless legs syndrome and pregnancy. Neurology 2004; 63:1065–1069.
19. Yasuda T, Nishimura A, Katsuki Y, et al. Restless legs syndrome treated successfully by kidney transplantation—a case report. Clin Transpl 1986; 86:138.
20. Winkelmann J, Stautner A, Samtleben W, et al. Long-term course of restless legs syndrome in dialysis patients after kidney transplantation. Mov Disord 2002; 17: 1072–1076.

21. Provini F, Vetrugno R, Meletti S, et al. Motor pattern of periodic limb movements during sleep. Neurology 2001; 57:300–304.
22. Entezari-Taher M, Singleton JR, Jones CR, et al. Changes in excitability of motor cortical circuitry in primary restless legs syndrome. Neurology 1999; 53:1201–1205.
23. Stiasny-Kolster K, Haeske H, Tergau F, et al. Cortical silent period is shortened in restless legs syndrome independently from circadian rhythm. Suppl Clin Neurophysiol 2003; 56:381–389.
24. Quatrale R, Manconi M, Gastaldo E, et al. Neurophysiological study of corticomotor pathways in restless legs syndrome. Clin Neurophysiol 2003; 114:1638–1645.

24a. Kutukcu Y, Dogruer E, Yetkin S, Ozgen F, Vural O, Aydin H. Evaluation of periodic leg movements and associated transcranial magnetic stimulation parameters in restless legs syndrome. Muscle Nerve 2006; 33:133–137.

25. Tergau F, Wischer S, Paulus W. Motor system excitability in patients with restless legs syndrome. Neurology 1999; 52:1060–1063.
26. Scalise A, Pittaro-Cadore I, Golob EJ, Gigli GL. Absence of postexercise and delayed facilitation of motor cortex excitability in restless legs syndrome: evidence of altered cortical plasticity? Sleep 2006; 29:770–775.
27. Alberts JL, Adler CH, Saling M, et al. Prehension patterns in restless legs syndrome patients. Parkinsonism Relat Disord 2001; 7:143–148.
28. Mrowka M, Jobges M, Berding G, et al. Computerized movement analysis and beta-CIT-SPECT in patients with restless legs syndrome. J Neural Transm 2004; 112:693–701.
29. Iannaccone S, Zucconi M, Marchettini P, et al. Evidence of peripheral axonal neuropathy in primary restless legs syndrome. Mov Disord 1995; 10:2–9.
30. Happe S, Zeitlhofer J. Abnormal cutaneous thermal thresholds in patients with restless legs syndrome. J Neurol 2003; 250:362–365.
31. Schattschneider J, Bode A, Wasner G, et al. Idiopathic restless legs syndrome: abnormalities in central somatosensory processing. J Neurol 2004; 251:977–982.
32. Martyn CN, Hughes RAC. Epidemiology of peripheral neuropathy. J Neurol Neurosurg Psychiatr 1997; 62:310–318.
33. Winkelmann J, Wetter TC, Collado-Seidel V, et al. Clinical characteristics and frequency of the hereditary restless legs syndrome in a population of 300 patients. Sleep 2000; 23:597–602.
34. Machtey I. Epidemiology of restless legs syndrome. Arch Int Med 2001; 161:484–485.
35. Ondo W, Jankovic J. Restless legs syndrome: clinicoetiologic correlates. Neurology 1996; 47:1435–1441.
36. Ondo W, Tan EK, Mansoor J. Rheumatologic serologies in secondary restless legs syndrome. Mov Disord 2000; 15:321–323.
37. Iannaccone S, Ferini-Strambi L, Zucconi M, et al. Peripheral nerve investigation in restless legs syndrome. J Neurol 1994; 24(suppl):S156.
38. Rutkove SB, Matheson JK, Logigian EL. Restless legs syndrome in patients with polyneuropathy. Muscle Nerve 1996; 19:670–672.
39. Gemignani F, Marbini A, Di Giovanni G, et al. Cryoglobulinaemic neuropathy manifesting with restless legs syndrome. J Neurol Sci 1997; 152:218–223.
40. Gemignani F, Melli G, Inglese C, et al. Cryoglobulinaemia is a frequent cause of peripheral neuropathy in undiagnosed referral patients. J Peripher Nerv Syst 2002; 7:59–64.
41. Melli G, Marbini A, Grosso R, et al. Restless legs syndrome in peripheral neuropathy. J Peripher Nerv Syst 2001; 6:52.
42. Gemignani F, Marbini A, Di Giovanni G, et al. Charcot-Marie-Tooth disease type 2 with restless legs syndrome. Neurology 1999; 52:1064–1066.
43. Gemignani F, Brindani F, Zinno L, et al. Frequency of clinically diagnosed small fiber neuropathy in a neuropathy population. J Peripher Nerv Syst 2004; 9:119.
44. Mold JW, Vesely SK, Keyl BA, et al. The prevalence, predictors, and consequences of peripheral sensory neuropathy in older patients. J Am Board Fam Pract 2002; 17:309–318.
45. Salvi F, Montagna P, Plasmati R, et al. Restless legs syndrome and nocturnal myoclonus: initial clinical manifestation of familial amyloid polyneuropathy. J Neurol Neurosurg Psychiatr 1990; 53:522–525.

46. Iannaccone S, Quattrini A, Sferrazza B, et al. Charcot-Marie-Tooth disease type 2 with restless legs syndrome. Neurology 2000; 54:1013–1014.
47. Akyol A, Kiylioglu N, Kadikoylu G, et al. Iron deficiency anemia and restless legs syndrome: is there an electrophysiological abnormality? Clin Neurol Neurosurg 2003; 106:23–27.
48. Wechsler LR, Stakes JW, Shahani BT, et al. Periodic leg movements of sleep (nocturnal myoclonus): an electrophysiological study. Ann Neurol 1986; 19:168–173.
49. Bliwise DL, Ingham RH, Date ES, et al. Nerve conduction and creatinine clearance in aged subjects with periodic movements in sleep. J Gerontol 1989; 44(5):M164–M167.
50. Harriman DGF, Taverner D, Woolf AL. Ekbom's syndrome and burning paraesthesiae. A biopsy study by vital staining and electron microscopy of the intramuscular innvervation with a note on age changes in motor nerve endings in distal muscles. Brain 1970; 93:393–406.
51. Ekbom KA. Restless legs: clinical study of hitherto overlooked disease in legs characterized by peculiar paresthesia ('anxietas tibiarum'), pain and weakness and occuring in two main forms, asthenia crurum paresthetica and asthenia crurum dolorosa; short review of paresthesias in general. Acta Med Scand 1945; 158:1–123.
52. Wagner ML, Walters AS, Coleman RG, et al. Randomized, double-blind, placebo-controlled study of clonidine in restless legs syndrome. Sleep 1996; 19:52–58.
53. Ausserwinkler M, Schmidt P. Erfolgreiche Behandlung des "restless legs"-Syndroms bei chronischer Niereninsuffizienz mit Clonidin. Schweiz Med Wschr 1989; 119:184–186.
54. Kanter AH. The effect of sclerotherapy on restless legs syndrome. Dermatol Surg 1995; 21:328–332.
55. Rajaram SS, Shanahan J, Ash C, et al. Enhanced external counterpulsation (EECP) as a novel treatment for restless legs syndrome (RLS): a preliminary test of the vascular neurologic hypothesis for RLS. Sleep Med 2005; 6:101–106.
56. Hattori C, Nishimura T, Suzuki K, et al. Therapeutic experience of deep vein thrombosis prevention system for restless legs syndrome. Sleep Biol Rhythms 2004; 2:125–128.
57. Berger K, Luedemann J, Trenkwalder C, et al. Sex and the risk of restless legs syndrome in the general population. Arch Int Med 2004; 164:196–202.
58. Phillips B, Young T, Finn L, et al. Epidemiology of restless legs symptoms in adults. Arch Int Med 2000; 160:2137–2141.
59. Ohayon MM, Roth T. Prevalence of restless legs syndrome and periodic limb movement disorder in the general population. J Psychosom Res 2002; 53:547–554.
60. Högl B, Kiechl S, Willeit J, et al. Restless legs syndrome. A community-based study of prevalence, severity, and risk factors. Neurology 2005; 64:1920–1924.
61. Ahlberg K, Ahlberg J, Könönen M, et al. Reported bruxism and restless legs syndrome in media personnel with or without irregular shift work. Acta Odontol Scand 2005; 63:94–98.
62. Rothdach AJ, Trenkwalder C, Haberstock J, et al. Prevalence and risk factors of RLS in an elderly population. The MEMO Study. Neurology 2000; 54:1064–1068.
63. Bradbury A, Evans CJ, Allan P, et al. The relationship between lower limb symptoms and superficial and deep venous reflux on duplex ultrasonography. The Edingburgh Vein Study. J Vasc Surg 2000; 32:921–931.
64. Langer RD, Ho E, Denenberg JO, et al. Relationships between symptoms and venous disease. The San Diego Population Study. Arch Int Med 2005; 165:1420–1424.
65. Ancoli-Israel S, Seifert AR, Lemon M. Thermal biofeedback and periodic movements in sleep: patients' subjective reports and a case study. Biofeedback Self Regul 1986; 11:177–188.
66. Ware JC, Blumoff R, Pittard JT. Peripheral vasoconstriction in patients with sleep related periodic leg movements. Sleep 1988; 11:182–186.
67. Coccagna G, Mantovani M, Brignani F, et al. Laboratory note. Arterial pressure changes during spontaneous sleep in man. Electroencephalogr Clin Neurophysiol 1971; 31:277–281.
68. Ekbom KA. Restless legs in amputees. Acta Med Scand 1961; 169:419–421.
69. Hedén S. Restless leg hos blodgivare. Sven Lakartidn 1957; 54:609–611.
70. Nordlander NB. Orsaker till "restless legs". Sven Lakartidn 1957; 54:1159–1165.

71. Estivill E, de la Fuente-Pañell V, Segarra-Isern F, et al. Restless legs syndrome in a patient with amputation of both legs. Rev Neurol 2004; 39:536–538.
72. Hanna PA, Kumar S, Walters AS. Restless legs symptoms in a patient with above knee amputations: a case of phantom restless legs. Clin Neuropharmacol 2004; 27:87–89.
73. Walters AS, Wagner M, Hening WA. Periodic limb movements as the initial manifestation of restless legs syndrome triggered by lumbosacral radiculopathy. Sleep 1996; 19:825–826.
74. Hemmer B, Riemann D, Glocker FX, et al. Restless legs syndrome after a borrelia-induced myelitis. Mov Disord 1995; 10:521–522.
75. Brown LK, Heffner JE, Obbens EA. Transverse myelitis associated with restless legs syndrome and periodic movements of sleep responsive to an oral dopaminergic agent but not to intrathecal baclofen. Sleep 2000; 23:591–594.
76. Tings T, Baier PC, Paulus W, et al. Restless legs syndrome induced by impairment of sensory spinal pathways. J Neurol 2003; 250:499–500.
77. Hartmann M, Pfister R, Pfadenhauer K. Restless legs syndrome associated with spinal cord lesions. J Neurol Neurosurg Psychiatr 1999; 66:688–689.
78. Högl B, Frauscher B, Seppi K, et al. Transient restless legs syndrome after spinal anesthesia: a prospective study. Neurology 2002; 59:1705–1707.
79. Winkelmann J, Wetter TC, Trenkwalder C, et al. Periodic leg movements in syringomyelia and syringobulbia. Mov Disord 2000; 15:752–755.
80. Schöls L, Haan J, Riess O, et al. Sleep disturbance in spinocerebellar ataxias: is the SCA3 mutation a cause of restless legs syndrome? Neurology 1998; 51:1603–1607.
81. Lee WY, Jin DK, Oh MR, et al. Frequency analysis and clinical characterization of spinocerebellar ataxia types 1, 2, 3, 6, and 7 in Korean patients. Arch Neurol 2003; 60: 858–863.
82. Abele M, Bürk K, Laccone F, et al. Restless legs syndrome in spinocerebellar ataxia types 1, 2, and 3. J Neurol 2001; 248:311–314.
83. Nogués M, Cammarota A, Leiguarda R, et al. Periodic limb movements in syringomyelia and syringobulbia. Mov Disord 2000; 15:113–119.
84. Duysens J, Van de Crommert HWAA. Neural control of locomotion: part 1: the central pattern generator from cats to humans. Gait Posture 1998; 7:131–141.
85. Esteves AM, de Mello MT, Lancellotti CLP, et al. Occurrence of limb movements during sleep in rats with spinal cord injury. Brain Res 2004; 1017:32–38.
86. Dickel MJ, Renfrow SD, Moore PT, et al. Rapid eye movement sleep periodic leg movements in patients with spinal cord injury. Sleep 1994; 17:733–738.
87. Lee MS, Choi YC, Lee SH, et al. Sleep-related periodic leg movements associated with spinal cord lesions. Mov Disord 1996; 11:719–722.
88. Yokota T, Hirose K, Tanabe H, et al. Sleep-related periodic leg movements (nocturnal myoclonus) due to spinal cord lesions. J Neurol Sci 1991; 104:13–18.
89. de Mello MT, Lauro FA, Silva AC, et al. Incidence of periodic leg movements and of the restless legs syndrome during sleep following acute physical activity in spinal cord injury subjects. Spinal Cord 1996; 34:294–296.
90. Watanabe S, Ono A, Naito H. Periodic leg movements during either epidural or spinal anesthesia in an elderly man without sleep-related (nocturnal) myoclonus. Sleep 1990; 13:262–266.
91. Smith RC. Relationship of periodic movements in sleep (nocturnal myoclonus) and the Babinski sign. Sleep 1985; 8:239–243.
92. Bara-Jimenez W, Aksu M, Graham B, et al. Periodic limb movements in sleep. State-dependent excitability of the spinal flexor reflex. Neurology 2000; 54:1609–1615.
92a. Clemens S, rye D, Hochman S. Restless legs syndrome: revisiting the dopamine hypothesis from the spinal cord perspective. Neurology 2006; 67:125–130.
92b. Ondo WG, He Y, Rajasekaran S, Le WD. Clinical correlates of 6-hydroxydopamine injections into A11 dopaminergic neurons in rats: a possible model for restless legs syndrome. Movement Disorders 2000; 15:154–158.
93. Smith RC. Confirmation of Babinski-like response in periodic movements in sleep (nocturnal myoclonus). Biol Psychiatr 1987; 22:1271–1273.

94. Fujiki A, Shimizu A, Yamada Y, et al. The Babinski reflex during sleep and wakefulness. Electroencephalogr Clin Neurophysiol 1971; 31:610–613.
95. Aksu M, Bara-Jimenez W. State dependent excitability changes of spinal flexor reflex in patients with restless legs syndrome secondary to chronic renal failure. Sleep Med 2002; 3:427–430.
96. Martinelli P, Coccagna G. Rilievi neurofisiologici sulla sindrome della gambe senza riposo. Riv Neurol 1974; 46:552–560.
97. Paradiso G, Khan F, Chen R. Effects of apomorphine on flexor reflex and periodic limb movement. Mov Disord 2002; 17:594–597.
98. de Weerd AW, Rijsman RM, Brinkley A. Activity patterns of leg muscles in periodic limb movement disorder. J Neurol Neurosurg Psychiatr 2004; 75:317–319.
99. Trenkwalder C, Bucher SF, Oertel WH. Electrophysiological pattern of involuntary limb movements in the restless legs syndrome. Muscle Nerve 1996; 19:155–162.
100. Bucher SF, Trenkwalder C, Oertel WH. Reflex studies and MRI in the restless legs syndrome. Acta Neurol Scand 1996; 94:145–150.
101. Connor JR, Boyer PJ, Menzies SL, et al. Neuropathological examination suggests impaired brain iron acquisition in restless legs syndrome. Neurology 2003; 61: 304–309.
102. Pittock SJ, Parrett T, Adler CH, et al. Neuropathology of primary restless legs syndrome: absence of specific $\tau$- and $\alpha$-Synuclein pathology. Mov Disord 2004; 19: 695–698.
103. Trenkwalder C, Walters AS, Hening WA, et al. Positron emission tomographic studies in restless legs syndrome. Mov Disord 1999; 14:141–145.
104. Smith RC, Gouin PR, Minkley P, et al. Periodic limb movement disorder is associated with normal motor conduction latencies when studied by central magnetic stimulation–successful use of a new technique. Sleep 1992; 15:312–318.
105. Adler CH, Gwinn KA, Newman S. Olfactory function in restless legs syndrome. Mov Disord 1998; 13:563–565.
106. Trenkwalder C, Paulus W. Why do restless legs occur at rest?—pathophysiology of neuronal structures in RLS. Neurophysiology of RLS (part 2). Clin Neurophysiol 2004; 115:1975–1988.
107. Lai YY, Siegel JM. Sensory-motor integration in the medial medulla. Curr Neuropharmacol 2005; 3:115–143.
108. Bucher SF, Seelos KC, Oertel WH, et al. Cerebral generators involved in the pathogenesis of the restless legs syndrome. Ann Neurol 1997; 41:639–645.
109. Allen RP, Barker PB, Wehrl F, et al. MRI measurement of brain iron in patients with restless legs syndrome. Neurology 2001; 56:263–265.
110. Haba-Rubio J, Staner L, Petiau C, et al. Restless legs syndrome and low brain iron levels in patients with haemochromatosis. J Neurol Neurosurg Psychiatr 2005; 76:1009–1010.
111. Briellmann RS, Rösler KM, Hess CW. Blink reflex excitability is abnormal in patients with periodic leg movements in sleep. Mov Disord 1996; 11:710–714.
112. Mosko SS, Nudleman KL. Somatosensory and brainstem auditory evoked responses in sleep-related periodic leg movements. Sleep 1986; 9:399–404.
113. Coleman RM. Periodic movements in sleep (nocturnal myoclonus) and restless legs syndrome. In: Guilleminault C, Lugaresi E, eds. Sleeping and Waking Disorders: Indications and Techniques. Addison-Wesley: Menlo Park, 1982:265–296.
114. Kim JS, Lee SB, Park SK, et al. Periodic limb movement during sleep developed after pontine lesion. Mov Disord 2003; 18:1403–1405.
115. Lavoie S, de Bilbao F, Haba-Rubio J, et al. Influence of sleep stage and wakefulness on spectral EEG activity and heart rate variations around periodic leg movements. Clin Neurophysiol 2004; 115:2236–2246.
116. Sforza E, Juony C, Ibanez V. Time-dependent variation in cerebral and autonomic activity during periodic leg movements in sleep: implications for arousal mechanisms. Clin Neurophysiol 2002; 113:883–891.
117. Winkelman JW. The evoked heart rate response to periodic leg movements of sleep. Sleep 1999; 22:575–580.

118. Sforza E, Pichot V, Barthelemy JC, et al. Cardiovascular variability during periodic leg movements: a spectral analysis approach. Clin Neurophysiol 2005; 116:1096–1105.
119. Eisensehr I, Wetter TC, Linke R, et al. Normal IPT and IBZM SPECT in drug-naive and levodopa-treated idiopathic restless legs syndrome. Neurology 2001; 57:1307–1309.
120. Linke R, Eisensehr I, Wetter TC, et al. Presynaptic dopaminergic function in patients with restless legs syndrome: are there common features with early Parkinson's disease? Mov Disord 2004; 19:1158–1162.
121. Michaud M, Soucy JP, Chabli A, et al. SPECT imaging of striatal pre- and postsynaptic dopaminergic status in restless legs syndrome with periodic leg movements in sleep. J Neurol 2002; 249:164–170.
122. Turjanski N, Lees AJ, Brooks DJ. Striatal dopaminergic function in restless legs syndrome. $^{18}$F-dopa and $^{11}$C-raclopride PET studies. Neurology 1999; 52:932–937.
122a. Cervenka S, Palhagen SE, Comley RA, et al. Support for dopaminergic hypoactivity in restless legs syndrome: a PET study on D2-receptor binding. Brain 2006; 129: 2017–2028.
123. Staedt J, Stoppe G, Kögler A, et al. Single photon emission tomography (SPET) imaging of dopamine D2 receptors in the course of dopamine replacement therapy in patients with nocturnal myoclonus syndrome (NMS). J Neural Transm 1995; 99: 187–193.
124. Tribl GG, Asenbaum S, Klosch G, et al. Normal IPT and IBZM SPECT in drug naive and levodopa-treated idiopathic restless legs syndrome. Neurology 2002; 59:649–650.
125. San Pedro EC, Mountz JM, Mountz JD, et al. Familial painful restless legs syndrome correlates with pain dependent variation of blood flow to the caudate, thalamus, and anterior cingulate gyrus. J Rheumatol 1998; 25:2270–2275.
126. von Spiczak S, Whone AL, Hammers A, et al. The role of opioids in restless legs syndrome: an [$^{11}$C]diprenorphine PET study. Brain 2005; 128:906–917.
127. Walters AS, LeBrocq C, Dhar A, et al. Validation of the International Restless Legs Syndrome Study Group rating scale for restless legs syndrome. Sleep Med 2003; 4:121–132.
128. Allen RP, Barker PB, Horská A, et al. Patients with restless legs syndrome (RLS) show reduced brain thalamic creatine on magnetic resonance spectroscopy (MRS)[abstr]. Sleep 2003; 26(suppl):A339.
129. Etgen T, Draganski B, Ilg C, et al. Bilateral thalamic gray matter changes in patients with restless legs syndrome. Neuroimage 2005; 24:1242–1247.
129a. Ondo WG. VIM deep brain stimulation does not improve pre-existing restless legs syndrome in patients with essential tremor. Park Dis Rel Disord. In press.
130. Saletu B, Anderer P, Saletu M, et al. EEG mapping, psychometric, and polysomnographic studies in restless legs syndrome (RLS) and periodic limb movement disorder (PLMD) patients as compared with normal controls. Sleep Med 2002; 3(suppl):S35–S42.
131. Lugaresi E, Cirignotta F, Coccagna G, et al. Nocturnal myoclonus and restless legs syndrome. In: Fahn S, Marsden CD, Van Woert M, eds. Myoclonus. Raven Press: New York, 1986:295–307.
132. Iriarte J, Urrestarazu E, Alegre M, et al. Oscillatory cortical changes during periodic limb movements. Sleep 2004; 27:1493–1498.
133. Trenkwalder C, Bucher SF, Oertel WH, et al. Bereitschaftspotential in idiopathic and symptomatic restless legs syndrome. Electroencephalogr Clin Neurophysiol 1993; 89:95–103.
134. Rau C, Hummel F, Gerloff C. Cortical involvement in the generation of "involuntary" movements in restless legs syndrome. Neurology 2004; 62:998–1000.
135. Karadeniz D, Ondze B, Besset A, et al. EEG arousals and awakenings in relation with periodic leg movements during sleep. J Sleep Res 2000; 9:273–277.
136. Ferrillo F, Beelke M, Canovaro P, et al. Changes in cerebral and autonomic activity heralding periodic limb movements in sleep. Sleep Med 2004; 5:407–412.
137. Sforza E, Nicolas A, Lavigne G, et al. EEG and cardiac activation during periodic leg movements in sleep: support for a hierarchy of arousal responses. Neurology 1999; 52:786–791.
138. Terzano MG, Parrino L. Origin and significance of the cyclic alternating pattern (CAP). Sleep Med Rev 2000; 4:101–123.

139. Parrino L, Boselli M, Buccino GP, et al. The cyclic alternating pattern plays a gate-control on periodic limb movements during non-rapid eye movement sleep. J Clin Neurophysiol 1996; 13:314–323.
140. El Ad B, Chervin RD. The case of a missing PLM. Sleep 2000; 23:450–451.
141. Boylan LS, Sackheim HA. Magnetoelectric brain stimulation in the assessment of brain physiology and pathophysiology. Clin Neurophysiol 2000; 111:504–512.
142. Rothwell JC. Techniques and mechanisms of action of transcranial stimulation of the human motor cortex. J Neurosci Methods 1997; 74:113–122.
143. Inghilleri M, Berardelli A, Cruccu G, et al. Silent period evoked by transcranial stimulation of the human cortex and cervicomedullary junction. J Physiol 1993; 466:521–534.
144. Lipton RE, Singleton JR, Entezari-Taher M, et al. Cortical and segmental excitability in restless legs syndrome associated with peripheral neuropathy. Neurology 2000; 54(suppl 3):A26.
145. Currá A, Modugno N, Inghilleri M, et al. Transcranial magnetic stimulation techniques in clinical investigation. Neurology 2002; 59:1851–1859.
146. Schober T, Wenzel K, Feichtinger M, et al. Restless legs syndrome: changes of induced electroencephalographic beta oscillations—an ERD/ERS study. Sleep 2004; 27:147–150.
147. Kaelin-Lang A, Luft AR, Sawaki L, et al. Modulation of human corticomotor excitability by somatosensory input. J Physiol 2002; 540:623–633.
148. Sailer A, Molnar GF, Cunic DL, et al. Effects of peripheral sensory input on cortical inhibition in humans. J Physiol 2002; 544:617–629.
149. Daskalakis ZJ, Paradiso GO, Christensen BK, et al. Exploring the connectivity between the cerebellum and motor cortex in humans. J Physiol 2004; 557:689–700.
150. Luft AR, Manto MU, Ben Taib NO. Modulation of motor cortex excitability by sustained peripheral stimulation: the interaction between motor cortex and the cerebellum. Cerebellum 2005; 4:90–96.
151. Hening WA, Allen RP, Earley CJ, et al. An update on the dopaminergic treatment of restless legs syndrome and periodic limb movement disorder. Sleep 2004; 27:560–583.
152. Fulda S, Wetter TC. Emerging drugs for restless legs syndrome. Expert Opin Emerg Drugs 2005; 10:537–552.
153. Wetter TC, Collado-Seidel V, Oertel H, et al. Endocrine rhythms in patients with restless legs syndrome. J Neurol 2002; 249:146–151.
154. Winkelmann J, Schadrack J, Wetter TC, et al. Opioid and dopamine antagonist drug challenges in untreated restless legs syndrome patients. Sleep Med 2001; 2:57–61.
155. Garcia-Borreguero D, Larrosa O, de la LY. Circadian aspects in the pathophysiology of the restless legs syndrome. Sleep Med 2002; 3(suppl):S17–S21.
156. Montplaisir J, Godbout R, Boghen D, et al. Familial restless legs with periodic movements in sleep: electrophysiologic, biochemical, and pharmacologic study. Neurology 1985; 35:130–134.
157. Stiasny-Kolster K, Möller JC, Zschocke J, et al. Normal dopaminergic and serotonergic metabolites in cerebrospinal fluid and blood of restless legs syndrome patients. Mov Disord 2004; 19:192–196.
158. Earley CJ, Hyland K, Allen RP. CSF dopamine, serotonin, and biopterin metabolites in patients with restless legs syndrome. Mov Disord 2001; 16:144–149.
159. Cohrs S, Guan Z, Pohlmann K, et al. Nocturnal urinary dopamine excretion is reduced in otherwise healthy subjects with periodic leg movements in sleep. Neurosci Lett 2004; 360:161–164.
159a. Earley CJ, Hyland K, Allen RP. Circadian changes in CSF dopaminergic measures in restless legs syndrome. Sleep Med 2006; 7:263–268.
160. Allen R. Dopamine and iron in the pathophysiology of restless legs syndrome (RLS). Sleep Med 2004; 5:385–391.
161. Krieger J, Schroeder C. Iron, brain and restless legs syndrome. Sleep Med Rev 2001; 5:277–286.
162. Earley CJ, Connor JR, Beard JL, et al. Abnormalities in CSF concentrations of ferritin and transferrin in restless legs syndrome. Neurology 2000; 54:1698–1700.
163. Davis BJ, Raiput A, Raiput ML, et al. A randomized, double-blind placebo-controlled trial or iron in restless legs syndrome. Eur Neurol 2000; 43:70–75.

164. Earley CJ, Heckler D, Allen RP. The treatment of restless legs syndrome with intravenous iron dextran. Sleep Med 2004; 5:231–235.
165. Allen RP, Picchietti D, Hening WA, et al. Restless legs syndrome: diagnostic criteria, special considerations, and epidemiology. A report from the restless legs syndrome diagnosis and epidemiology workshop at the National Institutes of Health. Sleep Med 2003; 4:101–119.
166. Bassetti CL, Mauerhofer D, Gugger M, et al. Restless legs syndrome: a clinical study of 55 patients. Eur Neurol 2001; 45:67–74.
167. Foley DJ, Ancoli-Israel S, Britz P, et al. Sleep disturbances and chronic disease in older adults. Results of the 2003 National Sleep Foundation Sleep in America Survey. J Psychosom Res 2004; 56:497–502.
168. Delgado JA, Murali G, Goldberg R. Sleep disorders in fibromyalgia [abstr]. Sleep 2004; 27(suppl):A339.
169. Khan S, Goldberg R, Haber A. Sleep disorders in fibromyalgia [abstr]. Sleep 2005; 28(suppl):A290.
170. Yunus MB, Aldag JC. Restless legs syndrome and leg cramps in fibromyalgia syndrome: a controlled study. Br Med J 1996; 312:1339.
171. Reynolds G, Blake DR, Pall HS, et al. Restless leg syndrome and rheumatoid arthritis. Br Med J 1986; 292:659–660.
172. Salih AM, Gray RE, Mills KR, et al. A clinical, serological and neurophysiological study of restless legs syndrome in rheumatoid arthritis. Br J Rheumatol 1994; 33:60–63.
173. Young WB, Piovesan EJ, Biglan KM. Restless legs syndrome and drug-induced akathisia in headache patients. CNS Spect 2003; 8:450–456.
174. Ulfberg J, Nyström B, Carter N, et al. Prevalence of restless legs syndrome among men aged 18 to 64 years: an association with somatic disease and neuropsychiatric symptoms. Mov Disord 2001; 16:1159–1163.
175. Ulfberg J, Nyström B, Carter N, et al. Restless legs syndrome among working-aged women. Eur Neurol 2001; 46:17–19.
176. Ulfberg J, Nyström B. Restless legs syndrome in blood donors. Sleep Med 2004; 5:115–118.
177. Banno K, Delaive K, Walld R, et al. Restless legs syndrome in 218 patients: associated disorders. Sleep Med 2000; 1:221–229.
178. Leutgeb U, Martus P. Regular intake of non-opioid analgesics is associated with an increased risk of restless legs syndrome in patients maintained on antidepressants. Eur J Med Res 2002; 7:368–378.
179. Leutgeb U, Schmelz M, Koppert W. Altered central excitability and analgesic treatment in patients with restless legs syndrome. Brain 2005; 128:E34.
180. Stiasny-Kolster K, Magerl W, Oertel WH, et al. Static mechanical hyperalgesia without dynamic tactile allodynia in patients with restless legs syndrome. Brain 2004; 127:773–782.
181. Chiu YH, Silman AJ, Macfarlane GJ, et al. Poor sleep and depression are independently associated with a reduced pain threshold. Results of a population based study. Pain 2005; 115:316–321.
182. Onen SH, Alloui A, Gross A, et al. The effects of total sleep deprivation, selective sleep interruption and sleep recovery on pain tolerance thresholds in healthy subjects. J Sleep Res 2001; 10:35–42.
183. Walters AS, Winkelmann J, Trenkwalder C, et al. Long-term follow-up on restless legs syndrome patients treated with opioids. Mov Disord 2001; 16:1105–1109.
184. Kaplan PW, Allen RP, Buchholz DW, et al. A double-blind, placebo-controlled study of the treatment of periodic limb movements in sleep using carbidopa/levodopa and propoxyphene. Sleep 1993; 16:717–723.
185. Walters AS, Wagner ML, Hening WA, et al. Successful treatment of the idiopathic restless legs syndrome in a randomized double-blind trial of oxycodone versus placebo. Sleep 1993; 16:327–332.
186. Walters AS. Review of receptor agonist and antagonist studies relevant to the opiate system in restless legs syndrome. Sleep Med 2002; 3:301–304.
187. Montplaisir J, Lorrain D, Godbout R. Restless legs syndrome and periodic leg movements in sleep: the primary role of dopaminergic mechanism. Eur Neurol 1991; 31:41–43.

188. Hening WA, Walters A, Kavey N, et al. Dyskinesias while awake and periodic movements in sleep in restless legs syndrome: treatment with opioids. Neurology 1986; 36:1363–1366.
189. Walters A, Hening W, Cote L, et al. Dominantly inherited restless legs with myoclonus and periodic movements of sleep: a syndrome related to the endogenous opiates? Adv Neurol 1986; 43:309–319.
190. Picchietti D, Winkelman JW. Restless legs syndrome, periodic limb movements in sleep, and depression. Sleep 2005; 28:891–898.
191. Winkelmann J, Prager M, Lieb R, et al. "Anxietas Tibiarum." Depression and anxiety disorders in patients with restless legs syndrome. J Neurol 2005; 252:67–71.
192. Sevim S, Dogu O, Kaleagasi H, et al. Correlation of anxiety and depression symptoms in patients with restless legs syndrome: a population based survey. J Neurol Neurosurg Psychiatr 2004; 75:226–230.
193. Cortese S, Konofal E, Lecendreux M, et al. Restless legs syndrome and attention-deficit/hyperactivity disorder: a review of the literature. Sleep 2005; 28:1007–1013.
194. Bakshi R. Fluoxetine and restless legs syndrome. J Neurol Sci 1996; 142:151–152.
195. Hargrave R, Beckley DJ. Restless leg syndrome exacerbated by sertraline. Psychosomatics 1998; 39:177–178.
196. Dimmitt SB, Riley GJ. Selective serotonin receptor uptake inhibitors can reduce restless legs symptoms. Arch Int Med 2000; 160:712.
197. Yang C, White DP, Winkelman JW. Antidepressants and periodic leg movements of sleep. Biol Psychiatr 2005; 58:510–514.
198. Trenkwalder C, Hening WA, Walters AS, et al. Circadian rhythm of periodic limb movements and sensory symptoms of restless legs syndrome. Mov Disord 1999; 14:102–110.
199. Hening WA, Walters AS, Wagner M, et al. Circadian rhythm of motor restlessness and sensory symptoms in the idiopathic restless legs syndrome. Sleep 1999; 22:901–912.
200. Michaud M, Dumont M, Selmaoui B, et al. Circadian rhythm of restless legs syndrome: relationship with biological markers. Ann Neurol 2004; 55:372–380.
201. Michaud M, Dumont M, Paquet J, et al. Circadian variation of the effects of immobility on symptoms of restless legs syndrome. Sleep 2005; 28:843–846.
202. Roth C, Clavadetscher S, Gugger M, et al. Restless legs syndrome: a circadian disorder? J Sleep Res 2004; 13(suppl 1):624.
203. Tribl GG, Waldhauser F, Sycha T, et al. Urinary 6-hydroxy-melatonin-sulfate excretion and circadian rhythm in patients with restless legs syndrome. J Pineal Res 2003; 35:295–296.
204. Kunz D, Bes F. Exogenous melatonin in periodic limb movement disorder: an open clinical trial and a hypothesis. Sleep 2001; 24:183–187.
205. Garcia-Borreguero D, Serrano C, Larrosa O, et al. Circadian effects of dopaminergic treatment in restless legs syndrome. Sleep Med 2004; 5:413–420.
206. Zisapel N. Melatonin-dopamine interactions: from basic neurochemistry to a clinical setting. Cell Mol Biol 2001; 21:605–616.
207. Allen RP, Walters AS, Montplaisir J, et al. Restless legs syndrome prevalence and impact. REST general population study. Arch Int Med 2005; 165:1286–1292.
208. Hedman C, Pohjasvaara T, Tolonen U, et al. Effects of pregnancy on mothers' sleep. Sleep Med 2002; 3:37–42.
209. Lee KA, Zaffke ME, Baratte-Beebe K. Restless legs syndrome and sleep disturbance during pregnancy: the role of folate and iron. J Womens Health Gend Based Med 2001; 10:335–341.
210. Goodman JDS, Brodie C, Ayida GA. Restless leg syndrome in pregnancy. Br Med J 1988; 297:1101–1102.
211. Suzuki K, Ohida T, Sone T, et al. The prevalence of restless legs syndrome among pregnant women in Japan and the relationship between restless legs syndrome and sleep problems. Sleep 2003; 26:673–677.
212. Fulda S, Dzaja A, Lancel M, et al. Sleep and periodic leg movements in late term pregnancy and postpartum in women with and without RLS. J Sleep Res 2004; 13(suppl 1): 252.

213. Polo-Kantola P, Rauhala E, Erkkola R, et al. Estrogen replacement therapy and nocturnal periodic limb movements: a randomized controlled trial. Obstet Gynecol 2001; 97:548–554.
214. Saletu-Zyhlarz G, Anderer P, Gruber G, et al. Insomnia related to postmenopausal syndrome and hormone replacement therapy: sleep laboratory studies on baseline differences between patients and controls and double-blind, placebo-controlled investigations on the effects of a novel estrogen- progesterone combination (Climodien Lafamme) versus estrogen alone. J Sleep Res 2003; 12:239–254.
215. Allen RP, Mignot E, Ripley B, et al. Increased CSF hypocretin-1 (orexin-A) in restless legs syndrome. Neurology 2002; 59:639–641.
216. Mignot E, Lammers GJ, Ripley B, et al. The role of cerebrospinal fluid hypocretin measurement in the diagnosis of narcolepsy and other hypersomnias. Arch Neurol 2002; 59:1553–1562.
217. Stiasny-Kolster K, Mignot E, Ling L, et al. CSF hypocretin-1 levels in restless legs syndrome. Neurology 2003; 61:1426–1429.
218. Schlienger JL. Syndrome des membres inférieurs impatients dû à une hypothyroïdie modérée. Presse Med 1985; 14:791.
219. Bon E, Rolland Y, Laroche M, et al. Hypothyroidism on colchimax® revealed by restless legs syndrome. Rev Rhum Engl Ed 1996; 63:304.
220. van de Vijver DAMC, Walley T, Petri H. Epidemiology of restless legs syndrome as diagnosed in UK primary care. Sleep Med 2004; 5:435–440.
221. Tan EK, Ho SC, Eng P, et al. Restless legs symptoms in thyroid disorders. Parkinsonism Relat Disord 2004; 10:149–151.
222. Collado-Seidel V, Kohnen R, Samtleben W, et al. Clinical and biochemical findings in uremic patients with and without restless legs syndrome. Am J Kidney Dis 1998; 31:324–328.
223. Takaki J, Nishi T, Nangaku M, et al. Clinical and psychological aspects of restless legs syndrome in uremic patients on hemodialysis. Am J Kidney Dis 2003; 41:833–839.
224. Rijsman RM, de Weerd AW, Kerkhof GA, et al. Periodic limb movement disorder and restless legs syndrome in dialysis patients. Nephrology 2004; 9:353–361.
225. Unruh ML, Levey AS, D'Ambrosio C, et al. Restless legs symptoms among incident dialysis patients: association with lower quality of life and shorter survival. Am J Kidney Dis 2004; 43:900–909.
226. Kraemer HC, Kadzin AE, Offord DR, et al. Coming to terms with the terms of risk. Arch Gen Psychiatr 1997; 54:337–343.

# 6 Progress in the Animal Models of Restless Legs Syndrome

**Weidong Le, Hongru Zhao, and William G. Ondo**

*Department of Neurology, Baylor College of Medicine, Houston, Texas, U.S.A.*

## INTRODUCTION

Restless legs syndrome (RLS) is a common disease with a prevalence up to 10% in the general population (1,2). The age of onset is variable, tending to be earlier in familial RLS, and it affects women somewhat more than men. This syndrome is a sensomotor disorder characterized by an intense urge to move the limbs, especially the legs. Some patients report an actual sensation whereas others only report the uncontrollable need or urge to move, referred to as an akathisia. This distinguishes it from paresthesias, hyperesthesias, and other pain-related syndromes (3). This urge has a circadian pattern and is most pronounced in the evening or during the night and often relieved by walking. At least 80% of RLS patients also suffer from the associated periodic limb movements of sleep (PLMS) and sleep disturbance (4). Sleep efficiency in RLS is reduced because the patients must continually move their legs to alleviate the irritating crawling sensations. Another supportive feature is that the symptoms usually improve with low doses of levodopa and other dopamine agonists (5,6).

The underlying pathophysiology of RLS, therefore, may involve dopamine transmission insufficiency, as demonstrated by modestly abnormal dopaminergic functional brain imaging studies, the worsening of symptoms with dopamine antagonists, and the improvement with dopamine agonists (7–9). There is also a growing body of literatures that suggests a robust role for iron in RLS. A strong inverse correlation between cerebrospinal fluid (CSFs) serum ferritin levels and RLS symptoms suggests that central nervous system (CNS) iron deficiency is culpable (10). Imaging studies and neuropathological examination also suggest impaired brain iron homeostasis in RLS (10–12). Anatomically, the spinal cord is implicated by the primary involvement of the legs. Finally, the strongly nocturnal pattern of symptoms suggests a connection to circadian control center.

To date, the pathophysiology of the syndrome has not been fully elucidated. In order to learn more about RLS, a few animal models have been developed based on current theories of pathogenesis of the disorder.

## 6-HYDROXYDOPAMINE–LESIONED RAT MODEL

Pathologic data of people with RLS are sparse. However, the clinical features of RLS provide evidence to postulate pathoanatomic pathways. Foremost is that RLS is extremely responsive to very low doses of dopaminergic agents. This indicates that dopaminergic system is implicated in the pathogenesis of RLS. The preponderance of sensomotor disturbance in the limbs suggests spinal cord or possibly peripheral nerve involvement. The circadian pattern reflects input from circadian control areas. The unpleasant sensory component suggests dysfunction of intrinsic antinociceptive mechanisms.

The anatomy of the diencephalic-spinal dopaminergic tract, originating from the A11 to A14 nuclei might explain all of the RLS features (13,14). The tract is near the suprachiasmatic nucleus, which controls circadian control, is dopaminergic, is involved in sensory control, and projects into the spinal cord.

In order to test this hypothesis, Ondo et al. (15) lesioned which controls circadian control, is dopaminergic, is involved in sensory control, and projects into the spinal cord rats in this area to determine if any subsequent behavioral responses were consistent with RLS. 6-Hydroxydopamine (6-OHDA) was stereotaxically injected into the bilateral diencephalic A11 dopaminergic nuclei of Sprague–Dawley rats. Control animals underwent sham surgeries. The behavior of these rats was observed several months later. Rat brains were sectioned and examined for the A11 lesion and possible extension to substantial nigra (SN) and ventral tegmental area (VTA). To examine the effect of the dopaminergic treatment on the rats, dopamine agonist pramipexole was used.

An overall reduction of about 50% of tyrosine hydroxylase (TH) -positive cells in the A11 region was found in rats after 6-OHDA lesions. Interestingly, these cells proved more resistant to 6-OHDA lesioning than other dopaminergic areas. The number of dopaminergic cells in the SN and VTA were not meaningfully reduced. Compared to controls, the 6-OHDA–lesioned rats demonstrated a longer latency to sleep, less sleep time, and more episodes of standing upright during short observation periods. Subsequently, pramipexole-treated rats showed less standing episodes and total standing time when compared with untreated lesioned rats. There were no movements that clearly resembled the PLMS seen in patients with RLS.

Overall, the rats showed sleep disturbance and motor restlessness, which were normalized with dopamine agonist. All of these observations were consistent with clinical RLS. This study, however, only focused on the movement symptoms and it could not assess the subjective aspects of RLS, such as "unpleasant sensations" or "an urge to move," and this preliminary study was limited by the lack of electrophysiological sleep measures, the intermittent observations, and the small sample size.

## 6-OHDA–LESIONED AND IRON-DEFICIENT MICE

In Qu et al.'s anatomical study (16), fluorescent tracer Fluoro-Gold (FG) was used to investigate the pathway of diencephalic dopaminergic innervation of the spinal cord in mice. The fluorescent tracer FG was stereotaxically injected into the lumbar spinal cord of C57BL mice. Then, the diencephalic sections were stained with TH antibodies and the FG tracer present in the diencephalic dopaminergic neurons were examined under fluorescence microscope. The results suggested that the diencephalic A11 dopaminergic neurons possessed long axons extending over several segments, possibly traversing the entire length of the spinal cord. It was shown for the first time that both A10 and A11 group dopaminergic neurons project into the spinal cord in mice. Although increasing evidence has demonstrated that dopaminergic diencephalic-spinal neurons are strongly implicated with RLS, lesioning this area may only partially mimic the clinical features of RLS.

There is robust evidence to suggest that the underlying pathophysiology of RLS involves CNS iron homeostatic dysregulation. CSF ferritin was lower in patients with RLS (10), and imaging studies (10,12) showed reduced iron stores in the striatum and red nucleus. Most importantly, pathological data in RLS autopsied brains showed reduced ferritin and iron staining, and increased transferrin staining, but decreased transferrin receptors density (17). No pathology aside from iron abnormalities has been identified (18). Subsequent studies have demonstrated a strong correlation between serum ferritin levels and RLS symptoms severity; decreasing ferritin was associated with increasing RLS severity. Open-label oral iron supplementation can improve RLS in some elderly patients (19). High-dose, intravenous iron therapy brought these patients marked relief of symptoms in a majority of RLS patients for periods of up to 3 to 9 months, even though these patients had a normal serum iron status before treatment (20).

The relationship between iron and the dopaminergic system is hard to disregard, given the obvious evidence that both are involved in the pathophysiology of RLS. There exist several possible associations between these two demonstrated abnormalities in RLS. Iron is a cofactor for TH, which is the rate-limiting enzyme for dopamine synthesis (Fig. 1). A decrease in iron may reduce dopamine synthesis and activity. Studies in iron-deficient animals, however, have also demonstrated a decrease in dopamine D2 receptors in the striatum (21), and a decrease in dopamine transporter function. Changes in basal ganglia dopamine metabolism associated with iron deficiency in rats are dependent on the time of day. Using microdialysis techniques, it was reported that the levels of dopamine and its metabolites were specifically increased at the beginning of the dark period (22). Iron also participates in the D2 receptor signal transduction dopamine synaptic stabilization and dopamine release. Therefore, both iron deficiency and diencephalic-spinal dopaminergic system dysfunction seem to play an important role in the pathogenesis of RLS.

In order to develop an ideal animal model of RLS, Qu et al. (23) performed stereotaxic bilateral 6-OHDA lesions into the A11 nucleus of C57BL/6 mice and

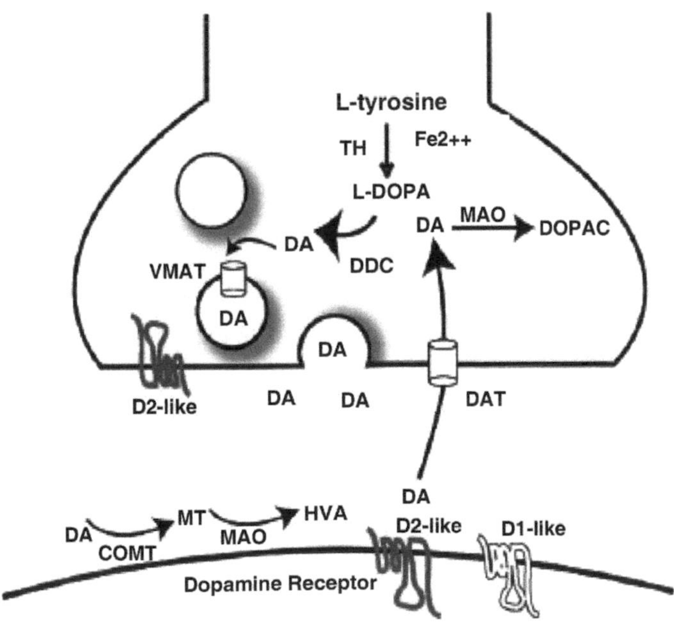


**FIGURE 1** The metabolic pathway of dopamine.

iron deprivation to observe whether these manipulations could induce animal behavioral changes that mimic clinical RLS.

Half of the mice received a regular diet (35 mg iron/kg) and the other half was fed a low-iron diet (3.5 mg iron/kg). One month after dietary manipulation, 6-OHDA was stereotaxically injected into the bilateral A11 nucleus in half of the dietary segregated group. The other half of the mice from both groups underwent sham surgeries. Iron levels in serum were measured and behaviors were observed at baseline, after dietary manipulation, and following 6-OHDA lesioning. Several pharmacological interventions of dopaminergic systems were subsequently performed.

Locomotor activities were carried out at different times in the mice using motion detecting laser cages. One month after surgery, the animals were challenged with three drugs known to improve or exacerbate human RLS. These drugs included dopamine receptors D2/D3 agonist ropinirole, D1 agonist SKF-38393, and D2 antagonist haloperidol. The locomotor activities of animals were recorded.

A serum iron assessment was obtained by tail vein in different periods. Brain and spinal cord samples were later autopsied to measure the tissue iron concentration. After behavioral observation in all groups of animals, the sections from diencephalic regions and mesencephalon were stained for TH immunohistochemistry.

Pathological examination demonstrated a marked reduction in A11 TH positive cells in the mice injected with 6-OHDA (Fig. 2). Iron levels in serum, brain, and spinal cord were significantly decreased after iron deprivation. Interestingly, the iron levels were more reduced in the spinal cord of animals that had A11 lesioning than those without lesioning, despite similar amounts of dietary iron and similar serum iron levels.

Locomotor activity was significantly increased in both iron-deprived mice and A11-lesioned mice compared to controls. The combination of iron deprivation and A11 lesioning further significantly augmented motor activity. In addition, the mice in the lesioned group were more aggressive and often attacked each other. Compared to controls, the increased activity in A11-lesioned mice with or without iron deprivation returned to baseline after treatment with the D2/D3 agonist ropinirole, which is

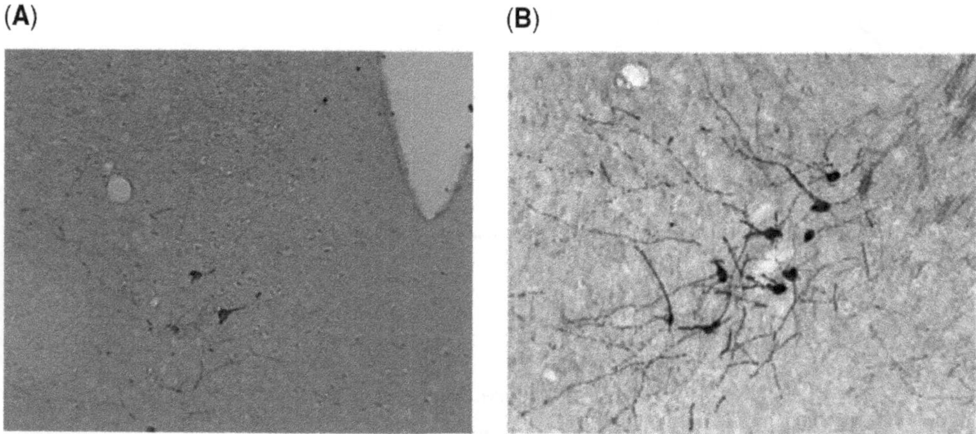


**FIGURE 2** (**A**) Tyrosine hydroxylase (TH)-cells in 6-OHDA–lesioned mice. (**B**) TH-cells in sham operation mice.

used to treat RLS, but was aggravated by the D1 agonist SKF38393. The D2 antagonist haloperidol also nonspecifically worsened the locomotor activity in all groups.

This study demonstrated that iron deprivation alone could increase the activity in mice. This behavior was significantly enhanced with 6-OHDA lesioned in A11 dopaminergic neurons.

The mRNA and protein levels as well as the affinity of dopamine receptor subtypes (D1, D2 and D3) were also examined in the lumbar spinal cord of C57BL/6 male mice after dietary iron deprivation and 6-OHDA lesion in the bilateral A11 nucleus. The specific binding of D1, D2 and D3 receptors was determined using [$^3$H]SCH23390, [$^3$H]Spiperone and [$^3$H]PD128907 radioligands respectively. The levels of D2/D3 mRNA and proteins in the spinal cord were significantly decreased by 6-OHDA lesions; while iron deprivation alone did not induce noticeable changes of the D2 and D3 expression. Furthermore, D2/D3 receptor binding was significantly decreased by 6-OHDA lesion, and iron deprivation with 6-OHDA lesion produced a synergistic decrease of D2 binding. Although iron deprivation increased D1 mRNA and protein expression in the spinal cord, it did not significantly change D1 receptor binding. This data shows that iron deprivation and A11 lesions differentially alter the D1, D2 and D3 receptors expression and binding capacity in the lumbar spinal cord of the RLS animal model.

Overall, this study supports that manipulation of iron and dopaminergic systems can result in animal behavioral changes, and combination of iron deficiency and A11 lesion could best mimic clinical RLS. This animal model provides a useful tool to study the pathophysiology of RLS and for the preclinical therape trials. However, we have yet to evaluate for the characteristic human symptom of PLMS commonly seen in RLS, and we have yet to assess sleep in this model.

Glover and Jacobs (24) had previously studied the activity pattern of iron-deficient rats. In marked contrast to our results, they found that iron-deficient rats appeared to decrease total activity. It also altered diurnal rhythm. These were reversed by the administration of iron. The discrepancy of these two studies may result from the different time of iron-deficiency diet and different animals.

## DOPAMINE D3 RECEPTOR KNOCKOUT (D3KO) MICE MODEL

Mammalian nervous system activity is under strong circadian control from the hypothalamic suprachiasmatic nuclei (SCN) (25,26). One SCN projection is to the dorsomedial hypothalamic (A11) dopaminergic nucleus (27,28). A11 neurons are the major source of spinal dopamine, with strong projections to the sympathetic preganglionic neurons in the intermediolateral nucleus (13,28). Spinal cord function is strongly modulated by monoamines (serotonin, dopamine, and noradrenalin); however, there are only a few studies on the modulatory actions of dopamine in the spinal cord. A11 dopaminergic neurons send collaterals throughout most of the spinal cord. There is extensive evidence for the existence of D1, D2, and D3 receptors in the spinal cord (29); however, the contribution of these receptors to spinal reflex excitability is not well known. Some previous data have demonstrated the presence of D3 dopamine receptors in rat spinal cord expressed in highest densities in the superficial layers of the dorsal horn of the cervical and lumbar regions (Fig. 3). The presence of D3 receptors in the superficial layers of the dorsal horn suggested that these receptors might play a role in sensory or nociceptive processing. The distribution of D3 receptors in the pars centralis suggested that the receptors might also contribute to sensory–motor integration.

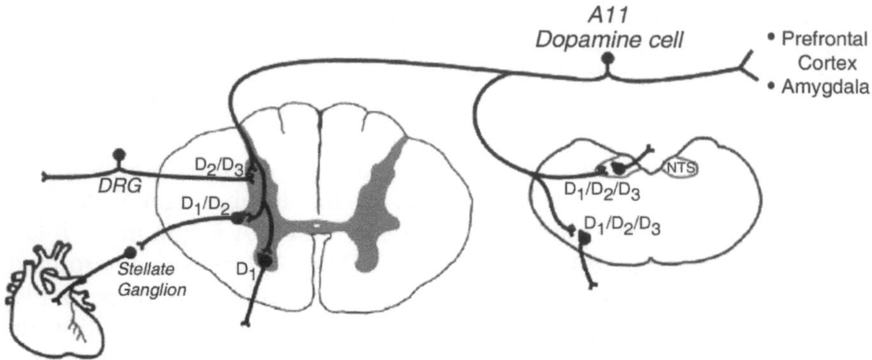


**FIGURE 3** Dopaminergic circuits originating from the A11 diencephalic cell cluster.

These potential functional roles for spinal D3 receptors are supported by pharmacological studies, which indicate that D2-like dopamine receptors modulate synaptic transmission in the spinal cord and contribute to nociception. The D3 receptor knockout (D3KO) mouse displayed hyperactivity of locomotion and hypertension. This phenotype resembles some features of patients with RLS (30,31). RLS manifests itself with abnormal sensations in the limbs that are reduced during motor activity and with a circadian pattern that peaks at night. Interestingly, the level of hypothalamic dopamine changes from day to night. It displays a circadian rhythm with lowest concentrations observed at night when RLS emerges (32,33). Finally, the dopamine agonists most widely used to treat RLS all have their strongest affinity for the D3 receptor.

Clemens and Hochman (33) studied the effects of dopamine and D2/D3 receptor agonists on spinal cord excitability as measured by electrophysiological recordings of spinal reflexes in the wild type (WT) and D3KO mice, to determine the contribution of spinal D3 receptors to dopamine-induced modulatory actions. The spinal cords from D3KO mice and WT mice were dissected out of the body cavity and placed in cooled artificial CSF. After the dura mater was opened, the ventral roots were identified. Glass suction electrodes were placed on the distal parts of dorsal and ventral roots of lumbar segments, then the dorsal roots were stimulated with various current pulses to achieve a maximal reflex response at interstimulus intervals. Reflexes were recorded from the corresponding ventral roots, amplified, and digitized.

To observe the effect of several drugs on reflex amplitude, comparisons were made between the averaged amplitudes measured before drug application and several consecutive reflex responses during the application. The dopamine receptor–selective ligands pergolide, bromocriptine, D3-selective agonist PD 128907, and antagonists GR 103691 were, respectively, applied at different concentrations.

The result showed that low doses of dopamine decreased the monosynaptic "stretch" reflex (MSR) amplitude in WT animals but increased it in D3KO animals. Higher doses of dopamine decreased MSR amplitudes in both D3KO mice and WT mice, but such effect was greater in WT mice. Like low-dose dopamine, the D3 receptor agonists pergolide and PD 128907 reduced MSR amplitude in WT but not in D3KO mice. Conversely, D3 receptor antagonists (GR 103691 and nafadotride) increased the MSR in WT but not in D3KO mice. In comparison, the D2-preferring agonists bromocriptine and quinpirole depressed the MSR in both groups. Thus, low-dose dopaminergic stimulation activates D3 receptors to limit reflex excitability. Moreover, in D3 ligand-insensitive mice, excitatory actions are unmasked, functionally converting the modulatory action of dopamine from depression to facilitation. Thus, D3 receptors are believed to involve in limiting spinal cord excitability. Given their observations in D3KO mice, their phenotype, and its correspondence to the RLS phenotype in patients, it is an intriguing possibility that a similar conversion in modulatory actions occurs in patients suffering from RLS. Because the modulatory action of low dopamine is converted from depression to facilitation in an animal that lacks a functional D3 receptor, the D3KO mouse identifies one explanation of how reduced D3 activity could contribute to the increased reflex excitability seen in RLS, thus representing a relevant model to address these questions in more detail. It is important to be aware, however, that in patients with RLS, D3 receptor agonists commonly have a therapeutic benefit, suggesting that RLS is not caused by D3 receptor dysfunction but rather by reduced D3 receptor activation.

Clemens et al. (34) also determined the local circadian expression of the TH in the murine spinal cord and compared these levels between WT and D3KO mice. The results suggested that TH and nitric oxide synthase (NOS) levels both displayed circadian patterns in WT and D3KO animals with overall reduced TH expression and increased NOS expression in the D3KO mice. TH expression was inverted in D3KO mice, with TH levels consistently lower than in WT throughout the day, but strongly increased temporarily prior to daylight. Their data on circadian TH expression were consistent with the observation that of brain dopamine content in mice (35). Because dopamine largely decreases spinal cord excitability (33,36), a reduction in descending inhibitory drive from the brain should result in increased spinal cord excitability. The observations in D3KO mice of circadian dopaminergic dysfunction are in concert with increased cord excitability in relation to RLS. Because hypothalamic dopamine levels are at their lowest in the early morning hours when RLS symptoms are present, it is easy to consider that a reduced dopaminergic activity in spinal cord is responsible for the increase in excitability observed in RLS patients and in D3KO mice.

In summary, these data demonstrate that dopamine synthesis in spinal sympathetic neurons is under circadian controls and is changed in D3KO mice. Importantly, an inverted circadian cycling in TH expression in D3KO mice could lead to changes in autonomic function and cord excitability, two observed features of the RLS phenotype in humans. These observations demonstrate that those alterations in circadian TH expression and a possible component of dopamine dysfunction in RLS patients support a circadian component to the spinal dopamine dysfunction observed in D3KO mice, further validating D3KO mice as a potential animal model of RLS.

Although this study has demonstrated that dopamine, specifically D3 receptors, plays an important role and proves the existence of circadian rhythms, it has not addressed iron deficiency, which is demonstrated in RLS. Assessment of this model in the setting of iron deficiency should be considered in future studies.

## AN ANIMAL MODEL OF PERIODIC LIMB MOVEMENTS OF SLEEP

PLMS are periodic leg, more than arm, movements that predominately occur in Stage I and Stage II of sleep. Their periodicity in humans ranges from 30 to 90 seconds. Similar movements, called periodic limb movements while awaking, can occur during drowsiness. PLMS can occur as an isolated phenomenon but are often associated with RLS and represent the only sign of this disorder that can be measured electrophysiologically (37).

It is known that the occurrence of PLMS and RLS in humans increases with age and many dopaminergic drugs can reduce them. It is not proven whether dopamine antagonists induce PLMS, or aggravate existing PLMS and clinically worsen RLS. Although these observations suggest that a dopaminergic system is involved in the genesis of PLMS and RLS, the pathophysiological mechanisms and biochemical interactions are not yet known. To elucidate the underlying causes, an animal model of PLMS would be of great value.

In order to delineate whether rats display periodic hindlimb movements (PHLM) while they are asleep, Baier et al. (38) assessed hindlimb movements and sleep–wake behavior in this species. They investigated the occurrence of PHLM in a group of animals and determined whether the dopamine antagonist haloperidol could induce PHLM.

The experiments were performed on Wistar rats. Stainless steel screws were implanted epidurally in the skull to derive the electroencephalogram (EEG). For electromyography (EMG) recording, stainless steel wires were inserted into the neck muscles bilaterally and attached to the skull. For movement detection, two magnets were implanted subcutaneously in both hindlimbs. The animals recovered from surgery before data acquisition.

EEG, EMG, and hindlimb movements were recorded from light onset to dark onset. Haloperidol was injected intraperitoneally at light onset. EEG and EMG signals were amplified, filtered, and digitized (39). A video recorder documented the animals' behavior for the entire time of data acquisition. Three vigilance stages, wakefulness, nonrapid eye movement (NREM) sleep, and rapid eye movement (REM) sleep, were determined by the visual assessment of EEG and EMG recordings, as described by the authors (40,41).

Hindlimb movements occurring during NREM were subdivided into those associated with an arousal (HLM) and those not associated with an arousal (HLM+). They defined PHLM in rats according to the modified human criteria (42) as at least four consecutive hindlimb movements with an intermovement interval of 5 to 60 seconds.

All animals exhibited comparable amounts of wakefulness and NREM, while young animals had significantly more REM sleep than the old ones. Haloperidol administration to the old animals did not affect the overall time spent in any of the vigilance stages.

All animals displayed occasional HLM and HLM+ in NREM but most did not meet criteria for PHLM. The young animals showed especially few PHLM. Haloperidol did not significantly influence any of these parameters. Interestingly, the percentage of old rats spontaneously displaying PHLM resembles the increased prevalence of PLMS in older humans.

Overall, this study demonstrated for the first time that hindlimb movements in sleep can occur spontaneously in rats. A clear effect of age on this phenomenon was seen, with old animals displaying more movements. To validate whether the observed PHLM constitute a good model for human PLMS or even RLS, their pharmacological properties need to be characterized in a large number of PHLM-positive animals. CNS iron metabolism or deprivation has not been evaluated in this model.

## ANIMAL MODELS OF OPIOID DOPAMINERGIC INTERACTIONS

RLS is successfully treated with opioids as well as dopaminergics, and is associated with iron deficiency. There is also clinical evidence that opioid drugs work through dopaminergic systems (43–45). Sun et al. are currently working a neuropathological model attempting to link these systems (46). They showed that decreasing iron by chelating resulted in dopaminergic cell death. This dopaminergic cell death was prevented by pretreating the cells with opioids (30). This research suggests that deprivation of iron, hypofunction dopamine and the endogenous opiates may be causally connected in RLS. It specifically suggests that opioid treatment may be neuroprotective against the symptoms of RLS.

In summary, several potential animal models for RLS have been developed, although not always for that intended purpose. The key features of these animal models involve iron deprivation and dopaminergic manipulation via genetic alterations or pharmacological intervention. The change in symptoms caused by dopamine agonists and antagonists has been proven to be consistent with the clinical RLS in some models. However, it is difficult to completely mimic all cardinal features of RLS in any animal model as the sensory component, or urge to move cannot be readily assessed. It will be a major challenge to develop a model in animals that can demonstrate this feature of the disorder. Future work on current models includes the evaluation of detailed sleep physiology and circadian patterns, such as PLMS, the assessment of other behavioral features, such as aggression, and the addition of pathoanatomical correlations as they become known. Continued research on human RLS genetics will eventually lead to specifically culpable proteins and altered protein function. This may result in similar genetically altered animals that may prove to be excellent animal models of RLS.

## REFERENCES

1. Phillips B, Young T, Finn L, Asher K, Hening WA, Purvis C. Epidemiology of restless legs syndrome in adults. Arch Intern Med 2000; 160:2137–2147.
2. Ulfberg J, Nystrom B, Carter N, Edling C. Prevalence of restless legs syndrome among men aged 18–64 years: an association with somatic disease and neuropsychiatric symptoms. Mov Disord 2001; 16:1159–1163.
3. Haskovec L. Akathisia. Arch Bohemes Med Clin 1902; 3:193–200.
4. Allen RP, Prichietti D, Hening WA, Treakwalker C, Walter, Mantplaisi J. Restless legs syndrome diagnosis and epidemiology workshop at the National Institute of Health. International restless legs syndrome study groups. Sleep Med 2003; 4:101–109.
5. Chesson AL, Wise M, Davila D, et al. Practice parameters for the treatment of restless legs syndrome and periodic limb movement disorder. Sleep 1999; 22:962–968.
6. Hening W, Allen R, Earley C, Kushida C, Picchietti D, Silber M. The treatment of restless legs syndrome and periodic limb movement disorder. Sleep 1999; 22:970–999.
7. Ondo WG, Jankovic J. Restless legs syndrome. In: Appel SH, ed. Current Neurology. Amsterdam: IOS Press, 1997:207–236.
8. Trenkwalder C, et al. Positron emission tomographic studies in restless legs syndrome. Mov Disord 1999; 14:141–145.
9. Turjanski N, Lees AJ, Brooks DJ. Striatal dopaminergic function in restless legs syndrome: 18F-dopa and 11C-raclopride PET studies. Neurology 1999; 127:2282–2288.
10. Earley CJ, Connor JR, Beard JL, Malecki EA, Epstein DK, Allen RP. Abnormalities in CSF concentrations of ferritin and transferrin in restless legs syndrome. Neurology 2000; 54:1698–1700.
11. Connor JR, Boyer PJ, Menzies BS, et al. Neuropathological examination suggests impaired brain iron acquisition in restless legs syndrome. Neurology 2003; 61:304–309.

12. Mizuno S, Mihara T, Miyaoka T, Inagaki T, Horiguchi J. CSF iron, ferritin and transferrin levels in restless legs syndrome. J Sleep Res 2005; 14:43–47.
13. Skagerberg G, Lindvall O. Organization of diencephalic neurons projecting to the spinal cord in the rat. Brain Res 1985; 342:340–351.
14. Takada M, Li ZK, Hattori T. Single thalamic dopaminergic neurons project to both the-neocortex and spinal cord. Brain Res 1988; 455:346–352.
15. Ondo WG, He Y, Rajasekaran S, Le WD. Clinical correlates of 6-hydroxydopamine injections into A11 dopaminergic neurons in rats: a possible model for restless legs syndrome? Mov Disord 2000; 15:154–158.
16. Qu S, Ondo WG, Zhang X, Xie WJ, Pan TH, Le WD. Projections of diencephalic dopamine neurons into the spinal cord in mice. Exp Brain Res. 2006; 168:152–156.
17. Allen RP, Earley CJ. Restless legs syndrome: a review of clinical and pathophysiologic features. J Clin Neurophysiol 2001; 18:128–147.
18. Pittock SJ, Parrett T, Adler CH, Parisi JE, Dickson DW, Ahlskog JE. Neuropathology of primary restless leg syndrome: absence of specific tau- and alpha-synuclein pathology. Mov Disord 2004; 19:695–699.
19. O'Keeffe ST, Gavin K, Lavan JN. Iron status and restless legs syndrome in the elderly. Age Aging 1994; 23:200–203.
20. Earley CJ, Heckler D, Allen RP. The treatment of restless legs syndrome with intravenous iron dextran. Sleep Med 2004; 5:231–235.
21. Ben-Shachar D, Finberg JP, Youdim MB. Effect of iron chelators on dopamine D2 receptors. J Neurochem 1985; 45:999–1005.
22. Chen Q, Beard JL, Jones BC. Abnormal rat brain monoamine metabolism in iron deficiency anemia. J Nutr Biochem 1995; 6:486–493.
23. Qu S, Le WD, Zhang X, Xie WJ, Ondo WG. Animal model for restless legs syndrome: A11 dopaminergic lesioning and iron deprivation. Mov Disord 2005; 20:1420.
24. Glover J, Jacobs A. Activity pattern of iron-deficient rats. Br Med J 1972; 2:627–628.
25. Moore RY. Entrainment pathways and the functional organization of the circadian system. Prog Brain Res 1996; 111:103–119.
26. LeSauter J, Silver R. Output signals of the SCN. Chronobiol Int 1998; 15:535–550.
27. Reuss S. Components and connections of the circadian timing system in mammals. Cell Tissue Res 1996; 285:353–378.
28. Abrahamson EE, Moore RY. Suprachiasmatic nucleus in the mouse: retinal innervation, intrinsic organization and efferent projections. Brain Res 2001; 916:172–191.
29. Levant B, McCarson KE. D(3) dopamine receptors in rat spinal cord: implications for sensory and motor function. Neurosci Lett 2001; 303:9–12.
30. Ali NJ,Davies RJ, Fleetham JA, Stradling JR. Periodic movements of the legs during sleep associated with rises in systemic blood pressure. Sleep 1991; 14:163–165.
31. Espinar SJ, Vela BA, Luque OM. Periodic leg movements in sleep in essential hypertension. Psychiatry Clin Neurosci 1997; 51:103–107.
32. Stiasny K, Oertel WH, Trenkwalder C. Clinical symptomatology and treatment of restless legs syndrome and periodic limb movement disorder. Sleep Med Rev 2002; 6:253–265.
33. Clemens S, Hochman S. Conversion of the modulatory actions of dopamine on spinal reflexes from depression to facilitation in D3 receptor knock-out mice. J Neurosci 2004; 24:11337–11345.
34. Clemens S, Sawchuk MA, Hochman S. Reversal of the circadian expression of tyrosine-hydroxylase but not nitric oxide synthase levels in the spinal cord of dopamine D3 receptor knockout mice. Neuroscience 2005; 133:353–357.
35. Huie JM, Sharma RP, Coulombe RA Jr. Diurnal alterations of catecholamines, indoleamines and their metabolites in specific brain regions of the mouse. Comp Biochem Physiol C 1989; 94:575–579.
36. Svensson E, Wikstrom MA, Hill RH, Grillner S. Endogenous and exogenous dopamine presynaptically inhibits glutamatergic reticulospinal transmission via an action of D2-receptors on N-type Ca2_ channels. Eur J Neurosci 2003; 17:447–454.
37. Montplaisir J, Boucher S, Poirier G, Lavigne G, Lapierre O, Lesperance P. Clinical, polysomnographic, and genetic characteristics of restless legs syndrome: a study of 133 patients diagnosed with new standard criteria. Mov Disord 1997; 12:61–65.

38. Baier PC, Winkelmann J, Höhne A, Lancel M, Trenkwalder C. Assessment of spontaneously occurring periodic limb movements in sleep in the rat. J Neurol Sci 2002; 198: 71–77.
39. Lancel M, Mathias S, Faulhaber J, Schiffelholz T. Effect of interleukin-1 beta on EEG power density during sleep depends on circadian phase. Am J Physiol 1996; 270:R830–R837.
40. Neckelmann D, Ursin R. Sleep stages and EEG power spectrum in relation to acoustical stimulus arousal threshold in the rat. Sleep 1993; 165:467.
41. Lancel M, Langebartels A. Gamma-aminobutyric Acid(A) (GABA(A)) agonist 4,5,6, 7-tetrahydroisoxazolo[4,5-c]pyridin-3-ol persistently increases sleep maintenance and intensity during chronic administration to rats. J Pharmacol Exp Ther 2000; 293: 1084–1090.
42. Force AT. Recording and scoring leg movements. Sleep 1993; 16:748–759.
43. Winkelmann J, Schadrack J, Wetter TC, Zieglgansberger W, Trenkwalder C. Opioid and dopamine antagonist drug challenges in untreated restless legs syndrome patients. Sleep Med 2001; 2:57–61.
44. Akpinar S. Restless legs syndrome: treatment with dopaminergic drugs. Clin Neuropharmacol 1987; 10:69–79.
45. Montplaisir J, Lorrain D, Godbout R. Restless legs syndrome and periodic leg movements in sleep: the primary role of dopaminergic mechanism. Eur Neurol 1991; 31:41–43.
46. Sun Y, Hoang-Lee T, Neubauer JA, Walters AS. Opioids protect against substantia nigra cell degeneration under conditions of iron deprivation: a possible model for restless legs syndrome. Sleep 2003; 26:A343.

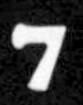

# Pathology of Restless Legs Syndrome

**James R. Connor and Xinsheng Wang**

*Department of Neurosurgery, Pennsylvania State University College of Medicine, Milton S. Hershey Medical Center, Hershey, Pennsylvania, U.S.A.*

## INTRODUCTION

This chapter will focus on the results of postmortem evaluations of brains from individuals with restless legs syndrome (RLS). The autopsy analyses involved standard histological evaluations of the brain and a more detailed focus on parameters associated with iron status in the substantia nigra. The substantia nigra was chosen because of magnetic resonance imaging (MRI) data, which suggested that this brain region contained relatively low iron levels in individuals with RLS (1). A connection between iron status and RLS has long been considered and is reviewed in greater detail in Chapter 17. Immunocytochemical and quantitative analyses were performed for iron management proteins and showed that there was insufficient iron in the RLS substantia nigra, and the data suggested that the insufficient iron levels might be traced to a defect in an iron regulatory protein (IRP) responsible for stabilizing the mRNA for the transferrin (Tf) receptor. We have developed a proposal, discussed in this chapter, that the consequences of an iron deficiency in the substantia nigra may lead to a loss of Thy-1 expression and a loss of integrity of dopaminergic (DA) synapses. The results of these studies provide compelling evidence that brain iron insufficiency is involved in RLS and indicate a possible mechanism by which iron deficiency compromises DA transmission in RLS. Taken together, the studies to date provide a link between decreased brain iron and the responsiveness to dopamine agents and iron supplementation treatment in RLS.

## NEUROPATHOLOGICAL EVALUATION

We conducted neuropathological evaluations on postmortem tissue to identify changes in the brains of individuals with RLS that could underlie the disorder. A total of seven brains from individuals with the clinical diagnosis of primary RLS and five age-matched control brains were evaluated. There were no gross abnormalities in any of the RLS brains examined. Alzheimer's type changes consistent with Braak & Braak stage I/II were found in four out of seven of the RLS brains, and the remaining brains were at stage III. Lewy bodies and Lewy neurites were observed in the substantia nigra in only one out of seven. The presence of Lewy bodies in an aged control population is around 8% (2) but has been reported as high as 30% (3). The percentage of RLS brains with Lewy bodies is well within the lower range for that reported in the brains of patients with non-neurodegenerative diseases. This finding distances RLS from neurodegenerative diseases that involve the DA system. Standard neuropathological evaluations did not reveal any histological abnormalities that were unique to the RLS brains (4,5). These findings were corroborated in a second study on four RLS brains, which also failed to

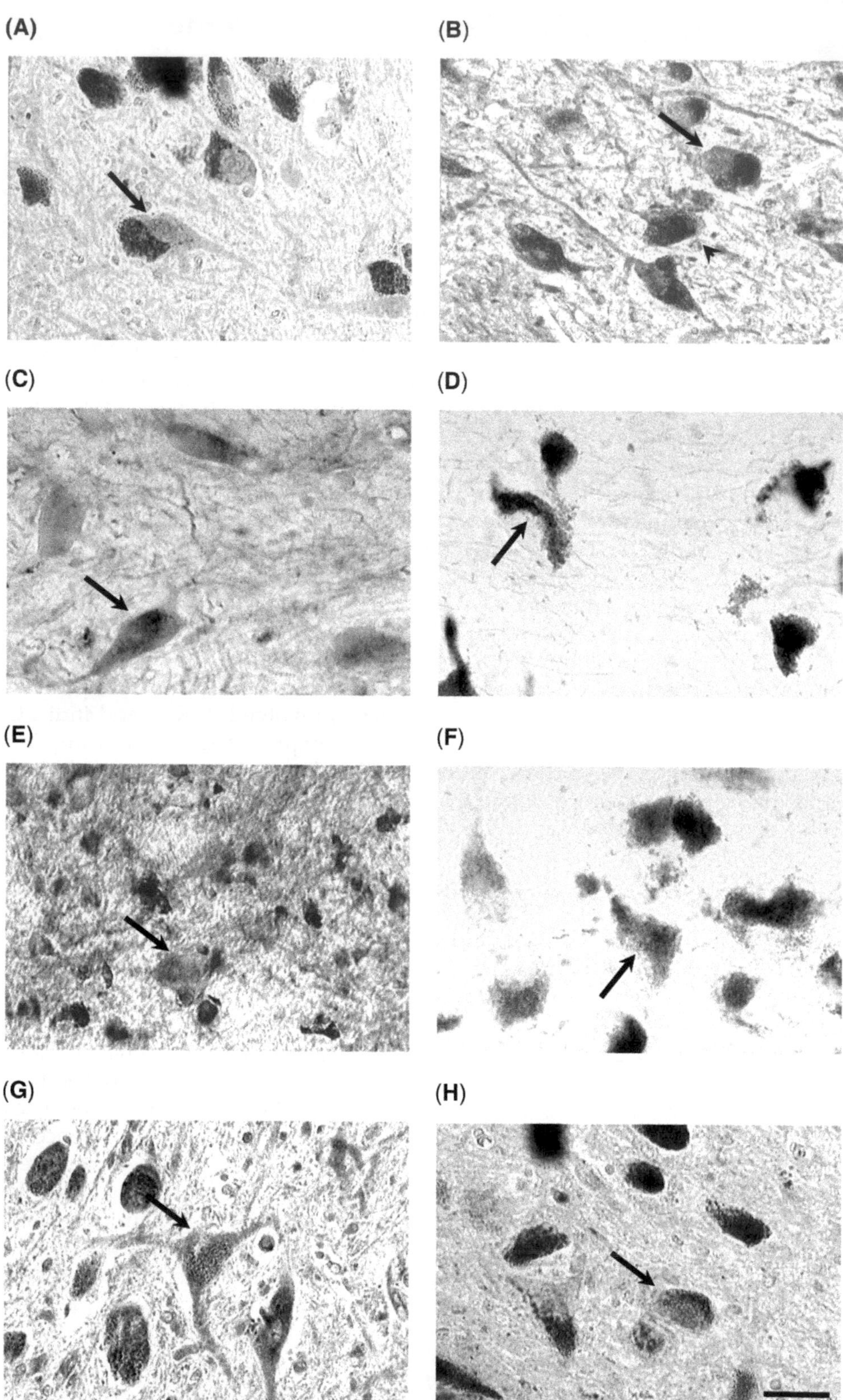


**FIGURE 1** (*Caption on facing page*)

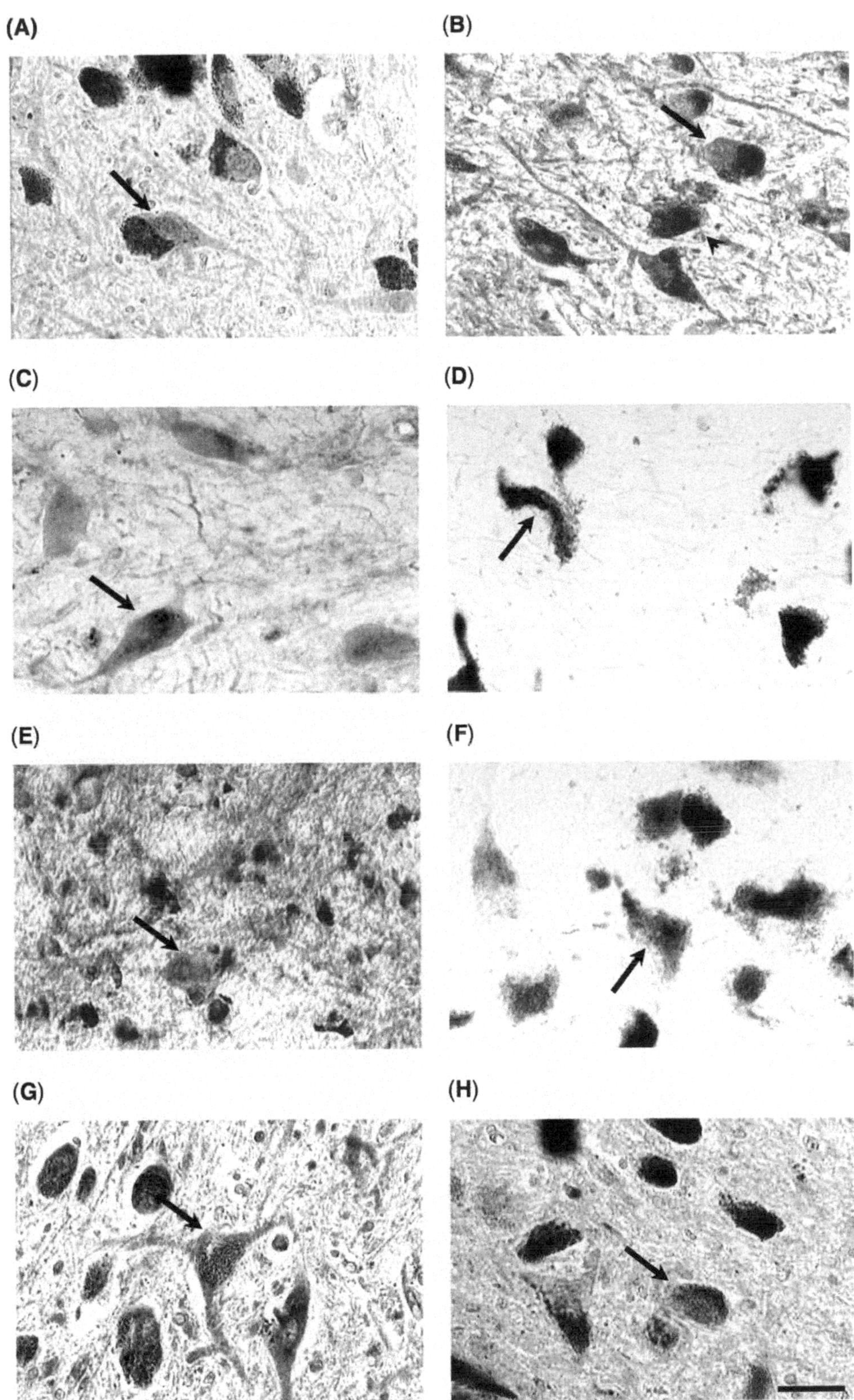


**FIGURE 7.1** The pictures represent the immunostaining patterns of the human substantia nigra in control brains (*left panels*) and restless leg syndrome (RLS) brains (*right panels*). (*See p. 102*)

ages of symptom onset (8). The earlier onset cases (< 45 years) more commonly had RLS among first-degree relatives, were observed to have a much slower progression of RLS symptoms with age, had less of a relationship between body iron stores and RLS severity (22), and demonstrated a lower rate of occurrence of small-fiber neuropathy (23). As a result, the age of onset criterion needs to be incorporated into genetic investigation.

## INHERITANCE MODELS AND SEGREGATION ANALYSIS

Studies with single RLS families suggested that transmission of RLS can be autosomal dominant (18,19,24–26) or recessive (10,27) with variable expressivity (18,19,26). A number of epidemiological studies suggested that different races may have variable susceptibilities to RLS. Whites generally have a much higher population prevalence rate of RLS than Asians and Africans. Furthermore, genetic anticipation was proposed to be a possible genetic transmission mode for RLS (18), in which individuals in successive generations presented at an earlier age and/or with more severe manifestations. Genetic anticipation is often observed in disorders resulting from the expression of a trinucleotide repeat mutation that tends to increase in size and have a more significant effect when passed from one generation to the next (28). Lazzarini et al. (18) analyzed five pedigrees with 81 RLS-affected members for age of onset, sex ratio, and transmission pattern. These pedigrees showed an autosomal-dominant mode of inheritance and a male:female ratio of 1:1.4 ($p = 0.15$). One of the five analyzed pedigrees showed some evidence of reduced penetrance. In two of five analyzed pedigrees, there is statistical support for anticipation ($p < 0.05$). The authors thus argued that these variations in penetrance and anticipation suggest possible genetic heterogeneity.

An accurate assumption of the model of inheritance in RLS and related genetic parameters such as penetrance and rate of phenocopies is critical for linkage analysis, which often resorts to complex segregation analysis. However, only one study for complex segregation analysis of RLS was reported (17). In this study, 238 RLS patients, 537 first-degree relatives, and 133 spouses were interviewed. Altogether, 908 interview records from 196 families were subject to segregation analysis. Two groups of families were stratified: mean age at onset up to 30 years of age (Group A) and older than 30 years (Group B). Nine inheritance models were compared using the program Pedigree Analysis Package: (i) no major gene; (ii) mixed model, dominant; (iii) mixed model, recessive; (iv) mixed model, codominant and mixed model, dominant; (v) recessive; (vi) codominant; (vii) environmental; (viii) environmental + multifactorial; and (ix) general (dominant). In Group A, segregation analysis strongly favored a single major gene acting autosomal dominant with a multifactorial component. Parameter estimates were 0.003 for the allele frequency, 1.0 for the penetrance, and 0.005 for the phenocopy rate. In Group B, no evidence for a major gene could be elucidated. The segregation pattern found in the studied families demonstrated an autosomal allele acting dominantly in the RLS families with an early age at onset of symptoms with an additional multifactorial component and suggested that RLS was a causative heterogeneous disease.

## FAMILIAL AGGREGATION ANALYSIS

Familial aggregation analysis is another common approach to determining genetic components of RLS. Chen et al. (10) conducted a familial aggregation analysis using identify any overt neurodegeneration in the spinal cord. Therefore, the underlying pathology in RLS is thought to result from a dysfunction in biochemical pathways rather than a deposition of a pathogenic agent [e.g., plaques in Alzheimer's disease, α-synuclein in Parkinson's disease (PD)].

### Tyrosine Hydroxylase Immunostaining

Because DA agents are used successfully in the treatment of many RLS cases (see Chapter 25), tyrosine hydroxylase immunostaining was used to evaluate the presence and morphological integrity of the DA neurons in the substantia nigra. None of the RLS cases had any histologic abnormality in this major DA region. No differences between the control and RLS brains were observed in the staining intensity or the appearance of these neurons and associated processes in any of the midbrain structures after staining with antiserum to tyrosine hydroxylase. In addition to the substantia nigra, we attempted to identify the DA cluster of neurons identified as A11 in the human diencephalon because this nucleus gives rise to the descending DA pathway and has been suggested as being involved in RLS (6) in animal studies. Although a cluster of DA neurons representing A11 could not be specifically identified in the human diencephalon, there were clearly tyrosine hydroxylase neurons present in this region in both controls and RLS, but they were too widely dispersed to generate data.

In general, the absence of Lewy bodies and α-synuclein positive staining, the intact appearance of DA neurons, and lack of gliosis further distance RLS from neurodegenerative diseases that include the DA system such as PD, Lewy body disease, and Alzheimer's disease.

## IRON MANAGEMENT PROTEINS

Because of the MRI data suggesting that there are lower levels of iron in the substantia nigra in the RLS brain (1), a detailed histochemical analysis for iron and

**FIGURE 1** (*Facing page*) (*See color insert*) The pictures represent the immunostaining patterns of the human substantia nigra in control brains (*left panels*) and restless leg syndrome (RLS) brains (*right panels*). In each of the micrographs, the dark gray substance is neuromelanin and the blue is the immunoreaction product for the antibody. (**A**) Transferrin. Relatively light staining for transferrin is identified in the neuromelanin cells (*arrow*) in the control brain. The immuno-product is mostly limited to the cytoplasm and few cells have processes that contain the immuno-product. Compared to the control brain, the RLS brain (**B**) has considerably more Tf reaction product in the neuromelanin cells (*arrow*) and the immuno-product extends to the neuronal processes in most of the cells. Small, round cells identified as oligodendrocytes are also present (*arrowhead*) in the RLS brain. (**C**) Ferroportin. Many intensely labeled neuromelanin cells are observed in the SN of the control brain (**C**). The immuno-product is present in the cell body (*arrow*) and proximal dendrites. In contrast, most of the neuromelanin cells are devoid of ferroportin reaction product (*cell at arrow*) in the RLS brain (**D**). H-ferritin. Lightly labeled neuromelanin cells (*arrow*) are observed in the SN of the control brain but there are multiple immunopositive oligodendrocytes visible (**E**). In the RLS brain (**F**), there is no detectable H-ferritin in the neuromelanin containing neurons (*arrow*). There are also almost no oligodendrocytes that are immunopositive for ferritin. Transferrin receptor. Strong staining is observed in the neuromelanin cells (*arrow*) of the control brains (**G**). The immunoreaction product is found on the soma and extends into a primary process in many of the cells (*cell at arrow*). In the RLS brains (**H**), the immunoreaction product for Tf receptor is minimal and cell processes are unlabeled (*cell at arrow*). Bar = 16 μm for all micrographs. *Abbreviation*: SN, substantia nigra.

immunocytochemical analysis for the iron management proteins was undertaken in this brain region (4). The immunostaining analysis revealed an increase in transferrin (Tf), the iron mobilization protein, in the neuromelanin cells in the RLS brains compared to control (Fig. 1A and B). There is a decrease in the neuromelanin cells in the RLS brain for ferroportin (Fig. 1C and D), which is also known as metal transport protein 1. Ferroportin is important for cellular iron export (7). We also observed a decrease in ferritin (Fig. 1E and F), normally considered an iron storage protein. This expression pattern is seen in experimental animal models of brain iron deficiency (8). Another consistent observation in cells that are iron deficient is an increase in expression of Tf receptors (9,10). However, in RLS, the neuromelanin cells immunostained less intensely for Tf receptors than controls (Fig. 1G and H). Tf receptors are only expressed on neurons in the brain. Therefore, relative differences in staining intensity for Tf receptors among the different cell types, which may have been informative about the iron status of non-neuronal cells, could not be determined. On the other hand, the ratio of H to L subunits of ferritin varies according to cell type in the brain (11), and the staining pattern for these subunits may suggest differences in iron status of the different cell populations. Neuromelanin cells express very little H- (Fig. 1E) or L-ferritin in control or RLS brains. L-ferritin is normally found in glial cells but not in neurons (11,12), and the presence of L-ferritin in microglia and astrocytes in the RLS brain is much more robust than in the control brains. Because there is no suggestion of gliosis in the RLS brains, the expression of L-ferritin in microglia and astrocytes in the RLS brains may indicate alterations in the iron delivery mechanism or misdirection of iron after it crosses the blood–brain barrier in the RLS brain, which could lead to the iron deficiency in neurons. The mechanisms of iron delivery into and within the brain are poorly understood, but iron delivery to the brain continues even when the normally targeted cells are compromised (13).

To more quantitatively and precisely evaluate the expression of iron management proteins, neuromelanin cells were harvested from the substantia nigra of four RLS brains and four control brains, using laser capture microdissection (LCM) (14). This approach allowed us to specifically determine the iron management profile of the neuromelanin cells without confounding input from the glial cells. This quantitative analysis confirmed the findings in the immunocytochemical study (4,14).

As with the immunocytochemical analysis, the inconsistent part of the puzzle is that the neuromelanin cells in RLS are iron insufficient, yet they show relatively diminished staining intensity for Tf receptors compared to that seen in the normal brains. There is a report that neuromelanin cells express receptors for lactoferrin, which could be an alternative iron source for these cells (15). However, the increase in Tf in the neuromelanin cells in the RLS brain, coupled with the decrease in H- and L-ferritin staining, strongly indicates that these cells do not have a sufficient iron supply. The lack of the expected increase in Tf receptor expression on neuromelanin cells suggests that there is a malfunction in the regulation of Tf receptors in RLS.

It should be noted that a typical treatment strategy for RLS includes DA agonists. Although there is considerable literature on the effects of iron status on the DA system (16,17), there is little information on how manipulations of the DA system may impact brain iron status, and, based on the relationship between the iron and the DA system and the evolving relationship among iron, RLS, and dopamine, determining if the DA interventions can impact iron status clearly warrants further investigation.

### Iron Regulatory Proteins and RLS

As mentioned, an exception to the protein profile that indicates iron insufficiency in the RLS neuromelanin cells is the decrease in TfR expression compared with control. TfR expression is posttranscriptionally regulated by IRPs. Therefore, the decrease in TfR expression could be due to a lack of transcription of the mRNA or a problem with the IRPs. To determine if the Tf receptor mRNA was being expressed, we performed in situ hybridization and detected mRNA in the neuromelanin cells from the RLS brains. Although the in situ hybridization was not quantitative, it did indicate that the Tf receptor mRNA was being expressed. Subsequently, we determined the concentration and activity of IRP1 and IRP2 in the neuromelanin cells that had been isolated by LCM. The amount and the activity of IRP1 were decreased in RLS compared with controls. The second IRP (IRP2) was slightly but significantly elevated.

Normally, total IRP1 levels in the cell do not change significantly when cellular iron status is altered. IRP1 is either in mRNA binding form or in cytosolic aconitase (18,19). When iron status is low, the functional mode of IRP1 is that of the mRNA binding protein. When iron status is sufficient, IRP1 does not bind mRNA and functions as a cytosolic aconitase. Therefore, cytosolic aconitase activity in the isolated neuromelanin cells was measured and found to be decreased in RLS compared with control. Thus, our data strongly suggest that total expression of IRP1 is decreased in neuromelanin cells from RLS brains compared to control.

IRPs stabilize TfR mRNA when cellular iron status is low (20,21). Therefore, the decreased expression of IRP1 could contribute to, or be the cause of, the cellular iron insufficiency in the neuromelanin cells by failing to stabilize the TfR mRNA. TfR mRNA does not increase in neurons in iron-deficient rat brains (22,23), but rather suggest that the failure of neuronal TfR mRNA to increase with iron deficiency indicates that IRP1 stabilizes the mRNA; one interpretation suggested that IRPs did not regulate TfR mRNA in neurons (23). In contrast, our data indicate that IRPs are present in neurons and do stabilize the TfR mRNA to promote translation.

The cause of the decrease in IRP1 is under investigation. Genetic mapping of RLS patients has identified a locus upstream of IRP1, which was initially promising but appears to have been excluded in this cohort (24). One study that did not find a linkage between RLS in an Asian family and a number of gene candidates in the iron metabolism pathway, including IRP1, has been reported (25).

## PROPOSED CONSEQUENCES OF INSUFFICIENT IRON IN THE RESTLESS LEGS SYNDROME SUBSTANTIA NIGRA

Deficient iron levels in the brain are frequently associated with disruptions in the DA system in animal models (26,27). Clinical data on RLS suggest that the DA system is involved in this disorder (28). Thus, the data reported here support the current management strategies for RLS and suggest that iron deficiency in neuromelanin cells may underlie the DA dysfunction in RLS. Analysis of the components of the DA system in RLS is currently in progress.

In addition to directly assessing the DA system in RLS, we performed a gene array analysis to identify genes that are responsive to iron as possible candidate genes that could be mutated in RLS (29). One of the genes we identified, Thy-1, is one of the most abundant mammalian neuronal surface glycoproteins on mature neurons, accounting for 7.5% of the surface proteins. Thy-1 is also present in synaptic vesicles (30,31) and plays a regulatory role in vesicular release of neurotransmitter at the synapse (32). It is also important for stabilization of synapses and suppression of neuritic outgrowth (33). We demonstrated in the autopsy samples that the concentration of Thy-1 in the substantia nigra of RLS patients is less than half that of controls (34). To directly demonstrate a relationship between Thy-1 protein expression and iron status, we treated PC12 cells with the iron chelator, Desferal, and showed decreased expression of Thy-1 in a dose- and time-dependent manner. We also found a significant decrease in Thy-1 in iron-deficient rat brains. These studies reveal a novel mechanism by which iron deficiency can affect brain function. They also indicate a possible mechanism by which iron deficiency compromises DA transmission in RLS.

The decrease in Thy-1 in RLS cases is not secondary to a loss of neurons in the RLS substantia nigra, because the number of Thy-1-positive cells in the substantia nigra appeared to be similar in RLS and controls (34). The normal number of Thy-1-positive cells in the RLS substantia nigra is consistent with the histological evaluation and the tyrosine hydroxylase immunostaining that did not find differences in neuronal cell density in the substantia nigra between RLS and control (4).

The studies with Thy-1 provide a potentially important link between decreased brain iron and the responsiveness to dopamine agonists and iron supplementation treatment in RLS. We have proposed the hypothesis that a deficiency in Thy-1, caused by insufficient iron levels, contributes to RLS by affecting the integrity of the DA system. This hypothesis is consistent with the considerable evidence for a central role for the DA system in RLS (35). In particular, this hypothesis that the problem with RLS is loss of efficacy of DA connections is consistent with clinical observations that there can be dramatic improvement in symptoms following treatment with relatively low doses of dopamine agonists and levodopa (36,37). Consistent with our autopsy findings, our interpretation of the positive effects of low doses of DA agents to treat the symptoms of RLS is that, unlike PD in which treatment is required to replenish a depleted neurotransmitter system, in RLS the problem is suboptimal synaptic contact. Studies on the relationship of Thy-1 to the DA system, using Thy-1 null mice (38,39), are in progress.

## CONCLUSION

The published analyses from RLS postmortem studies indicate that RLS is not rooted in pathologies associated with traditional neurodegenerative processes. There are probably several mechanisms involved in the pathophysiology of RLS. However, evidence continues to mount from multiple sources (MRI, cerebrospinal fluid, serum ferritin levels, and autopsy studies) that RLS brains have reduced relative availability of iron in the brain, and that this contributes to the symptoms. A relationship between the DA system and iron is well-established (40). Local iron insufficiency in the substantia nigra could impair DA functioning in a number of ways. First, iron is a cofactor for tyrosine hydroxylase, the enzyme that governs the rate-limiting step in the production of dopamine (41). Second, iron is involved in the activity and expression of dopamine transporters and receptors. Iron-deprived animals show a significant reduction in dopamine receptor density and impaired behavioral response to DA stimulation (26,42). There is no clinic data in humans to support either of these theories. Third, we have presented evidence that argues for a loss of efficacy in DA nerve terminals via a decrease in Thy-1 expression.

As a result of our animal and human postmortem studies, we generated the following working hypothesis: brain iron acquisition in neuromelanin cells is compromised in RLS brains through a decrease in function of IRP1 and subsequent failure to stabilize the mRNA for Tf receptors. The insufficient iron status of the neuromelanin cells may be the primary deficit, leading to a series of events (i.e., decreased synaptic efficacy leading to impaired DA activity) that ultimately manifest as RLS symptoms. The mechanisms by which this dopamine dysfunction actually result in clinical RLS are not known.

## ACKNOWLEDGMENTS

This work was supported by the National Institutes of Health (1 PO1 AG021190-01) and the Restless Legs Syndrome Foundation. The authors are particularly grateful to the Restless Legs Syndrome Foundation Brain Donation program for providing them with the autopsy tissue for their studies. The authors also express their profound gratitude to the individuals who participated in the brain donation program that made these studies and the resulting insights into the pathology of RLS possible. Sharon Menzies was a key contributor to the initial studies on the RLS brain tissue and died at the age of 38 after the first studies were performed.

## REFERENCES

1. Allen RP, Barker PB, Wehrl F, Song HK, Earley CJ. MRI measurement of brain iron in patients with restless legs syndrome. Neurology 2001; 56:263–265.
2. Mikolaenko I, Pletnikova O, Kawas CH, et al. Alpha-synuclein lesions in normal aging, Parkinson disease, and Alzheimer disease: evidence from the Baltimore Longitudinal Study of Aging (BLSA). J Neuropathol Exp Neurol 2005; 64:156–162.
3. Jellinger KA. Lewy body-related alpha-synucleinopathy in the aged human brain. J Neural Transm 2004; 111:1219–1235.
4. Connor JR, Boyer PJ, Menzies SL, Dellinger B, Allen RP, Earley CJ. Neuropathological examination suggests impaired brain iron acquisition in restless legs syndrome. Neurology 2003; 61:304–309.
5. Pittock SJ, Parrett T, Adler CH, Parisi JE, Dickson DW, Ahlskog JE. Neuropathology of primary restless leg syndrome: absence of specific tau- and alpha-synuclein pathology. Mov Disord 2004; 19:695–699.
6. Ondo WG, He Y, Rajasekaran S, Le WD. Clinical correlates of 6-hydroxydopamine injections into A11 dopaminergic neurons in rats: a possible model for restless legs syndrome. Mov Disord 2000; 15:154–158.
7. Burdo JR, Menzies SL, Simpson IA, et al. Distribution of divalent metal transporter 1 and metal transport protein 1 in the normal and Belgrade rat. J Neurosci Res 2001; 66:1198–1207.
8. Pinero DJ, Li NQ, Connor JR, Beard JL. Variations in dietary iron alter brain iron metabolism in developing rats. J Nutr 2000; 130:254–263.
9. Tong X, Kawabata H, Koeffler HP. Iron deficiency can upregulate expression of transferrin receptor at both the mRNA and protein level. Br J Haematol 2002; 116:458–464.
10. Barisani D, Conte D. Transferrin receptor 1 (TfR1) and putative stimulator of Fe transport (SFT) expression in iron deficiency and overload: an overview. Blood Cells Mol Dis 2002; 29:498–505.
11. Connor JR, Boeshore KL, Benkovic SA, Menzies SL. Isoforms of ferritin have a specific cellular distribution in the brain. J Neurosci Res 1994; 37:461–465.

12. Thompson K, Menzies S, Muckenthaler M, et al. Mouse brains deficient in H-ferritin have normal iron concentration but a protein profile of iron deficiency and increased evidence of oxidative stress. J Neurosci Res 2003; 71:46–63.
13. Connor JR, Menzies SL. Altered cellular distribution of iron in the central nervous system of myelin deficient rats. Neuroscience 1990; 34:265–271.
14. Connor JR, Wang XS, Patton SM, et al. Decreased transferrin receptor expression by neuromelanin cells in restless legs syndrome. Neurology 2004; 62:1563–1567.
15. Faucheux B, Nillesse N, Damier P, et al. Expression of lactoferrin receptors is increased in the mesenchephalon of patients with parkinson disease. Proc Natl Acad Sci USA 1995; 92:9603–9607.
16. Beard J, Erikson KM, Jones BC. Neonatal iron deficiency results in irreversible changes in dopamine function in rats. J Nutr 2003; 133:1174–1179.
17. Ward RJ, Dexter D, Florence A, et al. Brain iron in the ferrocene-loaded rat: its chelation and influence on dopamine metabolism. Biochem Pharmacol 1995; 49:1821–1826.
18. Toth I, Bridges KR. Ascorbic acid enhances ferritin mRNA translation by an IRP/aconitase switch. J Biol Chem 1995; 270:19,540–19,544.
19. Oshiro S, Nozawa K, Hori M, et al. Modulation of iron regulatory protein-1 by various metals. Biochem Biophys Res Commun 2002; 290:213–218.
20. Koeller DM, Casey JL, Hentze MW, et al. A cytosolic protein binds to structural elements within the iron regulatory region of the transferrin receptor mRNA. Proc Natl Acad Sci USA 1989; 86:3574–3578.
21. Mullner EW, Neupert B, Kuhn LC. A specific mRNA binding factor regulates the iron-dependent stability of cytoplasmic transferrin receptor mRNA. Cell 1989; 58:373–382.
22. Han J, Day JR, Connor JR, Beard JL. Gene expression of transferrin and transferrin receptor in brains of control vs. iron-deficient rats. Nutr Neurosci 2003; 6:1–10.
23. Moos T, Oates PS, Morgan EH. Expression of the neuronal transferrin receptor is age dependent and susceptible to iron deficiency. J Comp Neurol 1998; 398:420–430.
24. Chen S, Ondo WG, Rao S, Li L, Chen Q, Wang Q. Genomewide linkage scan identifies a novel susceptibility locus for restless legs syndrome on chromosome 9p. Am J Hum Genet 2004; 74:876–885.
25. Li J, Hu LD, Wang WJ, Chen YG, Kong XY. Linkage analysis of the candidate genes of familial restless legs syndrome. Yi Chuan Xue Bao 2003; 30:325–329.
26. Erikson KM, Jones BC, Hess EJ, Zhang Q, Beard JL. Iron deficiency decreases dopamine D1 and D2 receptors in rat brain. Pharmacol Biochem Behav 2001; 69:409–418.
27. Beard JL, Erikson KM, Jones BC. Neurobehavioral analysis of developmental iron deficiency in rats. Behav Brain Res 2002; 134:517–524.
28. Allen RP, Earley CJ. Restless legs syndrome: a review of clinical and pathophysiologic features. J Clin Neurophysiol 2001; 18:128–147.
29. Ye Z, Connor JR. Identification of iron responsive genes by screening cDNA libraries from suppression subtractive hybridization with antisense probes from three iron conditions. Nucleic Acids Res 2000; 28:1802–1807.
30. Morris RJ, Beech JN, Barber PC, Raisman G. Early stages of Purkinje cell maturation demonstrated by Thy-1 immunohistochemistry on postnatal rat cerebellum. J Neurocytol 1985; 14:427–452.
31. Seki M, Nawa H, Morioka T, et al. Establishment of a novel enzyme-linked immunosorbent assay for Thy-1; quantitative assessment of neuronal degeneration. Neurosci Lett 2002; 329:185–188.
32. Jeng CJ, McCarroll SA, Martin TF, et al. Thy-1 is a component common to multiple populations of synaptic vesicles. J Cell Biol 1998; 140:685–698.
33. Almqvist P, Carlsson SR, Hardy JA, Winblad B. Regional and subcellular distribution of Thy-1 in human brain assayed by a solid-phase radioimmunoassay. J Neurochem 1986; 46:681–685.
34. Wang X, Wiesinger J, Beard J, et al. Thy1 expression in the brain is affected by iron and is decreased in Restless Legs Syndrome. J Neurol Sci 2004; 220:59–66.

35. Montplaisir J, Lorrain D, Godbout R. Restless legs syndrome and periodic leg movements in sleep: the primary role of dopaminergic mechanism. Eur Neurol 1991; 31:41–43.
36. Chesson AL, Jr., Wise M, Davila D, et al. Practice parameters for the treatment of restless legs syndrome and periodic limb movement disorder. An American Academy of Sleep Medicine report. Standards of Practice Committee of the American Academy of Sleep Medicine. Sleep 1999; 22:961–968.
37. Hening W, Allen R, Earley C, Kushida C, Picchietti D, Silber M. The treatment of restless legs syndrome and periodic limb movement disorder. An American Academy of Sleep Medicine review. Sleep 1999; 22:970–999.
38. Nosten-Bertrand M, Errington ML, Murphy KP, et al. Normal spatial learning despite regional inhibition of LTP in mice lacking Thy-1. Nature 1996; 379:826–829.
39. Hollrigel GS, Morris RJ, Soltesz I. Enhanced bursts of IPSCs in dentate granule cells in mice with regionally inhibited long-term potentiation. Proc Biol Sci 1998; 265:63–69.
40. Beard JL, Connor JR. Iron status and neural functioning. Annu Rev Nutr 2003; 23:41–58.
41. Beard J. Iron biology in immune function, muscle metabolism, and neuronal functioning. J Nutr 2001; 131:568s–580s.
42. Erikson KM, Jones BC, Beard JL. Iron deficiency alters dopamine transporter functioning in rat striatum. J Nutr 2000; 130:2831–2837.

# 8 Genetics of Restless Legs Syndrome

**Shaoqi Rao**

*Department of Molecular Cardiology, Lerner Research Institute, Centers for Cardiovascular Genetics and Molecular Genetics, The Cleveland Clinic Foundation, and Department of Molecular Medicine, Cleveland Clinic Lerner College of Medicine of Case Western Reserve University, Cleveland, Ohio, U.S.A.*

**Juliane Winkelmann**

*Max Planck Institute of Psychiatry, RG Neurological Genetics, Institute of Human Genetics, Munich, Germany*

**Qing K. Wang**

*Department of Molecular Cardiology, Lerner Research Institute, Centers for Cardiovascular Genetics and Molecular Genetics, The Cleveland Clinic Foundation, and Department of Molecular Medicine, Cleveland Clinic Lerner College of Medicine of Case Western Reserve University, Cleveland, Ohio, U.S.A.*

## OVERVIEW

Recent advances in molecular and genetic epidemiological studies of restless legs syndrome (RLS) (MIM 102300) have led to a series of important discoveries that promise to greatly expand our knowledge of the molecular basis of this common disease. Several genetic epidemiological studies and twin studies have characterized the genetic components of RLS and suggest that it is a highly heritable trait. The accumulated evidence suggests that a single founder mutation(s) in an RLS pedigree can lead to a monogenic inheritance pattern; however, in most cases, RLS is a complex disease with mixed contributions of major genes, modifier genes, and environmental factors, reflecting its nature of genetic heterogeneity. The chromosomal positions of three putative RLS genes (9p, 12q, and 14q) have been determined by either model-based linkage analysis of single, large, and well-characterized pedigrees or model-free linkage analysis of multiple pedigrees. However, the causative or susceptibility genes within these linkage regions remain to be identified. A few population-based, case–control genetic studies have investigated several candidate genes for the pathogenesis of RLS. In this chapter, we describe these advances in the field of genetics of RLS.

## PREVALENCE AND ENVIRONMENTAL FACTORS

RLS is a common sensorimotor disorder that affects between 5% and 12% of White populations (1–4). Asian and African populations appear to be less affected (Chapter 12) (5–7). The etiology of RLS is poorly understood. Family studies, twin studies, and segregation analysis (discussed in detail later), all support the hypothesis that genetic factors contribute to the pathogenesis of RLS (8). However, as with other common diseases, RLS is expected to have a polygenic basis, possibly with mixed contributions of multiple major genes, modifier genes, and complex interactions of genes with genes, and genes with environmental factors. The environmental factors that increase the risk of RLS are discussed in this section.

Although clinical observations suggest that RLS may be associated with emotional distress, psychosocial dysfunction, and depression, several large-scale epidemiological studies (1,2,7) were undertaken to systematically identify the significant correlates with RLS. Berger et al. (7) performed a large-scale cross-section survey with face-to-face interviews and physical examinations of 4310 participants in the Study of Health in Pomerania in northeastern Germany. The overall prevalence rate of RLS was 10.6%; however, it increased with age, and women were twice as often affected as men. In addition, the risk of RLS increased gradually with women with more children. Thus, these epidemiological variables were implicated as important environmental factors for RLS. The 1996 Kentucky Behavioral Risk Factor Surveillance Survey collected data on the frequency of those experiencing RLS, self-rated general and mental health status, demographic, and behavioral risk factors, by telephone interviews with 1803 men and women, 18 years and older (1). After adjusting for age, body mass index, sex, smoking, diabetes, exercise, income, and alcohol consumption, the study found that RLS was significantly related to diminished general health and poor mental health. People with RLS were 2.4 times more likely to report diminished general health than those without the disease. Likewise, RLS was associated with poor mental health, with an odds ratio (OR) of 3.1 for having experienced all the days of the previous month in poor mental health (1). The health and lifestyle characters independently associated with RLS were higher BMI, greater age, cigarette smoking, history of nongestational diabetes, less exercise, and low alcohol consumption. Notably, having diabetes and getting almost no exercise (less than 3 hours per month) were particularly strong predictors of RLS, with adjusted ORs of 4.4 and 3.3, respectively (1).

Another large-scale epidemiological study (2), the Memory and Morbidity in Augsburg Elderly study conducted in Germany, focused on the prevalence and risk factors of RLS in an elderly population of 65 to 83 years of age. The study found that there was a significant gender difference ($p = 0.012$) for RLS, with a prevalence rate of 13.9% in women and 6.1% in men. Men showed a trend toward a decrease of RLS with age, whereas this age trend was not observed in women. Male RLS cases were on average taller but had the same weight as male non-RLS cases. In contrast to the Kentucky survey, RLS-positive subjects reported less diabetes and significantly ($p = 0.04$) lower rates of hypertension. A higher ($p = 0.06$) percentage were nonsmokers. No significant difference was observed on performance tests, including foot tapping and rising from chair. RLS-positive cases took more benzodiazepines and estrogen compared with non-RLS cases, but the difference was not statistically significant. However, participants with RLS had a higher incidence of depression ($p = 0.012$) and lower self-reported mental health scores ($p = 0.029$) than non-RLS subjects.

## FAMILY HISTORY

Determination of the genetic component of a complex human disease is a critical issue because human pedigrees are often ascertained from clinical settings, and the sampling schemes may not be defined by a single ascertainment scheme. The ascertainment biases can impose additional difficulty on obtaining accurate genetic parameter estimates. Nevertheless, genetic analysis of the collected RLS samples for evidence of genetic factors should be performed. Without familial aggregation, in which genetic factors play an important role, the expense and effort involved in further gene mapping and cloning of RLS genes would be wasted (9). Thus, there are a number of published studies that have attempted to collect genetic evidence using various approaches, including family history studies, complex segregation analysis, and other epidemiological studies to characterize inheritance models, and heritability analysis via either family aggregation analysis or twin studies. We summarized here recent genetic studies in Table 1, with aims to elucidate the genetic roles in RLS.

Seeking RLS cases with a clear family history is perhaps the most direct way to identify the evidence of genetic and common environmental contributions. A number of studies have documented families with a high occurrence of RLS (15–19), while in some cases RLS occurs sporadically and without strong evidence of familial aggregations (17). Montplaisir et al. (15) documented that 80 of 127 patients (63%) reported the presence of RLS in at least one of their first-degree relatives. In these families, 221 of 568 first-degree relatives (39%) were reported by the patients to be affected with RLS. Allen and Early (20) believed that RLS would have a high chance to occur commonly in some families because it is a common disorder. Up to date, several published studies (Table 1) addressed family histories of RLS in a systematic way. The first study finding that a positive family history is correlated with a younger age at disease onset was from Walters et al. in their Nightwalker survey (16). They found that 58% of patients with age at onset greater than 20 years had family history, while this number increased to 81% for earlier age at onset ($<20$ years). The relation between family history and age at onset was corroborated in later studies. In the study by Allen et al. (21), the frequency of occurrence of RLS in a family was found to relate to the age at onset of RLS symptoms. For RLS probands with RLS symptoms starting before age of 45 years, RLS occurred among 23.6% of the first-degree relatives compared with 3.5% for control probands. In contrast, RLS was reported for only 10% of the first-degree relatives of RLS patients reporting late onset of symptoms (after age 45). The authors thus suggested that the early onset RLS had stronger genetic components (21). The observation that familial RLS cases had younger ages at onset is also supported by other studies (13,14). Winkelmann et al. (13) analyzed the clinical data for 300 RLS patients. Family history was defined as definitely positive when at least one first-degree relative had the RLS phenotype according to the criteria of the International RLS Study Group. Of the 300 patients, 232 had idiopathic RLS and 68 had secondary RLS due to uremia. About 42.3% of the idiopathic RLS cases and 11.7% of the secondary RLS cases were classified as having definite positive hereditary RLS. Patients with definite hereditary RLS were significantly younger at the age of onset than those with a negative family history (34.45 vs. 47.17 years, $p < 0.05$). Ondo and Jankovic (14) studied the family histories of 54 RLS patients (29 women and 25 men). The mean age at onset was $34.13 \pm 20.30$ years. A family history of RLS was found in 92% of cases with idiopathic RLS (without neuropathy), but only 13% for neuropathic RLS cases. Interestingly, in about 30% of cases, patients with a family history of RLS were not aware of this history, attesting to the under recognition of RLS. Consistent with other studies, the sporadic/neuropathic RLS cases were older at symptom onset and tended to have a more rapid progression than the familial/idiopathic patients.

These data have fostered the refinement criteria for subtyping RLS phenotypes in terms of presence of a family history and age at symptom onset. Compared with familial cases, sporadic RLS cases had more neuropathy and later

a total of 15 large and extended multiplex RLS families, with a total of 453 subjects including 134 individuals affected with RLS collected from North America. Familial correlations were estimated using the statistical analysis for genetic epidemiology (S.A.G.E.) program Familial CORrelations (FCOR) (29) to quantify the genetic contributions in the ascertained multiplex families. Program FCOR calculates multivariate familial correlations and their asymptotic standard errors for all pair types available in the RLS pedigrees based on the equivalent count of independent pairs that could theoretically have been used to obtain the same standard error for a given correlation (29). The program estimates familial correlations for both subtypes and main types (groups of subtypes), together with the corresponding asymptotic standard errors derived from the variance–covariance matrices of the estimated correlations (29). Correlations for relative pairs at different levels (the first-degree relative pairs to the fourth-degree relative pairs, etc.) were averaged over all the types contained using a uniform weight (each pair was inversely proportional to the number of such pairs in the pedigrees) (29). These large extended families provide sufficient information to decompose genetic components from RLS phenotypic variations. Reliable estimates for various types of relative pairs can be obtained. The recruited pedigrees consist of one pedigree with two generations, five with three generations, seven with four generations, and two with five generations, which provide a maximum of 634 parent–offspring pairs, 399 sibling–sibling pairs, and 492 grandparent–grandchild pairs, respectively.

Technically, familial aggregation analysis is a more detailed version of the mixed linear model approach, in that each type of relative pairs is estimated separately instead of modeling them as a function of a few parameters in a single covariance matrix. Historically, familial aggregation analysis has been the most popular method for determining genetic causes for complex diseases. This method, in essence, is to estimate the correlations between various biological relatives and then similarly assume that they can be parsimoniously explained by an additive genetic contribution and a common household contribution, but without making other assumptions of the mixed linear model. The authors (10) obtained correlation coefficients ($r$) for pedigree relatives at four levels of degrees, consisting of 14 major relative types. The correlations for sibling relationship are intraclass correlations and those for other relationships are interclass correlations. Statistical tests against the null hypothesis of zero correlation were conducted by a $t$-test using the asymptotic standard error estimates given by the S.A.G.E. FCOR program (29). The correlation coefficients ($r$) are 0.17 (918 pairs) for the first-degree relative pairs, 0.04 (1205 pairs) for the second-degree relative pairs, 0.09 (1243 pairs) for the third-degree relative pairs, and 0.06 (1412 pairs) for the fourth-degree relative pairs (Table 1). These results suggest a strong familial aggregation of RLS in this ascertained cohort. The correlation estimates between the same-gender pairs of individuals were higher than those between individuals of the opposite sex, with brother–brother pairs having the highest $r$ of 0.48, sister–sister pairs with $r$ of 0.39, and sister–brother with $r$ of 0.19 only, which may suggest a sex-linked effect for the disorder. There is a considerable negative correlation between spouses ($r = -0.41$), which may reflect the lower risk of RLS among the married-in spouses (5–12%) than in the ascertained families (29.6 %). The study herein reports a formal familial aggregation analysis performed so far to elucidate the genetic architecture of this complex disease. A high positive correlation coefficient of 0.17 between the first-degree relatives suggests their strong phenotypic resemblance. Furthermore, the heritability of RLS was estimated to be a very high value of 0.60 with all types

**TABLE 1** Recent Evidence of Genetic Contribution in Restless Legs Syndrome

| Method | Parameter | Sample | Estimate | Reference |
|---|---|---|---|---|
| Familial correlation | First-degree relatives: | 918 pairs | $0.171^{a}$ | (10) |
| | Parent–offspring | 567 pairs | $0.096^{a} \pm 0.033$ | (10) |
| | Father–son | 135 pairs | $0.195^{b} \pm 0.088$ | (10) |
| | Mother–son | 134 pairs | $-0.182^{b} \pm 0.110$ | (10) |
| | Father–daughter | 148 pairs | $0.232^{a} \pm 0.087$ | (10) |
| | Mother–daughter | 150 pairs | $0.132 \pm 0.103$ | (10) |
| | Siblings | 351 pairs | $0.291^{a} \pm 0.096$ | (10) |
| | Brother–brother | 106 pairs | $0.480^{a} \pm 0.161$ | (10) |
| | Brother–sister | 166 pairs | $0.161 \pm 0.132$ | (10) |
| | Sister–sister | 79 pairs | $0.392^{a} \pm 0.122$ | (10) |
| | Second-degree relatives | 1205 pairs | 0.039 | (10) |
| | Third-degree relatives | 1243 | $0.090^{a}$ | (10) |
| | Fourth-degree relatives | 1412 | $0.064^{b}$ | (10) |
| | Unrelated spouse | 117 | $-0.412^{a} \pm 0.085$ | (10) |
| Relative risk ratios | Parent–offspring | | 10.25 | (10) |
| | Sibling | | 16.23 | (10) |
| | First-degree | | 5.7 | (11) |
| Twin studies | MZ twins | 12 twin pairs | 83.3% | (8) |
| | Twins | 933 MZ pairs; 1004 DZ pairs | Heritability of 54% | (12) |
| Family history (rate) | Idiopathic RLS | 232 cases | 42.3% | (13) |
| | Uremia RLS | 68 cases | 11.7% | (13) |
| | Idiopathic RLS | 25 cases | 92.0% | (14) |
| | Neuropathic RLS | 15 cases | 13.3% | (14) |
| | RLS | 127 cases | 63% | (15) |
| | RLS | 105 cases | 58–81% | (16) |
| | Early age-at-onset families | 196 cases | 45.4% | (17) |

[a] $p < 0.01$.
[b] $p < 0.05$.
*Abbreviations*: MZ, monozygotic; DZ, dizygotic.

of relative pairs. These results indicate that RLS is a highly heritable trait in this ascertained cohort. It is interesting that the correlations for relative pairs was higher for siblings than parent–offspring, and was the highest for siblings of same sex. This implicates the involvement of gender and other environmental factors in RLS, and that the estimate may represent an upper limit of the degree of heritability that may include a part of shared common environment. However, the authors (10) viewed that familial correlations and heritability were estimated in an ascertained cohort, and they may not be generalized to the RLS population at large.

A few studies such as shown in Table 1 have attempted to estimate the relative risk ($\lambda_R$) of the RLS patients using the epidemiological approach described by Risch (30). In brief, $\lambda_R$ is the risks of relatives of type R of RLS-affected individuals themselves being affected divided by the population prevalence frequency (K). If the frequency of affected pairs with relationship R is denoted by $K_2$, then $\lambda_R = K_2/K^2$. LaBuda (11) reported that the risk to first-degree relatives was 19.9%, which compared with 3.5% for first-degree relatives of control subjects, and provides an estimate of the relative risk in first-degree relative of 5.7. Chen et al. (10) also estimated familiar relative risk ratios for the first-degree relative pairs using Risch's model (30). To be conservative, a high population prevalence rate of 12% was used. The absolute risks in terms of the concordance rate of affection status between the pairs were 23% and 15% for parent–offspring and siblings, respectively. The relative risk ratio $\lambda_R$ was 10.25 for parent–offspring and 16.23 for siblings. These results are in agreement with the previous familial aggregation analysis, family history survey, and complex segregation analysis, and suggest strong familial components in RLS.

## TWIN STUDIES

Twin samples provide valuable materials for determining whether a disease has a genetic component. Monozygotic (MZ) twins present a fixed genetic background in humans against which one can compare and study the contributions of genetic origin vs. environmental sources. Low concordance rates between MZ twins, or equal concordance rates between MZ and dizygotic (DZ) twins, suggest a strong environmental component rather than a genetic one. To date, two twin studies (Table 1) of RLS were reported. Ondo et al. (8) described demographic, phenotypic, and serological evaluations of 12 identical twin pairs in which one or both members have RLS. A high concordance rate of 83.3% was found, i.e., both subjects in 10 pairs reported definite RLS. Despite the high concordance rate, the RLS symptom and age at onset varied markedly, which underscores the phenotypic variability noted in genetic RLS, even in identical twins. Furthermore, the majority of twin pairs were unaware that the other twin suffered from RLS. Recently, Desai et al. (12) performed a large-scale epidemiological study of self-reported symptoms of obstructive sleep apnea (OSA) and restless legs, using a total of 1937 female twin pairs (MZ:DZ = 933:1004) obtained from a national volunteer twin register of Britain. Concordance rates were higher for MZ than DZ twins for OSA and RLS. Genetic modeling suggests that both genetic and environmental factors contribute to the two phenotypes and the heritability of RLS was estimated to be 54% [95% confidence interval (CI) 36–68%], which is consistent with the previous estimate of 0.60 based on familial correlations (10). Overall, these twin studies again suggest that genetic factors are important in the pathogenesis of RLS.

## LINKAGE STUDIES

A genome-wide linkage scan is a comprehensive and unbiased approach for identifying RLS genes (31,32). It may lead to the identification of novel RLS genes and can define unrecognized genetic pathways for the pathophysiology of RLS. To date, three genetic susceptibility loci have been reported (Table 2, see over). A genome scan using a large French-Canadian family (27) identified a significant linkage to RLS on chromosome 12q (RLS1). A series of adjacent microsatellite markers yielded a maximum two-point logarithm-of-odds (LOD) score of 3.42 (point-wise $p$ value $= 6 \times 10^{-4}$) at a recombination fraction of 0.05, assuming an autosomal recessive mode of inheritance, whereas multipoint linkage calculations yielded a LOD score of 3.59. Haplotype analysis refined the disease gene in a 14.71-cM region between markers D12S1044 and D12S78. However, Kock et al. (33) could not confirm the locus for RLS on chromosome 12q in either of the South Tyrolean families. Winkelmann et al. (17) noted that the study of the single French-Canadian family by Desautels et al. (27) used an autosomal recessive model with very high allele frequency ($q = 0.75$), which is unlikely to be representative for RLS as a whole. Interestingly, Desautels et al. (34) published a confirmation of linkage to chromosome 12q using a total of 276 individuals from 19 families. Using a selection of markers spanning the identified candidate interval on chromosome 12q, two-point analyses of individual pedigrees indicated that five kindreds were consistent with linkage to chromosome 12q. When considering these five pedigrees along with the family in which linkage was originally reported, the authors observed a maximum two-point LOD score of 5.67 at a recombination fraction of 0.10, assuming an autosomal recessive mode of inheritance, and a maximum multipoint LOD score of 8.84 between the interval defined by markers D12S326 and D12S304. Furthermore, the study also suggests the presence of heterogeneity in RLS, as linkage was formally excluded across the region in six pedigrees.

Bonati et al. (37) reported the second RLS locus, RLS2, on 14q13-q21 using an Italian family in which at least 15 members spanning three generations had RLS inherited in an autosomal-dominant pattern. The mean age at onset was 26 years. The RLS gene at this locus was defined within a 9.1-cM region between markers D14S70 and D14S1068 (maximum two-point LOD score of 3.23 at D14S288). Later, Levchenko et al. (38) provided weak confirmation of the RLS locus in one of 14 French-Canadian families investigated.

The third RLS susceptibility locus was identified on chromosome 9p24–22 (RLS3). Chen et al. (10) characterized 15 large and extended multiplex pedigrees consisting of 453 subjects, of whom 134 were affected with RLS. Model-free linkage analysis identified one novel susceptibility locus for RLS on 9p24-p22 with a multipoint nonparametric linkage score of 3.22. Model-based linkage analysis, with the assumption of an autosomal-dominant mode of inheritance, validated the linkage of RLS to 9p24-p22 in two families (two-point LOD score of 3.77; multipoint LOD score of 3.91). This linkage was later confirmed by another group in a German RLS family under the assumption of intrafamilial heterogeneity (35,40). With a stratification according to the age at onset of 32 years, LOD scores of 3.78 (multipoint analysis) and 3.88 (two-point analysis) were obtained. The authors also analyzed transmission disequilibrium tests (TDTs) and affecteds-only linkage analysis in one large family of Bavarian origin, taking into account age at onset. $p$ values were 0.0054 for maker D9S1810 for TDT and 0.0009 for the affecteds-only linkage analysis, providing a confirmation of RLS3. This study narrows the region containing the autosomal dominant RLS3 locus to 11.1 cM (16.6 Mbp).

**TABLE 2** Genetic Loci for Restless Legs Syndrome

| Subjects | Inheritance | Location | Linkage evidence | References |
|---|---|---|---|---|
| An FC family | Autosomal recessive | 12q | Multipoint LOD score of 3.59 | (27) |
| Two South Tyrolean families | Autosomal dominant | 12q | No confirmation | (33) |
| 19 families (13 FC, 5 unknown origin) | Autosomal recessive | 12q | Confirmed, maximum multipoint LOD score of 8.84 | (34) |
| 12 German families | | 12q | Confirmed, TDT ($p$ value = 0.045) | (35) |
| A Chinese family | Autosomal dominant | 16 regions | No linkage | (36) |
| An Italian family | Autosomal dominant | 14q13–21 | Maximum two-point LOD score of 3.23 | (37) |
| 14 French-Canadian families | Autosomal recessive | 14q13–21 | Confirmed in one family, maximum multipoint LOD score of 2.51 | (38) |
| 12 German families | | 14q13–21 | Could not prove or disprove the linkage | (35) |
| 15 U.S. white families | Autosomal dominant | 9p24–22 | Maximum multipoint LOD score of 3.91; HLOD of 2.46 | (10,39) |
| 12 German families | Intrafamilial heterogeneity | 9p24–22 | Maximum multipoint LOD score of 3.78 | (40) |
| 2 Italian families | Autosomal dominant | The above 3 loci | No linkage | (41) |

*Abbreviations*: FC, French-Canadian; LOD, logarithm-of-odds; TDT, transmission disequilibrium test; HLOD, heterogeneity logarithm-of-odds.

In a Chinese (Han) RLS pedigree (36), microsatellite markers that cover the chromosomal regions flanking 16 candidate genes responsible for dopaminergic transmission or iron metabolism were genotyped. Results showed that the LOD scores at a recombination fraction of 0.00 are smaller than −2.00, which indicated that these loci were not linked to familial RLS of the pedigree. The known RLS loci were not analyzed in the Chinese study. Recently, Adel et al. (41) investigated whether a large multigenerational family (196 individuals spaning 7 generations) and a small family (5 members in 2 generations) are linked to the above 3 RLS loci, both originating in a small alpine village in the Western Alps of South Tyrol in northern Italy. Inheritance of RLS was consistent with autosomal dominant transmission, and linkage analysis excluded all three known loci for RLS. Several iron regulatory genes and spinal cerebellar atrophy genes are also reported to be normal in RLS population (36,42).

In summary, three genetic loci have been defined for RLS on chromosome 12q (RLS1), 14q (RLS2), and 9p (RLS3); however, the specific RLS gene at each locus remains to be identified or cloned.

## GENETIC ASSOCIATION STUDIES

Genetic association analysis is often used to establish a genetic link between a genetic determinant (variants in a candidate gene) and the target disease phenotype. Two association studies have been carried out for RLS.

The molecular mechanism for the pathogenesis of RLS remains largely unknown. A growing literature suggests the involvement of the dopaminergic system in the etiology of RLS. The clinical improvement observed with agents increasing the dopaminergic transmission (20) and evidence provided by brain imaging studies (43,44) support the hypothesis of a central dopaminergic dysfunction in RLS. Desautels et al. (45) analyzed eight candidate genes involved in dopaminergic transmission and metabolism for RLS using a population-based case–control study with a French-Canadian population. They studied dopaminergic receptors D1 to D5, dopamine transporter, tyrosine hydroxylase, and dopamine b-hydroxylase. However, comparison of allele and genotype frequencies between 92 patients with RLS and 182 controls matched for ethnic background suggests that these candidate genes are not associated with RLS. Further stratification analyses according to age at onset and periodic leg movements during sleep index found no significant differences for any of the genes examined. Nevertheless, the authors believe that the importance of dopamine in the pathogenesis of RLS cannot be ruled out, as other genes in the dopaminergic system have not yet been examined. Moreover, the possibility remains that other functional polymorphisms that are not in linkage disequilibrium with those investigated might affect the occurrence or the outcome of the syndrome.

A later study (46) from the same group claimed the finding for a genetic association between monoamine oxidase (MAO) A and RLS using a small sample size. MAO is a mitochondrial enzyme that catalyzes the degradation of several neuroactive amines, including dopamine, through oxidative deamination. Based on substrate selectivity and biochemical characteristics, two isoenzymes of MAO, designated MAOA and MAOB, have been described. MAOA preferentially deaminates serotonin and morepinephrine, whereas MAOB exhibits a higher affinity for phenylethylamine and benzylamine. Dopamine is a common substrate of both forms of the enzyme. The two MAO isoenzymes are encoded by two distinct, but closely linked genes on human chromosome Xp11. To investigate a possible role for the MAOA and MAOB genes in RLS, Desautels et al. (46) examined a dinucleotide repeat located within the second intron of the MAOB gene and a functional variable number of tandem repeat polymorphism in the MAOA gene promoter region (47). The study involved 96 extensively characterized RLS patients and 200 control subjects matched for ethnic background. The results indicate that females with the high-activity allele of the MAOA gene had a greater risk (OR: 2.0; 95% CI: 1.06 to 3.77) of being affected with RLS than females carrying the low-activity alleles. The authors (46) did not observe this association among the male subjects. No differences were observed regarding the MAOB gene in the samples. It will be interesting to determine whether the association of the MAOA gene and RLS can be replicated in another independent population.

## CONCLUSION AND OUTLOOK

Family history and twin studies suggest that genetic factors contribute to the pathogenesis of RLS. Epidemiological studies also identified several environmental factors that increase the risk to RLS, for example, poor general health and mental health status, gender, age, diabetes, BMI, and smoking. As a complex disease trait, RLS is expected to be caused by genetic factors, environmental factors, and the interactions among these factors. Genetic dissection of the RLS phenotype indicates that RLS is a highly inheritable trait. Genome-wide linkage analysis has defined three genetic loci for RLS: RLS1 on chromosome 12q, RLS2 on 14q, and RLS3 on 9p24–22. These studies provide a framework for the ultimate identification and cloning of the genes for RLS.

The future research in the field of RLS genetics will continue to focus on: (i) identification of new genetic loci for RLS, (ii) identification of the first gene for RLS and other RLS genes by positional cloning, and (iii) identification of candidate genes that are associated with RLS by population-based case–control studies. Identification of the first RLS gene will define the genetic pathway for the pathogenesis of RLS, which will provide fundamental understanding of the disease's process involved in the pathogenesis of RLS. Identification of the RLS genes promises to revolutionize the diagnosis and treatment of RLS. Genetic testing will make diagnosis more accurate. RLS genes can serve as targets for developing drugs that can prevent or treat RLS.

## REFERENCES


1. Phillips B, Young T, Finn L, et al. Epidemiology of restless legs symptoms in adults. Arch Intern Med 2000; 160(14):2137–2141.
2. Rothdach AJ, Trenkwalder C, Haberstock J, et al. Prevalence and risk factors of RLS in an elderly population: the MEMO study. Memory and morbidity in Augsburg elderly. Neurology 2000; 54(5):1064–1068.
3. Ulfberg J, Nystrom B, Carter N, et al. Prevalence of restless legs syndrome among men aged 18 to 64 years: an association with somatic disease and neuropsychiatric symptoms. Mov Disord 2001; 16(6):1159–1163.
4. Ulfberg J, Nystrom B, Carter N, et al. Restless legs syndrome among working-aged women. Eur Neurol 2001; 46(1):17–19.
5. Kageyama T, Kabuto M, Nitta H, et al. Prevalences of periodic limb movement-like and restless legs-like symptoms among Japanese adults. Psychiatry Clin Neurosci 2000; 54(3):296–298.

6. Tan EK, Ondo W. Restless legs syndrome: clinical features and treatment. Am J Med Sci 2000; 319(6):397–403.
7. Berger K, Luedemann J, Trenkwalder C, et al. Sex and the risk of restless legs syndrome in the general population. Arch Intern Med 2004; 164(2):196–202.
8. Ondo WG, Vuong KD, Wang Q. Restless legs syndrome in monozygotic twins: clinical correlates. Neurology 2000; 55(9):1404–1406.
9. Farrer LA, Cupples LA. Determining the genetic component of a disease. In: Haines JL, Pericak-Vance MA, eds. Approaches to Gene Mapping in Complex Human Diseases. New York: Wiley-Liss, 1998:93–129.
10. Chen S, Ondo WG, Rao S, et al. Genomewide linkage scan identifies a novel susceptibility locus for restless legs syndrome on chromosome 9p. Am J Hum Genet 2004; 74(5):876–885.
11. LaBuda MC. Epidemiology, family patterns and genetics of restless legs. RLS Foundation Conference, Washington, D.C., 1997.
12. Desai AV, Cherkas LF, Spector TD, et al. Genetic influences in self-reported symptoms of obstructive sleep apnoea and restless legs: a twin study. Twin Res 2004; 7(6):589–595.
13. Winkelmann J, Wetter TC, Collado-Seidel V, et al. Clinical characteristics and frequency of the hereditary restless legs syndrome in a population of 300 patients. Sleep 2000; 23(5):597–602.
14. Ondo W, Jankovic J. Restless legs syndrome: clinicoetiologic correlates. Neurology 1996; 47(6):1435–1441.
15. Montplaisir J, Boucher S, Poirier G, et al. Clinical, polysomnographic, and genetic characteristics of restless legs syndrome: a study of 133 patients diagnosed with new standard criteria. Mov Disord 1997; 12(1):61–65.
16. Walters AS, Hickey K, Maltzman J, et al. A questionnaire study of 138 patients with restless legs syndrome: the 'Night-Walkers' survey. Neurology 1996; 46(1):92–95.
17. Winkelmann J, Muller-Myhsok B, Wittchen HU, et al. Complex segregation analysis of restless legs syndrome provides evidence for an autosomal dominant mode of inheritance in early age at onset families. Ann Neurol 2002; 52(3):297–302.
18. Lazzarini A, Walters AS, Hickey K, et al. Studies of penetrance and anticipation in five autosomal-dominant restless legs syndrome pedigrees. Mov Disord 1999; 14(1):111–116.
19. Trenkwalder C, Seidel VC, Gasser T, et al. Clinical symptoms and possible anticipation in a large kindred of familial restless legs syndrome. Mov Disord 1996; 11(4):389–394.
20. Allen RP, Earley CJ. Restless legs syndrome: a review of clinical and pathophysiologic features. J Clin Neurophysiol 2001; 18(2):128–147.
21. Allen RP, LaBuda MC, Becker PM, et al. Family history study of RLS patients from two clinical population [abstr]. Sleep Res 1997; 26:309.
22. Allen RP, Earley CJ. Defining the phenotype of the restless legs syndrome (RLS) using age-of-symptom-onset. Sleep Med 2000; 1(1):11–19.
23. Polydefkis M, Allen RP, Hauer P, et al. Subclinical sensory neuropathy in late-onset restless legs syndrome. Neurology 2000; 55(8):1115–1121.
24. Montagna P, Coccagna G, Cirignotta F, et al. Familial Restless Legs Syndrome: Long-Term Evolution. New York: Raven Press, 1983.
25. Montplaisir J, Godbout R, Boghen D, et al. Familial restless legs with periodic movements in sleep: electrophysiologic, biochemical, and pharmacologic study. Neurology 1985; 35(1):130–134.
26. Walters AS, Picchietti D, Hening W, et al. Variable expressivity in familial restless legs syndrome. Arch Neurol 1990; 47(11):1219–1220.
27. Desautels A, Turecki G, Montplaisir J, et al. Identification of a major susceptibility locus for restless legs syndrome on chromosome 12q. Am J Hum Genet 2001; 69(6):1266–1270.
28. http://0-ghr.nlm.nih.gov.library.unl.edu/ghr/glossary/anticipation.
29. S.A.G.E. Statistical Analysis for Genetic Epidemiology, 4.4. A computer program package available from Statistical Solutions, Cork, Ireland, 2003.
30. Risch N. Linkage strategies for genetically complex traits. I. Multilocus models. Am J Hum Genet 1990; 46(2):222–228.
31. Olson JM, Witte JS, Elston RC. Genetic mapping of complex traits. Stat Med 1999; 18(21):2961–2981.

32. Wang Q, Chen Q. Cardiovascular disease and congenital defects. In: Encyclopedia of Life Sciences, 2000: A1907.
33. Kock N, Culjkovic B, Maniak S, et al. Mode of inheritance and susceptibility locus for restless legs syndrome, on chromosome 12q. Am J Hum Genet 2002; 71(1):205–208; author reply:208.
34. Desautels A, Turecki G, Montplaisir J, et al. Restless legs syndrome: confirmation of linkage to chromosome 12q, genetic heterogeneity, and evidence of complexity. Arch Neurol 2005; 62(4):591–596.
35. Winkelmann J, Lichtner P, Pütz B, et al. Evidence for further genetic locus heterogeneity and confirmation of RLS-1 in restless legs syndrome. Mov Disord 2005; 21(1):28–33.
36. Li J, Hu LD, Wang WJ, et al. Linkage analysis of the candidate genes of familial restless legs syndrome. Yi Chuan Xue Bao 2003; 30(4):325–329.
37. Bonati MT, Ferini-Strambi L, Aridon P, et al. Autosomal dominant restless legs syndrome maps on chromosome 14q. Brain 2003; 126(Pt 6):1485–1492.
38. Levchenko A, Montplaisir JY, Dube MP, et al. The 14q restless legs syndrome locus in the French Canadian population. Ann Neurol 2004; 55(6):887–891.
39. Chen S, Li L, Rao S, et al. Reply to ray and weeks: linkage for restless legs syndrome on chromosome 9p is significant. Am J Hum Genet 2005; 76(4):707–710.
40. Liebetanz KM, Winkelmann J, Trenkwalder C, et al. RLS3: fine-mapping of an autosomal dominant locus in a family with intrafamilial heterogeneity. Neurology 2006, 67(2), 320–321.
41. Adel S, Djarmati A, Kabakci K, et al. Co-occurrence of restless legs syndrome and Parkin mutations in two families. Mov Disord 2006; 21:258–263.
42. Konieczny M, Bauer P, Tomiuk J, et al. CAG repeats in restless legs syndrome. Am J Med Genet B Neuropsychiatr Genet 2006; 141:173–176.
43. Staedt J, Stoppe G, Kogler A, et al. Nocturnal myoclonus syndrome (periodic movements in sleep) related to central dopamine D2-receptor alteration. Eur Arch Psychiatry Clin Neurosci 1995; 245(1):8–10.
44. Turjanski N, Lees AJ, Brooks DJ. Striatal dopaminergic function in restless legs syndrome: 18F-dopa and 11C-raclopride PET studies. Neurology 1999; 52(5):932–937.
45. Desautels A, Turecki G, Montplaisir J, et al. Dopaminergic neurotransmission and restless legs syndrome: a genetic association analysis. Neurology 2001; 57(7):1304–1306.
46. Desautels A, Turecki G, Montplaisir J, et al. Evidence for a genetic association between monoamine oxidase A and restless legs syndrome. Neurology 2002; 59(2):215–219.
47. Deckert J, Catalano M, Syagailo YV, et al. Excess of high activity monoamine oxidase A gene promoter alleles in female patients with panic disorder. Hum Mol Genet 1999; 8(4):621–624.

# 9 Consequences of Sleep Deprivation

**Li Ling Lim**

*Department of Neurology, Sleep Disorders Unit, Singapore General Hospital, National Neuroscience Institute, Singapore, Republic of Singapore*

**Nancy Foldvary-Schaefer**

*Department of Neurology, Sleep Disorders Center, Cleveland Clinic Foundation, Cleveland, Ohio, U.S.A.*

## INTRODUCTION

With the invention of the light bulb and ready availability of electrical power, sleep loss has become increasingly prevalent in industrialized nations. Air travel across multiple time zones, globalization of commercial markets, shift work, 24/7 services, television, and the Internet have contributed to longer waking hours and reduced sleep. The mean number of hours of nocturnal sleep has fallen steadily in the last century from about 9 to 6.9 hours in 2005, based on the most recent National Sleep Foundation Poll (1). The proportion of Americans sleeping 8 or more hours on weekday nights has fallen steadily from 38% in 2001 to 26% in 2005. Therefore, sleep deprivation (SD) has become one of the most important yet understated public health issues of modern times.

Restless legs syndrome (RLS) can result in marked SD. In one tertiary center that specializes in RLS, the SD seen in RLS on polysomnography was greater than that of any illness except mania and fatal familial insomnia (Allen, personal communication). In this chapter, we will discuss the medical and neuropsychiatric consequences of SD.

### How Much Sleep Do We Need?

Sleep needs vary from one individual to another and with age. Most adults require 6 to 10 hours of sleep per night to function optimally. Experts often recommend at least 8 hours of sleep, estimating that 1 hour of sleep is needed for every 2 hours awake (2). A recent dose–response sleep restriction experiment showed that cumulative wakefulness in excess of 16 hours resulted in performance lapses, whereas cognitive performance remained stable with 8 hours of sleep (3). With the exception of "short sleepers" who function well with less sleep than expected for their age, most people sleeping fewer than 5 to 6 hours per night are not getting enough sleep (4). In the 2005 National Sleep Foundation Poll, adult Americans reported that a minimum of 6.5 hours of sleep on average was needed for optimal daytime functioning. The median sleep duration was 7 to 7.9 hours and 16% of respondents slept less than 6 hours on weekday nights.

Large epidemiological surveys have consistently demonstrated a U-shaped association between sleep duration and mortality, with a nadir at 7 hours (5,6). Life expectancy is significantly reduced in people sleeping less than 4.5 hours per night and the mortality risk is even greater in subjects sleeping over 7.5 hours per night, even after controlling for comorbidities. These findings strongly suggest that sleep needs should be individualized and that a standard recommendation of 8 hours of sleep per night should not be uniformly made.

### Sleep Deprivation vs. Sleep Fragmentation

While Dement has stated "all wakefulness is sleep deprivation," SD usually refers to the "failure to obtain sufficient nocturnal sleep to support normal alert wakefulness" (2). Volitional chronic partial SD with its detrimental effects, classified as behaviorally induced insufficient sleep syndrome by the International Classification of Sleep Disorders 2, is the most common form of SD in humans (7).

Sleep loss can be voluntary or produced by a variety of environmental factors, or medical, psychiatric, and sleep disorders which disrupt sleep, including chronic pain, depression, sleep apnea, and RLS. High-frequency sleep fragmentation due to repeated arousals from sleep produces nonrestorative sleep and results in similar neurobehavioral consequences and performance deficits as voluntary SD (8). Sleep fragmentation and SD both result in daytime sleepiness, decreased psychomotor performance, and comparable physiological changes (9). In combination, voluntary sleep restriction and sleep fragmentation due to underlying medical or sleep disorders, both individually common occurrences, are likely to have synergistic and therefore even greater negative impact.

### Behaviorally Induced Insufficient Sleep Syndrome

Volitional, but unintentional lack of sleep, is often chronic and a result of the excessive social and occupational demands of modern life and inadequate sleep hygiene. Excessive daytime sleepiness is the chief complaint, associated with a host of secondary symptoms such as fatigue, low energy, poor concentration, inattention, irritability, and dysphoria. The nocturnal habitual sleep period is shorter in duration than expected for age, leading to the common habit of sleeping in on weekends to "catch up." Polysomnographic features include a short sleep onset latency, high sleep efficiency, and prolonged total sleep time if allowed to sleep in. A short sleep latency with or without multiple sleep onset rapid eye movement (REM) sleep periods (SOREMPs) is typically observed on multiple sleep latency testing (MSLT).

SD can be acute or chronic, partial or total. While prolonged total sleep loss is rarely encountered in humans outside of a research setting, chronic partial sleep loss is a frequent occurrence, affecting an estimated one-third or more of normal adults, with especially severe sleep loss seen in night-shift workers (10).

## HUMAN EXPERIMENTAL SLEEP DEPRIVATION

Although the optimal duration and function of sleep remain unclear, the detrimental effects of SD have been studied for over a century. Human SD studies are discussed in detail below. Animal studies are also briefly reviewed for comparison. Experiments have addressed the effects of total, partial, and selective SD and recovery sleep.

The effects of total SD and partial SD in humans are qualitatively similar, with differences mainly in the time course of symptom evolution (3). Selective deprivation of specific stages, such as REM or slow wave sleep (SWS), has not consistently been shown to cause major psychological disturbances or performance decrements (11).

Total SD experiments, including one of the first in 1896 (90 hours) and the longest documented (264 hours or 11 days), have consistently produced the following effects (12,13):

1. Sleepiness, especially severe at night (circadian variation), which can be overcome with arousal (e.g., external stimulation and physical activity) and brief sleep episodes ("microsleep"), which are usually imperceptible to the subject.
2. Mild dysphoria and irritability.
3. Impaired performance in tasks requiring close attention such as vigilance testing, but not visually stimulating motor activity such as exciting arcade games. Performance can be transiently improved with motivation and incentives.
4. Neurological disturbances including visual illusions and hallucinations, blurred vision, ptosis, disorientation incoordination, slurred speech, memory lapses, delusions, slowed mentation, and difficulty in thinking.
5. Mild decrease in body temperature, but no major physical or metabolic abnormalities.
6. Relatively short recovery sleep over 1 to 3 nights with apparent return to baseline alertness and function, comprising approximately 25% of total sleep lost: two-thirds of lost SWS, one-third of lost REM sleep, and less than 10% of lost light non-REM (NREM) sleep.

A recent large-scale, dose–response chronic sleep restriction experiment compared the neurobehavioral and physiological effects of partial and total SD (3). Chronic partial SD of 4 to 6 hours per night over 14 days resulted in significant cumulative, dose-dependent deficits in cognitive performance and an increase in self-reported daytime sleepiness. The cognitive effects of chronic partial SD of 6 hours or less per night was equivalent to that produced by 2 nights of total SD. The rate of deterioration was inversely related to the duration of sleep time, with total SD producing more rapid decrements. Relatively moderate sleep restriction seriously impaired waking neurobehavioral functions in healthy adults. The subjects were largely unaware of these.

## Effect of Sleep Deprivation on Alertness, Mood, and Performance

### *Alertness*

Sleepiness is the most evident consequence of SD. Carskadon and Dement performed the earliest studies using the MSLT to measure the effects of total SD on young adults. A marked and persistent decline in mean sleep latency (MSL) approaching zero and returning to baseline after the second recovery night was observed. Performance and mood similarly declined following two nights of total SD (14). The same authors reported similar relative reductions in MSL with partial SD, when the normal sleep period was shortened by only 30 to 60 minutes (15). When partial SD was prolonged, the MSL was further reduced.

These early observations of the cumulative effect of partial sleep restriction on waking functions have since been confirmed in other studies and have led to the concept that SD results in the accumulation of a "sleep debt" that must be repaid in order to restore normal alertness (16).

### *Mood*

A meta-analysis of 19 studies reported over the last several decades concluded that mood is more vulnerable to SD than either cognitive or motor performance (17).

Mood ratings of sleep-deprived subjects were found to be more than three standard deviations worse than non–sleep-deprived individuals.

One study of partial SD for seven consecutive nights in healthy young adults reported increased mood disturbances and negative mood states, which the authors postulated may be exacerbated by the stresses of coping with daytime sleepiness, impaired cognition, and the compensatory effort required to stay awake and motivated during the day (16). In physician trainees who slept an average of only 5.95 hours daily, a higher incidence of depression was found in the internship year than expected for age group, with risk factors being female sex, unmarried status, and a past history of major depression (18). In another study, surgical residents whose sleep was acutely restricted to less than 4 hours per night were found to be more depressed, tense, and angry than in the rested state (19).

Interestingly, in depressed subjects, SD has the reverse effect (i.e., antidepressant), which is short-lived and reversible in most cases after a single night of recovery sleep (20). Although the mechanism remains unclear, partial, total, and selective SD have all been used successfully to treat depression (21).

*Performance*

Sleep loss has consistently been shown to significantly impair psychomotor performance. One meta-analysis found that the mean level of functioning of sleep-deprived subjects was comparable to that of only the ninth percentile of non–sleep-deprived subjects (17). Cognitive performance was found to be more affected than motor performance, and mood was much more affected than either cognitive or motor performance.

Performance deficits involving vigilance are evident after only two nights of mild sleep restriction to 5 hours (15,22). With longer duration (60 days) of comparable degrees of sleep loss, progressive decline in vigilance is seen (23). Similar cumulative deficits in alertness and performance have been shown in partial and total SD, with greater and more rapidly accumulating deficits with total SD.

In contrast to vigilance tasks, a controlled study of 11 male subjects showed that up to 60 hours of sleep loss did not significantly impair physical performance testing, including isometric and isokinetic muscular strength and endurance, and cardiovascular and respiratory responses to treadmill running (24). Military studies have also shown that physical performance remains relatively unaffected in spite of severe sleep restriction (0–3 hours of sleep) for up to nine days (25,26).

The impact of SD on performance is particularly relevant in everyday tasks such as driving and in certain occupations where chronic sleep restriction is common. The U.S. Department of Transportation recently identified fatigue as the number one safety problem in transportation operations, costing billions of dollars annually (27). In June 2003, the state of New Jersey was the first in the United States to pass legislation prohibiting driving a motor vehicle while impaired by lack of sleep (28).

Impairment in simulated driving tests after modest sleep loss has been shown to be comparable to that produced by alcohol. In one study, 18.5 and 21 hours of wakefulness produced deficits of the same magnitude as 0.05% and 0.08% blood alcohol concentration, respectively (29). The combined effect of sleep restriction and alcohol is additive, reducing alertness, and impairing simulated automobile driving in healthy young men, even with low alcohol intake and safe alcohol concentrations below 0.08% blood alcohol concentration, the legal intoxication level in most states (30,31). The effects of regular sleep loss on driving are further exacerbated by coexisting disorders like sleep apnea, the treatment of which with positive airway pressure therapy has been shown to reduce the risk of traffic accidents (32).

Certain high-risk occupations such as physician trainees are particularly vulnerable to chronic partial SD. One study showed that interns slept an average of less than 6 hours per night (18). Acutely sleep-deprived house officers exhibited significant deficits in mental tasks involving rote memory, language, numeric skills, and high-level cognitive tasks (33). A study of rested vs. fatigued anesthesia residents showed significant deterioration in tasks requiring vigilance in a simulated monitoring situation (34). Physician trainees were also shown to have a higher incidence of drowsy driving and sleep-related motor vehicle accidents, especially post-call, than a control group of rested physicians (35).

## Factors Affecting the Impact of SD on Alertness, Mood, and Performance

The impact of SD on alertness, mood, and performance is influenced by extrinsic factors such as those causing arousal, and intrinsic factors such as sleep homeostasis, circadian rhythm effects, and age.

### *Extrinsic Factors*

Because our propensity to sleep is a balance of sleep debt and level of arousal, it stands to reason that extrinsic factors that increase arousal can counteract and even mask the effects of sleep loss. Physical activity or exercise and stimulant drugs, including caffeine, are common examples.

In a study of 12 normal adults, a five-minute walk produced a significant elevation of heart rate, a measure of physiological arousal, and prolongation of mean sleep onset latency on the MSLT (36). The performance benefits of exercise are short-lived. Longer periods of physical activity do not improve overall performance in sleep deprived individuals (37). Bright light, noise, and ambient temperature are other extrinsic factors that have also been shown to increase arousal (38–42). For example, a driving simulator study using noise (radio) and cold air as a countermeasure to sleepiness in partially sleep-deprived young adults demonstrated improvement in subjective sleepiness scores and a trend toward reduction of "lane-drifting" incidents. The increased alertness was, however only marginal and transient, and comparatively less effective than a short nap (<15 minutes) or 150 mg of caffeine (42).

There is an extensive body of literature demonstrating the effects of stimulant drugs on mood, alertness, and performance following SD. Amphetamines reverse the effects of 48 hours SD on sleep latency and behavior in a dose-dependent manner (43). Methylphenidate increased MSL, improved performance on vigilance tasks, as well as depression and fatigue scores in a placebo-controlled study (44). Similar alerting and performance benefits have been demonstrated with modafinil (45,46). Caffeine has also been shown to reverse the effects of SD on alertness and mood. A double-blind study of normal subjects sleep deprived for 49 hours showed that a 600 mg dose of caffeine significantly increased sleep latency and decreased sleepiness, fatigue, and confusion to near resting levels (47).

Performance can also be affected by factors related to the test situation such as level of interest in a given task and by incentives such as financial rewards for good performance (48,49). Immediate feedback produces momentary arousal that can improve performance, while increasing task duration has the opposite effect (50). Increasing the difficulty and complexity of a task also adversely affects performance (51,52). Generally, the most profound deficits are observed on tasks that are long in duration, newly learned, difficult, externally paced, devoid of feedback, and have a memory component (51,53–55).

### *Sleep Homeostasis, Circadian Rhythm, and Other Intrinsic Factors*

Wakefulness accumulates sleep debt, which leads to increased sleepiness that, in turn, is discharged during sleep. This homeostatic process is modulated by the circadian pacemaker, which regulates level of alertness, usually lowest during the nocturnal hours and in the mid-afternoon (56) (Chapter 3).

A study of the effects of 72 hours of SD in 12 subjects, in whom levels of alertness, affect, motivation, and cognition were measured, showed that most of these variables were significantly affected by the number of days of sleep loss and all were significantly affected by the hour of the day (57). The peak time for self-reported complaints was in the early morning between 4:00 A.M. and 8:00 A.M., while the fewest symptoms were reported in the late afternoon between 4:00 P.M. and 8:00 P.M.

Sleep homeostasis is affected by daytime napping, which reduces sleep debt. Taking a nap before a period of prolonged wakefulness transiently improves alertness, mood, and performance in a dose-related manner (58). The beneficial effects of three- to four-hour prophylactic naps are comparable to a moderate dose of caffeine (300 mg), and the combined effect of naps and caffeine is additive (59).

Intrinsic factors such as age may have an impact, although relatively minor, on the effects of sleep loss. Tests of performance and alertness in normal older sleep-deprived subjects reveal loss of performance and alertness similar to that seen in younger individuals. However, older individuals may tolerate sleep loss with less decrease in ability compared to baseline than young adults, and may recover function faster than young adults (60).

## Neurologic Effects of Sleep Deprivation

Prolonged SD produces reversible neurologic signs such as slurred speech, hand tremor, ptosis, nystagmus and abnormal corneal, gag, and deep tendon reflexes (61,62). Sleep loss also affects immediate recall and short-term memory, causing memory deficits on testing similar to that seen with alcohol intoxication and aging, postulated to be due to impaired encoding and retrieval of information (55,63). On positron emission tomography studies, 24-hour SD resulted in a global decline in brain activity, most marked in the thalamus and prefrontal and posterior parietal cortices, areas mediating attention, and higher-order cognitive processes (64).

Electroencephalographic (EEG) studies have shown a progressive slowing of the waking alpha rhythm in proportion to the duration of sleep loss, with loss of alpha reactivity after prolonged SD (65). In one study, a correlation between theta and delta activity during wakefulness and impaired performance following SD was observed (66). Microsleep episodes lasting up to 10 seconds are also seen in the EEGs of healthy human subjects sleep deprived for 60 hours (67). Such microsleep episodes are ameliorated with stimulating agents such as modafinil (46).

SD has long been recognized as a precipitating factor for seizure recurrence in people with epilepsy. Patients with epilepsy frequently report SD as a seizure precipitant (68). SD is also often used as an activating procedure during routine EEG and long-term video EEG monitoring (69–71). Early studies in nonepileptic, mostly military populations who were profoundly sleep deprived, found a significantly higher incidence of seizures than in demographically similar populations who were not sleep deprived (72). EEG studies of both normal healthy subjects (65,73) and subjects with suspected epilepsy (74–77) have also demonstrated a clear increase in interictal epileptiform abnormalities following SD.

### Other Physiological Changes Associated with SD

Despite the vast body of evidence supporting the multitude of adverse consequences of SD on neurologic function, similarly marked changes in other organ systems have not been found (78). Accelerated metabolism (and premature death) following partial and total SD seen in animals has not been demonstrated in humans. However, sleep-deprived humans do exhibit similar declines in body temperature and increased sympathetic tone (12,79). The range of physiological changes associated with SD in cardiovascular, respiratory, endocrine, and immune function is discussed.

Several epidemiologic studies have found an association between cardiovascular morbidity and chronic sleep restriction (6,80). In the Nurses' Health Study, women sleeping less than 7 hours per night had an increased risk of coronary events compared to those averaging 8 hours. Precisely, how chronic SD affects cardiovascular morbidity remains unknown.

Respiratory testing in healthy adults has shown small but significant decreases in forced vital capacity, hypoxic and hypercapneic ventilatory responses after SD (81,82). SD has also been shown to cause reversible worsening of respiratory events in normal infants and adults with obstructive sleep apnea syndrome (83,84).

With the exception of thyroid hormones, appreciable hormonal alterations have not been observed after total SD, including catecholamine, cortisol, or sex hormone levels (85). With partial SD, impaired glucose tolerance, elevated evening cortisol levels, and thyroid function abnormalities have been reported (79). Sleep loss can alter the pattern of secretion of hormones under circadian influence. For example, selective deprivation of SWS can diminish the secretion of growth hormone (86).

Human studies have demonstrated a variety of changes in immune function following SD. However, firm evidence for increased susceptibility to infections is lacking. Some reported findings include

1. enhanced ability of lymphocytes to produce interferon (87),
2. impaired natural killer cell activity and T-cell cytokine production (88),
3. decreased DNA synthesis of blood lymphocytes (89),
4. altered antigen uptake (90), and
5. decreased antibody responses in humans to viral vaccines (91,92).

Although the studies examining the effect of SD on immune function in humans are difficult to compare due to differences in methodology, it is generally believed that sleep loss does influence the immune system. Short-term SD may enhance immune responses, while chronic sleep loss is probably detrimental.

### Selective Sleep Deprivation

The earliest REM SD experiments were conducted in an attempt to determine the function and necessity of REM sleep. Initial interest in this area of research was stimulated by the Freudian belief that subconscious impulses and desires, if unexpressed as dreams during REM sleep, would cause a buildup of "psychic pressure," and eventually lead to neurosis and psychosis. REM SD in rats induces hyperactivity, irritability, aggressiveness, stereotypy, and hypersexuality, which some authors consider a model for mania (93). In selective deprivation experiments in which human volunteers would be awoken at the first sign of REM sleep, REM sleep onset latency decreased and REM sleep duration increased progressively, eventually producing SOREMPs. REM SD caused confusion, bad temperedness, and severe sleepiness, but not psychosis (2). While animal studies have shown an association between REM sleep and memory and learning, firm evidence for this in humans is lacking. REM density has been reported to increase after training in humans, implicating REM sleep in memory processing (94). Yet, antidepressant drugs that suppress REM sleep are used commonly without apparent adverse effect on memory, suggesting that the role of REM sleep in human memory and learning is complex and poorly understood.

In comparison to selective REM deprivation, there are fewer studies addressing selective deprivation of SWS in humans. Selective SWS deprivation studies are difficult to perform and often affected by methodological problems. Selective SWS disruption, without reducing total sleep or sleep efficiency, has been associated with fatigue, decreased pain threshold, and reduced vigor (95). However, daytime performance testing following several nights of either REM or SWS deprivation has not been shown to result in apparent decrements (11).

### Changes in Sleep Architecture During and After SD

The effect of SD on sleep architecture was studied in healthy subjects who underwent partial sleep restriction (50% or 4 hours) for four nights followed by three recovery nights of 8 hours (96). During the period of SD, there was decreased light NREM sleep (stages 1, 2) and REM sleep, but SWS was mostly unaffected. On the first recovery night, there was shortening of the sleep onset latency and increased total sleep time, including enhanced SWS and REM sleep. On the second recovery night, SWS duration approached normal while REM sleep rebound continued. Sleep architecture subsequently normalized by the third recovery night.

### Recovery from Sleep Deprivation

The effects of SD on alertness and performance reverse after 1 to 3 nights of recovery sleep, regardless of the duration of prior wakefulness (63,97,98). Studies of prolonged total SD have shown that the amount of recovery sleep required to restore baseline performance is only about 25% of the amount of sleep loss incurred (12,13). It is unclear whether this means that accumulated sleep debt need not be repaid in full as originally thought, or if residual deficits may be too small to be measurable or difficult to measure in typical SD paradigms.

## ANIMAL SLEEP DEPRIVATION STUDIES

Animal models of SD, employing in some cases long periods of sleep loss, have demonstrated more pronounced abnormalities than observed in sleep-deprived humans (99,100). Rats subjected to SD experience weight loss and assume a malnourished appearance in spite of increased food intake. Skin lesions (ulcers and discolored fur), increased energy expenditure due to increased heat loss, decreased body temperature during the late stages of deprivation, biochemical changes including increased plasma norepinephrine and decreased plasma thyroxine are observed. Eventual death ensues after an average of 19 days of near-total SD. Animals subjected to selective REM or SWS deprivation survive longer. The mechanisms leading to death after total SD are unclear and confounded by the effect of stress, which accompanies profound sleep loss. Proposed mechanisms include hypothermia, hypermetabolism, and impaired immunity, but none have been firmly proven. For example, septicemia involving opportunistic microbes, implicating impaired immunity in the hypercatabolic, malnourished, and ultimately life-threatening state associated with prolonged SD was described (101). However, subsequent studies demonstrated that elimination of the bacterial invasion did not prevent hypothermia or early death in rats subjected to total SD (102).

Studies of recovery sleep in surviving rats have shown near-complete reversal of SD-related changes in appearance, metabolism, temperature, biochemistry, and high energy expenditure (103). Recovery sleep is characterized by immediate and prominent REM sleep rebound, which contrasts with the SWS rebound seen in humans.

## CONCLUSIONS

Human studies have consistently demonstrated significant detrimental effects of SD on alertness, mood, performance, and neurological function. Chronic SD has been associated with increased all-cause and cardiovascular mortality. Physiological effects are relatively minor and include changes in thermoregulation, respiratory, endocrine, and immune function. Chronic partial SD is often unrecognized and likely represents one of the most important public health issues in modern society. Dement considered "the pervasive lack of awareness about SD a national emergency" (2). The additive effects of alcohol, drugs, social and occupational demands, and the coexistence of common disorders that disrupt sleep, including chronic pain, depression, sleep apnea, and RLS, exacerbate the problem. The impact of SD on transportation and occupational safety, comparable to the effects of alcohol intoxication, are potentially catastrophic. Measures to address these concerns have included legislation against drowsy driving, later school start times, and restriction of duty hours for physician trainees. These measures underscore the serious health and socioeconomic consequences of sleep loss, but represent just a few of the initiatives required to manage this enormous problem.

## REFERENCES

1. National Sleep Foundation. 2005 Sleep in America Poll, 2005.
2. Dement WC, Vaughan C. The promise of sleep. The scientific connection between health, happiness, and a good night's sleep. 1999.
3. Van Dongen HP, Maislin G, Mullington JM, Dinges DF. The cumulative cost of additional wakefulness: dose-response effects on neurobehavioral functions and sleep physiology from chronic sleep restriction and total sleep deprivation. Sleep 2003; 26(2):117–126.
4. American Academy of Sleep Medicine. International Classification of Sleep Disorders, revised. Diagnostic and Coding Manual. 2001:87–90.
5. Tamakoshi A, Ohno Y. Self-reported sleep duration as a predictor of all-cause mortality: results from the JACC study, Japan. Sleep 2004; 27(1):51–54.

6. Kripke DF, Garfinkel L, Wingard DL, Klauber MR, Marler MR. Mortality associated with sleep duration and insomnia. Arch Gen Psychiatry 2002; 59(2):131–136.
7. Sateia MJ. ICSD-2-The International Classification of Sleep Disorders. In: Diagnostic and Coding Manual-2, Westchester. 2nd. Illinois: American Academy of Sleep Medicine, 2005:104–106.
8. Bonnet MH, Arand DL. Clinical effects of sleep fragmentation versus sleep deprivation. Sleep Med Rev 2003; 7(4):297–310.
9. Bonnet MH. Effect of sleep disruption on sleep, performance, and mood. Sleep 1985; 8(1):11–19.
10. Bonnet MH, Arand DL. We are chronically sleep deprived. Sleep 1995; 18(10):908–911.
11. Johnson LC, Naitoh P, Moses JM, Lubin A. Interaction of REM deprivation and stage 4 deprivation with total sleep loss: experiment 2. Psychophysiology 1974; 11(2):147–159.
12. Patrick GT, Gilbert JA. On the effects of loss of sleep. Psychol Rev 1896; 3:469.
13. Gulevich G, Dement W, Johnson L. Psychiatric and EEG observations on a case of prolonged (264 hours) wakefulness. Arch Gen Psychiatry 1966; 15(1):29–35.
14. Carskadon MA, Dement WC. Effects of total sleep loss on sleep tendency. Percept Mot Skills 1979; 48(2):495–506.
15. Carskadon MA, Dement WC. Cumulative effects of sleep restriction on daytime sleepiness. Psychophysiology 1981; 18(2):107–113.
16. Dinges DF, Pack F, Williams K, et al. Cumulative sleepiness, mood disturbance, and psychomotor vigilance performance decrements during a week of sleep restricted to 4–5 hours per night. Sleep 1997; 20(4):267.
17. Pilcher JJ, Huffcutt AI. Effects of sleep deprivation on performance: a meta-analysis. Sleep 1996; 19(4):318–326.
18. Ford CV, Wentz DK. The internship year: a study of sleep, mood states, and psychophysiologic parameters. South Med J 1984; 77(11):1435–1442.
19. Bartle EJ, Sun JH, Thompson L, Light AI, McCool C, Heaton S. The effects of acute sleep deprivation during residency training. Surgery 1988; 104(2):311–316.
20. Wu JC, Bunney WE. The biological basis of an antidepressant response to sleep deprivation and relapse: review and hypothesis. Am J Psychiatry 1990; 147(1):14–21.
21. Giedke H. The usefulness of therapeutic sleep deprivation in depression. J Affect Disord 2004; 78(1):85–86.
22. Wilkinson RT. Performance following a night of reduced sleep. Psychonom Sci 1966; 5:471.
23. Webb WB, Agnew HW, Jr. The effects of a chronic limitation of sleep length. Psychophysiology 1974; 11(3):265–274.
24. Symons JD, VanHelder T, Myles WS. Physical performance and physiological responses following 60 hours of sleep deprivation. Med Sci Sports Exerc 1988; 20(4):374–380.
25. Haslam DR. Sleep loss, recovery sleep, and military performance. Ergonomics 1982; 25(2):163–178.
26. Haslam DR. The military performance of soldiers in sustained operations. Aviat Space Environ Med 1984; 55(3):216–221.
27. Statistics. U.S. Department of Transportation. 2005; internet communication.
28. Senate and General Assembly of the State of New Jersey. An Act concerning vehicular homicide. Assembly, No. 1347 State of New Jersey 210th Legislature. 2003.
29. Arnedt JT, Wilde GJ, Munt PW, MacLean AW. How do prolonged wakefulness and alcohol compare in the decrements they produce on a simulated driving task?. Accid Anal Prev 2001; 33(3):337–344.
30. Roehrs T, Beare D, Zorick F, Roth T. Sleepiness and ethanol effects on simulated driving. Alcohol Clin Exp Res 1994; 18(1):154–158.
31. Horne JA, Reyner LA, Barrett PR. Driving impairment due to sleepiness is exacerbated by low alcohol intake. Occup Environ Med 2003; 60(9):689–692.
32. Cassel W, Ploch T, Becker C. Risk of traffic accidents in patients with sleep-disordered breathing: reduction with nasal CPAP. Eur Resp J 1996; 9:2606–2611.
33. Hawkins MR, Vichick DA, Silsby HD, Kruzich DJ, Butler R. Sleep and nutritional deprivation and performance of house officers. J Med Educ 1985; 60(7):530–535.

34. Denisco RA, Drummond JN, Gravenstein JS. The effect of fatigue on the performance of a simulated anesthetic monitoring task. J Clin Monit 1987; 3(1):22–24.
35. Marcus CL, Loughlin GM. Effect of sleep deprivation on driving safety in housestaff. Sleep 1996; 19(10):763–766.
36. Bonnet MH, Arand DL. Sleepiness as measured by modified multiple sleep latency testing varies as a function of preceding activity. Sleep 1998; 21(5):477–483.
37. Angus RG, Heslegrave RJ, Myles WS. Effects of prolonged sleep deprivation, with and without chronic physical exercise, on mood and performance. Psychophysiology 1985; 22(3):276–282.
38. Dijk DJ, Cajochen C, Borbely AA. Effect of a single 3-hour exposure to bright light on core body temperature and sleep in humans. Neurosci Lett 1991; 121(1–2):59–62.
39. Komada Y, Tanaka H, Yamamoto Y, Shirakawa S, Yamazaki K. Effects of bright light pre-exposure on sleep onset process. Psychiatry Clin Neurosci 2000; 54(3):365–366.
40. Tassi P, Nicolas A, Seegmuller C, Dewasmes G, Libert JP, Muzet A. Interaction of the alerting effect of noise with partial sleep deprivation and circadian rhythmicity of vigilance. Percept Mot Skills 1993; 77(3 Pt 2):1239–1248.
41. Poulton EC, Edwards RS, Colquhoun WP. The interaction of the loss of a night's sleep with mild heat: task variables. Ergonomics 1974; 17(1):59–73.
42. Reyner LA, Horne JA. Evaluation "in-car" countermeasures to sleepiness: cold air and radio. Sleep 1998; 21(1):46–50.
43. Newhouse PA, Belenky G, Thomas M, Thorne D, Sing HC, Fertig J. The effects of d-amphetamine on arousal, cognition, and mood after prolonged total sleep deprivation. Neuropsychopharmacology 1989; 2(2):153–164.
44. Bishop C, Roehrs T, Rosenthal L, Roth T. Alerting effects of methylphenidate under basal and sleep-deprived conditions. Exp Clin Psychopharmacol 1997; 5(4):344–352.
45. Pigeau R, Naitoh P, Buguet A, et al. Modafinil, d-amphetamine and placebo during 64 hours of sustained mental work. I. Effects on mood, fatigue, cognitive performance and body temperature. J Sleep Res 1995; 4(4):212–228.
46. Lagarde D, Batejat D, Van BP, Sarafian D, Pradella S. Interest of modafinil, a new psychostimulant, during a sixty-hour sleep deprivation experiment. Fundam Clin Pharmacol 1995; 9(3):271–279.
47. Penetar D, McCann U, Thorne D, et al. Caffeine reversal of sleep deprivation effects on alertness and mood. Psychopharmacology (Berl) 1993; 112(2–3):359–365.
48. Wilkinson RT. Effects of up to 60 hours' sleep deprivation on different types of work. Ergonomics 1964; 7:175–186.
49. Horne JA, Pettitt AN. High incentive effects on vigilance performance during 72 hours of total sleep deprivation. Acta Psychol (Amst) 1985; 58(2):123–139.
50. Steyvers FJ, Gaillard AW. The effects of sleep deprivation and incentives on human performance. Psychol Res 1993; 55(1):64–70.
51. Williams HL, Lubin A. Speeded addition and sleep loss. J Exp Psychol 1967; 73: 313–317.
52. Babkoff H, Mikulincer M, Caspy T, Kempinski D, Sing H. The topology of performance curves during 72 hours of sleep loss: a memory and search task. Q J Exp Psychol A 1988; 40(4):737–756.
53. Donnell JM. Performance decrement as a function of total sleep loss and task duration. Percept Mot Skills 1969; 29(3):711–714.
54. Light AI, Sun JH, McCool C, Thompson L, Heaton S, Bartle EJ. The effects of acute sleep deprivation on level of resident training. Curr Surg 1989; 46(1):29–30.
55. Nilsson LG, Backman L, Karlsson T. Priming and cued recall in elderly, alcohol intoxicated and sleep-deprived subjects: a case of functionally similar memory deficits. Psychol Med 1989; 19(2):423–433.
56. Richardson GS, Carskadon MA, Orav EJ, Dement WC. Circadian variation of sleep tendency in elderly and young adult subjects. Sleep 1982; 5(suppl 2):S82–S94.
57. Mikulincer M, Babkoff H, Caspy T, Sing H. The effects of 72 hours of sleep loss on psychological variables. Br J Psychol 1989; 80(Pt 2):145–162.
58. Bonnet MH, Gomez S, Wirth O, Arand DL. The use of caffeine versus prophylactic naps in sustained performance. Sleep 1995; 18(2):97–104.

59. Bonnet MH, Arand DL. The use of prophylactic naps and caffeine to maintain performance during a continuous operation. Ergonomics 1994; 37(6):1009–1020.
60. Bonnet MH, Arand DL. Sleep loss in aging. Clin Geriatr Med 1989; 5(2):405–420.
61. Kollar EJ, Namerow N, Pasnau RO, Naitoh P. Neurological findings during prolonged sleep deprivation. Neurology 1968; 18(9):836–840.
62. Ross JJ. Neurological findings after prolonged sleep deprivation. Arch Neurol 1965; 12:399–403.
63. Williams HL, Gieseking CF, Lubin A. Some effects of sleep loss on memory. Percept Mot Skills 1966; 23(3):1287–1293.
64. Thomas M, Sing H, Belenky G, et al. Neural basis of alertness and cognitive performance impairments during sleepiness. I. Effects of 24 h of sleep deprivation on waking human regional brain activity. J Sleep Res 2000; 9(4):335–352.
65. Rodin EA, Luby ED, Gottlieb JS. The electroencephalogram during prolonged experimental sleep deprivation. Electroencephalogr Clin Neurophysiol 1962; 14:544–551.
66. Naitoh P, Pasnau RO, Kollar EJ. Psychophysiological changes after prolonged deprivation of sleep. Biol Psychiatry 1971; 3(4):309–320.
67. Lagarde D, Batejat D. Evaluation of drowsiness during prolonged sleep deprivation. Neurophysiol Clin 1994; 24(1):35–44.
68. Nakken KO, Solaas MH, Kjeldsen MJ, Friis ML, Pellock JM, Corey LA. Which seizure-precipitating factors do patients with epilepsy most frequently report? Epilepsy Behav 2005; 6(1):85–89.
69. Gastaut H, Tassinari C. Triggering mechanisms in epilepsy. The electroclinical point of view. Epilepsia 1966; 7:85–138.
70. Dinner DS. Effect of sleep on epilepsy. J Clin Neurophysiol 2002; 19(6):504–513.
71. Mendez M, Radtke RA. Interactions between sleep and epilepsy. J Clin Neurophysiol 2001; 18(2):106–127.
72. Gunderson CH, Dunne PB, Feyer TL. Sleep deprivation seizures. Neurology 1973; 23(7):678–686.
73. Bennett DR. Sleep deprivation and major motor convulsions. Neurology 1963; 13: 953–958.
74. Bennett DR, Mattson RH, Ziter FA, Calverley JR, Liske EA, Pratt KL. Sleep deprivation: neurological and electroencephalographic effects. Aerosp Med 1964; 35:888–890.
75. Welch LK, Stevens JB. Clinical value of the electroencephalogram following sleep deprivation. Aerosp Med 1971; 42(3):349–351.
76. Mattson RH, Pratt KL, Calverley JR. Electroencephalograms of epileptics following sleep deprivation. Arch Neurol 1965; 13(3):310–315.
77. Pratt KL, Mattson RH, Weikers NJ, Williams R. EEG activation of epileptics following sleep deprivation: a prospective study of 114 cases. Electroencephalogr Clin Neurophysiol 1968; 24(1):11–15.
78. Horne JA. A review of the biological effects of total sleep deprivation in man. Biol Psychol 1978; 7(1–2):55–102.
79. Spiegel K, Leproult R, Van CE. Impact of sleep debt on metabolic and endocrine function. Lancet 1999; 354(9188):1435–1439.
80. Ayas NT, White DP, Manson JE, et al. A prospective study of sleep duration and coronary heart disease in women. Arch Intern Med 2003; 163(2):205–209.
81. Cooper KR, Phillips BA. Effect of short-term sleep loss on breathing. J Appl Physiol 1982; 53(4):855–858.
82. White DP, Douglas NJ, Pickett CK, Zwillich CW, Weil JV. Sleep deprivation and the control of ventilation. Am Rev Respir Dis 1983; 128(6):984–986.
83. Canet E, Gaultier C, D'Allest AM, Dehan M. Effects of sleep deprivation on respiratory events during sleep in healthy infants. J Appl Physiol 1989; 66(3):1158–1163.
84. Persson HE, Svanborg E. Sleep deprivation worsens obstructive sleep apnea. Comparison between diurnal and nocturnal polysomnography. Chest 1996; 109(3): 645–650.
85. Gary KA, Winokur A, Douglas SD, Kapoor S, Zaugg L, Dinges DF. Total sleep deprivation and the thyroid axis: effects of sleep and waking activity. Aviat Space Environ Med 1996; 67(6):513–519.

86. Beck U, Marquetand D. Effects of selective sleep deprivation on sleep-linked prolactin and growth hormone secretion. Arch Psychiatr Nervenkr 1976; 223(1):35–44.
87. Palmblad J, Cantell K, Strander H. Stressor exposure and immunological response in man: interferon producing capacity and phagocytosis. Psychosom Res 1976; 20: 193–199.
88. Irwin M, McClintick J, Costlow C, Fortner M, White J, Gillin JC. Partial night sleep deprivation reduces natural killer and cellular immune responses in humans. FASEB J 1996; 10(5):643–653.
89. Palmblad J, Petrini B, Wasserman J, Akerstedt T. Lymphocyte and granulocyte reactions during sleep deprivation. Psychosom Med 1979; 41(4):273–278.
90. Casey FB, Eisenberg J, Peterson D, Pieper D. Altered antigen uptake and distribution due to exposure to extreme environmental temperatures or sleep deprivation. J Reticuloendothel Soc 1974; 15(2):87–95.
91. Lange T, Perras B, Fehm HL, Born J. Sleep enhances the human antibody response to hepatitis A vaccination. Psychosom Med 2003; 65(5):831–835.
92. Spiegel K, Sheridan JF, Van CE. Effect of sleep deprivation on response to immunization. JAMA 2002; 288(12):1471–1472.
93. Gessa GL, Pani L, Fadda P, Fratta W. Sleep deprivation in the rat: an animal model of mania. Eur Neuropsychopharmacol 1995; 5(suppl):89–93.
94. Smith CT, Nixon MR, Nader RS. Posttraining increases in REM sleep intensity implicate REM sleep in memory processing and provide a biological marker of learning potential. Learn Mem 2004; 11(6):714–719.
95. Lentz MJ, Landis CA, Rothermel J, Shaver JL. Effects of selective slow wave sleep disruption on musculoskeletal pain and fatigue in middle aged women. J Rheumatol 1999; 26(7):1586–1592.
96. Brunner DP, Dijk DJ, Borbely AA. Repeated partial sleep deprivation progressively changes in EEG during sleep and wakefulness. Sleep 1993; 16(2):100–113.
97. Lubin A, Hord DJ, Tracy ML, Johnson LC. Effects of exercise, bedrest and napping on performance decrement during 40 hours. Psychophysiology 1976; 13(4):334–339.
98. Webb WB, Agnew HW, Jr. Effects on performance of high and low energy-expenditure during sleep deprivation. Percept Mot Skills 1973; 37(2):511–514.
99. Rechtschaffen A, Bergmann BM, Everson CA, Kushida CA, Gilliland MA. Sleep deprivation in the rat: I. Conceptual issues. Sleep 1989; 12(1):1–4.
100. Rechtschaffen A, Bergmann BM, Everson CA, Kushida CA, Gilliland MA. Sleep deprivation in the rat: X. Integration and discussion of the findings. Sleep 1989; 12(1):68–87.
101. Everson CA. Sustained sleep deprivation impairs host defense. Am J Physiol 1993; 265(5 Pt 2):R1148–R1154.
102. Bergmann BM, Gilliland MA, Feng PF, et al. Are physiological effects of sleep deprivation in the rat mediated by bacterial invasion? Sleep 1996; 19(7):554–562.
103. Everson CA, Gilliland MA, Kushida CA, et al. Sleep deprivation in the rat: IX. Recovery. Sleep 1989; 12(1):60–67.

# 10 History of Restless Legs Syndrome

**Wayne A. Hening**

*Department of Neurology, UMDNJ-RW Johnson Medical School, New Brunswick, New Jersey, U.S.A.*

## EARLY DESCRIPTIONS OF CONDITIONS RESEMBLING RESTLESS LEGS SYNDROME

When was the first description of restless legs syndrome (RLS)? Montaigne, the great French essayist, wrote about restlessness of the legs, sometimes aroused by sermons in church, "so that though I was seated, I was never settled" (1). Montaigne seems to catch the core feeling of RLS—the "never settled." Montaigne wrote that, "it may have been said of me from my infancy that I had either folly or quicksilver in my feet, so much stirring and unsettledness there is in them, wherever they are placed." But Montaigne recognized an even earlier sufferer, the third century B.C. Greek stoic philosopher, Chrysippus, who, at a dinner party, was said to have legs that moved about as if drunk (2).

The first medical description of RLS may have been due to Willis, the 17th century anatomist and physician, who described one case that many with RLS would probably endorse (3,4):

> "... whilst they would indulge sleep, in their beds, immediately follow leapings up of the Tendons, in their Arms and Legs, with Cramps, and such unquietness and flying about of their members, that the sick can no more sleep, than those on the Rack."

As Critchley noted (5), Willis seems to be clearly on point with many features of RLS—the leg discomfort (cramps), the periodic limb movement (PLM) while awake (leapings up), the onset at night (indulge sleep), and the very difficulty with sleeping that causes the greatest problem for many RLS patients. One reason to think that this disorder was RLS is that Willis was able to treat this patient with laudanum, which is a preparation of opium, and belongs to one class of medications still used for RLS today (Chapter 27).

Over the next few centuries, there are scattered references in the medical literature to conditions that sound like RLS. In most cases, these references suggested a condition with vague or uncertain cause, such as "anxietas tibiarum," an irritation of the lower legs (6). Beard suggested the spinal origin of these discomforts (7), while Oppenheim may have been the first to propose a familial tendency (8). Beginning around 1940, more precise characterizations of the disorder appeared.

Mussio Fournier and Rawak noted the association with pregnancy (9). Allison in 1943 made some truly important observations: that RLS was common, but unrecognized, that it typically presented as a sleep problem, and that it included "involuntary" movements (10). Allison called the condition "leg jitters," a term that has persisted in some locales as a dialectical name for RLS.

## THE WORK OF KARL EKBOM

But the real dawn of understanding came during World War II when, at night in kitchen in neutral and unoccupied Sweden, Karl Ekbom prepared the key, pioneering paper on RLS. After a small preliminary note (11), Ekbom's work was published as a separate, supplementary volume of Acta Medica Scandinavica (12). In this long essay, and later papers that were published, Ekbom sketched out a rather full and diverse clinical picture for the varieties and discomforts of this unknown medical condition. Ekbom noted that RLS was common and could be easily diagnosed—if the physician was aware of its typical symptoms. Ekbom described at length patients' difficulties with sleep—and the restlessness and reported movements in sleep—that these patients suffered and the difficulties they might have with leg discomfort if they remained seated for a sustained time. Ekbom noted that some, such as truck drivers, could have real difficulties with their jobs. Ekbom also noted that the disorder ran in families, could be increased in pregnancy or with anemia, and could be provoked by stomach surgery that reduced the ability of the body to absorb such vitamins as B12. Even today, it is profitable to re-read many of Ekbom's cases to get a clear picture of the various faces of RLS.

## THE NAMING OF RESTLESS LEGS

Ekbom also named the disorder. At first, a Latinate name was considered: Ekbom suggested either "asthenia crurum paraesthetica" or, for the kind of RLS with painful symptoms, "asthenia crurum dolorosa." As an alternative, Ekbom considered the term, "irritable legs." But after some thought, settled on the simple term of "restless legs," to which Ekbom later added the qualifier, "syndrome" (13). This term has become generally accepted, although the label, "Ekbom's syndrome" has been occasionally used to honor Ekbom's contribution.

Restless legs has been translated into a number of terms (such as the Italian "gambe senza reposo" or the French "jambes sans repos" or the German "ruhelose beinen"), but even in other literatures, the English "restless legs" often remains the accepted term. There have been various initiatives, spurred on by the seeming triviality of the name, "restless legs," to rename the condition. Unless there is some great breakthrough in understanding, so that we know the cause of the condition and could name it for that cause, the term RLS will probably continue to be used. Meanwhile, Ekbom's syndrome is the accepted term for a delusional condition (delusional psychosis) in which the patient actually believes that there are real, live ants or other organisms crawling around in the legs.

## NOCTURNAL MYOCLONUS, NOW CALLED PERIODIC LIMB MOVEMENTS

After Ekbom's initial contributions, RLS assumed a small niche in the medical literature and every year or so there was another study or paper written about it. Nordlander made a major contribution in 1953 by showing that patients with iron deficiency could be successively treated with intravenous iron supplementation (14). The next major advance, however, came from Italy where Lugaresi and Coccagna were helping develop the field of sleep medicine in the 1960s. They were recording sleep, using attended polysomnographic recordings in their laboratory. One patient, a monk, came to them complaining of difficulty with sleep and jerks in legs. Coccagna, staying up all night to monitor the patient, heard repeated scratches of the polygraph (15). Coccagna looked at the patient and found that every 20 or 30 seconds, the patient's legs would move. This continued for a sustained period. Starting with this one patient—and some of affected family members—the Bologna group discovered that in many patients with RLS they could find the same movements; in fact, these movements seemed a prominent feature of RLS (16,17). They designated these movements as "nocturnal myoclonus," but this was later found to be an inaccurate name (at the 1990 Movement Disorder meeting in Washington, D.C.), because myoclonus indicates a brief and rapid movement. Nocturnal myoclonus had been suggested as a term for various movements that occurred in sleep (18), but the repetitive movements often seen with RLS are not usually brisk. However, some of these involuntary movements, more often those that occur when the patient is awake, can have myoclonic speed (19,20). In the following decade, it became apparent that these movements also occurred in many individuals without RLS. Guilleminault, Weitzman, and Coleman developed a scheme for counting these movements (21,22), which they first called "periodic movements in sleep," then "periodic leg movements in sleep." Most recently, these movements are called periodic limb movements in sleep (PLMS). Because these movements can be observed and counted, they have played an important role in the study of RLS. They remain the key objective measure of RLS.

## EARLY THERAPEUTIC TRIALS OF RLS

PLMS were initially thought to cause major problems by disrupting sleep. The resulting condition was called PLM disorder (PLMD). Initial treatment for RLS was aimed at reducing these movements and sometimes little distinction was made between RLS and PLMD without RLS. In the 1980s, there began to be therapeutic studies for RLS alone, in which it was considered whether the leg discomforts of patients were reduced and whether their overall sleep was improved.

While Ekbom had suggested using vasodilating cholinomimetics for RLS, the early treatment of RLS and PLMS in sleep began with the use of clonazepam, a benzodiazepine that had come into favor for treatment of myoclonus (23,24). A major advance was made in the early 1980s with the discovery by Akpinar in Turkey that medications which increase the brain's dopamine activity could benefit RLS (25). Akpinar was consulted by a colonel in the Turkish military who could not sleep at night because of leg discomfort and leg jerks. The entire family would sleep seated together in one room of their house. Akpinar tried many different medications and found that levodopa and the dopamine agonist, pergolide, worked quite well. Akpinar was also impressed by the benefits of opioid medications, the narcotic pain killers. A few years later, it was discovered that anticonvulsant medications that suppress seizures, such as carbamazepine, could also benefit RLS (26,27). With this addition, the major classes of medications used to treat RLS (Chapter 24)—dopaminergics, opioids, anticonvulsants, and sedative hypnotics—were included in the therapeutic formulary.

## THE RLS FOUNDATION AND THE INTERNATIONAL RLS STUDY GROUP

In the 1990s, two organizations were founded that have had a major impact in moving forward education about and the study of RLS, the RLS Foundation (RLSF) and the International RLS Study Group (IRLSSG). Started as a small group exchanging a round-robin letter, the RLSF was legally established in 1992 as a nonprofit corporation by Virginia Wilson and Pickett Guthrie. In the following years, it has brought the passion and advocacy of patients to bear in raising public awareness, providing public advocacy, and sponsoring medical and scientific advances.

Around the same time, Arthur Walters founded the IRLSSG. Started with a couple of dozen RLS researchers in seven or so countries, by 2005 it had over 140 members worldwide in more than two dozen countries. The first major project of the group was a standardized definition of RLS. First published in 1995, this definition has been critical for both clinical medicine and research (28). This definition facilitated the recognition of RLS in the clinical setting and provided a basis for recognizing RLS in order to facilitate research. The two groups also collaborated, developing a medical advisory board soon after they were both founded. This board has worked closely with the lay members of the foundation. Board members, both current and prior, attend what are now national foundation meetings and share information about RLS. In 2004, under the direction of Michael Silber of the Mayo clinic, the medical advisory board published recommendations for how to treat RLS (29). Another collaboration that emerged from these organizations was the first book on RLS, written by Virginia Wilson, who provided the patient viewpoint on RLS, and Arthur Walters, who ensured that he and several colleagues could bring current medical knowledge to bear (30). The book was published in 1996 and was the first book whose sole topic was RLS.

## RECENT DEVELOPMENT ON MANY FRONTS

The mid-1990s were an exciting time. In many ways, 1994 was a benchmark year. For the first time, RLS was recognized as worthy of study. In 1994, the first U.S. symposium on RLS was held at the annual American Sleep Society meeting in Boston and the first international symposium was held at the European Sleep Research Society meeting in Florence, Italy. One RLSF board member, Robert Yoakum, wrote an article about RLS that appeared in Modern Maturity (31). The response was overwhelming, over 40,000 letters replied to the article and made it clear that RLS was both common and, for many sufferers, clearly devastating. The response also inspired Mr. Yoakum to begin a 10-year odyssey to write the second patient-oriented book on RLS that was published in 2006 (32).

Beginning in 1994, one study after another has demonstrated that RLS is indeed common and causes significant morbidity. The first study of a large population was performed across Canada by Lavigne and Montplaisir and published in that key year of 1994 (33). On average, almost one adult in six was found to have symptoms of RLS. Subsequent studies from the United States, Europe, and Chile have confirmed that RLS is common and that at least several percent of the population suffers from the condition (34–36). More recent studies have also found that the mental state and quality of life of RLS patients are impaired by the disorder (37,38). Sleep disruption, an immediate consequence of RLS, also impacts on daytime function, causing fatigue, inattention, and negative mood (39). It has even been found that adults and children with RLS are both quite likely to have attention-deficit disorder (40,41).

As it became apparent that RLS was not a rare condition, but instead one of the most common neurological disorders, pharmaceutical companies developed an interest in the condition. By the early 2000s, several companies had begun trials to see if medications they owned would be effective for RLS. By 2005, half a dozen companies had active research projects in RLS. Most trials focused on the dopamine-enhancing medications. The first to be approved for RLS was a levodopa compound (levodopa/benserazide) in Germany and Switzerland. In 2005, the dopamine agonist, ropinirole, was approved by the Food and Drug Administration in the United States for the treatment of RLS; in 2006, the dopamine agonist pramipexole was approved in Europe. At the time of this writing, it seems very likely that approvals for additional dopamine agonists should soon follow, while other types of medications are being studied with an eye to future approval. This entry of the pharmaceutical industry into the RLS field has led to a substantial increase in both public and professional education, which should improve diagnosis and treatment of RLS. The approval of different drugs for treatment of RLS gives a stamp of approval to the medical management of the condition. Before these recent registrations, every drug for RLS was prescribed "off label"; this had meant that those less expert in the condition were unlikely to prescribe the most effective, but less well-known medications. This was true even though there was evidence that some drugs were effective—in fact, the American Academy of Sleep Medicine first approved standards for treatment of RLS in 1999, recommending some drug therapies.

One factor that assisted in the performance of drug trials was the development of a rating scale for RLS. While several scales have been in use, one developed by the IRLSSG, the IRLSSG rating scale (IRLS), has been used to capture various aspects of RLS and its problems (42). Available generally since 2003, this scale has made it easier to do drug trials and establish drug benefits. It is not a perfect scale and, as time goes by, better ways of capturing the problems of RLS and their reduction by treatment should be developed.

The early 21st century has also provided exciting developments in the understanding of what causes RLS. Because so many RLS patients know of affected family members, it had long been thought that RLS shows familial aggregation. By 2006, several "regions of interest" had been detected on different chromosomes by a variety of genetic epidemiological methodologies. The first such linkage was reported in 2001 by the Montreal group (43). Two more sites have now been published while others have been reported informally. While no specific gene has yet been found to cause RLS, this is an area of great excitement and at least seven different research groups are working to uncover the genes involved.

Another recent development is an explanation of the connection between iron deficiency and RLS. Researchers from Johns Hopkins and Penn State Universities have been working together to find out why this connection occurs. In this search, they have been assisted by the development of the RLSF brain bank. A number of individuals suffering from RLS have been willing to have their brains harvested after death and saved for scientific researchers. Using these brains, the Hopkins and Penn State researchers have been able to show that brain iron is low in RLS brain cells (44), that the brain proteins that keep iron at the right level are not functioning correctly (45), and that the lack of iron may lead to deficiencies in a protein, Thy-1, needed to develop and maintain synaptic connectivity (46). There are clearly other pieces to the RLS puzzle—and any genes involved with RLS are likely to fit in here somewhere—but this is a promising start.

## SUMMARY THOUGHTS

What can we then say about this survey of RLS history? In several decades, RLS has leaped from being a rare disease known to few to what, in a few years from now, should become a standard part of medical practice. It has gone from being a condition, whose treatment some felt to be futile, to being a condition with multiple effective treatments, treatment recommendations, and approved drugs. It has gone from being an unknown mystery, to being a challenging disorder about which we now know quite a lot, but still have a great deal to learn.

## REFERENCES

1. Montaigne MD. On experience. In: Essays.
2. Laertius D. The Lives and Opinions of Eminent Philosophers. London: Henry G. Bohm, 1853.
3. Willis T. De Animae Brutorum. London: Wells and Scott, 1672.
4. Willis T. Two discourses concerning the soul of brutes. London: Dring, Harper and Leigh, 1683.
5. Critchley M. The pre-dormitum. Rev Neurol (Paris) 1955; 93:101–106.
6. Wittmaack T. Pathologie und Therapie der Sensibilität-Neurosen. Leipzig: E. Schäfer, 1861.
7. Beard G. A Practical Treatise on Nervous Exhaustion. New York City: William Wood, 1880.
8. Oppenheim H. Lehrbuch der Nervenkrankheiten. Berlin: Karger, 1923.
9. Mussio Fournier J, Rawak F. Familiäres auftreten von pruritus, urtikaria und parästhetischer hyperkinese der unteren extremitäten. Confin Neurol 1940; 3:110–114.
10. Allison F. Obscure pains in the chest, back or limbs. Can Med Assoc J 1943; 48:36–38.
11. Ekbom KA. Asthenia crurum paraesthetica (irritable legs). Acta Med Scand 1944; 118:197–209.
12. Ekbom KA. Restless legs: a clinical study. Acta Med Scand 1945; 158(suppl):1–122.
13. Ekbom KA. Restless legs syndrome. Neurology 1960; 10:868–873.
14. Nordlander NB. Therapy in restless legs. Acta Med Scand 1953; 145:453–457.
15. Coccagna G, Vetrugno R, Lombardi C, Provini F. Restless legs syndrome: an historical note. Sleep Med 2004; 5:279–283.
16. Lugaresi E, Coccagna G, Tassinari CA, Ambrosetto C. Relievi poligrafici sui fenomeni motori nella sindrome delle gambe senza riposo. Riv Neurol 1965; 35:550–561.
17. Lugaresi E, Coccagna G, Berti Ceroni G, Ambrosetto C. Restless legs syndrome and nocturnal myoclonus. In: Gastaut H, Lugaresi E, Berti Ceroni G, Coccagna G, eds. The Abnormalities of Sleep in Man. Bologna: Aulo Gaggi Editore, 1968:285–294.
18. Symonds CP. Nocturnal myoclonus. J Neurol Neurosurg Psychiatr 1953; 16:166–171.
19. Lugaresi E, Cirignotta F, Coccagna G, Montagna P. Nocturnal myoclonus and restless legs syndrome. In: Fahn S, Marsden CD, Van Woert M, eds. Myoclonus. Advances in Neurology. Vol. 43. New York: Raven Press, 1986:295–307.
20. Walters AS, Hening WA, Chokroverty S. Frequent occurrence of myoclonus while awake and at rest, body rocking and marching in place in a subpopulation of patients with restless legs syndrome. Acta Neurol Scand 1988; 77:418–421.
21. Guilleminault C, Raynal D, Weitzman ED, Dement WC. Sleep-related periodic myoclonus in patients complaining of insomnia. Trans Am Neurol Assoc 1975; 100:19–21.
22. Coleman RM, Pollack CP, Weitzman ED. Periodic nocturnal myoclonus in a wide variety of sleep-wake disorders. Trans Am Neurol Assoc 1979; 103:230–233.
23. Matthews WB. Treatment of restless legs syndrome with clonazepam. Br Med J 1979; 1:751.
24. Boghen D. Successful treatment of restless legs with clonazepam. Ann Neurol 1981; 8:341.
25. Akpinar S. Treatment of restless legs syndrome with levodopa plus benserazide. Arch Neurol 1982; 39:739.
26. Lundvall O, Abom PE, Holm R. Carbamazepine in restless legs: a controlled pilot study. Eur J Clin Pharmacol 1983; 25:323–324.
27. Telstad W, Sørensen O, Larsen S, Lillevold PE, Stensrud P, Nyberg-Hansen R. Treatment of the restless legs syndrome with carbamazepine: a double blind study. Br. Med J 1984; 288:444–446.

28. The International Restless Legs Syndrome Study Group (Arthur S. Walters MD—Group Organizer and Correspondent). Towards a better definition of the restless legs syndrome. Mov Disord 1995; 10:634–642.
29. Silber MH, Ehrenberg BL, Allen RP, et al. An algorithm for the management of restless legs syndrome. Mayo Clin Proc 2004; 79:916–922.
30. Wilson V. Sleep Thief: Restless Legs Syndrome. Orange Park, Florida: Galaxy Books, 1996.
31. Yoakum R. Night walkers: do your legs seem to have a life of their own? Your torment has a name. Modern Maturity 1994; 37:55, 82–84.
32. Yoakum R. Nightwalkers: Sleepless Victims of a Hidden Epidemic. New York: Simon and Schuster, 2006.
33. Lavigne GJ, Montplaisir JY. Restless legs syndrome and sleep bruxism: prevalence and association among Canadians. Sleep 1994; 17:739–743.
34. Hening W, Walters AS, Allen RP, Montplaisir J, Myers A, Ferini-Strambi L. Impact, diagnosis and treatment of restless legs syndrome (RLS) in a primary care population: the REST (RLS epidemiology, symptoms, and treatment) primary care study. Sleep Med 2004; 5:237–246.
35. Allen RP, Walters AS, Montplaisir J, et al. Restless legs syndrome prevalence and impact: REST general population study. Arch Intern Med 2005; 165:1286–1292.
36. Tison F, Crochard A, Leger D, Bouee S, Lainey E, El Hasnaoui A. Epidemiology of restless legs syndrome in French adults: a nationwide survey: the INSTANT Study. Neurology 2005; 65:239–246.
37. Winkelmann J, Prager M, Lieb R, et al. "Anxietas Tibiarum" Depression and anxiety disorders in patients with restless legs syndrome. J Neurol 2005; 252:67–71.
38. Abetz L, Allen R, Follet A, et al. Evaluating the quality of life of patients with restless legs syndrome. Clin Ther 2004; 26:925–935.
39. Kushida CA, Allen RP, Atkinson MJ. Modeling the causal relationships between symptoms associated with restless legs syndrome and the patient-reported impact of RLS. Sleep Med 2004; 5:485–488.
40. Picchietti DL, Walters AS. Restless legs syndrome and periodic limb movement disorder in children and adolescents: comorbidity with attention -deficit hyperactivity disorder. In: Dahl RE, ed. Child and Adolescent Psychiatric Clinics of North America: Sleep Disorders. Philadelphia: W.B. Saunders Company, 1996:729–740.
41. Wagner ML, Walters AS, Fisher BC. Symptoms of attention-deficit/hyperactivity disorder in adults with restless legs syndrome. Sleep 2004; 27:1499–1504.
42. The International Restless Legs Syndrome Study Group, Writing and central data collection and data analysis committee, Walters A, et al. Validation of the International Restless Legs Syndrome Study Group rating scale for restless legs syndrome. Sleep Med 2003; 4:121–132.
43. Desautels A, Turecki G, Montplaisir J, Sequeira A, Verner A, Rouleau GA. Identification of a major susceptibility locus for restless legs syndrome on chromosome 12q. Am J Hum Genet 2001; 69:1266–1270.
44. Connor JR, Boyer PJ, Menzies SL, et al. Neuropathological examination suggests impaired brain iron acquisition in restless legs syndrome. Neurology 2003; 61:304–309.
45. Connor JR, Wang XS, Patton SM, et al. Decreased transferrin receptor expression by neuromelanin cells in restless legs syndrome. Neurology 2004; 62:1563–1567.
46. Wang X, Wiesinger J, Beard J, et al. Thy1 expression in the brain is affected by iron and is decreased in restless legs syndrome. J Neurol Sci 2004; 220:59–66.

# 11 Restless Legs Syndrome: Diagnostic Criteria and Differential Diagnosis

**Shahul Hameed and E. K. Tan**

*Department of Neurology, Singapore General Hospital, National Neuroscience Institute, Singapore, Republic of Singapore*

## INTRODUCTION

Restless legs syndrome (RLS) is characterized by an urge to move the limbs, associated with unpleasant sensations deep inside the legs and sometimes the arms (1). RLS, first named in 1945 by the Swedish neurologist Ekbom (2), has a prevalence of about 5% to 15% in the White population (3,4), but is less common amongst Asians (5). In 1995, the International RLS Study Group (IRLSSG) proposed and published a set of clinical diagnostic criteria for RLS (6). In 2002, the RLS Foundation and the National Institute on Aging, in partnership with the National Center on Sleep Disorders Research, the National Institute of Neurological Disorders and Stroke, the National Institute of Mental Health, the National Institute of Nursing Research, and the National Institute of Child Health and Human Development, held a consensus meeting at the National Institutes of Health to update diagnostic criteria (6). Members of the IRLSSG also participated in this meeting, which discussed and improved upon the diagnostic criteria based on new scientific knowledge and clinical experience with RLS. The consensus was that four essential criteria are all required to make the diagnosis of RLS. Three other clinical features may support the diagnosis in uncertain clinical cases, and three additional features of the disorder deserve consideration when evaluating the patient with a potential diagnosis of RLS. The primary revision from the previously proposed criteria involves the substitution of criterion 3, "relief with movement," for the previous criterion of "motor restlessness" (7). In addition, criteria for the diagnosis of RLS in the cognitively impaired elderly and in children were developed and criteria for the identification of augmentation proposed (7).

In this paper, we provide a concise summary of the diagnostic criteria of RLS and discuss the differential diagnosis.

## DIAGNOSTIC CRITERIA

The four essential criteria for diagnosis of RLS are listed in Table 1 (7).

### Criterion 1

An urge to move the legs is usually accompanied or caused by an uncomfortable and unpleasant sensation in the legs (sometimes the urge to move is present without uncomfortable sensations and sometimes other body parts such as arms are involved in addition to the legs). The sensory symptoms of RLS are frequently unpleasant, and most commonly experienced in the lower extremities, especially in the calves, but may occur in any part of the leg. Patients may report foot

**TABLE 1** Essential Diagnostic Criteria for Restless Legs Syndrome

| |
|---|
| An urge to move the legs, usually accompanied or caused by uncomfortable and unpleasant sensations in the legs (sometimes the urge to move is present without the uncomfortable sensations and sometimes the arms or other body parts are involved in addition to the legs) |
| The urge to move or unpleasant sensations begin or worsen during periods of rest or inactivity, such as lying or sitting |
| The urge to move or unpleasant sensations are partially or totally relieved by movement, such as walking or stretching, at least as long as the activity continues |
| The urge to move or unpleasant sensations are worse in the evening or night than during the day, or only occur in the evening or night (when symptoms are very severe, the worsening at night may not be noticeable but must have been previously present) |

*Source*: From Ref. 7.

involvement but when interrogated will usually deny experiencing any urge to move the toes.

Arm involvement is common. Winkelmann and coworkers recently found that 34% of RLS patients in their population of 300 have symptoms in their arms as well as their legs (8). Michand et al. also showed that 50% of RLS patients have symptoms in the arms, with leg symptoms preceding these by several years (9). In general, arm involvement is associated with a longer duration and more severe disease. The head and probably the torso should not be involved.

The discomfort is often difficult to characterize and usually bilateral. In a study by Ondo and Jankovic (10), the most common reported symptoms included "need to move," "crawling," " tingling," "restless," and " crawling" sensation. The exact semantics are often colloquial and education dependent, so an unusual description, such as "maggots in my legs," "soda in my veins," and "Elvis (Presley) legs" should not deter a diagnosis as long as there is an urge to move. These sensations are usually deep seated "in my bones" and not on the surface of the leg. Bassetti et al. (11) reported that more than 50% of their 55 RLS patients described pain as a primary component of their RLS. However, it should be emphasized that isolated pain without an urge to move is not RLS. The reported sensations tend to transverse a spectrum from a pure urge to move without any pain to mostly pain with some urge to move. Pain is associated with neuropathy in some cases. In fact, some patients may experience a typical superficial neuropathic pain and a separate urge to move. Although these may represent two distinct phenomena, most patients will not segregate the two sensations. The response to an urge to move in RLS should not be confused with habitual motor behaviors such as foot tapping, which are performed without the acute and distressing awareness of an urge to move. For example, the individual rapidly dorsi-flexing and plantar-flexing (bouncing) their ankle as an alerting strategy is not manifesting an RLS motor sign.

### Criterion 2

The urge to move or unpleasant sensations begin or worsen during periods of rest or during inactivity, such as lying or sitting. Michaud et al. studied the effects of immobility on RLS using a Suggested Immobilization Test (12). Compared to controls, patients with RLS have more periodic leg movements and an increase in sensory disturbance during immobilization period. The motor and sensory symptoms increase with the duration of rest. Rest includes physical immobility as well as cognitive inactivity. Situations such as watching television or reading a book qualify as cognitive inactivity in this setting. In contrast, playing a demanding video game or having an argument can improve RLS. Presumably both factors (immobility and decreased central nervous system activity supporting alertness) contribute to the onset of the condition (13). No specific body position causes the symptoms in RLS. This contrasts with body positional discomfort syndrome, in which a certain supine condition: i.e., lying on your right side, is uncomfortable. Pain or discomfort from circulatory compromise or stiffness from prolonged sitting or lying in a fixed position should also not be confused with RLS symptoms.

### Criterion 3

The urge to move or unpleasant sensations are partially or totally relieved by activities, such as walking or stretching, at least as long as the actions continue. Patients with RLS often relieve the unpleasant sensations by engaging in motor activities, such as floor pacing, stretching, flexing, or applying a counterstimulus such as rubbing the legs or taking hot or cold shower baths. Winkelman et al. (8) found that changes of temperature can be an effective coping strategy in 82% of their 300 patients (5). The walking, stretching, or bending, which patients with RLS employ to relieve their sensations, is voluntary. Again, intense cognitive activity that is alerting can also improve symptoms, but this is a flawed strategy when patients are trying to obtain sleep. The relief with activity is not always complete and they usually recur as soon as the activity ends. As RLS progresses, patients may notice that relief with significant movement does not occur as consistently.

### Criterion 4

The urge to move or unpleasant sensations are worse in the evening or night than during the day, or may only occur in the evening or night. When symptoms are very severe, the worsening at night may not be as noticeable but must have been previously present. Likewise, RLS after drug-induced augmentation (Chapter 26) and RLS associated with renal failure may not have overt nocturnal worsening. It has been noted that RLS is worse in the evening/night, and that RLS is worse on lying and sitting during either day or night (14). The nighttime worsening of symptoms with the daytime amelioration seems to occur independently of sleep deprivation or fatigue (15). In two studies, researchers have been able to separate the circadian effects from the impact of both recumbence and rest on symptoms of RLS (16). This confirms that RLS has a true circadian pattern and does not occur in the evening/night just because people are less physically active at night. This often results in sleep deprivation, which may be relatively worse in women (16a).

### Supportive Clinical Features

Supportive clinical features are listed in Table 2. They are not required for diagnosis of RLS, but their presence can help resolve any diagnostic dilemma.

#### *Positive Family History of RLS*

Idiopathic RLS can occur sporadically, though in some studies more than 50% of patients report having a positive family history of RLS. An individual with RLS is much more likely to have family history of RLS compared to someone without RLS, especially if age of RLS onset is less than 45 (16,17).

**TABLE 2** Supportive Clinical Features of Restless Legs Syndrome

| |
|---|
| *Family history* |
| The prevalence of RLS among first-degree relatives of people with RLS is 3–5 times greater than in people without RLS. |
| *Response to dopaminergic therapy* |
| Nearly all people with RLS show at least an initial positive therapeutic response to either L-dopa or a dopamine-receptor agonist at doses lower than the traditional doses of these medications used for the treatment of Parkinson's disease. This initial response is not, however, universally maintained. |
| *Periodic limb movements (during wakefulness or sleep)* |
| PLMS occur in at least 85% of people with RLS; however, PLMS also commonly occur in other disorders and in the elderly. In children, PLMS are much less common than in adults |

*Abbreviation*: PLMS, periodic limb movements in sleep.

### *Response to Treatment*

Both open-labeled and controlled studies have demonstrated that most RLS patients have a robust therapeutic response to dopaminergic drugs (18–24). Recently, Stiasny-Kolster et al systematically confirmed that improvement with an initial dose of levodopa is both sensitive (80-88%) and specific (100%) for making a diagnosis of RLS (24a). This is so consistent that it is considered a supportive feature. Although other medications help RLS, their effects are probably less specific and also help other conditions in the differential diagnosis of RLS.

### *Periodic Leg Movements*

Periodic leg movements of sleep (PLMS) are usually characterized by rhythmic extension of the big toe and dorsiflexion of ankle, with occasional flexion at the knee and hip. Although they can vary somewhat, they usually resemble a triple flexion response. An index of greater than five periodic limb movements in sleep (PLMS) per hour for the entire night is considered to be abnormal, although as people age PLMS index tends to increase in the general population. An elevated PLMS index is supportive of RLS. At least 80% of patients with RLS have a PLMS index greater than 5, depending on the number of nights that are evaluated. The PLM while awake appears to be more specific for RLS, though the data for this finding remain limited (25,26).

## Associated Features of RLS

### *Natural Clinical Course of RLS*

RLS can be a primary disorder with a genetic predisposition (27) or secondary to iron deficiency (28,29), pregnancy (30–32), chronic renal failure (33–36), and possibly other conditions (Table 3). Primary RLS is generally a chronic condition and the severity and frequency of symptoms typically increases over time. Recent data have suggested that many patients with early onset symptoms of RLS will not develop persistent daily symptoms until about the age of 40 to 60 years. Interestingly, RLS may improve in very old age. Secondary RLS generally remits without evidence of reoccurrence when the secondary condition resolves.

### *Sleep Disturbance*

Many patients with RLS have sleep onset or sleep maintenance insomnia, which is due to limb discomfort. The patient with moderate to severe RLS may sleep an

**TABLE 3** Associated Features of Restless Legs Syndrome

*Natural clinical course*
The clinical course of the disorder varies considerably, but certain patterns have been identified that may be helpful to the experienced clinician. When the age of onset of RLS symptoms is less than 50 yr, the onset is often more insidious; when the age of onset is greater than 50 yr, the symptoms often occur more abruptly and more severely. In some patients, RLS can be intermittent and may spontaneously remit for many years.

*Sleep disturbance*
Disturbed sleep is a common major morbidity for RLS and deserves special consideration in planning treatment. This morbidity is often the primary reason that the patient seeks medical attention.

*Medical evaluation/physical examination*
The physical examination is generally normal and does not contribute much to the diagnoses except for those conditions that may be comorbid or secondary causes of RLS. Iron status, in particular, should be evaluated because decreased iron stores are a significant potential risk factor that can be treated. The best widely available serum measures for low iron stores are ferritin and iron binding percentage. It should be noted that values falling within the normal range may still contribute to RLS symptoms. The presence of peripheral neuropathy and radiculopathy should also be determined because these conditions have a possible, although uncertain association and may require different treatment.

average of less than 5 hours per night and may clinically have less sleep time than patients with almost any other persistent disorder of sleep (37).

### *Medical Evaluation and Physical Examination*

The neurological examination is frequently normal in patients with RLS. Some patients will demonstrate slow stereotypes, usually involving ankle rotation. This is often not noticed by the patient and it is completely suppressible when attention is drawn to it. Other examination abnormalities may reflect an underlying secondary cause of RLS, usually neuropathy.

### *Diagnostic Criteria for Probable RLS in the Cognitively Impaired Elderly*

Cognitively impaired elderly have language dysfunction so the ability to report sensory symptoms may be lacking (Table 4). Therefore, the newly revised diagnostic criteria for RLS have been modified for this population (Tables 4 and 5).

## Diagnostic Criteria in Children

RLS in children is discussed in detail in Chapter 13. Briefly, the diagnostic criteria for children are less well validated than for adults. A diagnosis of "definite RLS"

**TABLE 4** Essential Criteria for the Diagnosis of Probable Restless Legs Syndrome in the Cognitively Impaired Elderly

Signs of leg discomfort such as rubbing or kneading the legs and groaning while holding the lower extremities are present.
Excessive motor activity in the lower extremities such as pacing, fidgeting, repetitive kicking, tossing and turning in bed, slapping the legs on the mattress, cycling movements of the lower limbs, repetitive foot tapping, rubbing the feet together, and the inability to remain seated are present.
Signs of leg discomfort are exclusively present or worsen during periods of rest or inactivity.
Signs of leg discomfort are diminished with activity.
Criteria 1 and 2 occur only in the evening or at night or are worse at those times than during the day.

*Note*: All five are necessary for diagnosis.

**TABLE 5** Supportive or Suggestive Criteria for the Diagnosis of Probable Restless Legs Syndrome in the Cognitively Impaired Elderly

| |
|---|
| Dopaminergic responsiveness |
| Patient's past history (as reported by a family member, caregiver, or friend) is suggestive of RLS |
| A first-degree, biologic relative (sibling, child, or parents) has RLS |
| Observe periodic limb movements while awake or during sleep |
| Periodic limb movements of sleep recorded by polysomnography or actigraphy |
| Significant sleep onset problems |
| Better quality sleep in the day than at night |
| The use of restraints at night (for institutionalized patients) |
| Low serum ferritin level |
| End-stage renal disease |
| Diabetes |
| Clinical, electromyographic, or nerve-conduction evidence of peripheral neuropathy or radiculopathy |

requires the presence of all four adult features plus a description of an unpleasant sensation, not only an urge to move. This was included to differentiate from the general fidgetiness and increased motor activity often seen in children. "Probable RLS" in verbalizing children requires criteria 1 to 3 (excluding worsening at night) but also requires a family history of RLS in a sibling or parent. "Probable RLS" in a nonverbalizing child requires motor manifestations typical for RLS and the same family history. "Possible RLS" requires the presence of PLMS and a similar family history.

## DIFFERENTIAL DIAGNOSIS

Motor restlessness, characterized by an irresistible urge to move about can be confused with RLS (38). Because motor restlessness can be a manifestation of many medical disorders, a careful history and examination are needed for early diagnosis. Unfortunately, it is often poorly recognized and underdiagnosed in clinical practice, because patients do not seek medical attention or their complaints are thought to be secondary to anxiety. The two major conditions to consider for patients who present with motor restlessness are RLS and Neuroleptic-Induced Akathisia (NIA). Other differential diagnoses to consider include painful legs and moving toes syndrome, attention deficit hyperactivity disorder (ADHD), hyperactivity states due to hyperthyroidism and Tourette's syndrome (TS), anxiety disorders, levodopa-induced dyskinesias, orthostatic tremor, orthostatic hypotension, and nerve entrapment syndromes.

### Neuroleptic-Induced Akathisias

Exposure or withdrawal of neuroleptics (such as haloperidol, thioridazine) can produce symptoms of NIA. Other drugs such as serotonin reuptake inhibitors (e.g., fluoxetine), and lithium have also been implicated in NIA or are associated with motor restlessness as part of the "serotonin syndrome" (39,40). While motor restlessness is common to both NIA and RLS, there are differences between them (Table 6). The urge to move in NIA is often generated by an inner sense of restlessness, not specifically referable to the extremities. While sensory symptoms may occur in NIA, the unpleasant dysesthesias in RLS is almost invariably present in

**TABLE 6** Differences Between Akathisia and Restless Legs Syndrome

| | Akathisia | RLS |
|---|---|---|
| Movements | Whole body rocking, marching in place, general fidgetiness | Stereotypic feet and leg movements |
| Sensory symptoms | No true sensory component | Usually unpleasant sensations |
| Cognitive and behavioral changes | Often present | Usually absent |
| Subjective sleep disturbances | Absent or mild | Mild to severe |
| Sleep studies | PLMS sometimes present | PLMS almost always present |
| Neurologic examination | May have rocking, tremor or EPSE, tardive dyskinesia | Normal in idiopathic RLS |
| Onset | Related to dopamine blocking drugs | Very gradual in idiopathic RLS, may be subacute in secondary RLS |
| Course | Acute akathisia resolves with drug discontinuation, tardive and withdrawal akathisia have variable courses | Idiopathic RLS has gradual worsening with age but varies |
| Diurnal variation | No pattern, but may be modestly worse at night | Worse at night |
| Family history | Noncontributory | Autosomal dominant pattern in idiopathic RLS |
| Treatment | B-antagonists, benzodiazepines, anticholinergics | Dopaminergics, opioids, benzodiazepines, gabapentin |

*Abbreviations*: PLMS, periodic limb movements in sleep; EPSE, extra-pyramidal side effects.

the lower extremities. Motor restlessness in NIA is neither as dramatically worsened at night nor improved with activity compared to RLS. Sleep disturbances and PLMS tend to be less severe in NIA, and constant body rocking and marching-in space occur in severe NIA, but are only minor or transient in RLS. Finally, concurrent drug-induced dyskinesias (oro-facial-lingual stereotypes being the most common) may often be seen in NIA (41) but not in RLS patients.

### Attention Deficit Hyperactivity Disorder

ADHD is usually a childhood disorder characterized by motor, cognitive, and behavioral disturbances that frequently affect the learning of the child. Hyperactivity in these children may be misinterpreted as RLS symptoms. However, a recent study has shown that the prevalence of PLMS on polysomnography was higher in the children with ADHD than in the control subjects (42). It is possible that PLMS may directly lead to symptoms of ADHD through the mechanism of sleep disruption. The association between ADHD and RLS/PLMS may be genetically linked and represent different phenotype of the same or related condition in some cases (Chapter 13).

### Tourette's Syndrome

TS is defined by multiple motor and at least one vocal tics before the age of 21 without a definable secondary cause. Hyperactivity, attention deficit, and obsessive compulsive disorder are associated conditions. The motor tics are usually preceded by a sensory premonition and relieved after action of tic. Constant leg movements, which may persist during sleep, can be seen in children with TS. A recent study (43) examined RLS and other TS comorbidities in 144 probands with TS or chronic tics and their parents. RLS was present in 10% of probands and 23% of parents. RLS in probands was associated with maternal RLS but not paternal RLS, suggesting that a maternal RLS factor may contribute to the variable expression of TS. Hence, while motor tics and hyperactivity in TS patients need to be differentiated from RLS, TS and RLS may coexist in some TS patients, suggesting a possible etiologic link between these two conditions. However, it can be difficult to differentiate a leg tic from the urge to move associated with RLS.

### Metabolic Disorders

Patients with hyperthyroidism frequently present with loss of weight, anxiety, and motor restlessness. Unlike RLS, the motor restlessness does not affect the lower extremities predominantly. But because dopaminergic dysfunction is associated with both thyroid disorders and RLS, it has been suggested that motor restlessness in some patients with hyperthyroidism may simulate RLS symptoms. Tan et al. (44) evaluated for RLS in patients diagnosed biochemically with either hyper- or hypothyroidism, and in controls without thyroid disorders. Amongst 146 consecutive patients with biochemically confirmed thyroid disorders, none satisfied all the IRLSSG criteria of RLS, similar to the control population (0.2%, 1/434). However, interestingly, they found 8.2% (12/146) with RLS-like symptoms (satisfied the first three IRLSSG criteria) compared to 0.9% (4/434) in the controls ($p < 0.0001$). Four (33.3%) of these patients reported complete resolution of these symptoms after treatment of their thyroid condition. They concluded that while RLS-like symptoms were observed in some patients with thyroid disorders, there was no significant difference of RLS prevalence between patients with thyroid disorders and euthyroid controls. Despite these observations, there has been a case report of a hypothyroid patient with low serum ferritin who upon challenge and withdrawal of L-thyroxine, developed RLS (45). There was a correlation of L-thyroxine replacement with a change in the IRLSSG severity score, the PLMS, the number of arousals due to PLMS, and sleep efficiency. Hence, it is important to recognize that RLS symptoms can complicate thyroxine replacement in at-risk hypothyroid patients with low serum ferritin.

### Levodopa-Induced Dyskinesias and Motor Fluctuations in Parkinson's Disease

Because dopaminergic dysfunction and response to dopaminergic agents are consistent features in RLS and Parkinson's disease (PD), some authors have suggested that these two diseases may share common pathophysiology, while others debate their association (46,47). However, it is important to highlight that RLS, if present in PD, appears milder than in patients with idiopathic RLS (47). These symptoms can sometimes be difficult to subjectively differentiate from other sensory and motor symptoms in PD. Furthermore, RLS symptoms might be a manifestation of wearing-"off" phenomenon, a dopaminergic-related complication of PD (46). Levodopa-induced dyskinesias usually do not pose a diagnostic problem in PD patients, because a careful history would differentiate these from RLS symptoms.

### Painful Legs and Moving Toes

Painful legs and moving toes is characterized by continuous or semicontinuous undulating movements, typically of the toe flexors and extensors, adductors, and abductors (48). Occasionally, hands and fingers may be involved. These movements often disappear during sleep. Pain, rather than restlessness, is the predominant complaint and is often severe. This syndrome is associated with peripheral nerve lesions, secondary to causes such as trauma or infections or due to central nervous system dysfunction. Some cases are considered idiopathic. It can be easily distinguished from RLS by its characteristic undulating movements and associated pain, and may not be worse at night or relieved by activity.

### Neuropathies and Others

While the association of RLS with neuropathy is well-recognized, entrapment neuropathy could sometimes produce RLS-like symptoms. For instance, carpal tunnel syndrome (CTS) is a nerve entrapment disorder, involving the median nerve when it passes the carpal tunnel at the wrist. In a case–control study (49), 312 electrophysiologically confirmed CTS patients and 100 matched controls were examined utilizing a questionnaire similar to the clinical diagnostic criteria of RLS. Forty-four (14.1%) of the CTS patients have symptoms compatible with restless hand syndrome compared with none (0%) in the control group. Because hand symptoms may sometimes be observed in RLS, it is important to remember that entrapment syndromes such as CTS can be associated with a form of restlessness in the hands, analogous to RLS. Patients with small fiber and/or large fiber neuropathies (e.g., in diabetics) may complain of dysesthesia, which may worsen at night. Usually, the neuropathic sensation is superficial.

Nocturnal leg cramps are manifested by painful paroxysmal spasms of muscles of the feet and calves (50). They are usually relieved more by vigorous stretching against the cramp as opposed to general movement. They are more common in the middle of sleep rather than at sleep onset. There should be palpable intense muscle contraction with true cramps. Body positional discomfort syndrome simply refers to the inability to maintain subjective comfort in a specific supine body position while trying to obtain sleep. This results in frequent change of positions, which can improve the subjective discomfort.

Patients with degenerative spine disease can present with worsening of symptoms, such as low back pain, and nighttime arousals and restlessness. Vesper's curse manifests as leg and lumbosacral pain that may be associated with restlessness and nighttime arousals (50). It is presumably due to lumbar stenosis in the setting of congestive heart failure (CHF). The increased right heart filling pressure engorges the paraspinal vasculature while in a recumbent position, thus exacerbating the pre-existing spinal stenosis and leading to recumbent neurogenic claudication symptoms. Treatment of the CHF improves the condition. Patients with orthostatic tremor can mimic RLS because they feel much better while walking compared to standing. However, they should not have symptoms while lying down. Patients with rest tremor or internal tremor from PD or chorea patients could be mistaken for RLS, but neurological examination should differentiate these. Finally, rare cases of orthostatic hypotension may cause leg sensations and movement while sitting, which resolves upon standing. Usually there are no symptoms while supine.

## EVALUATION OF THE RESTLESS LEGS SYNDROME PATIENT

Clinically, typical RLS, especially when associated with a positive family history, requires only a minimal laboratory evaluation. Serum ferritin, electrolytes, and possibly more sophisticated iron studies, such as iron binding percentage, should be obtained. Nerve conduction velocities (NCV) and electromyogram (EMG) should be performed in cases without a family history of RLS, atypical presentations (i.e., sensations beginning in the feet or superficial pain), in cases that have a predisposition for neuropathy (i.e., diabetes) or when physical symptoms and signs are consistent with a peripheral neuropathy. If EMG/NCV abnormalities are found they should be further evaluated. Polysomnographic evaluation is usually reserved for patients in whom the diagnosis is in doubt, in cases where PLMS are suspected to be severe and result in arousals, or if other sleep disorders are suspected. Radiographic evaluation, vascular studies, and other electrophysiological tests are seldom warranted.

## CONCLUSIONS

A high index of suspicion, supported by a careful history and examination, is frequently needed to diagnose RLS. It is important to recognize the common medical conditions that may be confused with RLS and to remember that in some instances RLS could coexist with medical diseases associated with dopaminergic dysfunction. The current proposed clinical diagnostic criteria are simple, practical, and encompassing enough for clinicians to apply them in their practice and for research purposes. Early diagnosis of RLS will prevent unnecessary morbidity and improve quality of life for those suffering from the condition.

## REFERENCES

1. Tan EK, Ondo W. Restless legs syndrome: clinical features and treatment. Am J Med Sci 2000; 319(6):397–403.
2. Ekbom KA. Restless legs. Acta Med Scand 1945; 158(suppl):1–124.
3. Ondo W. Epidemiology of restless legs syndrome. Sleep Med 2002(suppl 3):S13–S15.
4. Rothdach AJ, Trenkwalder C, Haberstock J, Keil U, Berger K. Prevalence and risk factors of RLS in an elderly population: the memory and morbidity in Augsburg elderly. Neurology 2000; 54:1064–1068.
5. Tan EK, Koh KK, Seah A, See SJ, Lim E, Wong MC. Restless legs syndrome in an Asian population: a study in Singapore. Mov Disord 2001; 16(3):577–579.
6. The International Restless Legs Syndrome Study Group, Walter AS. Towards a better definition of the restless legs syndrome. Mov Disord 1995; 10:634–642.
7. Allen RP, Picchietti D, Hening WA, Trenkwalder C, Walters AS, Montplaisi J. Restless legs syndrome diagnosis and epidemiology workshop at the National Institutes of Health; International Restless Legs Syndrome Study Group. Restless legs syndrome: diagnostic criteria, special considerations, and epidemiology. A report from the restless legs syndrome diagnosis and epidemiology workshop at the National Institutes of Health. Sleep Med 2003; 4(2):101–119.
8. Winkelmann J, Wetter TC, Collado-Seidek V, et al. Clinical characteristics and frequency of the hereditary restless legs syndrome in a population of 300 patients. Sleep 2000; 23:597–602.
9. Michaud M, Chabli A, Lavigne G, Montplaisir J. Arm restlessness in patients with RLS. Mov Disord 2000; 15:289–293.
10. Ondo WG, Jankovic J. RLS:clinico-radiologic correlates. Neurology 1996; 47:1435–1441.
11. Bassetti CL, Mauerhofer D, Gugger M, et al. RLS: a clinical study of 55 patients. Eur Neurology 2001; 45:67–74.
12. Michaud M, Lavigne G, Desautels A, et al. Effects of immobility on sensory and motor symptoms of RLS. Mov Disord 2002; 17:112–115.
13. Montplaisir J, Lapierre O, Lavigne G. The RLS: a condition associated withperiodic or aperiodic slowing of the EEG. Neurophysiol Clin 1994; 24:131–140.
14. Bornstein B. Restless legs. Psyhciatr Neurol 1961; 141:165–201.

15. Trenkwalder C, Walters AS, Hening W, Campbell S, Rahman K, Chokroverty S. Circadian rhythm of patients with the idiopathic RLS. Sleep Res 1995; 24:360.
16. Walters AS, Hickey K, Maltzman J, et al. A questionnaire study of survey Neurology 1996; 46:92–95.
16a. Bentley AJ, Rosman KD, Mitchell D: Gender differences in the presentation of subjects with restless legs syndrome. Sleep Med 2006; 7:37–41.
17. Lavigne GJ, Montplaisir JY. RLS and sleep bruxism; prevalence and associationamong Canadians. Sleep 1994; 17:739–743.
18. Benes H, Kurella B, Kummer J, et al. Rapid onset of action of Levodopa in restless legs syndrome: a double-blind, randomized, multicenter, Crossover trial. Sleep 1995; 22: 1073–1081.
19. Trenkwalder C, Stiasny K, Pollmacher T, et al. L-dopa therapy of uremic and idiopathic restless legs syndrome: a double blind crossover trial. Sleep 1995; 24:455–458.
20. Walters AS, Hening WA, Kavey N, et al. A double-blind randomized crossover trial of bromocriptine and placebo in RLS. Ann Neurol 1988; 24:455–458.
21. Earley CJ, Yaffee JB, Allen RP. Randomized, double-blind, placebo-controlled trial of pergolide in RLS. Neurology 1998; 51:1599–1602.
22. Ondo W, Romanyshyn J, Vuong KD, Lai D. Long-term treatment of restless legs syndrome with dopamine agonists. Arch Neurol 2004; 61(9):1393–1397.
23. Walters AS, Ondo WG, Dreykluft T, Grunstein R, Lee D, Sethi K. TREAT RLS 2 Therapy with Ropinirole: Efficacy And Tolerability in RLS 2 Study Group. Ropinirole is effective in the treatment of restless legs syndrome. TREAT RLS 2: a 12-week, double-blind, randomized, parallel-group, placebo-controlled study. Mov Disord. 2004; 19(12): 1414–1423.
24. Montplaisir J, Nicolas A, Denesle R, Gomez-Mancilla B. RLS improved by pramipexole: a double blind randomized trial. Neurology 1999; 52:938–943.
24a. Stiasny-Kolster K, Kohnen R, Carsten Moller J, Trenkwalder C, Oertel WH: Validation of the "L-DOPA test" for diagnosis of restless legs syndrome. Mov Disord 2006. (in press).
25. Montplaisir J, Boucher S, Nicolas A, et al. Immobilization tests and periodic leg movements in sleep for the diagnosis for RLS. Mov Disord 1998; 13:324–329.
26. Nicolas A, Michaud M, Lavigne G, Montplaisir J. The influence of sex, age and sleep/wake state on characteristics of periodic leg movements in RLS. Clin Neurophysiol 1999; 110:1168–1174.
27. Desautels A, Turecki G, Montplaisir J, et al. Identification of a major susceptibility locus for restless legs syndrome on chromosome 12q. Am J Hum Gent 2001; 69: 1266–1270.
28. O' Keefffe ST, Gaviv K, Lavan JN. Iron status and RLS in the elderly. Age Ageing 1994; 23:200–203.
29. Sun ER, Chen CA, Ho G, et al. Iron and the RLS. Sleep 1998; 21:371–379.
30. Goodman JD, Brodie C, Ayida GA. RLS in pregnancy. Br Med J 1988; 297:1101–1102.
31. Lee KA, Zaffke ME, Baratte-Beebe K. RLS and sleep disturbance during pregnancy: the role of folate and iron. J Women Health Gend Based Med 2001; 10:335–341.
32. McParland P, Pearce JM. RLS in pregnancy. Case reports. Clin Exp Obstet Gynecol 1990; 17:5–6.
33. Roger SD, Harris DC, Stewart JH. Possible relation between RLS and anemia in renal dialysis patients. Lancet 1991; 337:1551.
34. Collado-Seidel V, Kohnen R, Samtleben W, et al. Clinical and biochemical findings in uremic patients with and without RLS. Am J Kidney Dis 1998; 28:372–378.
35. Winkelman JW, Chertow GM, Lazarus JM. RLS in end stage renal disease. Am J Kidney Dis 1996; 28:372–378.
36. Walker S, Fine A, Kryger MH. Sleep complaints are common in a dialysis unit. Am J Kidney Dis 1995; 26:751–756.
37. Allen RP, Earley CJ. RLS: a review of clinical and pathophysiologic features. J Clin Neurophysiol 2001; 18:128–147.
38. Tan EK, Ondo WG. Motor restlessness. Int J Clin Pract 2001; 55(5):320–322.
39. Walters AS, Hening W, Rubinstein M, Chokroverty S. A clinical and Polysomnographic comparison of NIA and RLS: Sleep 1991; 14:339–345.

40. Lang AE. Akathisia and RLS. In: Jankovic J, Tolosa E, eds. Parkinson's Disease and Movement Disorders. 2nd ed. Baltimore, MD: Williams and Wilkins, 1993:399–418.
41. Tan EK, Jankovic J. Tardive and idiopathic oromandibular dystonia: a clinical comparison. J Neurol Neuro Surg Psychiatry 2000; 68(2):186–190.
42. Picchietti DL, Underwood DJ, Farris WA, et al. Further studies on periodic limb movement disorder and restless legs syndrome in children with attention-deficit hyperactivity disorder. Mov Disord 1999; 14(6):1000–1007.
43. Lesperance P, Djerroud N, Diaz Anzaldua A, Rouleau GA, Chouinard S, Richer F; Montreal Tourette Study Group. Restless legs in Tourette syndrome. Mov Disord 2004; 19(9):1084–1087.
44. Tan EK, Ho SC, Eng P, et al. Restless legs symptoms in thyroid disorders. Parkinsonism Relat Disord 2004; 10(3):149–151.
45. Tan EK, Ho SC, Koh L, Pavanni R. An urge to move with L-thyroxine: clinical, biochemical, and polysomnographic correlation. Mov Disord 2004; 19(11):1365–1367.
46. Tan EK, Lum SY, Wong MC. Restless legs syndrome in Parkinson's disease. J Neurol Sci 2002; 196(1–2):33–36.
47. Ondo WG, Vuong KD, Jankovic J. Exploring the relationship between Parkinson disease and restless legs syndrome. Arch Neurol 2002; 59(3):421–424.
48. Schoenen J, Gonce M, Delwiade PJ. Painful legs and moving toes: a syndrome with different pathophysiologic mecahnisms. Neurology 1984; 34:1108–1112.
49. Tan EK, Koh KK, Arulanandam S, Lo YL. Restless hand symptoms in carpal tunnel syndrome. Int J Clin Pract 2004; 58(11):1000–1002.
50. Laban NK, Viola SL, Femminineo AF, et al. RLS associated with diminished Cardiopulmonary compliance and lumbar spinal stenosis- motor concomitant of Vesper's curse. Arch Phys Med Rehabil 1990; 71:384–388.

# 12 Occurrence of Restless Legs Syndrome

**Jan Ulfberg**
*Sleep Disorders Center, Avesta Hospital, Avesta, Sweden*

**Bjørn Bjorvatn**
*Department of Public Health and Primary Health Care, University of Bergen, Bergen, Norway*

## INTRODUCTION

Epidemiology is the study of the distribution and determinants of diseases, health-related states, or events in a specified population (Epi = "on, upon, among"; Demos = "the people, population, man"; Ology = "the study of"). Evaluations of distributions of a disease may include the investigation of geographical distributions.

In statistical terms, a random sample is a set of items that have been drawn from a population in such a way that each time an item was selected every item in the population had an equal opportunity to appear in the sample. The only factor operating when a given item is selected must be chance. Actually, only a few studies on the occurrence of restless legs syndrome (RLS) are based on a random sample of the general population.

Data on the occurrence of RLS are historically quite variable, which may be due to several possible reasons. It is important to define the study population; i.e., whether the sample studied represents a clinical patient population or sole epidemiological data on RLS, which are harvested in the general population. Thus, the selection and the definition of the study population are important factors influencing prevalence. Moreover, the instruments used for the diagnosis of RLS vary among different epidemiological studies. Clearly, these aspects influence the result.

Different strategies of data collection may influence the results. Using mailed questionnaires is an often-used method in this context. Its strength is that with this method you may reach many participants, but its drawback may be that different participants interpret the questions in different ways. Telephone interviews may be more precise, but are more expensive. In these situations, it is important that the interviewer is trained. Face-to-face interviews and examinations by trained physicians are the most sensitive and specific way to acquire the data, but are limited by the time and expense, which can limit the number of participating subjects.

In 1995, the International Restless Legs Syndrome Study Group (IRLSSG) published a consensus report for the diagnosis of RLS (1). Data from studies performed before 1995, and even some studies performed after 1995 as well, used different diagnostic instruments in order to make a diagnosis of RLS. Mainly the investigators used only one or a few questions to make the diagnosis. Thus, reports on the occurrence of RLS not using the criteria from 1995 or the revised criteria from 2003, are not directly comparable to each other (2).

## THE OCCURRENCE OF RESTLESS LEGS SYNDROME—STUDIES ON POPULATIONS

In 1945, the thesis "Restless Legs. A Clinical Study of a Hitherto Overlooked Disease in the Legs" was published by the Swedish neurologist Ekbom (3). Thus, Ekbom coined the name of this disorder and wrote what is still considered to be the most substantial and comprehensive work on RLS. Ekbom questioned both what he called "normal series" of 503 persons about restlessness in their legs and a sample of 503 from the neurologic outpatient service. The normal series was composed partly of friends and acquaintances, medical students, nurses, hospital assistants, and the like, altogether 280 persons, and partly of 223 patients from the surgical outpatient department of the Serafimer Hospital in Stockholm, Sweden. Patients with the main complaint of paralysis, pain, or paresthesia in the legs were excluded from the neurologic outpatient group.

Ekbom reported a prevalence of 5.2% of restless legs in the "normal series." There was a slight female predominance. Among the neurologic patients, 7.8% of the cases suffered from restlessness in their legs (3).

Decades later, a survey conducted through written questionnaire was performed in Canada to estimate the prevalence of subjective symptoms related to RLS and to sleep bruxism. Of the 2019 respondents, all over 18 years of age, 15% reported "leg restlessness at bedtime" and 10% reported "unpleasant leg sensations." In this study, a female preponderance for RLS was found, as well as a progression of the leg restlessness with age (4).

A question reflecting clinical features of RLS was added to the 1996 Kentucky Behavioral Risk Factor Surveillance by Phillips and collaborators: "Do you have unpleasant feelings in your legs—for example, creepy-crawling or tingling feelings—when you, lie down at night that make you feel restless and keep you from getting a good nights sleep?" Data were collected by telephone interview from 1803 men and women. The prevalence of RLS for Kentucky adults was estimated to 10.0% (5). In this study, the RLS prevalence did not vary significantly with sex, but the prevalence of RLS increased clearly with age.

In a door-to-door personal interview of 369 people over the age of 65 in Augsburg, Germany, using IRLSSG criteria, Rothdach et al. found an RLS prevalence of 9.8%. RLS was more common in women compared with men (13.9% vs. 6.1%) (6). Patients with RLS also reported a higher prevalence of depression and had lower self-reported mental health scores compared to normal controls.

In two Swedish epidemiological studies, performed by sending questionnaires to a random sample of the population in Dalarna County in the middle of the country, the four symptom questions, accepted as minimal diagnostic criteria for RLS, were used to diagnose RLS. A total of 5.8% of the men, 18 to 64 years of age, suffered from RLS (7). Correspondingly, 11.4% of the women suffered from RLS (8). Among the men, the RLS prevalence increased with age (7).

Ohayon and Roth reported on cross-sectional studies performed in the United Kingdom, Germany, Italy, Portugal, and Spain. Overall, 18,980 subjects aged 15 to 100 years, representative of the general populations of these five European countries, underwent telephone interviews with the Sleep-EVAL system. The diagnosis of RLS was based on the minimal criteria provided by the International Classification of Sleep Disorders. The prevalence of RLS, as defined by this now little used criteria, was 5.5% (9). In this study, the prevalence of RLS significantly increased with age.

Berger et al. performed a large-scale study with the contribution of randomly selected individuals in northeast Germany (10), where 4310 subjects with ages between 20 and 79 years were interviewed using the IRLSSG criteria for RLS. The overall prevalence of RLS was 10.6% and increased with age. Women were twice as often affected as men. The RLS prevalence in women increased with the number of pregnancies; thus, parity may be one factor explaining the sex difference in the prevalence of RLS.

In order to estimate the prevalence of RLS among 2005 randomly selected adults (>18 years) among the population in Norway and Denmark, joint Scandinavian RLS researchers used telephone interviews and employed the IRLSSG criteria to diagnose the RLS (11). In Norway, 14.3%, and in Denmark, 8.8% of the respondents fulfilled the diagnostic criteria for RLS. Half of these reported the symptoms as moderate to very severe, based on the severity scale developed by IRLSSG (IRLS) (12). Mean duration of the complaint was 10 years. Prevalence was higher in females than males (13.4% vs. 9.4%), and lowest in the youngest age group (18–29 years). From the age of 30 years and above, no clear age-related difference was seen. The main predictors of RLS were insomnia and symptoms of periodic limb movements in sleep.

Hogl et al. conducted a cross-sectional study of a sex- and age-stratified random sample of the general population (50–89 years; $n = 701$) in Austria (13). The diagnosis of RLS was established by face-to-face interviews. The prevalence of RLS was 10.6% (14.2% in women, 6.6% in men); 33.8% of all patients with RLS had mild, 44.6% had moderate, and 21.6% had severe disease expression based on the IRLS, a validated scale often used in clinical trials. None had been previously diagnosed or was on dopaminergic therapy. Free serum iron, transferrin, and ferritin concentrations were similar in subjects with and without RLS; however, soluble transferrin receptor concentrations were higher in subjects with RLS (1.48 mg/L vs. 1.34 mg/L; $p < 0.001$).

In a recent substantial and comprehensive population-based survey, face-to-face home interviews were conducted among a random sample of 10,263 French adults (14). The four features defined by the IRLSSG in 1995 were used to assess the prevalence of symptoms consistent with a diagnosis of RLS. The 12-month prevalence of RLS symptoms in the French adult population was estimated to be 8.5%, with a higher prevalence observed in women (10.8%) than in men (5.8%). Prevalence increased with age until 64 years and decreased thereafter in both sexes. RLS was often underdiagnosed and few subjects received recommended RLS drug treatment.

Nichols et al. reported a population-based study from a single primary care center in rural Idaho, U.S.A. (15). A written questionnaire given to 2099 patients revealed that 24% of these patients were positive for all four of the essential symptoms of RLS and that 15.3% reported these symptoms at least weekly. RLS symptoms were significantly more common in women. The prevalence of symptoms increased with age until about 60 years and then showed a steady decrease thereafter.

The largest epidemiological study of RLS involved 23,052 persons from five countries: United States, United Kingdom, Germany, France, and Spain (16). Similar to most other reports, 9.6% of all people met criteria for RLS and reported at least weekly symptoms. About one-third of these patients had RLS more than twice per week and thus probably justified regular treatment. In general, northern European countries demonstrated higher prevalence compared to Mediterranean countries. Out of 551 RLS sufferers, 357 (64.8%) reported consulting a physician about their RLS symptoms, but only 46 of these 357 (12.9%) reported having been given a diagnosis. The primary physician records reported that 209 (37.9%) of these RLS sufferers consulted them about RLS symptoms, and 52 (24.9%) of these were given an RLS diagnosis.

The prevalence of RLS may be less in Asian populations. Tan et al. in Singapore personally interviewed and examined 157 consecutive individuals aged 55 years and older, selected from the general population of Singapore, and 1000 consecutive individuals from a primary health care center, aged 21 years and older (17). Based on IRLSSG criteria, the prevalence of restless leg syndrome was only 0.6% and 0.1%, respectively. Thus, a low prevalence was found in this study in an Asian population.

Kageyama et al. in Japan examined the sleep habits among 4612 adult subjects using written questionnaires (18). They used a single question in order to assess restlessness in the legs in relation to sleep. The prevalence of this was reported to be about 5% to 10% in regard to age groups. In contrast to almost all other studies, RLS was reported to be more prevalent among men.

In another Japanese study, Itoga et al. examined the sleep quality of the 4003 elderly (mean age 75 years) in Izumo City in Japan (19). The diagnostic questionnaire on RLS published by IRLSSG in 1995 was administered. The results showed that 150 of the subjects (3.7%) suffered from RLS.

Recently, a large-scale epidemiological study from Turkey was published by Sevim et al. (20). They found a prevalence of 3.2% in a sample of 3234 Turkish subjects, also showing higher frequencies in women, cigarette smokers, and individuals residing at high altitudes.

In South America, there is one study on the occurrence of RLS in the population (21). In order to evaluate the frequency of RLS in a sample of 100 adults in Chile, the investigators used the four IRLSSG diagnostic questions to make the RLS diagnosis. The authors reported that 13% of the subjects were affected by RLS.

There are no epidemiological reports of RLS in people of African descent. Anecdotally African Americans only rarely present with RLS, but it is unclear whether this represents a true lower prevalence, or rather differences in medical sophistication and referral patterns. Two reports have found a lower rate of RLS in African Americans than in white Americans in uremic patients (22,22a).

In summary, the majority of surveys on the occurrence of RLS study North American and European populations. The prevalence of RLS in this population usually ranges between 5% and 15%, with an average of about 10%. RLS that occurs at least three days a week, and likely justifies nightly treatment, probably occurs in about 3% to 4% of these populations. There seems to be evidence for a female preponderance in the prevalence of RLS, and RLS increases with age, at least until the eighth decade. Data harvested on the occurrence of RLS from other parts of the world are less exhaustive, but RLS may be less common in Asian and African populations. A summary of RLS population studies is presented in Table 1.

## RESTLESS LEGS SYNDROME IN PREGNANCY

There are a growing number of studies showing that RLS seems to be a substantial ailment among pregnant women (Chapter 20). The first actual case report on an association between pregnancy and RLS originated from Montevideo, Uruguay (28). It was first reported in Ekbom's thesis that RLS was common among pregnant

**TABLE 1** Studies on the Occurrence of Restless Legs Syndrome

| First author | Country | Year | *N* | Occurrence (%) |
|---|---|---|---|---|
| Ekbom (3) | Sweden | 1945 | 503 | 5.2 |
| Strang (23) | Sweden | 1967 | 320 | 2.5 |
| Oboler (24) | United States | 1991 | 453 | 29 |
| Lavigne (4) | Canada | 1994 | 2019 | 15 |
| Phillips (5) | United States | 2000 | 1803 | 10 |
| Kageyama (18) | Japan | 2000 | 4612 | 5–10 |
| Rothdach (6) | Germany | 2000 | 369 | 9.8 |
| Schmitt (25) | Switzerland | 2000 | 1473 | 4 |
| Ulfberg (9) | Sweden (men) | 2001 | 4000 | 5.8 |
| Ulfberg (8) | Sweden (women) | 2001 | 200 | 11.4 |
| Tan (17) | Singapore | 2001 | 1000 | 0.1 |
| Miranda (21) | Chile | 2001 | 100 | 13 |
| Ohayon (9) | Europe | 2002 | 18,980 | 5.5 |
| Itoga (19) | Japan | 2002 | 4003 | 3.7 |
| Sevim (20) | Turkey | 2003 | 3234 | 3.2 |
| Krishnan (26) | India | 2003 | 128 | 0.8 |
| Rijsman (27) | The Netherlands | 2004 | 1437 | 7.1 |
| Berger (10) | Germany | 2004 | 4310 | 10.6 |
| Bjorvatn (11) | Norway/Denmark | 2005 | 2005 | 14.3/8.8 |
| Tison (14) | France | 2005 | 10,263 | 8.5 |
| Nichols (15) | United States | 2004 | 2099 | 24 |
| Hogl (13) | Austria | 2005 | 701 | 10.6 |
| Hening (16) | United States/ Europe | 2004 | 23,052 | 9.6 |
| Wenning (22d) | Austria | 2005 | 206 | 10.8 |
| Vogl (22b) | Tyrolean | 2006 | 530 | 8.9 |
| Phillips (22c) | U.S.A. | 2006 | 1506 | 9.7 |

women. Ekbom not only surveyed the symptoms of restless legs in a sample of healthy people in the city of Stockholm but also asked 486 pregnant women about restlessness in their legs and found that 11.3% of them were suffering from this ailment during their pregnancy (3). Thus, the prevalence of RLS in pregnancy was twice that reported by Ekbom among a sample of 230 healthy women (5.7%).

In 1960, these data were corroborated by Karl Ekbom Jr., who investigated the occurrence of restlessness in the legs among 202 pregnant women and found that 25 cases (12%) suffered from restless legs (29). Ekbom Jr. also reported that the leg restlessness among these pregnant women who were iron deficient usually disappeared when prescribed oral or intravenous iron therapy. Goodman et al. surveyed 500 consecutive pregnant women attending a clinic in London (30). They found that 97 (19%) of the women reported symptoms consistent with RLS. During the four weeks before delivery, there was a reduction in the numbers of subjects suffering from restless legs. In the four weeks after delivery, the symptoms stopped in all but three women.

Lee et al. investigated the occurrence of RLS among 30 women before, during, and after pregnancy, and found that RLS increased from 0 during preconception to 23% during the third trimester of pregnancy (31). Only one subject continued to experience RLS after delivery. Compared with those without complaints of RLS, those with RLS had low serum ferritin at preconception and significantly lower folate levels during preconception and at each trimester.

Hedman et al. in Finland surveyed the sleep in 325 pregnant women and noted that as many as 37.7% of these women complained of RLS in late pregnancy,

**TABLE 2** Studies on the Occurrence of Restless Legs Syndrome in Pregnancy

| First author | Country | Year | *N* | Occurrence (%) |
|---|---|---|---|---|
| Ekbom KA (3) | Sweden | 1945 | 485 | 11.3 |
| ten Berge (35) | The Netherlands | 1953 | 54 | 13 |
| Jolivet (36) | France | 1953 | 100 | 27 |
| Ekbom K (29) | Sweden | 1960 | 202 | 12 |
| Goodman (30) | United Kingdom | 1988 | 500 | 19 |
| Lee (31) | United States | 2001 | 30 | 23 |
| Hedman (32) | Finland | 2002 | 325 | 37.7 |
| Suzuki (33) | Japan | 2003 | 16,528 | 19.9 |
| Manconi (34) | Italy | 2004 | 642 | 26 |

but this figure returned to the initial pre-pregnant level after delivery (32). Actually, that level was high as well, as much as 18%.

In a large cross-sectional survey, approaching 16,528 pregnant women in Japan, Suzuki et al. used self-administered questionnaires with one single question in order to diagnose those affected by possible RLS (33). As many as 19.9% of this group of pregnant women were considered to suffer from restless legs. This is particularly high, because population-based studies in Japan reveal relatively little RLS.

Manconi et al. used a structured clinical interview in order to assess symptoms of RLS from the beginning of pregnancy in a population of 642 pregnant women (34). This was the first study to use the IRLSSG criteria for RLS diagnosis among pregnant women as a diagnostic instrument. Twenty-six percent of the women were affected during their pregnancy. The disease was strongly related to the third trimester of pregnancy and tended to disappear reaching the time of delivery; thus, these results corroborated the data presented by Goodman et al. (30).

In summary, the higher prevalence of RLS during pregnancy seems to be real (Table 2). The risk for a pregnant woman to be affected by RLS is at least two- to three-fold compared to the risk among nonpregnant women and returns to baseline shortly after delivery.

## RLS and Iron Deficiency

Ekbom, in 1955, reported on two male cases with malignancies (cancer in the urinary bladder and cancer in the gut), who were severely iron deficient and also suffered from RLS (37). In the same paper, Ekbom reported on 34 cases (25 females, 9 males) with RLS, where 13 (38%) were suffering from low serum iron values, all below the lower limit for normal distribution. Thus, it seems as though Ekbom was also the first to report the occurrence of iron deficiency in subjects presenting with RLS.

In a population study of individuals 25 years old or more, all subjects with a suspicion of iron deficiency were questioned in 1964 by Aspenstrom about symptoms of restless legs (38). During one month, 80 cases of verified iron deficiency were found. Restless legs were reported in 30 of the 64 women (47%) and in 4 of the 16 men (25%).

In 1966, Karl Ekbom Jr., approached 317 patients by doing follow-up examinations 7 to 9 years after partial gastrectomy by the Billroth I or II method for gastric or duodenal ulcer (39). RLS was found to have developed postsurgically in 40 cases (12.6%). The hemoglobin and serum iron values were found to be low in all 13 cases in which this was assessed.

In 1994, O'Keeffe carried out a study of 18 elderly patients with RLS and 18 matched control subjects (40). Serum ferritin levels were reduced in the RLS patients compared with control subjects. The hemoglobin levels did not differ between the two groups.

In a Swedish survey consisting of 946 consecutive blood donors, 14.7% of the male blood donors and 24.7% of the female blood donors were affected by RLS (41). The mean intake of iron among the blood donors after each blood donation was much lower than recommended. Among the women, 7.4% demonstrated an iron deficiency. In this group of women, 37.5% were affected by RLS. In this study, the intake of iron was higher among women than among men, but irrespective of that, the women showed a higher frequency of RLS than the men. Moreover, a relationship between iron deficiency and RLS was only shown among the female blood donors. More of the RLS sufferers than the non-RLS subjects showed signs of impairment of the red blood cell production.

Low-density lipoprotein apheresis (LA) is an extracorporeal procedure to treat severe hyperlipidemia in patients with coronary heart disease who fail to respond to lipid-lowering diet and drug therapy. LA treatment may induce iron deficiency. Tings et al. in Goettingen, Germany, explored the occurrence of RLS in a group of LA patients (42). Of 25 LA patients, 12 (48%) were found to have RLS. Laboratory investigations showed that 11 of 12 patients with RLS had ferritin levels below or at the lower limit of the normal range, indicating a depletion of body iron stores.

In summary, there is an increasing bulk of data showing that RLS seems to be common among subjects with iron deficiency.

## RESTLESS LEGS SYNDROME AND PARKINSON'S DISEASE

It could be hypothesized that an association between RLS and Parkinson's disease (PD) is possible because both of these neurological conditions respond to dopaminergic treatment (Chapter 21). Hence, some studies have investigated an eventual association between RLS and PD.

Ekbom, who was the first to report on a large series of RLS patients, did not find any PD cases in his cohort (43). Moreover, Lang and Johnson did not find any RLS symptoms in 100 consecutive PD patients (44). However, a Swedish neurologist, Strang, a contemporary to Ekbom, reported in 1967 that in a group of 600 patients with PD, 40 (6.7%) were affected by restless legs (23).

In a study on the occurrence of PD in RLS patients, Banno et al. found extrapyramidal dysfunction in 17% of men and 23% of women, out of a total of 218 patients presenting with RLS (45). Corresponding figures in the control (non-RLS population) was 0.2%.

One study that evaluated 125 consecutive PD outpatients in Singapore found that only 0.8% fulfilled IRLSSG criteria for RLS (46). The prevalence rate found in PD was not significantly different compared with the 0.6% RLS reported in the general population in Singapore (17).

In a study by Ondo et al. of 303 Parkinson's patients, 20.8% had RLS (47). In 68% of patients with both PD and RLS, the PD symptoms preceded the RLS symptoms. Accordingly, the authors found no evidence that RLS symptoms early in life predisposed to the subsequent development of PD.

This observation has been supported by a recent study performed in India by Krishnan and associates who reported an occurrence of 7.9% of RLS among PD patients (26). Compared with only 0.8% in the Indian controls, the occurrence of RLS in PD patients in this sample of patients represents a high figure.

Taken together, some studies suggest an association between PD and RLS. However, the number of studies is still small. Further studies in this area are warranted.

## RESTLESS LEGS SYNDROME IN END-STAGE RENAL DISEASE

End-stage renal disease (ESRD) is probably the most investigated secondary condition associated with RLS (Chapter 18). Since 1966, when Callaghan reported on five patients with RLS out of 20 patients with renal damage (48), numerous reports have recognized that RLS is common in patients with ESRD, and that RLS occurs both before and after institution of dialysis treatment. This is also supported by the fact that RLS improves after renal transplantation in most cases of ESRD (49).

Prevalence ranges from 6.6% to 83% (50,51). However, one has to consider that the inclusion criteria have varied among these populations. Some studies have included several dialysis centers that led to a heterogeneous population mix, and control populations were used in only a few studies. In addition, the reliability of self-administered questionnaires to diagnose RLS in ESRD patients may be low, because of confusion with other causes of leg pain in this patient population. Moreover, there are many possible causes of ESRD, such as diabetes mellitus in late stage, which in itself may even cause neurological symptoms. Overall, these studies have failed to identify any consistent risk factors for the development of RLS in the uremic population. Table 3 only reports the occurrence of RLS in ESRD patients with samples of at least 200 subjects.

One survey on 308 patients with chronic renal failure undergoing maintenance hemodialysis examined the issue of racial differences in the prevalence of RLS (22). In this study, more Caucasian patients than African-American patients reported experiencing RLS symptoms during the past six months (68% vs. 48%). Hence, further studies on the racial differences in the prevalence of the RLS are warranted.

In summary, the data from the large numbers of studies exploring the relationship between ESRD and RLS strongly support the hypothesis that there is an association between these two conditions.

**TABLE 3** Studies with Samples of More Than 200 Subjects on the Prevalence of Restless Legs Syndrome in End-Stage Renal Disease

| First author | Country | Year | *N* | Occurrence (%) |
|---|---|---|---|---|
| Winkelman (52) | United States | 1996 | 204 | 20 |
| Sanner (53) | Germany | 1996 | 232 | 41.8 |
| Hui (54) | China | 2000 | 201 | 62 |
| Sabbatini (55) | Italy | 2002 | 694 | 52 |
| Kutner (22) | United States | 2002 | 308 | 68/48 |
| Takaki (56) | Japan | 2003 | 490 | 12.2 |
| Unruh (57) | United States | 2004 | 894 | 15 |
| Gigli (58) | Italy | 2004 | 601 | 21.5 |

## REFERENCES

1. Walters AS. Toward a better definition of the restless legs syndrome. The International restless legs syndrome study group. Mov Disord 1995; 10(5):634–642.
2. Allen RP, Picchietti D, Hening WA, Trenkwalder C, Walters AS, Montplaisir J. Restless legs syndrome: diagnostic criteria, special considerations, and epidemiology. A report from the restless legs syndrome diagnosis and epidemiology workshop at the National Institutes of Health. Sleep Med 2003; 4(2):101–119.
3. Ekbom KA. Restless legs. Acta Med Scand 1945; 158(suppl):1–123.
4. Lavigne GJ, Montplaisir JY. Restless legs syndrome and sleep bruxism: prevalence and association among Canadians. Sleep 1994; 17:739–743.
5. Phillips B, Young T, Finn L, Asher K, Hening WA, Purvis C. Epidemiology of restless legs symptoms in adults. Arch Intern Med 2000; 160:2137–2141.
6. Rothdach AJ, Trenkwalder C, Haberstock J, Keil U, Berger K. Prevalence and risk factors of RLS in an elderly population: The MEMO study. Neurology 2000; 54:1064–1068.
7. Ulfberg J, Nyström B, Carter N, Edling C. Prevalence of restless legs syndrome among men aged 18 to 64 years: an association with somatic disease and neuropsychiatric symptoms. Mov Disord 2001; 16:1159–1163.
8. Ulfberg J, Nyström B, Carter N, Edling C. Restless legs syndrome among working-aged women. Eur Neurol 2001; 46:17–19.
9. Ohayon MM, Roth T. Prevalence of restless legs syndrome and periodic limb movement disorder in the general population. J Psychosom Res 2002; 53:547–554.
10. Berger K, Luedemann J, Trenkwalder C, John U, Kessler C. Sex and the risk of restless legs syndrome in the general population. Arch Intern Med 2004; 164:196–202.
11. Bjorvatn B, Leissner L, Ulfberg J, et al. Prevalence, severity and risk factors of restless legs syndrome in the general adult population in two Scandinavian countries. Sleep Med 2005; 6(4):307–312.
12. Allen RP, Kushida CA, Atkinson MJ. Factor analysis of the International Restless Legs Syndrome Study Group's scale for restless legs severity. Sleep Med 2003; 4:133–135.
13. Högl B, Kiechl S, Willeit J, et al. Restless legs syndrome: a community-based study of prevalence, severity, and risk factors. Neurology 2005; 64(11):1920–1924.
14. Tison F, Crochard A, Legér D, Bouée S, Lainey E, El Hasnaoui A. Epidemiology of restless legs syndrome in French adults: a nationwide survey. The INSTANT study. Neurology 2005; 65:239–246.
15. Nichols DA, Allen RP, Grauke JH, Brown JB, Rice ML, Hyde PR, et al. Restless legs syndrome symptoms in primary care: a prevalence study. Arch Intern Med 2003; 163(19):2323–2329.
16. Hening W, Walters AS, Allen RP, Montplaisir J, Myers A, Ferini-Strambi L. Impact, diagnosis and treatment of restless legs syndrome (RLS) in a primary care population: the REST (RLS epidemiology, symptoms, and treatment) primary care study. Sleep Med 2004; 5(3):237–246.
17. Tan EK, Seah A, See SJ, Lim E, Wong MC, Koh KK. Restless legs syndrome in an Asian population: a study in Singapore. Mov Disord 2001; 16:577–579.
18. Kageyama T, Kabuto M, Nitta H, et al. Prevalences of periodic limb movement-like and restless legs-like symptoms among Japanese adults. Psychiatry Clin Neurosci 2000; 54:296–298.
19. Itoga M. Izumo project (report 1): Sleep quality questionnaire on the elderly in Izumo City. Seishin Igaku 2002; 44:401–408 [Japanese].
20. Sevim S, Dogu O, Camdeviren H, et al. Unexpectedly low prevalence and unusual characteristics of RLS in Mersin, Turkey. Neurology 2003; 61:1562–1569.
21. Miranda M, Araya F, Castillo JL, Duran C, Gonzalez F, Aris L. Restless legs syndrome: a clinical study in an adult general population and in uremic patients. Rev Med Chil 2001; 129:179–186.
22. Kutner NC, Bliwise DL. Restless legs complaint in African-American and Caucasian hemodialysis patients. Sleep Med 2002; 3:497–500.

22a. Lee J, Parker K, Ansari F, Bliwise D. A secondary analysis of racial differences in periodic limb movements in sleep and ferritin in hemodialysis patients sleep medicine 2006 (in press).

22b. Vogl FD, Pichler I, Adel S, Pinggera GK, Bracco S, De Grandi A, Volpato CB, Aridon P, Mayer T, Meitinger T, Klein C, Casari G, Pramstaller PP: Restless legs syndrome: Epidemiological and clinicogenetic stydy in a South Tyrolean population isolate. Mov Disord 2006.
22c. Phillips B, Hening W, Britz P, Mannino D: Prevalence and correlates of restless legs syndrome: results from the 2005 National Sleep Foundation Poll. Chest 2006; 129:76–80.
22d. Wenning GK, Kiechl S, Seppi K, Muller J, Hogl B, Saletu M, Rungger G, Gasperi A, Willeit J, Poewe W: Prevalence of movement disorders in men and women aged 50-89 years (Bruneck Study cohort): a population-based study. Lancet Neurol 2005; 4:815–820.
23. Strang RR. The symtom of restless legs. Med J Aust 1967; 1:1211–1213.
24. Oboler SA, Prochazka AV, Meyer TJ. Leg symptoms in outpatient veterans. West J Med 1991; 155:256–259.
25. Schmitt BE, Gugger M, Augustiny K, Bassetti C, Radanov BP. Prevalence of sleep complaints: a questionnaire-based study of a Swiss working population. Schweiz Med Wochenschr 2000; 130:772–778.
26. Krishnan PR, Bhatia M, Behari M. Restless legs syndrome in Parkinson's disease: a case-controlled study. Mov Disord 2003; 18:181–185.
27. Rijsman R, Knuistingh Neven A, Graffelman W, Kemp B, de Weerd A. Epidemiology of restless legs in the Netherlands. Eur J Neurol 2004; 11:607–611.
28. Mussio-Fournier JC, Rawak F. Familiäres auftreten von pruritus, urticaria und parästhetischer hyperkinese der unteren extremitäten. Confin Neurol 1940; 3:110–114. /German/.
29. Ekbom K. Akroparestesier och restless legs under graviditet. Lakartidningen 1960; 57:2597. /Swedish/.
30. Goodman JDS, Brodie C, Ayida GA. Restless leg syndrome in pregnancy. BMJ 1988; 297:1101–1102.
31. Lee KA, Zaffke ME, Baratte-Beebe K. Restless legs syndrome and sleep disturbance during pregnancy: the role of folate and iron. J Womens Health Gend Based Med 2001; 10:335–341.
32. Hedman C, Pohjasvaara T, Tolonen U, Suhonen-Malm AS, Myllylä VV. Effects of pregnancy on mothers' sleep. Sleep Med 2002; 3:37–42.
33. Suzuki K, Ohida T, Sone T, et al. The prevalence of restless legs syndrome among pregnant women in Japan and the relationship between restless legs syndrome and sleep problems. Sleep 2003; 26:673–677.
34. Manconi M, Govoni V, De Vito A, et al. Restless legs syndrome and pregnancy. Neurology 2004; 63:1065–1069.
35. ten Berge BS. Kuitkrampen en restless legs (anxietas tibiarum) in de zwangerschap. Geneeskd Gids 1953; 31:11–19 [Dutch].
36. Jolivet B. Paresthesies agitantes nocturnes des membres inferieurs impatiences. These de Paris 1953 [French].
37. Ekbom KA. Restless legs as an early symptom of cancer. Lakartidningen 1955; 52 (30):1875 [Swedish].
38. Aspenstrom G. Pica and restless legs in iron deficiency. Lakartidningen 1964–1961: 1174–1177 [Swedish].
39. Ekbom K. Restless legs syndrome after partial gastrectomy. Acta Neurol Scand 1966; 42:79–89.
40. O'Keeffe ST, Gavin K, Lavan JN. Iron status and restless legs syndrome in the elderly. Age Ageing 1994; 23:200–203.
41. Ulfberg J, Nystrom B. Restless legs syndrome in blood donors. Sleep Med 2004; 5:115–118.
42. Tings T, Schettler V, Canelo M, Paulus W, Trenkwalder C. Impact of regular LDL apheresis on the development of restless legs syndrome. Mov Disord 2004; 19:1072–1075.
43. Ekbom KA. Restless legs syndrome. Neurology 1960; 10:868–873.
44. Lang AE, Johnson K. Akathisia in idiopathic Parkinson's disease. Neurology 1987; 37:477–481.
45. Banno K, Delaive K, Walld R, Kryger MH. Restless legs syndrome in 218 patients: associated disorders. Sleep Med 2000; 1:221–229.

46. Tan EK, Lum SY, Wong MC. Restless legs syndrome in Parkinson's disease. J Neurol Sci 2002; 196:33–36.
47. Ondo WG, Vuong KD, Jankovic J. Exploring the relationship between Parkinson disease and restless legs syndrome. Arch Neurol 2002; 59:421–424.
48. Callaghan N. Restless legs syndrome in uremic neuropathy. Neurology 1966; 16: 359–361.
49. Winkelmann J, Stautner A, Samtleben W, Trenkwalder C. Long-term course of restless legs syndrome in dialysis patients after kidney transplantation. Mov Disord 2002; 17:1072–1076.
50. Bhowmik D, Bhatia M, Gupta S, Agarwal SK, Tiwari SC, Dash SC. Restless legs syndrome in hemodialysis patients in India: a case controlled study. Sleep Med 2003; 4:143–146.
51. Holley JL, Nespor S, Rault R. Characterizing sleep disorders in chronic hemodialysis patients. ASAIO Trans 1991; 37:M456–M457.
52. Winkelman JW, Chertow GM, Lazarus JM. Restless legs syndrome in end-stage renal disease. Am J Kidney Dis 1996; 28:372–378.
53. Sanner B, Schilken P, Konermann M, Burmann-Urbanek M, Sevecke-Herbst A, Hecking E. Sleep disturbances in end-stage renal disease. Nieren-und Hochdruckkrankheiten 1996; 25:27–30 [German].
54. Hui DS, Wong TY, Ko FW, et al. Prevalence of sleep disturbances in chinese patients with end-stage renal failure on continuous ambulatory peritoneal dialysis. Am J Kidney Dis 2000; 36:783–788.
55. Sabbatini M, Minale B, Crispo A, et al. Insomnia in maintenance haemodialysis patients. Nephrol Dial Transplant 2002; 17:852–856.
56. Takaki J, Nishi T, Nangaku M, et al. Clinical and psychological aspects of restless legs syndrome in uremic patients on hemodialysis. Am J Kidney Dis 2003; 41:833–839.
57. Unruh ML, Levey AS, D'Ambrosio C, Fink NE, Powe NR, Meyer KB. Restless legs symptoms among incident dialysis patients: association with lower quality of life and shorter survival. Am J Kidney Dis 2004; 43:900–909.
58. Gigli GL, Adorati M, Dolso P, et al. Restless legs in end-stage renal disease. Sleep Med 2004; 5:309–315.

# 13 Childhood-Onset Restless Legs Syndrome

**Suresh Kotagal and Michael H. Silber**

*Department of Neurology and the Sleep Disorders Center, Mayo Clinic, Rochester, Minnesota, U.S.A.*

## HISTORY

In 1832, Duchamp (1) observed that children may suffer aches and pains around puberty and labeled them as "growing pains." It was not until 1994 that Walters et al. (2) first described restless legs syndrome (RLS) in a mother and three children, aged six, four, and one years, as well as a 16-year old from an unrelated family. The disorder exhibited autosomal dominant transmission. The patients experienced leg discomfort and nocturnal motor restlessness, with temporary relief by voluntary movement. Earlier, in 1985, Kotagal et al. (3) had noted that as compared to sibling controls, leukemic children in remission who had received central nervous system radiation and intrathecal methotrexate were prone to exhibit "nocturnal myoclonus" or periodic limb movements of sleep (PLMS), but they failed to recognize that the limb discomfort in their patients might have represented RLS. PLMS are defined as a series of four or more limb electromyographic discharges of 0.5 to 5 second duration that are separated by intervals of 4 to 90 seconds (4). Walters et al. (2) had observed that children with RLS showed PLMS on nocturnal polysomnography. The presence of PLMS is not essential to the diagnosis of RLS, although around 80% of RLS patients do exhibit PLMS on nocturnal polysomnography (5). Owing to the subjective nature of the sleep complaints, it may be difficult to accurately diagnose RLS in young or nonverbal children. Clinical and epidemiological research into childhood RLS has therefore been limited. The recognition of childhood RLS has been facilitated by the recently published diagnostic criteria that were established at a Consensus Conference of the National Institutes of Health (NIH) (5). These diagnostic guidelines have been made intentionally more stringent than the criteria used for diagnosing RLS in adults.

## CLINICAL FEATURES

Preschool-age children may be unable to verbalize discomfort from RLS, which may be an unrecognized contributor to their bedtime resistance. Onset of symptoms of RLS can be as early as one to two years (6). An anecdotal recollection by the parent of a child with RLS (Table 1, subject #6) was that as a toddler, this patient was very difficult to put to sleep, and that the patient would fling legs so hard at bedtime that the patient almost "broke the crib."

A more reliable history of sleep initiation and sleep maintenance difficulties can be provided by older children who may describe a "creepy" or "crawling" feeling in their limbs that appears in the late evening or at night. Some children have described a feeling of "bugs crawling on the legs" or of "walking through snow." There is also an irresistible urge to move the legs. This sensorimotor

**TABLE 1** Diagnostic Criteria for Adult and Childhood Restless Legs Syndrome

*Essential Diagnostic Criteria (adults)*

- An urge to move the legs, usually accompanied or caused by uncomfortable and unpleasant sensations in the legs.
- The urge to move or unpleasant sensations begin or worsen during periods of rests or inactivity such as lying down or sitting
- The urge to move or unpleasant sensations are partially or totally relieved by movement, such as walking or stretching, at as long as the activity continues
- The urge to move or unpleasant sensations are worse in the evening or night than during the day, or only occur during the evening or night.

*Definite Childhood Results Legs Syndrome (RLS)*

- The child meets all four essential adult criteria, and
- The child relates a description in his or hen own words that is consistent with leg discomfort
  *OR*
- The child meets all four essential adult criteria, and two of three following
  - Sleep disturbance for age
  - A biologic parent or sibling has definite RLS
  - The child has polysomnographically documented periodic limb movement index of 5 or more per hour of sleep

*Probable Childhood Restless Less Syndrome (RLS)*

- The child meets all four essential adult criteria for RLS except criterion #4 (the urge to move or sensations are worse in the evening or at night than during the day), *and*
- The child has a biologic parent or sibling has definite RLS,
  OR
- The child is observed to have behavior manifestations of lower extremity discomfort when sitting or lying, accompanied by motor movement of the affected limbs; the discomfort has characteristics of adult criteria 2,3, and 4, and
- The child has a biologic parent or sibling has definite RLS

*Source*: From Ref. 5.

disturbance shows a circadian variation, and is most prominent in the evenings and at night. It is relieved by movement and exacerbated by rest. Some parents have observed that symptoms are more prominent while school is in session rather than during the summer vacation when children are more likely to be involved with vigorous outdoor physical activities. Although childhood RLS is now subclassified into *probable* and *definite* categories (5), both groups seem to be likely defining the same condition (6). Inheritance patterns, PLMS indices, levels of serum ferritin, and clinical response to therapeutic agents appear to be similar in both groups. The increased nocturnal arousals consequent to RLS may provoke parasomnias such as confusional arousals and sleepwalking. The child may appear unrefreshed upon awakening in the morning. Daytime fatigue, inattentiveness, hyperactivity, and oppositional behavior may coexist. Lower limb motor restlessness as measured by actigraphy may mimic RLS and has been documented in Asperger syndrome (7). It is not clear whether this represents RLS, because these noncommunicative children are unable to provide adequate history. RLS in childhood secondary to uremia has also been reported (8). RLS secondary to polyneuropathy has not been reported, though it probably does occur.

## PATHOGENESIS

### Genetic Predisposition

Childhood RLS most likely develops when genetic predisposition interacts with environmental factors that have yet to be fully identified. Winkelmann et al. carried out complex segregation analysis on 238 (predominantly adult) patients with RLS and 537 relatives (9). They found that patients with an age of onset of symptoms below 30 years most likely had single gene, autosomal dominant transmission with a multifactorial component. The lower end of the age range in their study population was 12 years. In those with onset after the age of 30 years, however, no genetic predisposition could be established.

Jing et al. (10) performed genetic linkage analysis in a Han family. They evaluated for known RLS linkage and 16 candidate genes responsible for dopaminergic transmission or iron transmission. Candidate genes examined included those for dopamine receptors D1 to D5, neuronal-specific transcription factor, tyrosine hydroxylase, dopamine beta hydroxylase, ferritin light and heavy peptides, transferrin, transferrin receptor (TfR), and aconitase and iron responsive element binding protein 2. None of the loci examined could be linked to familial RLS. When Bonati et al. (11) carried out linkage studies in a 30-member, three-generation Italian family, however, they observed a significant logarithm of odds score for marker D14S288 that is localized on chromosome region 14q13 to 21. There appears to be considerable genetic heterogeneity, however, because Desautels et al. had earlier observed an autosomal recessive inheritance pattern in the study of a 25-member French Canadian family in which 14/25 were considered to be affected (12). Haplotype analysis revealed the RLS predisposing gene to be located between markers D12S1044 and D12S78 on chromosome 12q.

In a series of 32 children with RLS, Kotagal and Silber (6) found a positive family history in 23 of 32 (72%) subjects. Mothers were four times more likely to be the affected parent than fathers. A predilection for mother–child transmission has also been observed in other studies as well. In 1994, Walters et al. had reported the occurrence of RLS in a mother and three children (2). The significance of the mother–child predilection is uncertain. It may represent genetic imprinting or simply be an artifact stemming from the fact that mothers are more likely to accompany their children to doctor visits than fathers, and women have RLS more often than men.

### Iron Deficiency

The reasons for iron deficiency in children with RLS have not been established. Nutritional factors may be important (13) as might genetic factors that regulate iron absorption. In our study, close to three-fourths of 32 children with RLS showed low levels of serum ferritin, the cellular storage protein for iron (6). Ferritin is composed of 24 subunits, which are a mixture of heavy chains (H) and light chains (L). The gene for the H-chains is localized to chromosome 11 while the gene for the L-chains is localized to chromosome 19. H-ferritin has strong ferro-oxidase activity that is required for the uptake of iron by the ferritin molecule (14). Mice lacking H-ferritin show a high lethality rate (15). There is close correspondence between the serum and intracellular levels of ferritin level and total body iron stores. There is, however, no correlation between serum ferritin and hematological indices of iron deficiency (low hemoglobin, hematocrit, and red blood cell mean corpuscular volume), because ferritin levels have to generally drop below 10 μg/dL before bone marrow stores of iron are affected (14).

In a prospective study of 39 children with a mean age of 7.5 years (SD = 3.1 years), Simakajornboon et al. (16) found a probable, though not statistically significant association between lowering of the serum ferritin and the periodic limb movement index (PLMI). Patients with serum iron levels less than 50 μg/dL showed significantly higher PLMI as compared to those with serum iron levels greater than 50 μg/dL (42.8 ± 18.3 vs. 23.1 ± 10.1; $p = 0.02$). Furthermore, the PLMI was reduced following oral iron replacement therapy.

Connor et al. examined the brains of seven adults with RLS and compared them with those of five age-matched controls who had no neurological disease (17). They noted that RLS patients showed a marked decrease in staining for iron and H-ferritin in the neuromelanin cells of substantia nigra, which are the major sites of synthesis of dopamine. More recently, Connor et al. (18) have suggested that the primary disturbance in RLS is a reduction in the level of iron regulatory protein-1 in these neuromelanin cells, which in turn leads to a lowering of intracellular levels of TfR. The lack of TfR hampers the binding of iron within the cell. Iron may affect dopamine in several ways. It is a cofactor for tyrosine hydroxylase synthesis, which is the rate-limiting step in the synthesis of dopamine, part of the dopamine-2 receptor, and is required for Thy-1 production, which stabilizes dopamine synapses.

## The Link Between Inattentiveness, Hyperactivity, and RLS

A significant association between childhood-onset RLS and hyperactivity and inattentiveness was observed by Chervin et al. when they compared 27 children with hyperactivity and inattention to 43 non-ADHD (attention deficit hyperactivity disorder) controls from a child psychiatry clinic ($p = 0.01$), but not when they compared these RLS subjects with another set of controls that was derived from a general pediatric clinic (19). There was no clear explanation for this disparity in comparison with the two sets of controls. It is possible that the study was insufficiently powered to satisfactorily address the issue. Also, the authors acknowledge that their results may have been different had they used a more detailed, validated questionnaire addressing RLS and also that larger, epidemiologic studies are needed to study the potential relationship between RLS and ADHD. Picchietti et al. have also observed a similar association between RLS and ADHD (20,21). They found that 8 of 25 biological parents of children with ADHD gave a history consistent with RLS as compared to none of the parents of control subjects ($p = 0.011$).

Although the association between RLS and ADHD is highly likely but not definitively established, the link between ADHD and PLMD (periodic limit movement disorder) is firmly established. Picchietti et al. (21) conducted a polysomnographic study of 14 consecutive children with ADHD and 10 control children without ADHD. About 9 of the 14 (64%) children with ADHD showed PLMD, with PLMI > 5/hr, as compared to none of the controls ($p < 0.0015$). The ADHD subjects also gave a history of significant sleep initiation and maintenance difficulty that was not observed in the controls.

## Do "Growing Pains" Represent RLS?

Walters (22) points out the heterogeneous nature of "growing pains" and suggests that a subset of children with "growing pains" may actually have RLS. The term "growing pains" is applied to a conglomeration of symptoms of discomfort in the limbs that are seen in children, usually at night, which may be secondary to arthritic or nonarthritic conditions. Walters provides a comprehensive and thoughtful discussion of this issue (22). His review mentioned that Ekbom reported an adult patient with RLS who recalled having "growing pains" during childhood, but that nature of the discomfort from these two conditions was different, thus leading Ekbom to conclude that RLS and growing pains were unrelated conditions (23). On the other hand, Brenning, a contemporary of Ekbom, studied 112 children and noticed a similarity between the symptoms of "growing pains" and RLS (24). Rajaram et al. (25) have also applied the RLS diagnostic criteria to a set of 11 children with growing pains (mean age = 10.4 years). They observed that 10/11 children with growing pains actually met the diagnostic criteria for RLS. Also, in 4 of 8 families of these 10 children, one of the parents had RLS. They once again concluded that a subset of children with "growing pains" actually had RLS. The strict application of the NIH Consensus Conference diagnostic criteria for childhood RLS (5) should help further clarify the relationship between RLS and growing pains. Walters also correctly observes that the bulk of literature on "growing pains" appeared quite some years before establishment of the current diagnostic criteria for RLS (21). For now, therefore, the comparison between the two conditions is likely to remain imprecise.

### How Do Age and Gender Impact Childhood RLS/PLMS?

In the recent series of Rajaram et al. (25), none of the 10 children who met diagnostic criteria for RLS exhibited a PLMI of over 5. On the other hand, a relationship between these two phenomena does become apparent over decades, because around 80% of adult RLS patients exhibit PLMS (5). While there is a general assumption that the PLMI increases gradually with age, longitudinal studies of this phenomenon through infancy and childhood are lacking.

Gender and age are important determinants of the serum ferritin levels in adolescents, with reference values in females being lower than those of age-matched males. In a longitudinal survey of dietary habits, physical activity, energy metabolism, iron status, and body composition in Sweden, Samuelson et al. (26) reported that the mean serum ferritin level was lower in both boys and girls at an age of 15 years than at an age of 17 years. For boys, the mean serum ferritin level at an age of 15 years was 36.3 μg/dL (SD = 17.8, $n = 103$), while at an age of 17 years the mean serum ferritin level was 53.6 μg/dL (SD = 32.8, $n = 103$). For girls, the mean serum ferritin level at an age of 15 years was 30 μg/dL (SD = 19, $n = 124$), while at 17 years it had risen to 33 μg/dL (SD = 30.6, $n = 124$). Unfortunately, age and gender differences in serum ferritin have not been adequately considered in the study of childhood RLS and PLMD.

## DIAGNOSIS

As in adults, childhood RLS is a clinical diagnosis that is based upon historical information (Table 2) and a detailed family history. Clinicians resort to polysomnography to document an elevated PLMI of greater than 5 more often in children than in adults simply because children are often unable to provide reliable history. An inexpensive and useful diagnostic aid is a review of a videotape of the child's sleep in the home environment, which may show periodic limb movements. Because a serum ferritin level below 50 μg/L is seen in close to three-fourths of children with RLS (6), it should receive consideration in the future as a supportive diagnostic criterion. ADHD appears to be an important comorbidity that necessitates neuropsychological assessment.

## TREATMENT

Systematic, prospective studies on the treatment of childhood RLS are lacking. Drugs commonly used to treat adults with RLS have been prescribed for children

**TABLE 2** Clinical Features in 32 Children with Restless Legs Syndrome

| Patient number | RLS type | Gender | Onset age/ diagnosis age | PLM/hr of sleep (index) | Serum ferritin μg/L | Affected parent | Treatment |
|---|---|---|---|---|---|---|---|
| 1 | Probable | Female | 5/8 | 1.8 | – | Mother | Pramipexole |
| 2 | Probable | Female | 13/15 | – | 11 | Mother | Oral iron |
| 3 | Probable | Male | 11/15 | 33.1 | – | Father | Gabapentin |
| 4 | Probable | Female | 11/13 | 0 | 10 | Mother | Oral iron |
| 5 | Probable | Male | 11/13 | – | – | Mother | – |
| 6 | Probable | Male | 1/5 | 21.5 | – | Mother | Gabapentin |
| 7 | Probable | Female | 2/14 | 5.3 | 16 | Mother | Gabapentin |
| 8 | Probable | Male | 5/6 | 20.8 | 20 | Father | Pramipexole |
| 9 | Probable | Female | 8/13 | – | 47 | Mother | Exercise |
| 10 | Definite | Male | 11/13 | 0 | 21 | None | Oral iron |
| 11 | Definite | Female | 14/16 | – | 71 | Mother | Gabapentin |
| 12 | Definite | Female | 13/15 | 42.9 | 10 | None | Oral iron |
| 13 | Definite | Male | 7/13 | 41 | 17 | Mother | Pramipexole |
| 14 | Definite | Male | 12/15 | 30.8 | 6 | None | Levodopa-carbidopa |
| 15 | Definite | Male | 8/13 | 1 | – | None | Clonazepam |
| 16 | Definite | Male | 8/11 | 10 | 50 | None | – |
| 17 | Definite | Female | 4/16 | 5.5 | – | Mother | Gabapentin |
| 18 | Definite | Female | ?/14 | – | 17 | Mother | Gabapentin |
| 19 | Definite | Female | 11/13 | – | 27 | None | Pramipexole |
| 20 | Definite | Female | 12/14 | 25 | 25 | None | Pramipexole |
| 21 | Definite | Male | 15/16 | 13.1 | – | Father | Gabapentin |
| 22 | Definite | Female | 2/16 | 0 | – | Mother | Pramipexole |
| 23 | Definite | Male | 4/16 | 11.5 | 51 | Father | Gabapentin |
| 24 | Definite | Female | 11/11 | 3.5 | 15 | Father | Clonazepam |
| 25 | Definite | Male | 6/6 | 13.6 | 23 | Mother | Pramipexole |
| 26 | Definite | Female | 13/17 | 0 | 29 | None | Gabapentin |
| 27 | Definite | Female | 16/17 | 50.3 | 60 | Mother | Pramipexole |
| 28 | Definite | Female | 14/17 | – | 11 | Mother | Pramipexole, oral iron |
| 29 | Definite | Female | 1/5 | 0 | 12 | None | Pramipexole |
| 30 | Definite | Female | 15/17 | – | 36 | Mother | Pramipexole |
| 31 | Definite | Male | 12/14 | 23.2 | 23 | Father | Pramipexole, oral iron |
| 32 | Definite | Male | 5/15 | 61.3 | 28 | Mother | Pramipexole |

*Abbreviation*: PLM, periodic limb movement.
*Source*: From Ref. 6.

as well on an off-label basis, with a generally favorable response. Agents that can potentially be prescribed include levodopa–carbidopa, dopamine agonists such as pramipexole and ropinirole; benzodiazepines, such as clonazepam or alprazolam; alpha-adrenergic agonists such as clonidine; and anticonvulsants such as gabapentin or carbamazepine (27).

Walters et al. (28) described the response of six children with ADHD and RLS to treatment with levodopa/carbidopa or pergolide. All six subjects showed subjective improvement in their sleep as well as significantly reduced PLMI and arousals from sleep. The daytime behavior also improved to the point that three of six no longer met the diagnostic criteria for ADHD. Also, a welcome development was the resolution of associated oppositional defiant disorder, as verified on the Conners subscale and on an Oppositional Defiant Disorder Scale.

In our series of 32 patients with RLS, 16 had been treated with the dopamine agonist, pramipexole (6). Doses used were 0.125 to 0.375 around bedtime. Of the 16 (37.5%), 6 showed no benefit from pramipexole, whereas 10 of 16 (62.5%) improved. Side effects were encountered in 3 of 16, consisting of tremor, confusion, and augmentation (one each). The augmentation that was seen in one patient resolved upon switching to an alternate dopaminergic agent, ropinirole. There was no correlation between favorable response to pramipexole and the presence or absence of PLMS, or the serum ferritin level. Konofal et al. (29) have recently reported a beneficial effect of ropinirole 0.25 mg at bedtime in treating a child with combined RLS and ADHD. They documented progressive resolution of both disorders over time. There is anecdotal evidence of gabapentin being helpful in treating childhood RLS. Clinical experience suggests that the observation of Garcia-Borreguero et al. (30) that gabapentin is most beneficial to patients who have RLS combined with pain also applies to children.

Iron replacement therapy may also lead to amelioration of RLS symptoms over time, as observed by Kryger et al. (31). The fact that improvement in RLS symptoms with oral iron replacement is gradual (taking months) should be emphasized to the patient and the family lest they develop unrealistic expectations about a prompt response. Combining oral iron with a dopamine agonist is a reasonable option for providing quick symptomatic relief and definitive resolution of symptoms over time. The long-term outcome of childhood RLS remains unknown, especially in terms of characteristics that predict its resolution or persistence.

## FUTURE DIRECTIONS

The clinical and polysomnographic manifestations in preschool-age children need better delineation, because at present one is unable to reliably verify the clinical features. Studies are needed to evaluate serial changes, if any, in the PLMI over the first two decades of life. Do probable and definite RLS need to be maintained as distinct diagnostic categories or should they be merged? The possible association between RLS/PLMS and ADHD needs to be studied both epidemiologically and in depth in the sleep laboratory. More extensive genetic linkage studies in multiplex families of different ethnicities are badly needed. We know that "growing pains" resolve gradually over time but the long-term outcome of childhood RLS remains uncertain. Drug treatment trials designed specifically for children are at the threshold of being launched. These issues will hopefully be addressed in the near future.

## REFERENCES

1. Duchamp M. Maladies de la croissance. In: Levrault FG, ed. Memories de medicine practique. Paris: Jean-Frederic Lobstein, 1832.
2. Walters AS, Picchietti DL, Ehrenberg DL, Wagner ML. Restless legs syndrome in childhood and adolescence. Pediatr Neurol 1994; 11:241–245.
3. Kotagal S, Rathnow SR, Chu JY, et al. Nocturnal myoclonus—a sleep disturbance in children with leukemia. Dev Med Child Neurol 1985; 27:124–126.
4. The Atlas Task Force of the American Sleep Disorders Association. Recording and scoring leg movements. Sleep 1993; 16:748–759.
5. Allen RP, Picchietti D, Hening WA, et al. Restless legs syndrome: diagnostic criteria, special considerations, and epidemiology. A report from the restless legs syndrome diagnosis and epidemiology workshop at the National Institutes of Health. Sleep Med 2003; 4:101–119.

6. Kotagal S, Silber MH. Childhood-onset restless legs syndrome. Ann Neurol 2004; 56:803–807.
7. Tuisku K, Tani P, Nieminen-von Wendt T, et al. Lower limb motor restlessness in Asperger's disorder measured using actometry. Psychiatry Res 2004; 128:63–70.
8. Davis I, Baron J, O'Riordan M. Sleep disturbances in pediatric dialysis patients. Pediatr Nephrol 2005; 20:69–75.
9. Winkelmann J, Muller-Myhsok B, Wittchen HU, et al. Complex segregation analysis of restless legs syndrome provides evidence for an autosomal dominant mode of inheritance in early age at onset families. Ann Neurol 2002; 52:297–302.
10. Jing LI, Lan-Dian HU, Wang WJ, Chen YG, Kong XY. Linkage analysis of the candidate genes of familial restless legs syndrome. Acta Genetica Sinica 2003; 30(4):325–329.
11. Bonati MT, Ferini-Strambi L, Aridon P, Oldani A, Zuconi M, Casari G. Autosomal dominant restless legs maps on chromosome 14q. Brain 2003; 126(6):1485–1492.
12. Desautels A, Turecki G, Montplaisir J, Sequeira A, Verner A, Rouleau GA. Identification of a major susceptibility locus for restless legs syndrome on chromosome 12q. Am J Hum Genet 2001; 69:1266–1270.
13. Hallberg L, Hulthen L. Perspectives on iron absorption. Blood Cells, molecules, and diseases. 2002; 29(3):562–573.
14. Harrison PM, Arosio P. The ferritins: molecular properties, iron storage function and cellular regulation. Biochem Biophys Acta 1996; 1275(3):161–203.
15. Ferreira C, Bucchini D, Martin ME, et al. Early embryonic lethality of H-ferritin gene deletion in mice. J Biol Chem 2000; 275:3021.
16. Simakajornboon N, Gozal D, Vlasic V, Mack C, Sharon D, McGinley BM. Periodic limb movements and iron status in children. Sleep 2003; 26(6):735–738.
17. Connor JR, Boyer PJ, Menzies SL, Dellinger B, Allen RP, Ondo WG. Neuropathological examination suggests impaired brain iron acquisition in restless legs syndrome. Neurology 2003; 61(3):304–309.
18. Connor JR, Wang XS, Patton SM, et al. Decreased transferring receptor expression by neuromelanin cells: a putative mechanism for restless legs syndrome. First Congress of the International BioIron Society, Prague, Czech Republic, May 22–26, 2005:195.
19. Chervin RD, Dillon JE, Basetti C, Ganoczy DA, Pituch KJ. Symptoms of sleep disorders, inattention and hyperactivity in children. Sleep 1997; 20(12):1185–1192.
20. Picchietti DL, England SJ, Walters AS, Willis K, Verrico T. Periodic limb movement disorder and restless legs syndrome in children with attention deficit hyperactivity disorder. J Child Neurol 1998; 13:588–594.
21. Picchietti DL, Walters AS. Moderate to severe periodic limb movement disorder in childhood and adolescence. Sleep 1999; 22:297–300.
22. Walters AS. Is there a subpopulation of children with growing pains who really have Restless Legs Syndrome. A review of the literature. Sleep Med 2002; 3(2):93–98.
23. Ekbom KA. Growing pains and restless legs. Acta Pediatr Scand 1975; 64:264–266.
24. Brenning R. Growing pains. Acta Soc Med-Upsalien 1960; 65:185–201.
25. Rajaram SS, Walters AS, England SJ, Mehta D, Nizam F. Some children with growing pains may actually have restless legs syndrome. Sleep 2004; 27(4):767–773.
26. Samuelson G, Lonnerdal B, Kempe B, Elverby J-E, Bratteby L-E. A follow-up study of serum ferritin and transferring receptor concentrations in Swedish adolescents at age 17 years compared to age 15. Acta Pediatr 2000; 89:1162–1168.
27. Tan E-K, Ondo W. Restless legs syndrome: Clinical features and treatment. Am J Med Sciences 2000; 319(6):397–403.
28. Walters AS, Mandelbaum DE, Lewin DS, Kugler S, England SJ, Miller M. Dopaminergic therapy in children with restless legs/periodic limb movements in sleep and ADHD. Pediatr Neurol 2000; 22:182–186.
29. Konofal E, Arnulf I, Lecendreux M, Mouren M-C. Ropinorole in a child with attention deficit hyperactivity disorder and restless legs syndrome. Pediatr Neurol 2005; 32:350–351.
30. Garcia-Borreguero D, Larossa O, de la Llave Y, Verger K, Masramon X, Hernandez G. Treatment of restless legs syndrome with gabapentin. A double-blind, cross-over study. Neurology 2002; 59:1573–1579.
31. Kryger MH, Otake K, Foerester J. Low body stores of iron and restless legs syndrome: a correctable cause of insomnia in adolescents and teenagers. Sleep Med 2002; 3:127–132.

# 14 Periodic Limb Movements and Periodic Limb Movement Disorder

**Margaret Park**
*Department of Behavioral Sciences, Sleep Disorders Service and Research Center, Rush University Medical Center, Chicago, Illinois, U.S.A.*

**Cynthia L. Comella**
*Section on Movement Disorders, Department of Neurological Sciences, Rush University Medical Center, Chicago, Illinois, U.S.A.*

## INTRODUCTION

Periodic limb movements (PLMs) are spontaneous, involuntary limb movements that occur during sleep. These movements typically consist of repetitive stereotypical movements of the lower extremities, such as dorsiflexion of the big toe or ankle with occasional knee and hip flexion, reminiscent of a flexion-withdrawal reflex (1,2). PLMs can also involve the upper extremities, usually a flexion motion at the elbow, although these occur more rarely (3).

### History and Significance

Due to the involuntary clonic nature of the movements, PLMs were originally thought to be an epilepsy variant and were referred to as *nocturnal myoclonus* (4). PLMs were eventually recognized as distinct events apart from physiological phenomena and from epileptic events, mainly due to the growing association between PLMs and restless legs syndrome (RLS) (5,6). Because of its common association with RLS, most of the initial studies regarding PLMs are derived from polysomnography studies of RLS patients. However, since its initial description, PLMs are now known to occur in a wide range of sleep disorders, including narcolepsy, rapid eye movement (REM) sleep behavior disorder, obstructive sleep apnea syndrome (OSA), insomnia, and hypersomnia (7–10).

PLMs can also occur in patients without any sleep complaints. Although less common in young individuals, asymptomatic PLMs increase in frequency with age and are common in older individuals (11,12). As a result, the clinical significance of isolated PLMs is unknown (13,14). However, it is presumed that if the PLMs are numerous enough, and associated with enough sleep disruption that cannot be explained by another disorder, then the patient likely has a sleep disorder associated with the PLMs, aptly named periodic limb movement disorder (PLMD) (15). The assumption then is that the PLMs can cause enough nocturnal sleep fragmentation to impair nocturnal sleep consolidation, causing nonrestorative sleep and/or daytime impairment.

## Evaluation and Diagnosis

Clinically, bed partners may report kicking, leg jerking, or twisted bed sheets and bed covers in the morning, but most patients themselves are unaware that PLMs are occurring. As a result, PLMD remains a polysomnographic diagnosis. They can also be reliably diagnosed by actigraphy, using accelerometers attached to the legs (16,17). This has the advantage of portability and lower cost, but does not collect any other information about sleep. Currently, actigraphy is usually reserved for investigational trials.

Overall, PLMs show a triple flexion of the ankle, knee, and hip. Variations on this triple flexion pattern are also seen. The anterior tibialis muscle is almost always involved but most major leg muscles can also contract (Fig. 1A and B) (3). Even within the same individual, actual muscle patterns vary markedly (18,19). Initial guidelines for scoring and recording PLMD were first developed in 1982, during an overnight study of a patient with RLS (20). The American Sleep Disorders

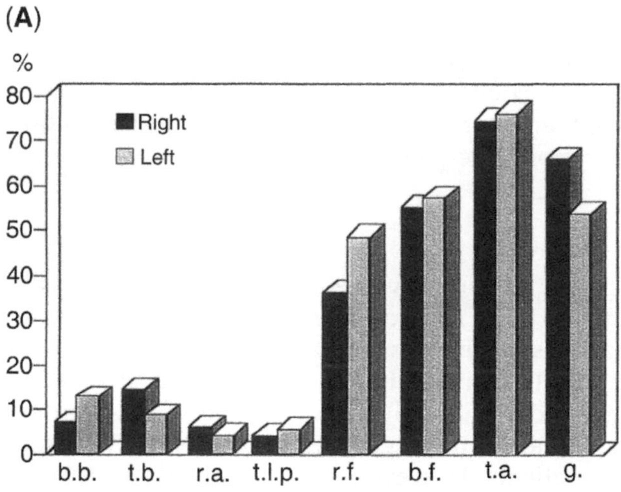


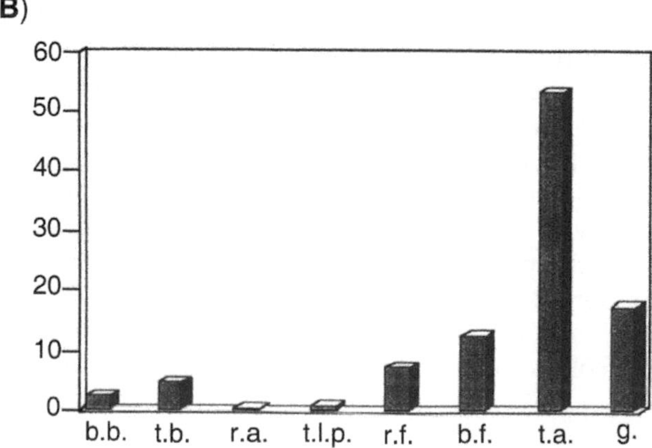


**FIGURE 1** (**A**) Anatomical distribution of PLMs. (**B**) Anatomical distribution of initial muscle involved in PLMs. *Abbreviations*: PLMs, periodic limb movements; bb, biceps brachii (arm); tb, triceps brachii (arm); ra, rectus abdominus; tlp, thoracolumbar paraspinals; rf, rectus femoris; bf, biceps femoris; ta, tibialis anterior; g, gastoc.

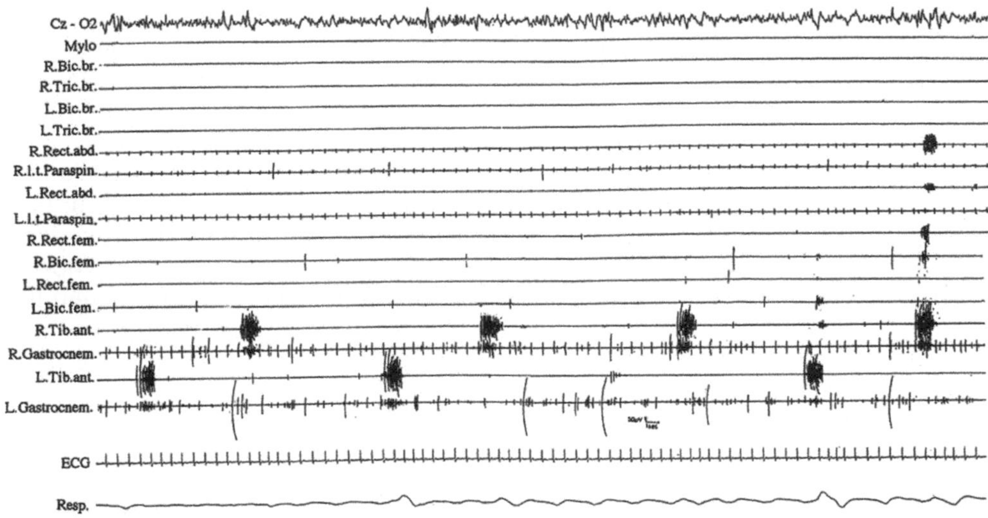


**FIGURE 2** Standard polysomnograph montage demonstrates periodic limb movements with electromyography attached to the anterior tibialis.

Association Task Force has minimally modified Coleman's original description, adding a minimum separation time of 5 seconds per successive movement and a movement amplitude requirement of 25% of electromyography (EMG) great toe dorsiflexion signal (15). According to current standard criteria, PLMs are scored if a series of four or more consecutive movements are recorded overnight, typically by EMG of the anterior tibialis muscles, with a duration of 0.5 to 5 seconds and an intermovement interval of 4–90 seconds (Fig. 2) (15). The significance of PLMs during wake (PLMW) continues to be debated, but some specialists do consider PLMW when evaluating RLS. Recent criteria have proposed to increase the burst duration of PLMW to 10 seconds, because the involuntary muscle movement may be prolonged by a voluntary component that lengthens the burst (21). However, traditional practice typically considers PLMs that only occur during sleep. PLMs are scored as the number occurring per hour of sleep, called the PLMs index (PLM-I). PLMs associated with arousal (PLM-AI) are evaluated and scored separately if associated with signs of electroencephalogram (EEG) arousal. A PLM-I greater than 5 is considered pathologic and diagnostic for PLMD in adults (15); however, some studies have shown that a PLM-I greater than 5 can be seen in normal, asymptomatic adults, highlighting the necessity of establishing normative criteria across age and gender, with a possible need to change existing criteria for diagnosing PLMD (5,11,22,23). Although PLMs can occur throughout the entire night during any stage of sleep, they tend to occur more frequently during light sleep [non-REM (NREM) stages 1 and 2], decrease during deep sleep (NREM stages 3 and 4), and generally disappear during REM sleep (24). The severity of PLMD is considered mild if the PLM-I is 5 to 25, moderate if the PLM-I is 25 to 50, and severe if the PLM-I is greater than 50 or if the PLM-AI is greater than 25 (15).

PLMs are often associated with other polysomnographic phenomena, such as EEG signs of arousal as described above, transient tachycardia (decreased R-R intervals for 5–10 beats) followed by bradycardia, and respiratory disturbances (25). When associated with sleep-disordered breathing, PLMs are considered incidental and secondary to this sleep disturbance. In these instances, it is crucial to evaluate the respiratory events as a cause for the sleep disturbance and/or daytime dysfunction before assigning a diagnosis of PLMD (22,26).

Despite polysomnographic guidelines, PLMD can be extremely difficult to qualify in terms of severity of nocturnal disruption and consequent disruption to daytime function. Further, the PLM-I can vary from night to night in any given individual and tends to cluster into episodes that can last from minutes to hours. As a result, polysomnography alone may not be able to accurately determine the severity of the disorder, or whether treatment is resolving the complaints of sleep disruption. However, despite difficulties in diagnosis, many patients can respond well to this method of evaluation and treatment.

### Differential Diagnosis

Differential diagnosis of PLMs generally includes physiologic phenomena, movement disorders, epilepsy, and other disorders of motor restlessness. Some of the more common of these will be discussed here.

Hypnic myoclonus is short, massive body movements that may involve the limbs in a symmetric fashion. However, they do not have the periodicity witnessed in PLMD. Although these movements are occasionally witnessed in transition between sleep stages, they are generally absent during sleep. As a result, these "sleep starts" are considered to be a normal phenomena associated with the normal transition from wake into sleep (25).

Unlike PLMs, most pathological movement disorders are suppressed during sleep. However, some motor disorders can be associated with sleep or appear during specific sleep stages. For example, fragmentary myoclonus is a limb twitch that occurs predominantly during the phasic bursts of REM sleep, but can persist throughout NREM sleep as well. If the movements are repetitive and semicontinuous, then the "painful legs and moving toes" syndrome should be considered. A careful history will usually reveal severe pain in one or both feet, occasionally associated with a burning sensation, not necessarily relieved by movements, and without a predominantly circadian component (27). This occurs while awake and asleep.

Movements secondary to myoclonic epilepsy are usually associated with abnormal synchronous EEG phenomena, but conventional EEG leads used in a standard polysomnography (PSG) study may not be sufficient to definitively conclude whether the "arousals" are epileptiform in origin. Careful history may elicit an underlying neurological disorder or early morning episodes of sudden limb movements.

Neuroleptic-induced akathisia may cause movements during sleep that fit criteria as PLMs. This is less prominent than with RLS. In addition, movements due to akathisia are not as responsive to dopaminergic treatment and are not limited to the limbs (28).

## EPIDEMIOLOGY OF PERIODIC LIMB MOVEMENTS DISORDER

The prevalence of PLMD in the general population is difficult to ascertain because evaluation of this disorder usually includes an evaluation of an associated comorbid disease state. In conjunction with other disorders, PLMD is estimated to be present in approximately 80% to 90% of RLS patients, 45% to 60% of patients with narcolepsy, approximately 70% of REM-behavior disorder patients, and between 22% and 45% of uremic patients (29–31).

Prior studies have estimated that PLMs alone are present in up to 6% of the general population, affecting 58% of adults over the age of 60 and greater than 44% of adults aged 65 and older (10,12,32,33). However, these studies do not differentiate between PLMs and PLMD. Ohayon et al. evaluated the prevalence of PLMD separately from RLS in the general population; approximately 3.9% of their sample subjectively reported PLMD, with a higher prevalence in women and in subjects aged 20 to 29 years (30). In direct contradiction to this study, other epidemiological studies reveal increased prevalence of PLMD with older age, affecting approximately 4% to 11% in the elderly (34). This inconsistency reflects the considerable variability of PLMs from night to night (34), making prevalence studies of PLMD difficult to evaluate at any given time. In general, PLMs' prevalence does increase with advanced age.

## ASSOCIATED DISEASE STATES

PLMD remains a diagnosis of exclusion. History and physical examination may reveal an underlying medical or neurological disorder associated with PLMD, such as a renal disorder, myelopathy, neuropathy, iron deficiency anemia, pregnancy, and medications. In some cases, remission of the patients' complaints may involve evaluating and treating the comorbid disease state associated with PLMD as well as the PLMD itself. A review of some of the more common disease states will be presented here.

### Restless Legs Syndrome

PLMD is a commonly witnessed occurrence in the polysomnography studies of RLS patients. A recent study found that 84% of RLS patients had a PLM-I greater than 5, with a higher PLM-AI compared to 36% of control subjects (35). Overall, it is estimated that 80% to 90% of RLS patients have a polysomnographic diagnosis of PLMD (29,30), although it is difficult to ascertain whether sleep disturbance and/or daytime dysfunction are due to RLS symptoms, PLMD, or a combination of both.

### Iron Deficiency

Iron-deficient states are extensively reported in RLS patients and generally hold true for PLMD without RLS as well. Low normal ferritin levels, with a cut-off value below 50 μg/L, are inversely correlated to the subjective severity of RLS symptoms and are also accompanied by more PLMs (36). One study evaluated children with PLMD and found that low serum iron rather than ferritin level was associated with the occurrence of PLMs. Treatment with iron reduced the frequency of PLMs in 76% of these children (37). Further, RLS can be induced by blood donation, and studies evaluating repeat blood donors have found a 4.4 times higher odds ratio of having RLS or PLMs when compared to nonrepeat blood donors (38,39). Other reports regarding iron-deficient states such as thalassemia, pregnancy, and anemia are also commonly associated with the occurrence of PLMs (40,41).

Iron has been extensively evaluated in RLS and PLMD in an attempt to clarify the pathophysiology underlying these diseases. Iron deficiency may explain why these disorders are so responsive to dopamine treatment. Tyrosine hydroxylase, the enzyme that catalyses the transformation from tyrosine to levodopa, relies on iron. D2 receptors require iron and synapse integrity relies on iron.

### Attention Deficit/Hyperactivity Disorder

In children, there is a bidirectional association between PLMs and attention deficit/hyperactivity disorder (ADHD), with 26% to 64% of children with ADHD having a PLM-I greater than 5 and approximately 44% of children with PLMs having symptoms of ADHD (42–44). This relationship suggests that a possible genetic link may coexist between the two disorders, further corroborated by data suggesting that dopaminergic agents improve both PLMs and ADHD symptoms in children with these disorders.

### Uremia and End-Stage Renal Disease

RLS has a known relationship with uremia, affecting as many as 15% to 40% of patients undergoing hemodialysis (45,46). However, RLS, RLS with PLMD, and PLMD independent of RLS are all common complaints in patients receiving dialysis (47). Further, the severity of both RLS and PLMD in patients receiving dialysis seems to be greater when compared to patients with idiopathic forms of RLS/PLMD (48,49). In a study by Benz et al. the severity of PLMD was a sensitive predictor of mortality in dialysis patients, equal to or better than serum albumin, urea reduction ratio, or other comorbid medical disease states (50).

It is unclear whether uremia itself is an independent contributor to the pathophysiology underlying RLS and/or PLMD. Several studies have attempted to analyze whether improvement in blood urea nitrogen and/or creatinine, particularly during hemodialysis, improves the frequency of PLMs; in one case, RLS symptoms resolved after successful renal transplantation, although PLMs were not evaluated (51). Criticism of these studies included the observation that transient improvement in renal status during the day may not necessarily address the possibility of nocturnal build-up of uremia. One study evaluated the frequency of nocturnal PLMs in patients treated with conventional hemodialysis during the day vs. those treated with nocturnal hemodialysis; results did not find a significant difference between treatment modalities, indirectly indicating that uremia itself has minimal contribution to the occurrence of PLMs (52). Further, the use of human erythropoietin has successfully decreased the frequency of PLMs in uremic patients treated by hemodialysis, confirming prior suspicion that uremia, and to some extent hemodialysis, may worsen the occurrence of PLMs by mechanisms related to an alteration in iron production and metabolism (53). Other studies have attempted to correlate blood concentrations of parathyroid hormone (PTH) levels, calcium, and phosphate to PLMs in patients with end-stage renal disease. Interestingly, PTH levels were lower in uremic patients suffering from RLS compared to uremic patients without RLS, but higher serum PTH levels were found in dialysis patients with PLMD compared to dialysis patients without PLMD (54). Calcium levels have not correlated with either condition, and the PTH data have not been replicated by other investigators.

Despite the discrepancies underlying the pathophysiologic relationship between PLMD and uremia, it is clear that the quality of life of patients can be improved by addressing their sleep–wake complaints (48). Therefore, the recognition and diagnosis of RLS with and without PLMD is important to assess in this chronically ill patient population.

### Neuropathy and Radiculopathy

There is a suggestion that PLMs are the motor manifestation of the sensory complaints in RLS. To that end, several studies have attempted to evaluate whether a neuropathic component exists in RLS and PLMD. Electrophysiologic evaluations in the past have found a mixture of small-fiber neuropathy, large-fiber neuropathy, axonal neuropathy, and radiculopathy in RLS patients with PLMD (55–57). In PLMD without RLS, there has been less evidence of neuropathy, although there is a suspicion that abnormal axonal pathology may exist (58).

Most studies evaluating PLMD with and without RLS focus on a theorized diminished inhibition at the spinal level. Diminished central inhibition, if present in patients with PLMD, theoretically causes an altered function of the descending spinal tracts that lead to movements mimicking an uninhibited flexion-withdrawal reflex (59). Abnormal incoming sensory stimuli then induce inappropriate activation of movement generators, located either in the medullary formation reticularis or within motor spinal dopaminergic cells (60). Despite these theories, research has yet to confirm whether neuropathic diseases cause increased frequency of PLMD.

### Depression

Both depression and the use of antidepressants have a known relationship with RLS and PLMs. However, patients with PLMD without RLS also have higher depression scores (61). One study found that approximately 58% of PLMD patients have elevated depression scale scores on the minnesota multiphasic personality inventory, and even higher scores when controlling for age, body mass index, and multiple sleep latency test sleep latencies; 32% of these patients reported prior treatment for depression (62). Although it is suspected that depression itself has a link to PLMD, the inherent pathophysiologic connection is difficult to evaluate because most patients are concomitantly treated with antidepressant medications that are known to cause PLMs, such as tricyclic antidepressants, selective serotonin reuptake inhibitors, lithium, and venlafaxine (63). However, there is also an increased prevalence of PLMD in patients treated with antidepressants that are unlikely to induce or exacerbate PLMs, such as bupropion, trazodone, and nefazodone (64), suggesting that the relationship between depression and PLMD exists independent of medication effect.

### Parkinson's Disease

Poor sleep quality with daytime dysfunction is a common complaint in patients with Parkinson's disease (PD). Recent interest has grown with regard to the relationship between sleep and PD, as sleep disorders often precede motor symptoms (65). Known sleep disorders in PD patients include OSA and central sleep apneas, REM-behavior disorder, and RLS with and without PLMD (66). Clinical evaluation of this patient population is further complicated by the use of dopaminergic medication for their PD symptoms, which is known to also induce sleepiness but improves PLMD (66,67).

RLS, RLS and PLMD, and PLMD in PD patients have an assumed pathophysiologic relationship because all of these disorders are highly responsive to dopaminergic medications (68,69). The suspicion that a common mechanism exists amongst these diseases is endorsed by reports that PLMs are increased in patients with PD, occurring in 30% to 80% of this patient population (45,56,70–73), and may possibly be more common with advancing disease stage (72,74,75).

Because dopaminergic cell loss is the key pathology in PD, and PLM respond to dopaminergics, nigrostriatal dysfunction has been theorized to be the generator of PLMs in PD patients. Single photon emission computed tomography (SPECT) studies evaluating idiopathic PLMD have shown a lower number of striatal D2 receptors (76) but with normal binding capacity of these receptors (77). However, no studies to date have evaluated functional imaging or autopsy studies in PD patients with PLMD to confirm or refute these theories.

Electrophysiologically, PLMs resemble propiospinal myoclonus (78–80), and their relation to PD is further corroborated by the fact that spinal dopaminergic cells are an inherent part of the motor system (60). However, other electrophysiological evidence postulates that the brainstem, rather than spinal cells, is responsible for the periodicity of PLMs, speculating that the appearance of PLMs may actually represent the earliest sign of brainstem involvement in PD (81).

In summary, PD is frequently associated with multiple sleep disorders, including RLS and PLMD. The differential diagnoses should include evaluation for nocturnal dyskinesias as well as other underlying sleep disorders that may account for movements in this population. Overall, studies are too few to conclude whether there is a pathophysiological difference between idiopathic PLMD and PLMD in PD, but there is some evidence that a relationship exists.

## PATHOPHYSIOLOGY

### Neurotransmitter and Neural Substrates

The pathophysiology of PLMs and PLMD has been assumed to be linked to RLS. In RLS, there is a presumption that the central nervous system has dopaminergic dysfunction, which has been indirectly validated by worsening RLS symptoms after administration of medications that block dopamine receptors (82). However, no studies have demonstrated dopamine abnormalities in pathways other than the nigrostriatal system. Further, cerebrospinal fluid (CSF) metabolite studies have not found differences in homovanillic acid levels between normal controls and patients with RLS (83).

Recent studies have evaluated the possibility that abnormal use and storage of iron may underlie deficiencies in dopaminergic pathways (76,84). There is a relative depletion in the iron storage protein, ferritin, in the CSF of RLS patients, which corresponds to magnetic resonance imaging (MRI) findings of substantia nigra abnormalities and is confirmed on autopsy studies (83,85). These hypotheses regarding iron-related dopamine deficiencies in RLS have been transposed onto PLMD, indirectly validated by the increase of PLMs seen in disorders with Lewy body pathology (7) and less commonly seen in disorders of dopamine excess, such as schizophrenia (86).

Despite the relationship among iron, dopamine, RLS, and PLMs, the exact pathophysiologic mechanism for PLMs remains unclear. Studies evaluating iron-related dopamine deficiency have not been replicated in patients who have

PLMD independent of RLS. As a result, some practitioners have argued that PLMD with RLS and PLMD without RLS may have different underlying pathophysiological mechanisms. There are several arguments in favor of separating these disease states. For example, prior studies of RLS have noted differing levels of neuropathy (55–57). However, studies of PLMD without RLS have failed to disclose a neuropathic abnormality and, instead, argue in favor of a relative disinhibition that may occur at a spinal level (59). In addition, spontaneous arousals found in PSG may be more clinically relevant in RLS with PLMD than in PLMD alone (87). These findings establish different central and peripheral mechanisms, thus contradicting the idea that PLMs are the motor manifestation to the sensory symptoms of RLS. Further complicating matters are reports that treating PLMD with dopamine agonist medication can induce RLS symptoms, possibly an augmentation phenomenon (88). In general, greater doses of dopaminergics are required to completely eliminate PLMs than are needed to completely eliminate RLS symptoms. These responses both indicate that, despite possible pathophysiological differences, a fundamental relationship exists between the two disorders.

### Anatomical Sites of Involvement

Studies evaluating the origin of PLMD have assessed cortical inhibition (89,90), impairment of motor inhibitory pathways in the cortical–subcortical motor system (91), reticular sites, pontine mechanisms (92), and spinal cord origin (93–96), all with conflicting results. The following is intended to be a general summary regarding the possibility of a PLM generator at these various levels.

#### *Cortical–Subcortical*

Loss of cortical or subcortical inhibition of the motor tracts theoretically leads to diminished control over motor limb movements during sleep. This theory is supported by reports of cortical and subcortical ischemia that subsequently cause the appearance of PLMs (97,98). However, studies have failed to disclose cortical potentials preceding PLMs, and the absence of synchronous generators at this level makes a cortical origin unlikely (5,89,99). Transcranial magnetic stimulation and cortical silent period (CSP) was reduced in patients with RLS, and dopaminergic treatment normalized this duration. However, there was no correlation between the PLM index and CSP duration (99). Although central mechanisms of iron and dopamine dysfunction are thought to underlie PLMs, this effect may be more prevalent at other levels involved in the motor pathway, such as the spinal level.

#### *Pontine*

Briellman et al. evaluated blink reflex excitability in patients with PLMD and found markedly enhanced excitability of the R2 response during PLMs (100). These results lend credence to the theory of altered motor control in PLMs, located within the subcortex and possibly related to the dopaminergic striatopallidal system. Standard MRI studies could not find anatomic lesions in RLS patients to support this finding. However, functional MRI studies have shown that RLS sensory complaints were associated with activation at the thalamic and cerebellar levels, while PLMW movements were associated with activation at the level of the pons and red nucleus (101,102). No cortical potentials were found in any of these studies. These results support the argument that RLS and PLMs may be generated at different anatomic sites, but an inherent link exists at the pontine level between iron, dopamine, and PLMs.

### Spinal Cord

Several pathological disease states involving the spinal cord have been reported to cause PLMs, including myelopathy, cervical spondylosis, spinal vascular accidents, and animal lesion studies. These reports suggest that activation (i.e., disinhibition) of skeletal muscles at this level is involved in generating PLMs (3,93,95,103). Because of their similarity to the Babinski response, studies have evaluated facilitation of the late component of the flexion reflex, indicating motor neuron hyperexcitability at the level of the spinal cord (1,2,12,93). These electrophysiological components are similar in duration and activate the same muscles as the flexion reflex, supporting proponents for a PLMs generator at the level of the spinal cord (2). Furthermore, this is consistent with dopaminergic involvement in PLMD, because dopamine cells transcend the spinal cord (2,3).

### Autonomic Involvement

Transient autonomic phenomena commonly occur in PLMD. Cardiac changes in particular have been found to occur in 99% of all PLMs (104), which can consist of tachycardia followed by bradycardia (8,104,105). Because these cardiac changes occur approximately one second prior to the onset of PLMs, autonomic activation is likely part of the arousal process and may be involved in the motor response to autonomic activity. Cerebral blood flow, assessed by transcranial Dopplers, also increases just prior to the PLM (106). These responses are likely specific to an underlying sleep mechanism, supported by the fact that EEG and heart rate responses to PLMs differ between the wake and sleep states (107).

The significant activity of heart rate and delta EEG supports a common brainstem mechanism that generates PLMs during sleep. In theory, the brainstem receives peripheral inputs from the vascular, cardiac, and respiratory systems, which, in turn, synchronizes these signals to the cortical EEG oscillation that occurs during sleep (108). PLMs with cardiac and cerebral changes can occur without the appearance of microarousals (109), suggesting that arousals occur only when the brainstem is unable to accurately coordinate the incoming peripheral signals to the cortical oscillators. This theory is supported by improvement in PLM-AI with hypnotic medications, which dampen the fast activity of the cortex, allowing fewer disruptions.

## IMAGING STUDIES

In general, brain imaging studies have been inconclusive. In RLS, MRI studies have shown reduced brain iron content in the substantia nigra and putamen, despite normal peripheral iron status (110); however, no standard MRI studies have evaluated PLMD independent of RLS. SPECT studies have found decreased striatal dopamine receptor occupancy in RLS with PLMD as well as in PLMD alone (111), and positron emission tomography (PET) studies have shown a mild reduction of 6-[$^{18}$F] fluoro-L-dopa ($^{18}$F-dopa) uptake in the caudate nucleus and putamen in patients with RLS and PLMD (112). These results highlight dopaminergic abnormalities that likely exist in PLMD, perhaps through decreased D2 receptor activity, increased intracellular dopamine, or both. Interestingly, studies regarding $^{18F}$DOPA uptake in RLS patients report variable findings in the striatum (84), which may indicate that dopaminergic dysfunction may differ between RLS with PLMD and PLMD alone. All studies, however, suffer from small patient populations, do not study dopaminergic function outside of the nigrostriatal system, and have not been performed in the evening or night when RLS and PLMD appear, making definitive conclusions regarding these studies difficult.

In some contradiction to the above PET and SPECT studies, functional MRI (fMRI) studies suggest anatomic involvement of nondopaminergic areas. During the sensory symptoms of RLS, fMRI shows contralateral thalamic activation with bilateral activation of the cerebellum (101). This pattern is similar to the histological distribution of opioid mu receptors found in human brains (113). When PLMs occur in conjunction with the sensory symptoms of RLS, additional activation is seen in the red nuclei and brainstem near the reticular formation. These results are consistent with PET findings of cerebellar involvement in sensorimotor processing (114), although the cerebellum may be more active in RLS with PLMD than in PLMD alone. Pharmacologically, a positive treatment response occurs when using opioids in RLS and PLMs, which reverses with naloxone. This medication effect favors the idea of an endogenous opiate system dysfunction underlying the appearance of PLMs in RLS patients. If true, then dopamine efficacy may be due to the action of L-dopa on opiate receptors. However, one study showed that blockade of opiate receptors by naloxone did not alter the effect of L-dopa on RLS, whereas pimozide, which is a dopamine receptor antagonist, partially blocked the effect of codeine in RLS (115). This result argues that the effect of opiates in RLS/PLMD is likely through the dopaminergic system rather than the reverse. However, other than pharmacologic data, no studies have been able to elucidate the interaction between dopamine and opiate systems in the generation of PLMs.

## TREATMENT

Four medication classes are commonly used to treat PLMD: dopaminergic medications, opioids, anticonvulsants, and benzodiazepines.

### Dopaminergic Medications

Initially, L-dopa with a dopa-decarboxylase inhibitor was considered the treatment of choice for RLS/PLMs (116). Several studies have found a significant reduction of PLMs throughout the night, with persistent efficacy of approximately 85% after two years; however, efficacy decreased soon thereafter, with only 31% after a mean of 31 months (117,118). Adverse side effects of L-dopa include nausea, vomiting, tachycardia, orthostatic hypotension, hallucinations, and daytime fatigue and sleepiness. Hallucinations and orthostatic hypotension, however, appear to only occur with parkinsonian conditions, not RLS. Morning rebound of PLMs can also occur with L-dopa treatment, with increased PLMs frequency during the last part of the night despite treatment at bedtime.

As a result of these adverse effects, as well as the phenomena of augmentation that can occur with L-dopa, dopaminergic agonists are now considered first-line treatment for RLS patients and are thus used as first-line treatment for PLMD. The D2 receptor agonist bromocriptine was initially studied and was effective in reducing PLMs, but due to adverse side effects, particularly nausea, this medication is now rarely used for treatment of RLS/PLMD. Pergolide is also a

D2 receptor agonist that has been shown to have persistent efficacy in 79% of patients (119,120); however, adverse effects were noted in 71%, with recent reports of cardiac valve dysfunction associated with ergot medications (121). Dopamine agonists appear to reduce PLM throughout the night. In contrast levodopa improves PLM more during the first half of sleep (122). This may be due to the fast onset of action and short half life with levodopa. During the second half of the night, the dopamine agonist with a longer half-life continues to suppress PLMs.

Pramipexole and ropinirole are two non-ergot derivative medications with dopamine agonist properties. Pramipexole has a high affinity for the D3 receptor and has proved extremely effective in suppressing PLMs (123). Sustained efficacy with this medication has been found in over 90% of patients (124,125). Ropinirole has a similar mechanism of action to pramipexole and has been recently approved by the Food and Drug Administration for treatment of RLS, with significant reduction in PLMs (126). Improvement in PLMs with dopamine agonists appears to be linearly dose dependent. With large dose (1.5 mg of pramipexole or 4 mg of ropinirole), PLMs will completely resolve in most subjects. This is usually larger than the dose needed to entirely suppress the sensory component of RLS. The major side effects of both ropinirole and pramipexole are similar to those of L-dopa and the ergot dopaminergic medications, including nausea and other gastrointestinal disturbances, but are generally better tolerated with less severity of side effects. In patients with PD, "sleep attacks," or sudden episodes of sleepiness have been associated with the use of dopaminergic agonists (127–129), although this is much less problematic when used in RLS (130). Increased impulsivity and gambling also seems less common.

## Opiates

Studies regarding the effects of opiates and other sedative/hypnotic medications on PLMD are fewer than those evaluating dopamine medications. Oxycodone and propoxyphene have been shown to improve both subjective and objective measures of PLMs, with decreased arousals and improved sleep efficiency, which persists over time (131–133). Similar results have been found in open-label trials with methadone and codeine (21). Opioids can be useful in the management of PLMD when dopaminergic medication cannot be tolerated, particularly in patients with severe augmentation induced by that class of medication. However, despite little evidence in the literature regarding abuse potential in PLMD patients, caution should be used with patients who have a history of substance abuse. There is also potential for this class of medications to worsen obstructive sleep apnea (133).

## Anticonvulsants

Only carbamazepine and gabapentin have been evaluated in controlled trials as treatment options for RLS and/or PLMD. Carbamazepine has not been found to be useful in the treatment of PLMD, regardless of subjective improvement of RLS symptoms (134). Garcia published a 24-patient, controlled, cross-over trial of gabapentin for RLS (135). The mean daily dose was 1855 mg/day. PLMs on placebo were $31 \pm 3$ vs. $12 \pm 3$ while on gabapentin ($p = 0.05$). RLS symptoms robustly improved.

XP13512 (Xenoport, Inc.) is a transported prodrug of gabapentin designed to facilitate oral absorption. A 2-week, 38-patient, multicenter, placebo-controlled, cross-over trial reported improved IRLSSG questionnaire scores (Xenoport, data on file). Polysomnography demonstrated improved total sleep time, improved slow wave sleep, and reduced awakenings from PLMs.

### Benzodiazepines

Benzodiazepines, including clonazepam and temazepam, improve the PLM-I and/or the PLM-AI (136–139). Although the general consensus seems to indicate that benzodiazepines are useful in the treatment of PLMD, research is limited by small sample sizes and the modest effect of treatment on PLMs (140). In fact, Saletu found that 1 mg of clonazepam improved subjective sleep and awakening quality in 10 RLS and 16 PLMD patients, and improved some sleep parameter in polysomnography, but failed to reduce the PLM-I at all (141). Similar to opioid treatment for PLMD, sleep-disordered breathing may worsen with benzodiazepine treatment, and repeat PSG studies may be indicated on a periodic basis.

### Other

Oral iron supplementation may be indicated if the ferritin level is below 50 µg/L, although good data are lacking. Intravenous iron improved PLM in a group of RLS patients (142). There is a single review article studying the effect of baclofen in PLMD, indicating increased PLM-I but decreased PLM-AI, with an improvement in sleep parameters (143). No long-term studies are available for review.

## REFERENCES


1. Smith RC. Relationship of periodic movements in sleep (nocturnal myoclonus) and the Babinski sign. Sleep 1985; 8(3):239–243.
2. Bara-Jimenez W, Aksu M, Graham B, et al. Periodic limb movements in sleep: state-dependent excitability of the spinal flexor reflex. Neurology 2000; 54(8):1609–1616.
3. Provini F, Vetrugno R, Meletti S, et al. Motor pattern of periodic limb movements during sleep. Neurology 2001; 57(2):300–304.
4. Symonds CP. Nocturnal myoclonus. J Neurol Neurosurg Psychiatry 1953; 16(3): 166–171.
5. Lugaresi E, Cirignotta F, Coccagna G, Montagna P. Nocturnal myoclonus and restless legs syndrome. Adv Neurol 1986; 43:295–307.
6. Lugaresi E, Coccagna G, Tassinari CA, Ambrosetto C. Polygraphic data on motor phenomena in the restless legs syndrome. Riv Neurol 1965; 35(6):550–561.
7. Montplaisir J, Michaud M, Denesle R, Gosselin A. Periodic leg movements are not more prevalent in insomnia or hypersomnia but are specifically associated with sleep disorders involving a dopaminergic impairment. Sleep Med 2000; 1(2):163–167.
8. Fantini ML, Michaud M, Gosselin N, et al. Periodic leg movements in REM sleep behavior disorder and related autonomic and EEG activation. Neurology 2002; 59(12): 1889–1894.
9. Fry JM, DiPhillipo MA, Pressman MR. Periodic leg movements in sleep following treatment of obstructive sleep apnea with nasal continuous positive airway pressure. Chest 1989; 96(1):89–91.
10. Coleman RM, Pollak CP, Weitzman ED. Periodic movements in sleep (nocturnal myoclonus): relation to sleep disorders. Ann Neurol 1980; 8(4):416–421.
11. Ancoli-Israel S, Kripke DF, Mason W, Kaplan OJ. Sleep apnea and periodic movements in an aging sample. J Gerontol 1985; 40(4):419–425.
12. Dickel MJ, Mosko SS. Morbidity cut-offs for sleep apnea and periodic leg movements in predicting subjective complaints in seniors. Sleep 1990; 13(2):155–166.

13. Karadeniz D, Ondze B, Besset A, Billiard M. Are periodic leg movements during sleep (PLMS) responsible for sleep disruption in insomnia patients? Eur J Neurol 2000; 7(3):331–336.
14. Bastuji H, Garcia-Larrea L. Sleep/wake abnormalities in patients with periodic leg movements during sleep: factor analysis on data from 24-h ambulatory polygraphy. J Sleep Res 1999; 8(3):217–223.
15. Diagnostic Classification Steering Committee of the American Sleep Disorders Association. (Thorpy MJ, chairperson). In: The International Classification of Sleep Disorders: Diagnostic and Coding Manual; Rochester, MN: American Sleep Disorders Association, 1997.
16. King MA, Jaffre MO, Morrish E, Shneerson JM, Smith IE. The validation of a new actigraphy system for the measurement of periodic leg movements in sleep. Sleep Med 2005; 6:507–513.
17. Sforza E, Johannes M, Claudio B. The PAM-RL ambulatory device for detection of periodic leg movements: a validation study. Sleep Med 2005; 6:407–413.
18. De Weerd AW, Rijsman RM, Brinkley A. Activity patterns of leg muscles in periodic limb movement disorder. J Neurol Neurosurg Psychiatry 2004; 75:317–319.
19. Plazzi G, Vetrugno R, Meletti S, Provini F. Motor pattern of periodic limb movements in sleep in idiopathic RLS patients. Sleep Med 2002; 3(Suppl):S31–S34.
20. Coleman RM. Periodic movements in sleep (nocturnal myoclonus) and restless legs syndrome. In: Guilleminault C, ed. Sleeping and Walking Disorders: Indications and Techniques. Menlo Park, CA: Addison-Wesley Publishing Co, 1982.
21. Michaud M, Poirier G, Lavigne G, Montplaisir J. Restless legs syndrome: scoring criteria for leg movements recorded during the suggested immobilization test. Sleep Med 2001; 2(4):317–321.
22. Nicolas A, Lesperance P, Montplaisir J. Is excessive daytime sleepiness with periodic leg movements during sleep a specific diagnostic category?. Eur Neurol ; 40(1): 22–26.
23. Carrier J, Frenette S, Montplaisir J, et al. Effects of periodic leg movements during sleep in middle-aged subjects without sleep complaints. Mov Disord 2005; 20(9):1127–1132.
24. Pollmacher T, Schulz H. Periodic leg movements (PLM): their relationship to sleep stages. Sleep 1993; 16(6):572–577.
25. Montplaisir J, Allen RP, Walters S, Ferini-Strambi L. Restless legs syndrome and periodic limb movements during sleep. In: Kryger MH, Roth T, Dement WC, eds. Principles and Practice of Sleep Medicine. 4th ed. Philadelphia: Elsevier, 2005:839–852.
26. Exar EN, Collop NA. The association of upper airway resistance with periodic limb movements. Sleep 2001; 24(2):188–192.
27. Spillane JD, Nathan PW, Kelly RE, Marsden CD. Painful legs and moving toes. Brain 1971; 94(3):541–556.
28. Walters AS, Hening W, Rubinstein M, Chokroverty S. A clinical and polysomnographic comparison of neuroleptic-induced akathisia and the idiopathic restless legs syndrome. Sleep 1991; 14(4):339–345.
29. Wetter TC, Pollmacher T. Restless legs and periodic leg movements in sleep syndromes. J Neurol 1997; 244(4 Suppl 1):S37–S45.
30. Ohayon MM, Roth T. Prevalence of restless legs syndrome and periodic limb movement disorder in the general population. J Psychosom Res 2002; 53(1):547–554.
31. Holley JL, Nespor S, Rault R. A comparison of reported sleep disorders in patients on chronic hemodialysis and continuous peritoneal dialysis. Am J Kidney Dis 1992; 19(2):156–161.
32. Bixler EO, Kales A, Vela-Bueno A, et al. Nocturnal myoclonus and nocturnal myoclonic activity in the normal population. Res Commun Chem Pathol Pharmacol 1982; 36(1):129–140.
33. Ancoli-Israel S, Kripke DF, Klauber MR, et al. Periodic limb movements in sleep in community-dwelling elderly. Sleep 1991; 14(6):496–500.
34. Hornyak M, Trenkwalder C. Restless legs syndrome and periodic limb movement disorder in the elderly. J Psychosom Res 2004; 56(5):543–548.

35. Michaud M, Paquet J, Lavigne G, et al. Sleep laboratory diagnosis of restless legs syndrome. Eur Neurol 2002; 48(2):108–113.
36. Sun ER, Chen CA, Ho G, et al. Iron and the restless legs syndrome. Sleep 1998; 21(4):371–377.
37. Simakajornboon N, Gozal D, Vlasic V, et al. Periodic limb movements in sleep and iron status in children. Sleep 2003; 26(6):735–738.
38. Kryger MH, Shepertycky M, Foerster J, Manfreda J. Sleep disorders in repeat blood donors. Sleep 2003; 26(5):625–626.
39. Silber MH, Richardson JW. Multiple blood donations associated with iron deficiency in patients with restless legs syndrome. Mayo Clin Proc 2003; 78(1):52–54.
40. Goodman JD, Brodie C, Ayida GA. Restless leg syndrome in pregnancy. BMJ 1988; 297(6656):1101–1102.
41. Rijsman RM, deWeerd AW. Secondary periodic limb movement disorder and restless legs syndrome. Sleep Med Rev 1999; 3(2):147–158.
42. Picchietti DL, England SJ, Walters AS, et al. Periodic limb movement disorder and restless legs syndrome in children with attention-deficit hyperactivity disorder. J Child Neurol 1998; 13(12):588–594.
43. Picchietti DL, Underwood DJ, Farris WA, et al. Further studies on periodic limb movement disorder and restless legs syndrome in children with attention-deficit hyperactivity disorder. Mov Disord 1999; 14(6):1000–1007.
44. Crabtree VM, Ivanenko A, O'Brien LM, Gozal D. Periodic limb movement disorder of sleep in children. J Sleep Res 2003; 12(1):73–81.
45. Wetter TC, Stiasny K, Kohnen R, et al. Polysomnographic sleep measures in patients with uremic and idiopathic restless legs syndrome. Mov Disord 1998; 13(5):820–824.
46. Winkelman JW, Chertow GM, Lazarus JM. Restless legs syndrome in end-stage renal disease. Am J Kidney Dis 1996; 28(3):372–378.
47. Rijsman RM, de Weerd AW, Stam CJ, et al. Periodic limb movement disorder and restless legs syndrome in dialysis patients. Nephrology (Carlton) 2004; 9(6):353–361.
48. Trenkwalder C, Stiasny K, Pollmacher T, et al. L-dopa therapy of uremic and idiopathic restless legs syndrome: a double-blind, crossover trial. Sleep 1995; 18(8):681–688.
49. Trenkwalder CSA, Wetter T, Stiasny K, et al. Classification of idiopathic and uremic restless legs syndrome: Results of a database of 134 patients. Neurology 1996; 46:A199.
50. Benz RL, Pressman MR, Hovick ET, Peterson DD. Potential novel predictors of mortality in end-stage renal disease patients with sleep disorders. Am J Kidney Dis 2000; 35(6):1052–1060.
51. Yasuda T, Nishimura A, Katsuki Y, Tsuji Y. Restless legs syndrome treated successfully by kidney transplantation—a case report. Clin Transpl 1986; 138.
52. Hanly PJ, Gabor JY, Chan C, Pierratos A. Daytime sleepiness in patients with CRF: impact of nocturnal hemodialysis. Am J Kidney Dis 2003; 41(2):403–410.
53. Benz RL, Pressman MR, Hovick ET, Peterson DD. A preliminary study of the effects of correction of anemia with recombinant human erythropoietin therapy on sleep, sleep disorders, and daytime sleepiness in hemodialysis patients (The SLEEPO study). Am J Kidney Dis 1999; 34(6):1089–1095.
54. Stepanski E, Faber M, Zorick F, et al. Sleep disorders in patients on continuous ambulatory peritoneal dialysis. J Am Soc Nephrol 1995; 6(2):192–197.
55. Iannaccone S, Zucconi M, Marchettini P, et al. Evidence of peripheral axonal neuropathy in primary restless legs syndrome. Mov Disord 1995; 10(1):2–9.
56. Ondo W, Jankovic J. Restless legs syndrome: clinicoetiologic correlates. Neurology 1996; 47(6):1435–1441.
57. Polydefkis M, Allen RP, Hauer P, et al. Subclinical sensory neuropathy in late-onset restless legs syndrome. Neurology 2000; 55(8):1115–1121.
58. Martinez-Mena JM, Pastor J. (Polyneuropathy in patients with periodic leg movements during sleep). Rev Neurol 1998; 27(159):745–749.
59. Rijsman RM, Stam CJ, de Weerd AW. Abnormal H-reflexes in periodic limb movement disorder; impact on understanding the pathophysiology of the disorder. Clin Neurophysiol 2005; 116(1):204–210.

60. Lindvall O, Bjorklund A, Skagerberg G. Dopamine-containing neurons in the spinal cord: anatomy and some functional aspects. Ann Neurol 1983; 14(3):255–260.
61. Saletu B, Anderer P, Saletu M, et al. EEG mapping, psychometric, and polysomnographic studies in restless legs syndrome (RLS) and periodic limb movement disorder (PLMD) patients as compared with normal controls. Sleep Med 2002; 3 (Suppl):S35–S42.
62. Aikens JE, Vanable PA, Tadimeti L, et al. Differential rates of psychopathology symptoms in periodic limb movement disorder, obstructive sleep apnea, psychophysiological insomnia, and insomnia with psychiatric disorder. Sleep 1999; 22(6): 775–780.
63. Yang C, White DP, Winkelman JW. The effects of antidepressants on leg movements. Sleep 2004; 27(Suppl 2):A311.
64. Picchietti D, Winkelman JW. Restless legs syndrome, periodic limb movements in sleep, and depression. Sleep 2005; 28(7):891–898.
65. Abbott RD, Ross GW, White LR, et al. Excessive daytime sleepiness and subsequent development of Parkinson disease. Neurology 2005; 65(9):1442–1446.
66. Ondo WG, Dat Vuong K, Khan H, et al. Daytime sleepiness and other sleep disorders in Parkinson's disease. Neurology 2001; 57(8):1392–1396.
67. Comella CL. Sleep disturbances in Parkinson's disease. Curr Neurol Neurosci Rep 2003; 3(2):173–180.
68. Arnulf I, Konofal E, Merino-Andreu M, et al. Parkinson's disease and sleepiness: an integral part of PD. Neurology 2002; 58(7):1019–1024.
69. Hogl B, Rothdach A, Wetter TC, Trenkwalder C. The effect of cabergoline on sleep, periodic leg movements in sleep, and early morning motor function in patients with Parkinson's disease. Neuropsychopharmacology 2003; 28(10):1866–1870.
70. Garcia-Borreguero D, Odin P, Serrano C. Restless legs syndrome and PD: a review of the evidence for a possible association. Neurology 2003; 61(6 Suppl 3):S49–S55.
71. Ondo WG, Vuong KD, Jankovic J. Exploring the relationship between Parkinson disease and restless legs syndrome. Arch Neurol 2002; 59(3):421–424.
72. Wetter TC, Collado-Seidel V, Pollmacher T, et al. Sleep and periodic leg movement patterns in drug-free patients with Parkinson's disease and multiple system atrophy. Sleep 2000; 23(3):361–367.
73. Chokroverty S. Sleep and degenerative neurologic disorders. Neurol Clin 1996; 14(4):807–826.
74. Wetter TC, Brunner H, Hogl B, et al. Increased alpha activity in REM sleep in de novo patients with Parkinson's disease. Mov Disord 2001; 16(5):928–933.
75. Young A, Home M, Churchward T, et al. Comparison of sleep disturbance in mild versus severe Parkinson's disease. Sleep 2002; 25(5):573–577.
76. Staedt J, Stoppe G, Kogler A, et al. Nocturnal myoclonus syndrome (periodic movements in sleep) related to central dopamine D2-receptor alteration. Eur Arch Psychiatry Clin Neurosci 1995; 245(1):8–10.
77. Tribl GG, Asenbaum S, Happe S, et al. Normal striatal D2 receptor binding in idiopathic restless legs syndrome with periodic leg movements in sleep. Nucl Med Commun 2004; 25(1):55–60.
78. Brown P, Rothwell JC, Thompson PD, Marsden CD. Propriospinal myoclonus: evidence for spinal "pattern" generators in humans. Mov Disord 1994; 9(5):571–576.
79. Chokroverty S. Propriospinal myoclonus. Clin Neurosci 1995; 3(4):219–222.
80. Trenkwalder C, Bucher SF, Oertel WH. Electrophysiological pattern of involuntary limb movements in the restless legs syndrome. Muscle Nerve 1996; 19(2):155–162.
81. Clouston PD, Lim CL, Fung V, et al. Brainstem myoclonus in a patient with non-dopa-responsive parkinsonism. Mov Disord 1996; 11(4):404–410.
82. Winkelmann J, Trenkwalder C. (Pathophysiology of restless-legs syndrome. Review of current research). Nervenarzt 2001; 72(2):100–107.
83. Earley CJ, Hyland K, Allen RP. CSF dopamine, serotonin, and biopterin metabolites in patients with restless legs syndrome. Mov Disord 2001; 16(1):144–149.
84. Turjanski N, Lees AJ, Brooks DJ. Striatal dopaminergic function in restless legs syndrome: 18F-dopa and 11C-raclopride PET studies. Neurology 1999; 52(5):932–937.

85. Connor JR, Boyer PJ, Menzies SL, et al. Neuropathological examination suggests impaired brain iron acquisition in restless legs syndrome. Neurology 2003; 61(3):304–309.
86. Ancoli-Israel S, Martin J, Jones DW, et al. Sleep-disordered breathing and periodic limb movements in sleep in older patients with schizophrenia. Biol Psychiatry 1999; 45(11):1426–1432.
87. Eisensehr I, Ehrenberg BL, Noachtar S. Different sleep characteristics in restless legs syndrome and periodic limb movement disorder. Sleep Med 2003; 4(2):147–152.
88. Santamaria J, Iranzo A, Tolosa E. Development of restless legs syndrome after dopaminergic treatment in a patient with periodic leg movements in sleep. Sleep Med 2003; 4(2):153–155.
89. Tergau F, Wischer S, Paulus W. Motor system excitability in patients with restless legs syndrome. Neurology 1999; 52(5):1060–1063.
90. Entezari-Taher M, Singleton JR, Jones CR, et al. Changes in excitability of motor cortical circuitry in primary restless legs syndrome. Neurology 1999; 53(6):1201–1205.
91. Tugnoli V, Manconi M, Quatrale R, et al. Neurophysiological study of corticomotor pathway in patients with primary restless legs syndrome (RLS). Neurology 2000; 54(suppl 3):26–27.
92. Wechsler LR, Stakes JW, Shahani BT, Busis NA. Periodic leg movements of sleep (nocturnal myoclonus): an electrophysiological study. Ann Neurol 1986; 19(2): 168–173.
93. Yokota T, Hirose K, Tanabe H, Tsukagoshi H. Sleep-related periodic leg movements (nocturnal myoclonus) due to spinal cord lesion. J Neurol Sci 1991; 104(1):13–18.
94. Lee MS, Choi YC, Lee SH, Lee SB. Sleep-related periodic leg movements associated with spinal cord lesions. Mov Disord 1996; 11(6):719–722.
95. de Mello MT, Lauro FA, Silva AC, Tufik S. Incidence of periodic leg movements and of the restless legs syndrome during sleep following acute physical activity in spinal cord injury subjects. Spinal Cord 1996; 34(5):294–296.
96. Hartmann M, Pfister R, Pfadenhauer K. Restless legs syndrome associated with spinal cord lesions. J Neurol Neurosurg Psychiatry 1999; 66(5):688–689.
97. Kang SY, Sohn YH, Lee IK, Kim JS. Unilateral periodic limb movement in sleep after supratentorial cerebral infarction. Parkinsonism Relat Disord 2004; 10(7):429–431.
98. Kim JS, Lee SB, Park SK, et al. Periodic limb movement during sleep developed after pontine lesion. Mov Disord 2003; 18(11):1403–1405.
99. Kutukcu Y, Dogruer E, Yetkin S, Ozgen F, Vural O, Aydln H. Evaluation of periodic leg movements and associated transcranial magnetic stimulation parameters in restless legs syndrome. Muscle Nerve 2005; 33:133–137.
100. Briellmann RS, Rosler KM, Hess CW. Blink reflex excitability is abnormal in patients with periodic leg movements in sleep. Mov Disord 1996; 11(6):710–714.
101. Bucher SF, Seelos KC, Oertel WH, et al. Cerebral generators involved in the pathogenesis of the restless legs syndrome. Ann Neurol 1997; 41(5):639–645.
102. Bucher SF, Trenkwalder C, Oertel WH. Reflex studies and MRI in the restless legs syndrome. Acta Neurol Scand 1996; 94(2):145–150.
103. Esteves AM, de Mello MT, Lancellotti CL, et al. Occurrence of limb movement during sleep in rats with spinal cord injury. Brain Res 2004; 1017(1–2):32–38.
104. Sforza E, Nicolas A, Lavigne G, et al. EEG and cardiac activation during periodic leg movements in sleep: support for a hierarchy of arousal responses. Neurology 1999; 52(4):786–791.
105. Winkelman JW. The evoked heart rate response to periodic leg movements of sleep. Sleep 1999; 22(5):575–580.
106. Droste D, Krauss J, Hagedorn G, Kaps M. Periodic leg movements are part of the B wave rhythm and cyclic alternating pattern. Acta Neurol Scand 1996; 94:347–353.
107. Lavoie S, de Bilbao F, Haba-Rubio J, et al. Influence of sleep stage and wakefulness on spectral EEG activity and heart rate variations around periodic leg movements. Clin Neurophysiol 2004; 115(10):2236–2246.
108. Ferrillo F, Beelke M, Canovaro P, et al. Changes in cerebral and autonomic activity heralding periodic limb movements in sleep. Sleep Med 2004; 5(4):407–412.

109. Sforza E, Juony C, Ibanez V. Time-dependent variation in cerebral and autonomic activity during periodic leg movements in sleep: implications for arousal mechanisms. Clin Neurophysiol 2002; 113(6):883–891.
110. Allen RP, Barker PB, Wehrl F, et al. MRI measurement of brain iron in patients with restless legs syndrome. Neurology 2001; 56(2):263–265.
111. Staedt J, Stoppe G, Kogler A, et al. Dopamine D2 receptor alteration in patients with periodic movements in sleep (nocturnal myoclonus). J Neural Transm Gen Sect 1993; 93(1):71–74.
112. Ruottinen HM, Partinen M, Hublin C, et al. An FDOPA PET study in patients with periodic limb movement disorder and restless legs syndrome. Neurology 2000; 54(2): 502–504.
113. Schadrack J, Willoch F, Platzer S, et al. Opioid receptors in the human cerebellum: evidence from (11C)diprenorphine PET, mRNA expression and autoradiography. Neuroreport 1999; 10(3):619–624.
114. Jueptner M, Rijntjes M, Weiller C, et al. Localization of a cerebellar timing process using PET. Neurology 1995; 45(8):1540–1545.
115. Montplaisir J, Lorrain D, Godbout R. Restless legs syndrome and periodic leg movements in sleep: the primary role of dopaminergic mechanism. Eur Neurol 1991; 31(1): 41–43.
116. Hening WA, Allen RP, Earley CJ, et al. An update on the dopaminergic treatment of restless legs syndrome and periodic limb movement disorder. Sleep 2004; 27(3): 560–583.
117. Earley CJ, Allen RP. Pergolide and carbidopa/levodopa treatment of the restless legs syndrome and periodic leg movements in sleep in a consecutive series of patients. Sleep 1996; 19(10):801–810.
118. Brodeur C, Montplaisir J, Godbout R, Marinier R. Treatment of restless legs syndrome and periodic movements during sleep with L-dopa: a double-blind, controlled study. Neurology 1988; 38(12):1845–1848.
119. Stiasny K, Wetter TC, Winkelmann J, et al. Long-term effects of pergolide in the treatment of restless legs syndrome. Neurology 2001; 56(10):1399–1402.
120. Wetter TC, Stiasny K, Winkelmann J, et al. A randomized controlled study of pergolide in patients with restless legs syndrome. Neurology 1999; 52(5):944–950.
121. Chaudhuri KR, Dhawan V, Basu S, et al. Valvular heart disease and fibrotic reactions may be related to ergot dopamine agonists, but non-ergot agonists may also not be spared. Mov Disord 2004; 19(12):1522–1523.
122. Earley CJ, Yaffee JB, Allen RP. Randomized, double-blind, placebo-controlled trial of pergolide in restless legs syndrome. Neurology 1998; 51(6):1599–1602.
123. Montplaisir J, Nicolas A, Denesle R, Gomez-Mancilla B. Restless legs syndrome improved by pramipexole: a double-blind randomized trial. Neurology 1999; 52(5):938–943.
124. Silber MH, Girish M, Izurieta R. Pramipexole in the management of restless legs syndrome: an extended study. Sleep 2003; 26(7):819–821.
125. Winkelman JW, Johnston L. Augmentation and tolerance with long-term pramipexole treatment of restless legs syndrome (RLS). Sleep Med 2004; 5(1):9–14.
126. Allen R, Becker PM, Bogan R, et al. Ropinirole decreases periodic leg movements and improves sleep parameters in patients with restless legs syndrome. Sleep 2004; 27(5):907–914.
127. Comella C. Sleep episodes in Parkinson's disease: more questions remain. Sleep Med 2003; 4(4):267–268.
128. Comella CL, Nardine TM, Diederich NJ, Stebbins GT. Sleep-related violence, injury, and REM sleep behavior disorder in Parkinson's disease. Neurology 1998; 51(2): 526–529.
129. Moller JC, Stiasny K, Cassel W, et al. ("Sleep attacks" in Parkinson patients. A side effect of nonergoline dopamine agonists or a class effect of dopamine agonists?). Nervenarzt 2000; 71(8):670–676.
130. Stiasny K, Moller JC, Oertel WH. Safety of pramipexole in patients with restless legs syndrome. Neurology 2000; 55(10):1589–1590.

131. Kaplan PW, Allen RP, Buchholz DW, Walters JK. A double-blind, placebo-controlled study of the treatment of periodic limb movements in sleep using carbidopa/levodopa and propxyphene. Sleep 1993; 16:717–723.
132. Walters AS, Wagner ML, Hening WA, et al. Successful treatment of the idiopathic restless legs syndrome in a randomized double-blind trial of oxycodone versus placebo. Sleep 1993; 16(4):327–332.
133. Walters AS, Winkelmann J, Trenkwalder C, et al. Long-term follow-up on restless legs syndrome patients treated with opioids. Mov Disord 2001; 16(6):1105–1109.
134. Zucconi M, Coccagna G, Petronelli R, et al. Nocturnal myoclonus in restless legs syndrome effect of carbamazepine treatment. Funct Neurol 1989; 4(3):263–271.
135. Garcia-Borreguero D, Larrosa O, de la Llave Y, et al. Treatment of restless legs syndrome with gabapentin: a double-blind, cross-over study. Neurology 2002; 59(10):1573–1579.
136. Bonnet MH, Arand DL. Chronic use of triazolam in patients with periodic leg movements, fragmented sleep and daytime sleepiness. Aging (Milano) 1991; 3(4):313–324.
137. Mitler MM, Browman CP, Menn SJ, et al. Nocturnal myoclonus: treatment efficacy of clonazepam and temazepam. Sleep 1986; 9(3):385–392.
138. Ohanna N, Peled R, Rubin AH, et al. Periodic leg movements in sleep: effect of clonazepam treatment. Neurology 1985; 35(3):408–411.
139. Peled R, Lavie P. Double-blind evaluation of clonazepam on periodic leg movements in sleep. J Neurol Neurosurg Psychiatry 1987; 50(12):1679–1681.
140. Hening W, Allen R, Earley C, et al. The treatment of restless legs syndrome and periodic limb movement disorder. An American academy of sleep medicine review. Sleep 1999; 22(7):970–999.
141. Saletu M, Anderer P, Saletu-Zyhlarz G, et al. Restless legs syndrome (RLS) and periodic limb movement disorder (PLMD): acute placebo-controlled sleep laboratory studies with clonazepam. Eur Neuropsychopharmacol 2001; 11:153–161.
142. Earley CJ, Heckler D, Allen RP. The treatment of restless legs syndrome with intravenous iron dextran. Sleep Med 2004; 5:231–235.
143. Guilleminault C, Flagg W. Effect of baclofen on sleep-related periodic leg movements. Ann Neurol 1984; 15(3):234–239.

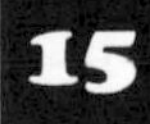

# Restless Legs Syndrome Effects on Quality of Life

**Richard P. Allen**

*Department of Neurology, Johns Hopkins University, Baltimore, Maryland, U.S.A.*

## INTRODUCTION

Restless legs syndrome (RLS) does not increase the risk of mortality nor does it have other serious health consequences aside from that associated with sleep loss. It only involves some peculiar sensori-motor symptoms that occur for a short period of the day and do not even occur every day. So why bother treating the disorder? The clinically significant morbidity of RLS involves its disruption of quality of life (QoL) more than any of its specific symptom features. RLS patients complain of sleep disruption (1) and sensory problems involving pain and discomfort (2). They may have some possible cognitive impairments (3). The first two of these clinical features, however, represent the large majority of patient complaints. In a large survey of the general population in the United States, those with moderate to severe RLS symptoms reported two types of major complaints: discomfort and pain for 88% and sleep disturbance for 76% (4). But such complaints, even when dramatic, may not be clinically significant. What indication do we have that these symptoms reported by RLS patients adversely affect normal living, thereby justifying considerable treatment efforts? Health-related QoL studies address this critical question of the clinical significance of disease-related complaints. RLS is not known to shorten life but does it significantly disrupt life? The answer for this question comes best from the QoL evaluations.

Three broad approaches are used to evaluate health-related QoL status: a disease-specific assessment of the impact of symptoms on QoL, a nondisease-specific assessment related generally to health and QoL, and various bench marks of life functioning (e.g., employment status, absenteeism, work productivity assessments, etc.). The first two of these have been used to evaluate QoL in RLS.

## DISEASE-SPECIFIC QUALITY OF LIFE EVALUATIONS OF RLS

Two disease-specific QoL scales have been developed and evaluated. The first of these, commonly referred to as either RLSQoL or the Hopkins RLSQoL, obtained significant items for RLS symptom effects on life functioning from expert opinion and patient groups. This 18-item patient-completed questionnaire was found to have one primary summary scale assessing QoL. The Hopkins RLSQoL summary score has good psychometric properties (e.g., Chronbach's alpha = 0.92 and test-retest for patients with stable symptoms = 0.84) and is responsive to changes in severity of the disorder (5). This scale has been used in some large clinical trials and is now available, translated into several different languages from MAPI Research Institute, Lyon, France. A second scale (referred to as the RLS-Quality of Life Questionarre-1) was developed using expert opinion and a large patient population accessed via the Internet with the cooperation of the Restless Legs Syndrome Foundation. This 17-item scale provided both a general summary score and four factors labeled: daily function, social function, sleep quality, and emotional well-being. It had good psychometric properties (6). This scale was used to demonstrate that RLS patients' sleep complaints related strongly to a negative impact on health-related QoL, supporting the clinical significance of the sleep disturbance with RLS. The amount of daytime sleepiness, however, was less than might have been expected for the degree of sleep loss (7). These findings not only demonstrated the clinically significant impact on QoL for the sleep disturbance symptoms of RLS, but also revealed a remarkable failure of the homeostatic drive for sleep to produce daytime sleepiness in RLS. Thus, those with RLS have the adverse QoL consequences from sleep loss, but are unable to sleep during the day to reduce these disruptions of life quality.

Most of the work with disease-specific scales for RLS has, however, used the Hopkins QoL. The summary score of the Hopkins QoL relates strongly to the patients' independent subjective rating of disease severity. Thus, it provides a good tool for evaluating treatment benefits for RLS on this important morbidity of decreased QoL. The disease-specific scales relating QoL issues to the effects of the disease symptoms will generally better capture treatment effects than a general QoL scale. Many factors other than changes in the disease severity can affect QoL and these nonspecific effects operate to reduce sensitivity to treatment effects in the more general scales. Thus, for treatment trials, the better measures are the disease-specific scales. The more general scale, however, provides a better evaluation of the disorder's impact on QoL because it allows comparisons with normative samples and with other disorders.

## GENERAL HEALTH-RELATED QUALITY OF LIFE EVALUATIONS

The Short-Form (SF)-36 has become the most commonly used general scale for evaluating health-related QoL. It has gained wide acceptance and has been used to produce normative data and data evaluating QoL in a variety of diseases. These existing data sources permit appropriate comparisons. One survey of 375 Americans, who reported at least moderately severe RLS symptoms, showed they had worse SF-36 scores on all eight of the questionnaire's dimensions (Fig. 1). The areas of greatest impact relate to energy/vitality, as expected for the sleep disruption, and both physical (how much physical problems disturb functioning) and bodily pain (how much pain disturbs functioning), again as expected for the commonly reported sensory symptoms of the patients. When compared to other medical conditions, these RLS sufferers had as much or more impairment of QoL than those with chronic disorders such as type 2 diabetes, osteoarthritis, hypertension, and depression (Fig. 2). Almost identical results were obtained from a sample of 85 patients diagnosed with RLS in a major treatment center (8). It is important to appreciate that these results come from those who had the RLS symptoms at least twice a week over the past year, reported moderate to severe distress with the symptoms, and sought medical care. The wider range of RLS patients with much milder or more intermittent symptoms are likely to show less disruption of their QoL, but these milder patients may not even come to medical attention for treatment of their RLS. In contrast, the more severe patients with the impaired QoL noted above are those likely to need treatment. Thus, moderate

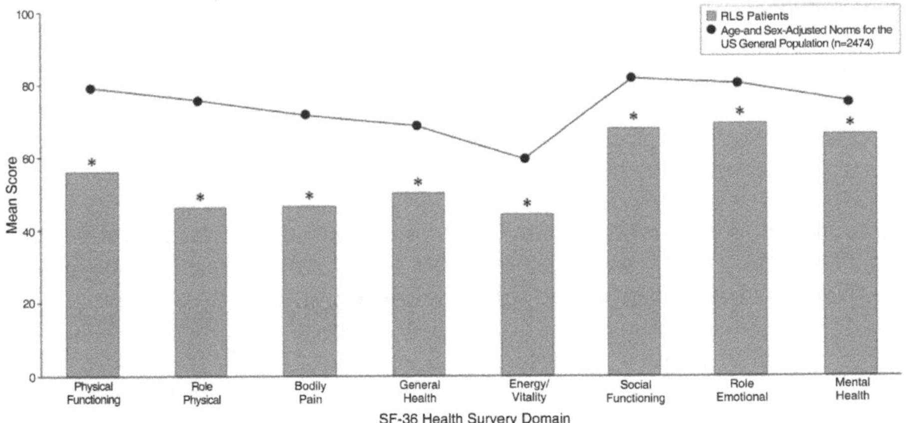


**FIGURE 1** Comparison of mean SF-36 Health Survey scores of patients with restless legs syndrome ("RLS sufferers") with age- and sex-adjusted U.S. population norms. Asterisks indicate that the scores of the RLS sufferer group were significantly below the norms for all eight dimensions. *Abbreviation*: SF-36, Short-Form 36. *Source*: From Ref. 4.

to severe RLS clearly and dramatically disturbs the life of the patient as much or more than other recognized chronic medical disorders.

## TREATMENT BENEFITS FOR QUALITY OF LIFE

Because RLS worsening in the QoL represents a primary morbidity for the disorder, treatment should improve QoL. Here the evaluation is somewhat hampered by the short-term nature of most treatment trials. It may take several weeks before the benefits of reduced symptoms translate into improvements in daily functioning

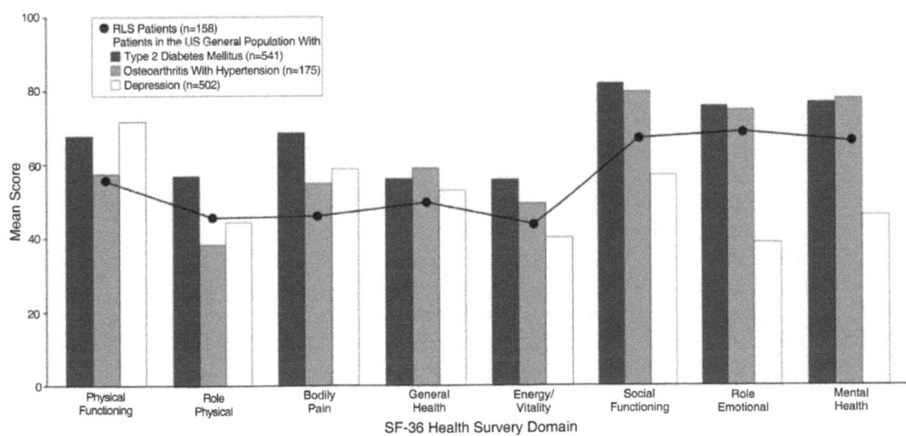


**FIGURE 2** Comparison of mean SF-36 Health Survey scores of U.S. patients with restless legs syndrome ("RLS sufferers") with those of U.S. patients with common chronic medical conditions. *Abbreviation*: SF-36, Short-Form 36. *Source*: From Ref. 4.

or lifestyle patterns. The disease-specific scales are, however, more likely to detect treatment effects, possibly even in short-term studies. Two large 12-week placebo-controlled clinical trials evaluating a dopamine agonist (ropinirole) reported statistically significant improvement in the Hopkins RLSQoL (9,10). Both of these studies reported about 25% greater improvement on ropinirole than placebo and the degree of improvement in both studies reached a clinically meaningful effect size (change in score/standard deviation) of approximately 1 (11). The SF-36 scales did not show significant differences between ropinirole and placebo for one of the studies (10). The other study, however, reported statistically significant improvement for ropinirole over placebo for three of the eight domains of the SF-36: mental health, social functioning, and vitality (9). Given the multiple factors that could affect the SF-36, besides change in RLS severity and the relatively short duration of this study, the limited positive results support the findings from the disease-specific RLSQoL scales. Dopaminergic treatment of RLS appears to significantly improve the QoL for these patients.

## SUMMARY

Evaluating QoL of RLS patients revealed a surprising degree of impairment. These patients with moderate to severe RLS suffer a disruption of their life as great as other serious chronic medical disorders. Even clinicians dealing daily with RLS patients often find these results surprising. They forget that when the patients are seen in the clinic they may have few or no symptoms. They may look and sound perfectly normal, making it hard to recognize the life disruption they are experiencing. These patients at home or work have marked discomfort and profound loss of energy; moreover, this occurs later in life when patients may want to be able to decrease activity slightly. It is important to remember that for a severe RLS patient, the disorder begins to dominate all aspects of life with thoughts focused on avoiding or reducing these RLS sensations.

RLS is often considered a trivial condition; marginally worthy of medical attention. Nothing could be further from the truth. RLS may be a thief of sleep, but it is even more a destroyer of the QoL.

## REFERENCES

1. Allen RP, Earley CJ. Validation of the Johns Hopkins restless legs severity scale. Sleep Med 2001; 2:239–242.
2. Bassetti CL, Mauerhofer D, Gugger M, Mathis J, Hess CW. Restless legs syndrome: a clinical study of 55 patients. Eur Neurol 2001; 45(2):67–74.
3. Pearson VE, Allen RP, Dean T, Gamaldo CE, Lesage SR, Earley CJ. Cognitive deficits associated with restless legs syndrome (RLS). Sleep Med 2006; 7(1):25–30.
4. Allen RP, Walters AS, Montplaisir J, et al. Restless legs syndrome prevalence and impact: REST general population study. Arch Intern Med 2005; 165(11):1286–1292.
5. Abetz L, Vallow SM, Kirsch J, Allen RP, Washburn T, Earley CJ. Validation of the restless legs syndrome quality of life questionnaire. Value Health 2005; 8(2):157–167.
6. Atkinson MJ, Allen RP, DuChane J, Murray C, Kushida CA, Roth T. Validation of the restless legs syndrome quality of life instrument (RLS-QLI): findings of a consortium of national experts and the RLS Foundation. Qual Life Res 2004; 13(3):679–693.
7. Kushida CA, Allen RP, Atkinson MJ. Modeling the causal relationships between symptoms associated with restless legs syndrome and the patient-reported impact of RLS. Sleep Med 2004; 5:485–488.

8. Abetz L, Allen R, Follet A, et al. Evaluating the quality of life of patients with restless legs syndrome. Clin Ther 2004; 26(6):925–935.
9. Walters AS, Ondo WG, Dreykluft T, Grunstein R, Lee D, Sethi K. Ropinirole is effective in the treatment of restless legs syndrome. TREAT RLS 2: a 12-week, double-blind, randomized, parallel-group, placebo-controlled study. Mov Disord 2004; 19(12):1414–1423.
10. Trenkwalder C, Garcia-Borreguero D, Montagna P, et al. Ropinirole in the treatment of restless legs syndrome: results from the TREAT RLS 1 study, a 12 week, randomised, placebo controlled study in 10 European countries. J Neurol Neurosurg Psychiatry 2004; 75(1):92–97.
11. Abetz L, Arbuckle R, Allen R, Mavraki E, Kirsch J. The reliability, validity, and responsiveness of the Restless Legs Syndrome Quality of Life questionnaire (RLSQoL) in a trial population. Health Qual Life 2005; 3:79.

# 16 Restless Legs Syndrome: Personal Perspectives

**Georgianna Bell**

*Restless Legs Syndrome Foundation, Rochester, Minnesota, U.S.A.*

## THE FACES OF RESTLESS LEGS SYNDROME

While most often diagnosed in middle-aged individuals, restless legs syndrome (RLS) does not limit itself to a certain generation of people. Children, teenagers, and young adults can find themselves affected by the symptoms of RLS as readily as their grandparents. And it is not just the patients themselves who are affected. Friends and family members are also integrally involved in living with RLS.

As you will read in the stories that follow, RLS is a *real* disorder. It affects a wide assortment of individuals in a wide assortment of ways. Each story is unique and individualized; however, the frustrations are always very similar. Lack of sleep, not being able to share a bed with your spouse, the inability to travel or attend concerts—these are always at the forefront. As Harriet Forman, an RN from New York City explained it: "I have suffered with RLS for decades, as did my mother, my son, and even my husband (by virtue of sleeping in the same bed with me). I've 'walked' enough in bed and out to have circumnavigated the globe several times." While unique, Harriet's story sounds remarkably similar to so many others.

## THE RLS FOUNDATION

These are real stories and real people that have found their way through the doors of the RLS Foundation, a nonprofit organization located in Rochester, Minnesota. Founded in 1992, the Foundation works to increase awareness, improve treatments, and through research, find a cure for RLS. With the help of more than 100 support groups across the United States and Canada, the RLS Foundation strives to provide educational resources for both patients and physicians, while funding research projects in search of a cause and cure for RLS.

Patient members of the RLS Foundation receive free shipping on RLS publications including the quarterly *NightWalkers* newsletter and a variety of other helpful medical tools. For physicians, the Foundation funds research grants each year and offers a health care provider membership that entitles all members to a scientific bulletin, automatic mailing of new education materials, free copies of patient brochures for use in their offices, a secure discussion board, PowerPoint presentations for use as a teaching tool, and much more.

In addition, the RLS Foundation maintains a website (www.rls.org) that provides the latest links to RLS resources, an online discussion board, copies of publications, a searchable database, and a health care provider directory that provides the names of physicians interested in treating patients with RLS.

The nine staff members at the Foundation are busy throughout the year creating publications for the public and physicians, answering phone calls from patients who need direction, and traveling across the country and the world to medical symposiums and events. All of this is done to promote awareness of RLS so that another generation does not have to combat RLS as their parents and grandparents have.

The following individuals have graciously shared the stories of how their lives have been forever altered by RLS. *They* are the faces of RLS.

## MARLENE'S STORY: "GOOD PHYSICIANS MAKE ALL THE DIFFERENCE"

I am currently 36 years old and have been living my life with the urge to move my legs and with pain in the calf muscle area since I was at least five years old. After I almost fell asleep at the wheel one night, I actually mentioned my frustrations to my doctor. He is a great man who knew everything about my life (except this), and I was glad to benefit from his service. When I told him, I did not get the reactions I usually do from other people. He completely understood and said his secretary had RLS and told me how many patients he treated with RLS.

During this difficult time, the RLS Foundation and the online discussion board were my only support besides him. My doctor and I are working to treat the symptoms. Through maintenance, I am now able to stay up about 0.5 to 1 hour longer before symptoms appear, and on a good day, I can sit through a movie without too much disruption. Of course there are a plentitude of treatments, lifestyle changes, and activities to try or items to buy, and each person who suffers has to find what works the best for him or her. I pray for research to back up this quite common condition and more medical choices or even a cure.

## LYNNE'S STORY: "I WANT TO LIVE WITH THEM, NOT THEM LIVE AROUND ME"

Ever think about a kid waking up in the dark and in pain? I am that face of RLS. Four years old and it is my first memory of life—dark, tears, and pain. I took charge of my disorder even at that early age. I was a kid that didn't ask for help. It just wasn't me. It's not me now either, but RLS changed that portion of my personality. I had to seek help some 2 years ago. I could no longer live with the lack of healing sleep, the pain, or the hopelessness. Seeking help has been every bit the challenge that RLS is.

I have changed my life many times in the past 10 years. RLS made sure of that. It's the finer points of life that really make it worth it, and the finer points often get lost in a fury of pain and sleep deprivation. It's no longer insulting when a friend calls to remind me of a lunch date. It's no longer a shock to my children that I have forgotten an appointment. It's no longer an issue to make all things happen after lunch. Everyone knows that I've only gone to bed just hours before. It's never an issue that I will need medication when I travel. Most of my family and friends know that I will not sleep. They have gotten used to the great attacks that leave me unable to join in the fun. The insult is that this is not the person I want to be. I want to live with them, not them live AROUND me.

Doctors and researchers, when you go to work and listen to the problems of the people who suffer with RLS, put my face in your mind. See what life I live day to day. Know that my children, my husband, my family, and my friends want me to be a part of my life. Not just a statement here and there. When you go to work and help me, you help us—the larger RLS community. We want goals and dreams.

We want the power to control our symptoms and not have them control us. We want a life outside of this disorder. If you need a face to bring it all home, think of me. I am the face of RLS.

## CLARE'S STORY: "I FOUND A WAY OF SHUTTING IT ALL OUT"

This is hard for me to do—to face up to my past and understand the path that I have let RLS, alcohol abuse and drug abuse steer me.

Since finding out about RLS, I have spent much of my time thinking about my past and how this illness has affected me from an early age. Childhood memories have flooded back to me ... things I have blanked out of my mind because of years of drug and alcohol abuse.

It starts from early memories of struggling to get out of my "buggy" as a toddler because I just had to get out of it and move. Then there are countless times I got into trouble at school for not sitting still and for fidgeting even though I tried explaining it was because my legs felt funny and hurt if I didn't move them. My teachers used to tell me not to be so silly and there was no such thing as "can't" sit still, and it was just that I was deliberately disturbing the class to get attention. No I wasn't! I just could not sit still because my legs felt funny and hurt if I didn't move them. I was classified as hyperactive and dismissed as a problem child.

I became isolated and introverted. I spent hours immersed in books to find an escape but could only read if I was lying flat on the front of my bed with my legs bouncing alternatively. The vibrations were enough to soothe my arms too. Even going to the doctor was no help; he told me and my mother it was growing pains. I was then labeled as a hypochondriac, malingerer, and attention seeker because everyone thought I was just putting it on.

But then I found a way of shutting it all out—teachers, doctors, parents, siblings, friends, school, everyone, and everything—alcohol! Thirteen years old and turning to alcohol to find escape from this joke called life. I believed I had nowhere to turn to but the bottle, and I became more and more introverted and unable to "grow" emotionally. As I became an adult, this did not change.

The abuse spiraled into drug abuse. After years of mild dabbling, I started to take amphetamines on the weekends, but then I started using them for work. I would take enough to get me through—a little bit everyday—but then I had to take downers to sleep. This continued for 3 years; it covered up my symptoms, and it allowed me to convince myself that it all really was in my head.

Fast forward a few years. By this time I had become aware that RLS existed, but I still didn't know anything about it, and I still hadn't made the connection with all my symptoms. I thought: *Well, that explains the funny feelings in my legs, but what about my arms and body? What about the pain? What about the sensitiveness? Why can't I sleep? Why don't my legs work properly when I get up sometimes? Why am I so exhausted?* It wasn't until I had access to the Internet and the information and the RLS Foundation support groups on it that I started to understand what had been happening to me all my life. Finally, I found the answers that I had been searching for in all the wrong places.

I'm now in the first stage of drug therapy and awaiting an appointment with a neurologist, and for the first time in my life, I feel I can begin to move forward and build a life. A sense of calm has come to me from knowing it really is not in my head and that this really is happening. RLS has had a devastating effect on my life and the quality of it—not only physically, but also emotionally. I know that my life is never going to be perfect and I have a long way to go, but I know that at least I can have a life now.

## MIKE'S STORY: "SLEEP DEPRIVATION AND WORK ARE AN INCOMPATIBLE COMBINATION"

My experience with RLS is a familiar one. I've suffered with the sleep deprivation RLS is famous for since 1992, but it wasn't until just last year that my physician diagnosed it as RLS. With this very belated diagnosis, I immediately went to the Internet and found the RLS Foundation website. This is when things started to improve. It was a relief in itself to find out the reason for my suffering. However, the major relief came from the information on the website explaining how massaging and stretching can help. Over time, I have developed a personalized routine of massaging and stretching that helps significantly. As a supplement, my physician prescribed hydrocodone. I use this about once every 10 days for those really bad nights.

RLS degrades the quality of my life through sleep deprivation. The many miseries associated with sleep deprivation are well known so I won't list them all. For me, sleep deprivation and the need to work for a living are an incompatible combination that has caused me great misery over the years. Simply put, RLS "lets" you sleep just when it's time to go to work. Fortunately, I just made the early retirement age of 55 when our plant closed this July. So for now, I can get some relief. I can sleep in longer. I really should work a few years longer—not a pleasant thought with RLS.

## SUE'S STORY: "I WANT BETTER FOR THEM"

"It's like an electrical current—maybe like a cattle prod," I tell my nephew. He asks more questions. "Is it like when your leg falls asleep?" he asks. "No," I say. I try to explain again and again. He wants to know, but what he really wants is to have "me" back—the "me" that doesn't need to leave before a certain time because I can't stand the long ride home in the car. The "me" that isn't always whining about how tired she is or how little sleep she got, or how the meds don't work, or how it's affecting work. I want that "me" back too.

RLS and periodic limb movement disorder have affected my life for as long as I can remember. When I would spend the night with my grandmother, I would watch her shake her legs while sitting, then hit them with her fists, then start to pace, back and forth, back and forth. Late at night, while my dreams were swirling in my head, she would still be up. Her doctors thought she was crazy—that she had mental instabilities. But I knew she wasn't, because if she was, then so was my mom, and my uncle, and me too.

My sister has children now. So far, there are no signs of RLS, but chances are high as the rest of us all have it to varying degrees. I wish for them something different should they end up with this. I wish for them to watch the sunrise because they wanted to, not because it hails the end of a dark, lonely, and long night. I wish for them to be taken seriously when they see their doctors. I wish for them to fall into a peaceful sleep when they are terribly tired instead of thrashing in bed, pacing the floor, doing stretches, or beating their thighs with their fists.

I want something elusive, at least to me. I find myself wondering what I would do if I had something truly horrible. I ask myself how bad can this be, this electrical current that keeps me on my toes and away from my slumber. Surely, I must be making it out to be worse than it is. But I am not. It is insidious. The lack of sleep day after day after day is like water wearing away at a stone. It affects everything around me, my career, my outlook on life, my mental health.

Maybe, just maybe, we're getting ready to change all of that. Maybe, as a group, we've had enough. I'm choosing this time to wave my hand and get someone's attention. I want someone to listen to us. Hear our stories and offer us some hope.

## JOCELLE'S STORY: "NEVER GIVE UP!"

I am 26 years old. I was diagnosed with RLS when I was 18. I had the chance to meet a great specialist in Montreal. He did a polysomnographic study and diagnosed RLS. He has been following me ever since. He's not a miracle man, and I'm not waiting for a miracle cure. I know that someone believes in my condition and is trying to help me with it. This is what he does, and I'm grateful. When something doesn't work, I don't get disappointed. At least my doctor tried something! I appreciate that he's honest and very open-minded. I talk to him about new treatments that I read in *NightWalkers* newsletters or on the Internet. We really work well together, and I'm an active partner in my treatment. That's important.

In life, I think we should always focus on positive things. I've found a positive thing with my RLS: my nieces and nephews like to sit on my legs because it's like sitting on a horse! Next time you can't sleep and you feel like you're the only person in the world who can't sleep, think of those who have the same condition and battle each day and every night. You are not alone. Never give up!

These stories were collected over several years and communicate the frustrations and difficulties that many people who have RLS have faced. Foremost is the frustration created by the lack of awareness in the public and the medical community. Fortunately, this is changing. The RLS Foundation continues to encourage people with RLS to seek better treatments and hopes that someday, many of these stories of frustration become stories of success.

# 17 Iron Deficiency–Associated Restless Legs Syndrome

**William G. Ondo**
*Department of Neurology, Baylor College of Medicine, Houston, Texas, U.S.A.*

## INTRODUCTION

Restless legs syndrome (RLS) is extremely common, affecting between 5% and 10% of Caucasian populations, although it appears less common in Asian and African populations (1). In roughly 60% of cases, a family history of RLS can be found, although this is often not initially reported by the patient (2). Three gene loci have been published, although specific causative proteins remain elusive (3–5). Given the wide distribution of RLS; however, it is likely that additional specific genetic etiologies are yet to be discovered. Despite the appropriate attention given to RLS genetics, between 2% and 6% of the population probably suffer from RLS without any identifiable highly penetrant genetic pattern. It is not known whether some "genetic" forms of RLS could express low penetrance, and mimic a sporadic pattern of onset. Therefore, patients without a positive family history are classified as either primary RLS, if no other explanation is found, or secondary RLS, if they concurrently posses a condition known to be associated with RLS. Because the exact pathophysiology of RLS is unknown, the relationship between "idiopathic" RLS and "secondary" RLS is not elucidated in any case. It is not known why some persons with an associated medical condition develop RLS symptoms while others, usually most others, do not. Furthermore, it is not established whether persons with a genetic predisposition for RLS may be symptom free without an additional insult caused by an associated condition, or if subclinical or mild genetic RLS is exacerbated by the coincidental occurrence of a secondary cause.

The most common causes of secondary RLS include systemic iron deficiency, renal failure, neuropathy, myelopathy, pregnancy, and possibly Parkinson's disease. There is some evidence to support an association of RLS with tremor, some genetic ataxias, sleep apnea, fibromyalgia, and rheumatological diseases. This chapter will discuss the role of systemic iron deficiency and RLS.

## CENTRAL NERVOUS SYSTEM IRON DEFICIENCY IN RLS

Recent evidence strongly implicates brain iron abnormalities in all cases of RLS. Cerebrospinal fluid (CSF) ferritin is lower in RLS cases (6,7). Magnetic resonance imaging (8) and transcranial ultrasound (9) show reduced iron stores in the striatum and red nucleus. Pathologic data in RLS show not only reduced ferritin, iron staining, and increased transferrin stains, but also reduced transferrin receptors (10,11). This is important because globally reduced iron stores would normally upregulate transferrin receptors. Therefore, it appears that primary RLS has reduced intracellular iron indices secondary to a perturbation of homeostatic mechanisms that regulate iron influx and/or efflux from the cell. Several proposed mechanisms for this dysregulation are discussed in detail elsewhere (Chapter 7).

The relationship between reduced central nervous system (CNS) iron stores and dopaminergic systems, also strongly implicated in RLS, is not clear. There are several interactions between iron and dopamine. First, iron is a cofactor for tyrosine-hydroxylase, which is the rate-limiting step in the production of dopamine. Second, iron is a component of the dopamine type-2 (D2) receptor. Iron deprivation in rats results in a 40% to 60% reduction of D2 postsynaptic receptors (12). The effect is quite specific, because other neurotransmitter systems including dopamine type-1 receptors are not affected. Third, iron is involved in Thy1 protein regulation. This cell adhesion molecule, which is robustly expressed on dopaminergic neurons, is reduced in brain homogenates in iron-deprived mice (13). Thy1 regulates vesicular release of monoamines, including dopamine (14). It also stabilizes synapses and suppresses dendritic growth (15). Although most suspect that the iron deficiency results in dopaminergic dysfunction, there is also animal model evidence to suggest that dopamine neuron ablation results in reduced iron storage capacity (Chapter 6).

Nevertheless, if low CNS intracellular iron incurred by some unknown genetic regulatory perturbation somehow causes RLS symptoms, it is intuitive to suggest that reduced body stores of iron could also result in low CNS intracellular iron and also cause RLS symptoms.

Low serum ferritin levels are the best indicator of low iron stores, although high ferritin levels do not necessarily indicate adequate iron stores because ferritin is an acute phase reactant. Therefore, in some inflammatory settings, such as renal failure, low iron stores can be difficult to identify. Each ferritin molecule, which is basically shaped like a hollow ball, can hold 2000 to 4000 iron atoms (Fig. 1). Serum-free elemental iron levels fluctuate markedly throughout the day, with their lowest levels at night, and are, therefore, not an accurate measure (16). Transferrin helps identify excessive iron but does not accurately identify reduced iron stores. Therefore, when screening for low systemic iron stores in RLS, ferritin is the most meaningful test. Serum iron binding percentage and soluble transferrin receptor (sTR) concentrations also can be used, but to date less data associates these with RLS.

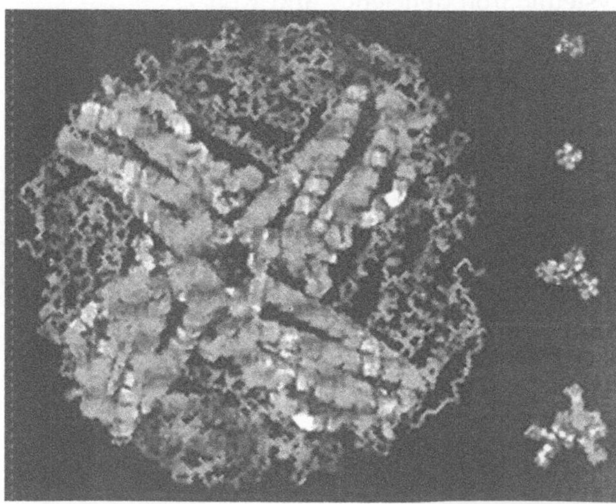

**FIGURE 1** Electron microscopy showing a large ferritin molecule, compared to other iron transport proteins.

## CLINICAL EXPERIENCE

A possible association between RLS symptoms and systemic iron deficiency has long been recognized (17–21). Ekbom originally reported that about 25% of his RLS patients were iron deficient, although he tended to emphasize the role of vascular insufficiency (18) Norlander was the first to emphasize the possible etiologic role of iron deficiency and treated RLS successfully with intravenous iron 50 years ago (21). Unfortunately, the importance of this groundbreaking research was only realized in the past decade after this association was "rediscovered."

A series of recent reports have associated low serum ferritin levels with RLS (22–27). In the modern era, O'keeffe et al. were the first to report on ferritin levels in 18 elderly patients with symptomatic RLS and compare them to age-matched controls (24). They discovered significantly lower ferritin levels in affected patients. Serum iron, hemoglobin levels, B12, and folate did not differ between the groups. Serum ferritin levels and symptom severity (determined by a simple 10 point subjective scale) were also inversely correlated (Spearman's rho −0.53, $p < 0.05$). Two months of oral iron supplementation improved the subjective scores in most affected patients. The authors suggested that all RLS patients with ferritin levels below 50 μg/L (a level within the normal range) should receive iron supplementation. These authors have also emphasized that iron deficiency can exist in the setting of normal serum ferritin levels (25).

Sun et al. reported that subjective RLS severity and awakening from PLMS were greater in RLS patients with lower serum ferritin levels (≤50 mcg/L) compared to those with higher serum ferritin (total $N = 27$) (27). Total PLMS was not different. RLS has been reported in blood donors (26,28). Silber et al. reported on eight patients in whom their RLS started shortly after donating blood (26). All had low serum ferritin and some were anemic. They suggested that RLS might be a relative contraindication against donating blood.

RLS and periodic limb movements associated with iron deficiency have also been reported in children. Kryger et al. reported RLS with low ferritin and iron binding percentage in three consecutive teenagers, who presented with sleep onset insomnia (29). All three had PLMS. After oral supplementation, both subjective and objective sleep measures improved along with iron indices. Seventy two percent of 39 children (mean age 7.5 ± 3.1) demonstrating pathological PLMS had serum ferritin levels of less than 50 μg/L (30). No correlation between ferritin level and PLMS was found, but lower serum iron levels did correlate ($r = 0.43$, $p < 0.01$) with PLMS. Some patients responded to iron supplementation.

In contrast, the MEMO study was a population based survey of 365 German subjects, aged 65 to 83. Serum ferritin, as evaluated by quartile analysis, was not significantly different in the 9.8% (36 subjects with RLS) who met criteria for RLS, compared to the remaining population (31). Although this data represents a superior design to study this question, a possible association may have been missed because of the relatively low number of RLS cases. The serum ferritin levels of both RLS subjects and non-RLS subjects were generally higher than other studies, perhaps suggesting an iron-rich diet in Augsburg, Germany. The number of RLS subjects with a family history of RLS was not reported.

Hogl et al. also evaluated iron status in a cross-sectional study involving 701 age-stratified participants. RLS was found in 10.6% (14.2% of women and 6.6% of men). Free serum iron, transferrin, and ferritin concentrations were similar in subjects with and without RLS. However, sTR concentrations were different in subjects with and without RLS (1.48 vs. 1.34 mg/L; $p < 0.001$).

Low serum iron may only be associated with certain populations of RLS patients. We have reported that serum ferritin is lower in patients with RLS who lack a family history but not-in those with familial RLS (2,32). Serum ferritin in RLS patients with a positive family history was $96.4 \pm 64.5$ ($N = 64$) compared to $61.5 \pm 54.1$ ($N = 26$) in patients without a family history of RLS.

Earley et al. have made the same general observation but segregated the groups based upon age of RLS onset (33). The patients with an older age of RLS onset had lower serum ferritin levels compared to patients with a younger age of onset. These groups, however, generally represent the same dichotomy as genetic-based segregations because there is a very strong correlation between a younger age of onset of RLS and the presence of a family history of RLS. An older age at onset and nonfamilial RLS appear to be strongly associated with low serum ferritin levels, whereas a younger age at onset and familial RLS generally are not associated with low serum ferritin levels. Therefore, the clinical epidemiology correlates nicely with the known basic science. Familial or primary RLS may be caused by CNS iron dysregulation; however, it can also be secondarily caused by systemic iron deficiency in people without a genetic cause for RLS. This is further highlighted by the observation that CSF ferritin, when sampled at night (6), but not during the day (7), is actually lower in patients with young onset RLS. Therefore, the serum to CSF ferritin ratio is markedly different in these two groups.

There is very little data evaluating the prevalence of RLS in populations of iron-deficient patients. One study that evaluated a population of 80 iron-deficient patients reported that 43% of them reported symptoms of RLS, using their own RLS criteria (20). RLS has been reported in subjects with systemic iron overload caused by hemochromotosis (34,35). However, this condition, seen in almost 0.5% of European descendents, does not usually cause CNS iron overload.

## IRON DEFICIENCY AND OTHER ASSOCIATIONS OF RESTLESS LEGS SYNDROME

The two most consistently identified secondary causes of RLS (renal failure and pregnancy) are also associated with iron deficiency. Roger et al. correlated RLS in dialysis patients with a lower hematocrit (36). However, numerous other studies have failed to clearly associate low iron with RLS in the renal failure population (Chapter 18).

Manconi et al. reported that 26% of pregnant women suffered from RLS, usually in the last trimester (37). The authors could find no significant differences in age, pregnancy duration, mode of delivery, tobacco use, the woman's body mass index, baby weight, or iron/folate supplementation in those with RLS. Hemoglobin, however, was significantly lower in the RLS group, and plasma iron tended to be lower compared to those without RLS. Lee et al. reported that 23% of 29 third trimester women developed RLS during pregnancy (38). Women with RLS in their population demonstrated lower preconception levels of ferritin, but had similar levels to women without RLS during pregnancy.

It is less clear that iron deficiency is causal in either condition because both improve with definitive treatments, (delivery or termination of the pregnancy, and renal transplant, for renal failure) more rapidly than serum iron deficits, would be restored. It is also difficult to accurately measure serum iron levels in either condition. Most dialysis patients take iron and erythropoietin, and have elevated ferritin as a marker of inflammation. Pregnancy redistributes tissue iron, serum iron, and fetal iron in a poorly understood ratio. CSF iron studies have not been done in either condition.

Parkinsons disease (PD) has also been associated with RLS and iron deficiency. In a survey of 303 consecutive PD patients, we found that 20.8% of all patients with PD met the diagnostic criteria for RLS (23). RLS did not correlate with duration of PD, age, H&Y, gender, dementia, use of levodopa, use of dopamine agonists, history of pallidotomy, or history of deep brain stimulation. The serum ferritin, however, was significantly lower in the PD/RLS group compared to the PD/no RLS group, or idiopathic RLS group. PD usually preceded RLS symptoms and these patients mostly lacked a family history of RLS. Overall, this suggested that a "double hit" (dopamine deficiency and iron deficiency) produced RLS in this population.

Ondo and Jankovic showed that RLS patients with neuropathy were less likely to have a family history of RLS than those without neuropathy (2). Many of these "neuropathic" RLS patients also had low ferritin levels, again suggesting that two separate precipitants (deafferentation and iron deficiency) could combine to result in RLS symptoms.

Using their own criteria for RLS, Salih et al. reported that RLS was present in 25% of 46 patients with rheumatoid arthritis vs 4% of 30 osteoarthritis controls (39). RLS patients appeared to have had significantly lower ferritin levels than controls, and a mildly higher rate of neuropathy. This, however, was not commented upon by the authors and is complicated by intrinsic inflammatory changes seen in arthritic conditions.

Overall, systemic iron deficiency remains the most common denominator among the accepted secondary causes of RLS. It does appear to be a true "secondary cause" in that it only seems to correlate with RLS in patients that lack a family history and/or have an older age of onset, and may combine with other risk factors to elicit symptoms. In contrast, population studies looking at all RLS subjects have not demonstrated a clear association of reduced serum ferritin and RLS, but this may result from the fact that genetic forms of RLS, usually a majority in most populations, are not actually associated with lower serum iron measures. The exact role of systemic iron deficiency in RLS remains unknown.

## IRON REPLACEMENT

The role of iron replacement in iron deficiency associated RLS, and for idiopathic RLS, is discussed in detail in Chapter 28. Although open label oral iron supplementation has been reported to improve RLS (93), the only controlled study of oral iron supplementation failed to improve RLS symptoms (94). Oral iron, however, has numerous limitations. It is very poorly absorbed and poorly tolerated. Absorption can be modestly improved when the iron is taken within a moderately acidic milieu, which is practically achieved by the concurrent addition of ascorbic acid. Even with ideal compliance, only modest augmentations of serum ferritin levels are usually achieved with oral supplementation in adult RLS populations. Pediatric supplementation may be more effective.

In contrast, the administration of intravenous iron can dramatically increase serum ferritin levels. Norlander first reported the benefit of intravenous iron. He reported that 21/22 subjects reported complete relief of RLS following high dose intravenous infusions (21). More recently, an open label study of high dose intravenous iron has also demonstrated robust efficacy (40,41). Intravenous iron also has limitations. High doses are required to increase CNS iron levels. This requires a long duration infusion and carries the risk of anaphylactic reactions. Additional controlled studies of at least two different intravenous preparations are ongoing.

In summary, most researchers feel that systemic iron deficiency can independently result in RLS symptoms. The role that low systemic iron may play in exacerbating symptoms in those genetically predisposed to RLS has not been explored. There is also some evidence to suggest that iron replacement can improve RLS symptoms, especially with high dose intravenous iron. Because iron entry into the CNS is highly regulated, very high serum doses may be required to "overrun" this system. Dose finding studies, however, are lacking. The role of oral iron replacement is not established but often recommended.

## REFERENCES


1. Ondo W. Epidemiology of restless legs syndrome. Sleep Med 2002; 3(suppl):S13–S15.
2. Ondo W, Jankovic J. Restless legs syndrome: clinicoetiologic correlates. Neurology 1996; 47:1435–1441.
3. Bonati MT, Ferini-Strambi L, Aridon P, Oldani A, Zucconi M, Casari G. Autosomal dominant restless legs syndrome maps on chromosome 14q. Brain 2003; 126:1485–1492.
4. Chen S, Ondo WG, Rao S, Li L, Chen Q, Wang Q. Genome wide linkage scan identifies a novel susceptibility locus for restless legs syndrome on chromosome 9p. Am J Hum Genet 2004; 74:876–885.
5. Desautels A, Turecki G, Montplaisir J, et al. Restless legs syndrome: confirmation of linkage to chromosome 12q, genetic heterogeneity, and evidence of complexity. Arch Neurol 2005; 62:591–596.
6. Earley CJ, Connor JR, Beard JL, Clardy SL, Allen RP. Ferritin levels in the cerebrospinal fluid and restless legs syndrome: effects of different clinical phenotypes. Sleep 2005; 28:1069–1075.
7. Earley CJ, Connor JR, Beard JL, Malecki EA, Epstein DK, Allen RP. Abnormalities in CSF concentrations of ferritin and transferrin in restless legs syndrome. Neurology 2000; 54:1698–1700.
8. Allen RP, Barker PB, Wehrl F, Song HK, Earley CJ. MRI measurement of brain iron in patients with restless legs syndrome. Neurology 2001; 56:263–265.
9. Schmidauer C, Sojer M, Seppi K, et al. Transcranial ultrasound shows nigral hypoechogenicity in restless legs syndrome. Ann Neurol 2005; 58:630–634.
10. Connor JR, Boyer PJ, Menzies SL, et al. Neuropathological examination suggests impaired brain iron acquisition in restless legs syndrome. Neurology 2003; 61:304–309.
11. Connor JR, Wang XS, Patton SM, et al. Decreased transferrin receptor expression by neuromelanin cells in restless legs syndrome. Neurology 2004; 62:1563–1567.
12. Ben-Shachar D, Finberg JP, Youdim MB. Effect of iron chelators on dopamine D2 receptors. J Neurochem 1985; 45:999–1005.
13. Ye Z, Connor JR. Identification of iron responsive genes by screening cDNA libraries from suppression subtractive hybridization with antisense probes from three iron conditions. Nucleic Acids Res 2000; 28:1802–1807.
14. Jeng CJ, McCarroll SA, Martin TF, et al. Thy-1 is a component common to multiple populations of synaptic vesicles. J Cell Biol 1998; 140:685–698.
15. Shults CW, Kimber TA. Thy-1 immunoreactivity distinguishes patches/striosomes from matrix in the early postnatal striatum of the rat. Brain Res Dev Brain Res 1993; 75: 136–140.
16. Borel MJ, Smith SH, Brigham DE, Beard JL. The impact of varying degrees of iron nutriture on several functional consequences of iron deficiency in rats. J Nutr 1991; 121: 729–736.
17. Apenstrom G. Pica och restless legs vid jardbist. 1964; 61:1174–1177.
18. Ekbom KA. Restless legs: a report of 70 new cases. 1950; 246:64.
19. Ekbom KA. Restless legs syndrome. 1960; 10:868–873.

20. Matthews WB. Letter: iron deficiency and restless legs. Br Med J 1976; 1:898.
21. Nordlander NB. Therapy in restless legs. Acta Med Scand 1953; 145:453–457.
22. Aul EA, Davis BJ, Rodnitzky RL. The importance of formal serum iron studies in the assessment of restless legs syndrome. Neurology 1998; 51:912.
23. Ondo WG, Vuong KD, Jankovic J. Exploring the relationship between Parkinson disease and restless legs syndrome. Arch Neurol 2002; 59:421–424.
24. O'Keeffe ST, Gavin K, Lavan JN. Iron status and restless legs syndrome in the elderly. Age Ageing 1994; 23:200–203.
25. O'Keeffe ST. Iron deficiency with normal ferritin levels in restless legs syndrome. Sleep Med 2005; 6:281–282.
26. Silber MH, Richardson JW. Multiple blood donations associated with iron deficiency in patients with restless legs syndrome. Mayo Clin Proc 2003; 78:52–54.
27. Sun ER, Chen CA, Ho G, Earley CJ, Allen RP. Iron and the restless legs syndrome. Sleep 1998; 21:371–377.
28. Kryger MH, Shepertycky M, Foerster J, Manfreda J. Sleep disorders in repeat blood donors. Sleep 2003; 26:625–626.
29. Kryger MH, Otake K, Foerster J. Low body stores of iron and restless legs syndrome: a correctable cause of insomnia in adolescents and teenagers. Sleep Med 2002; 3:127–132.
30. Simakajornboon N, Gozal D, Vlasic V, Mack C, Sharon D, McGinley BM. Periodic limb movements in sleep and iron status in children. Sleep 2003; 26:735–738.
31. Berger K, von Eckardstein A, Trenkwalder C, Rothdach A, Junker R, Weiland SK. Iron metabolism and the risk of restless legs syndrome in an elderly general population–the MEMO-Study. J Neurol 2002; 249:1195–1199.
32. Ondo W, Tan EK, Mansoor J. Rheumatologic serologies in secondary restless legs syndrome. Movement Disorders 2000; 15:321–323.
33. Earley CJ, Allen RP, Beard JL, Connor JR. Insight into the pathophysiology of restless legs syndrome. J Neurosci Res 2000; 62:623–628.
34. Earley CJ. Hemochromatosis and iron therapy of restless legs syndrome. Sleep Med 2001; 2:181–183.
35. Shaughnessy P, Lee J, O'Keeffe ST. Restless legs syndrome in patients with hereditary hemochromatosis. Neurology 2005; 64:2158.
36. Roger SD, Harris DC, Stewart JH. Possible relation between restless legs and anaemia in renal dialysis patients [letter]. Lancet 1991; 337:1551.
37. Manconi M, Govoni V, De Vito A, et al. Restless legs syndrome and pregnancy. Neurology 2004; 63:1065–1069.
38. Lee KA, Zaffke ME, Baratte-Beebe K. Restless legs syndrome and sleep disturbance during pregnancy: the role of folate and iron. J Womens' Health Gender-Based Med 2001; 10:335–341.
39. Salih AM, Gray RE, Mills KR, Webley M. A clinical, serological and neurophysiological study of restless legs syndrome in rheumatoid arthritis. Br J Rheumatol 1994; 33:60–63.
40. Earley CJ, Heckler D, Allen RP. Repeated IV doses of iron provide effective supplemental treatment of restless legs syndrome. Sleep Med 2005; 6:301–305.
41. Earley CJ, Heckler D, Allen RP. The treatment of restless legs syndrome with intravenous iron dextran. Sleep Med 2004; 5:231–235.

# 18 Restless Legs Syndrome and Renal Failure

**Kai Ming Chow and David Shu Cheong Hui**

*Department of Medicine and Therapeutics, Prince of Wales Hospital, Chinese University of Hong Kong, Shatin, New Territories, Hong Kong, P.R. China*

## INTRODUCTION

Since the detailed description of restless legs syndrome (RLS) by the Swedish neurologist Professor Axel Ekbom in 1945 (1), the condition has been known to be associated with various secondary causes including renal failure. The core feature of RLS is a distressing, irresistible need or urge to move the legs (focal akathisia). The akathisia often coexists with an uncomfortable, although not usually painful, sensation deep within the legs. These symptoms are brought on by rest (sitting or lying down). The more comfortable the patient becomes, the more likely that the symptoms will occur. The reverse is also true—the less comfortable the patient is, the less likely that he or she will have the symptoms. This review focuses on RLS that occurs in the renal failure population.

## EPIDEMIOLOGY

The largest corpus of literature about secondary RLS focuses on renal patients receiving dialysis therapy. There is a paucity of data on patients with milder degrees of renal insufficiency, except a single report of "restless legs" showing an incidence of less than 20% among a group of chronic kidney disease patients with plasma creatinine concentration between the range of 124 and 1280 μmol/L (2). In this chapter, we refer to "renal failure" and "uremia" interchangeably to denote the stage 5 chronic kidney disease patients requiring dialysis. Population-based screening studies have shown that RLS, mostly based on questionnaire survey, is present in up to 62% of patients undergoing dialysis (Table 1) (3), as compared with the quoted prevalence of between 2.5% and 15% in the general population (4). Studies of the Chinese dialysis population, for instance, found that 62% of peritoneal dialysis subjects and 70% of hemodialysis subjects fulfilled the diagnostic criteria of RLS (20,30). Our clinical observation concurs with other investigators, who found no difference in prevalence of RLS between patients on peritoneal dialysis and hemodialysis renal replacement therapy (31). The prevalence of RLS in pediatric dialysis patients is less well established; one study reported symptoms of restless legs in 6 out of 20 pediatric dialysis patients (30%) based on questionnaire survey (7).

For unknown reasons, there was a low prevalence (6.6%) of RLS in a study of Indian hemodialysis patients (15), again using the diagnostic criteria of the International RLS Study Group (IRLSSG) (32,33). This is thought to indicate racial or ethnic difference because the prevalence is much less than that in similar studies conducted in developed countries by the same diagnostic methods. Arguably, the best population-based epidemiological study thus far involved 308 maintenance hemodialysis patients in the United States. Based on personal interview,

**TABLE 1** Highlights of RLS in Renal Failure Patients as Opposed to Idiopathic[a]

| Author (year) | Cohort | RLS diagnosis | Number and percentage with RLS | RLS predictors |
|---|---|---|---|---|
| Merlino (5) (2006) | HD, HDF, Italy | IRLSSG, written, interview | 152/826 (18.4%) | Excessive daytime sleepiness, insomnia |
| Siddiqui (6) (2005) | HD, UK | IRLSSG, interview | 127/277 (45.8%) | Female, $P=0.01$, dialysis duration, $P=0.03$, increasing body weight, $P=0.02$ |
| Davis (7) (2005) | PD/HD, U.S.A. | PLMS only | 29% of 21 children with PLMS | NR |
| Mucsi (8) (2005) | HD, Hungary | NIH criteria | 14% of 333 | Association with insomnia |
| Unruh (9) (2004) | HD, U.S.A. | Single question for "severe" RLS | 15% of 894 | Association with increased mortality |
| Mucsi (10) (2004) | HD/PD, Hungary | | 15% | NR |
| Gigli (11) (2004) | HD/PD, Italy | Written IRLSSG | 21.5% of 601 | Greater duration of dialysis |
| Bhowmik (12) (2004) | India | | 1.5% of 65 | NR |
| Takaki (13) (2003) | HD, Japan | IRLSSG (4/4), IRLSSG ($\geq$2/4) | 60/490 (12.2%), 112/490 (22.9%) | Hyperphosphatemia, stress |
| Goffredo (14) (2003) | HD, Brazil | IRLSSG, interview | 26/176 (14.8%) | Caucasian > non-Caucasian |
| Bhowmik (15) (2003) | HD, India | | 6.6% | NR |
| Kutner (16) (2002) | HD, U.S.A. | IRLSSG, interview | 308, 68% Caucasian 48% African American | Caucasian > African American, no other significant predictors |
| Cirignotta (17) (2002) | HD, Italy | IRLSSG, written, interview | 38/114 (33.3%) | NR |
| Sabbatini (18) (2002) | HD, Italy | RLS question | 257/694 (37%) | None |
| Miranda (19) (2001) | HD, Chile | Interview | 43/166 (26%) | None |
| Hui (20) (2000) | PD, Hong Kong | Written question | 124/201 (62%) | Insomnia |
| Virga (21) (1998) | HD | RLS | (27.4%) | None |
| Collado-Seidel (22) (1998) | HD, Germany | IRLSSG (4/4), IRLSSG ($\geq$3/4) | 32/138 (23%) 44/138 (32%) | Inc. parathyroid hormone |
| Winkelmann (23) (1996) | HD, U.S.A. | IRLSSG (3/4) | 40/204 (20%) | Dec. Hct poor sleep |
| Walker (24) (1995) | HD, Canada | ICSD | 31/54 (57%) | Inc. BUN, $P=0.04$, Inc. Cr, $P=0.08$ |
| Stepanski (25) (1995) | PD | "Leg twitching" | 26/81 (32%) | NR |
| Holley (26) (1992) | HD/PD | RLS | 30/70 (42%) | NR |
| Roger (27) (1991) | HD/PD, U.K. | RLS | 22/55 (40%) | Hct, $P=0.03$, female |
| Bastani (28) (1987) | HD | RLS | 6/42 (17%) | NR |
| Nielson (29) (1971) | None | RLS | 43/109 (39%) | NR |

[a]Studies evaluating RLS in renal failure.

*Abbreviations*: HDF, hemodiafiltration; IRLSSG, International Restless Legs Syndrome Study Group; PLMS, periodic limb movements in sleep; NIH, National Institutes of Health; ICSD, International Classification of Sleep Disorders; BUN, blood urea nitrogen; NR, not reported.

symptoms of RLS was less frequently reported by African-American patients than Caucasians, with estimated prevalence 48% vs. 68% in the latter ($p = 0.0006$). An independent association of African-American patients with reduced risk of RLS was confirmed by multivariate logistic regression analysis in that study (14).

Although an autosomal dominant mode of inheritance has been suggested by studies of large kindreds and several major susceptibility loci have been identified, a positive family history is less common among renal failure patients with RLS as compared with those with idiopathic RLS. This observation has been made in 232 idiopathic RLS patients and another 68 patients with secondary RLS due to uremia. All of the index cases were diagnosed according to the IRLSSG criteria (32). A definitive positive family history, defined as having at least one first-degree relative who was examined by the investigators and verified according to the IRLSSG criteria, occurred in 42.3% of the patients with idiopathic RLS, as compared with only 11.7% in those with uremic RLS (34).

## PATHOGENESIS

The pathogenesis of RLS is complex and remains incompletely elucidated. Broadly speaking, recent research supports the primary role of the central nervous system and interaction at the spine level, instead of a pure peripheral origin.

Anemia and possibly iron deficiency, in particular, may play a prominent causal role in RLS in general and among dialysis patients. An association between restless legs and anemia was initially reported among 55 dialysis patients (27). Patients with restless legs were reported to have lower hemoglobin levels than those without restless legs, 8.2 g/dL vs. 9.5 g/dL ($P = 0.03$). The authors further demonstrated the therapeutic benefit with epoetin alfa in another group of 27 hemodialysis patients with restless legs. It should be noted, however, that there existed no relationship between the presence of symptoms and the initial ferritin concentration (34).

Molnar et al. recently queried for risk factors in a dialysis population of 177 patients who were waiting for renal transplantation (35). They confirmed an association with lower hemoglobin and iron deficiency. The estimated glomerular filtration rate (eGFR) was also a risk factor for RLS: eGFR greater than 60 mL/minutes/1.73 $m^2$ was 1.8%, eGFR 30 to 59 mL/minutes/1.73 $m^2$ was 5.1%, eGFR 15 to 29 mL/minutes/1.73 $m^2$ was 6.5%, and eGFR less than 15 mL/minutes/1.73 $m^2$ was 23.5% ($p < 0.001$). RLS was significantly less frequent in patients taking steroids than in patients not taking this medication (4% vs. 9%, $p < 0.05$). Dialysis treatment was also associated with an increased risk for RLS (odds ratio 2.2; 95% confidence interval 1.11–4.35; $p < 0.05$) even after adjusting for serum hemoglobin and comorbidity.

In contrast, the absence of an association between uremic RLS and serum iron, ferritin, and total iron binding capacity was noted in another two studies, where the criteria of IRLSSG were strictly adhered to. In the first study involving 32 hemodialysis patients with a definite diagnosis of RLS (fulfilling all four minimal diagnostic criteria of IRLSSG) and 88 unaffected hemodialysis patients, there was again no significant difference between the two groups in serum ferritin, serum transferring, and iron concentrations (22). They did find an association with low parathyroid hormone, but not calcium. This has not been corroborated in any other study. The second study involved 48 patients undergoing hemodialysis and peritoneal dialysis; serum iron, ferritin, and total iron binding capacity were similar for patients with and without RLS (36). High serum phosphorus appeared to predict the occurrence of RLS in one multivariate analysis according to a recent study of Japanese hemodialysis patients (37).

Overall, studies have not clearly confirmed an association between RLS and baseline serum iron deficiency in renal failure. This is complicated by the fact that serum ferritin is an acute phase reactant and often is artificially elevated in uremic patients, and thus is not always an accurate measure of iron stores.

In fact, the only randomized placebo-controlled trial showing a proven benefit of intravenous iron dextran administration was performed in 25 dialysis patients without iron deficiency by biochemical standards (38). Similarly, the effect of human recombinant erythropoietin on RLS cannot be inferred from observational investigations (27,39). Even if therapeutic benefit of erythropoietin could be established, the etiopathogenic factors underlying any implicated benefit might not necessarily derive from the correction of anemia alone. This is particularly intriguing because recent experimental data have shown neuroprotective effects of erythropoietin in the brain, spinal cord, and peripheral nervous system (39), all of which have been implicated in the pathogenesis of RLS.

The rationale for the potential role of iron in the pathogenesis of uremic RLS remains because iron homeostatic abnormalities certainly occur in uremia and are postulated to cause idiopathic RLS. One caveat is that neither brain iron nor cerebrospinal fluid iron was evaluated in any of these studies; we are left with the unanswered question of whether low brain iron plays a more important causative role.

## DIAGNOSIS

The diagnosis of RLS among the renal-failure population is a subject of confusion. Much of the confusion stems from the symptoms of peripheral neuropathy, which might mimic those of RLS. A high prevalence of false positive results from a self-administered questionnaire had been highlighted by a recent validation study involving 127 hemodialysis subjects who confused other leg symptoms (such as pain, paresthesia, nocturnal, or diurnal cramps) or peripheral polyneuropathy with those of RLS (17). The authors concluded that written surveys were inadequate to make a diagnosis of RLS in this population.

As discussed in the other chapters, the diagnosis of RLS hinges on the clinical history or patient interview in order to fulfill four core clinical features (32,33). Additional supportive diagnostic features, however, may not be present in uremic RLS. For example, a positive family history of RLS is a particularly common diagnostic clue for idiopathic RLS patients but is less prevalent among uremic RLS (Table 2) (34).

The presence of semirhythmic, repetitive, stereotypic leg movements on polysomnography, referred to as periodic limb movements in sleep, is often associated with, albeit not pathognomonic of, RLS (40). Although polysomnography identification of these movements (Fig. 1) is not absolutely necessary for diagnostic purposes, the diagnosis of RLS should be made with caution among renal-failure patients in their absence (33). According to a polysomnographic study comparing 10 patients with uremic RLS and 17 idiopathic RLS patients, the total number of periodic leg movements and the periodic leg movement index were significantly higher in uremic patients (41). The relationship between RLS and periodic limb movement disorder among dialysis patients has been evaluated by 48-hour polysomnography, comparing 28 dialysis subjects with RLS and 20 unaffected patients.

**TABLE 2** Highlights of RLS in Renal Failure Compared to Idiopathic RLS

| | RLS in renal failure patients | Idiopathic RLS |
|---|---|---|
| Epidemiology | Lower frequency of familial clustering | High familial tendency and high concordance in identical twins |
| Pathophysiology | Similar to idiopathic RLS; additional factors of anemia, psychological issues | Dopaminergic pathways and neuronal iron handling |
| Diagnosis | Potential diagnostic pitfalls using self-administered questionnaire; confusion with other leg symptoms or peripheral polyneuropathy. Marked PLMS | Classic criteria, relatively less PLMS |
| Treatment | Less data of pharmacotherapy confined to L-dopa, pergolide, ropinirole, clonazepam, clonidine, gabapentin; renal transplant remains definitive treatment | Dopamine precursors and agonists, antiepileptics, sedative-hypnotic agents, opiates |
| Prognostic implications | Potential markers of high-risk dialysis patients with increased mortality | |

*Abbreviation*: PLMS, periodic limb movements in sleep.

The median periodic limb movement index was 87 in those with RLS as compared to 16 in the dialysis patients without RLS ($P = 0.003$). Furthermore, nearly 90% of dialysis patients with RLS were found to have periodic limb movement disorder, the combination of which was associated with significantly worse sleep quality and quality of life (36).

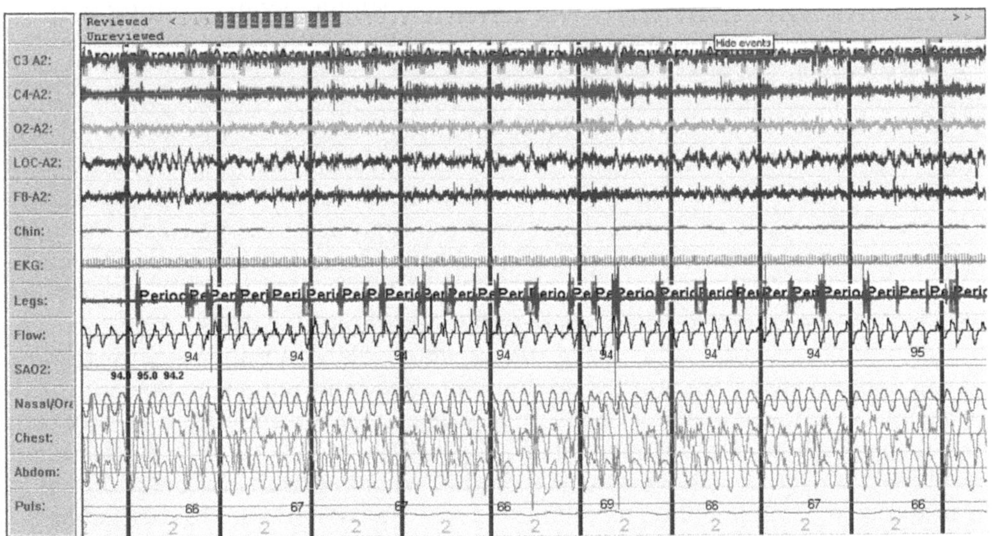


**FIGURE 1** Polysomnography profile from a 65-year-old end-stage renal disease patient with symptoms of restless legs syndrome and daytime sleepiness. Obstructive sleep apnea was excluded by overnight sleep study, which showed an apnea-hypopnea index of 1.3 events/hour of sleep. However, she had an arousal index of 49.1/hour with 21 arousals per hour related to periodic limb movements.

## TREATMENT

Actual dialysis does not seem to improve RLS symptoms. Although no comparison between nondialyzed severely uremic vs. dialyzed uremic patients has ever been attempted, patients do not report improvement of RLS after dialysis. In fact the only study to correlate dialysate loads with RLS actually showed a positive correlation, such that those that were dialyzed more had higher rates of RLS (42). Causality, of course, cannot be determined in such a study.

There are only a few reported studies of drug therapy for RLS in the dialysis population. In general, the dopaminergic agents are considered to be the treatment of first choice for patients with both idiopathic and uremic RLS. Although formal treatment comparisons to idiopathic RLS have not been reported, uremic RLS may be more refractory and require higher doses of dopaminergic medications.

Based on two double-blind crossover studies of uremic RLS, a bedtime dose of 100 to 200 mgL-dopa standard plus decarboxylase inhibitor appears to be effective, although results were contradictory in terms of overall sleep quality and disrupted sleep (43,44). Walker et al, reported improved PLMS and improved slow wave sleep on 100 mg of extended release levodopa (a relatively small dose) compared to placebo in five subjects, but sleep architecture was still markedly abnormal (44). Furthermore, augmentation may occur; this relates to the development of RLS features earlier during the day, a more rapid onset of symptoms with inactivity, together with increased symptom severity and additional involved anatomy. To overcome the problems of symptom augmentation after the long-term use of levodopa, dopamine agonists have been used with variable success. One small randomized double-blind crossover study with pergolide, involving eight dialysis patients, demonstrated subjective improvement in symptoms of restless legs despite a similar degree of sleep disturbance, objectively (45). PLMS were not significantly improved compared to placebo [$53.7 \pm 22.3$ vs. $35.8 \pm 11.8$ ($P = 0.2$)].

The only randomized trial comparing a dopamine agonist, ropinirole, and L-dopa (using a crossover open-label study design with 6 week arms separated by a 1 week washout in 11 hemodialysis patients) favored ropinirole (46). The 10 patients who completed the study reported a 33.5% improvement (from $16.7 \pm 3.2$ to $11.1 \pm 4$; $P < 0.001$) of the six-item IRLS scores during levodopa sustained release (SR) treatment and a 73.5% improvement (from $16.6 \pm 2.8$ to $4.4 \pm 3.8$; $P < 0.001$) during ropinirole treatment. By the end of the study, the mean levodopa SR dosage was 190 mg/d and the mean ropinirole dosage was 1.45 mg/d. Ropinirole was superior to levodopa SR in reducing six-item IRLS scores ($P < 0.001$) and in increasing sleep time ($P < 0.001$). The patient clinical global impression scale showed a significant difference favoring ropinirole ($P < 0.01$).

By and large, most other drug treatments of dialysis patients with restless legs are extrapolated from studies in idiopathic RLS, and remain to be confirmed. Currently, evidence of alternative pharmacotherapy for uremic RLS is mostly confined to clonazepam (in an open-label study) (47), clonidine (in a double-blind study) (48), as well as gabapentin. The efficacy of gabapentin has been shown in a randomized double-blind placebo-crossover study among 16 hemodialysis patients (49) and another open-label study comparing with L-dopa among 15 hemodialysis patients (50). Gabapentin has also been used successfully in another open label report (51).

Second-line treatments such as methadone have also been shown to reduce symptoms, without augmentation, in small case series involving dialysis patients (52). The precise role of high-dose intravenous iron supplementation remains undefined. In one double-blind placebo-controlled study involving 25 dialysis patients, symptom improvement, albeit significant, only lasted for 4 weeks (35).

On the basis of available data, the only definitive treatment strategy of uremic RLS is renal transplantation. After the initial case report of successful treatment of RLS following kidney transplant (53), long-term results had been reported in a series of 11 hemodialysis patients with RLS who underwent kidney transplantation (54). Remarkably, all 11 patients reported complete resolution of restless legs symptoms within 21 days of receiving a kidney transplant. After kidney graft failure and return to dialysis, recurrent RLS symptom ensued, but again resolved in one subject, who underwent a second successful kidney transplant. Most important of all, in a large cross-sectional European sample of 992 chronic kidney disease patients, it has recently been shown that the prevalence of RLS (questionnaire-based diagnosis) was significantly lower in the transplanted patients than a comparable group of dialysis subjects wait-listed for transplant, 4.8% vs. 11.4% respectively ($P < 0.001$). Furthermore, there was a graded increase in RLS prevalence according to the eGFR of transplanted recipients. In other words, the frequency of RLS increased as the transplant kidney function declined (35). Taken together, these observations suggest that restless legs symptoms are largely derived from kidney failure or uremia-related factor(s).

## PROGNOSIS

In general, dialysis patients with RLS have worse sleep quality, more insomnia complaints, impaired quality of life, and lower mental health (6,7,53). A problem with emotion-oriented coping (using the Coping Inventory for Stressful Situations) and high anxiety levels (using the Hospital Anxiety and Depression Scale) are associated with RLS in one multivariate analysis, according to a recent study of Japanese hemodialysis patients (55). Causal relationships, nevertheless, cannot be established in a cross-sectional study.

Recently, 333 patients on chronic maintenance dialysis were queried for RLS and assessed with the Athens Insomnia Scale (AIS) and Kidney Disease Quality-of-Life Questionnaire among other scales (8). The overall prevalence of RLS was 14%. RLS patients were twice as likely to have significant insomnia (35% vs. 16%; $P < 0.05$), worse overall sleep (median AIS score: 8 vs. 4; $P < 0.01$), and poorer QoL, even after adjusting for other clinical and socio-demographic factors.

Recent observational investigations have also emphasized the association of uremic RLS with many more adverse clinical outcomes. Notably, a previous study of 41 hemodialysis patients with restless legs symptoms highlighted the increased risk of RLS for premature discontinuation of dialysis and risk of increased mortality (23). Although that particular study did not adjust for the severity of illness, its intriguing observation hypothesized the putative association between RLS and nonadherence to dialysis—and hence potential causal relationship with mortality risk. Sleep fragmentation is another possible reason for increased cardiovascular mortality. This was suggested by another study, involving a selected cohort of 29 end-stage renal failure patients, who reported disturbed sleep or daytime sleepiness, among whom periodic limb movements were significantly predictive of patient mortality (56).

The best evidence for survival prognostic implication of uremic RLS comes from a prospective follow up of 894 incident peritoneal dialysis and hemodialysis patients. Severe restless legs symptoms were found to be associated with a 39% greater hazard of death after controlling for comorbidity, demographic variables, and potential clinical confounders (9). Even though these studies cannot address putative mechanisms of shorter survival among RLS patients, the clinical or prognostic importance of RLS is beyond doubt.

Despite the increasing body of evidence to suggest the prognostic significance of RLS on dialysis patient outcome, little is known about the potential modifiers of treating RLS. There are no published data to suggest that drug treatment of RLS improves patient mortality.

## SUMMARY

With the recognition of secondary RLS in the setting of renal failure, it has become clear that its prevalence is far greater than hitherto recognized. Differences in uremic RLS and idiopathic RLS have been highlighted in this chapter (Table 2). Drug treatment of dialysis patients with RLS remains controversial because the body of scientific evidence available to guide clinical decisions is mostly extrapolated from idiopathic RLS. In general, similar medication strategies are employed to treat uremic RLS as idiopathic RLS, however uremic patients may be more refractory. Renal clearance issues, especially with pramipexole, must also be considered. Fundamental questions such as the pathophysiological basis of RLS in uremia, its intriguing interplay with iron status, and occurrence in earlier stages of chronic kidney disease, remain largely unanswered.

## REFERENCES

1. Ekbom KA. Restless legs syndrome. Acta Med Scand 1945; 158(suppl):4–122.
2. Neundörfer B, Kayser-Gatchalian C, Huber W, Werner W. Neuropsychiatric symptomatology with chronic renal insufficiency in the stage of compensated and decompensated retention. II. Peripheral nerve disturbances. J Neurol 1976; 211:263–274.
3. Kavanagh D, Siddiqui S, Gedds CC. Restless legs syndrome in patients on dialysis. Am J Kidney Dis 2004; 43:763–771.
4. Allen RP, Earley CJ. Restless legs syndrome: a review of clinical and pathophysiologic features. J Clin Neurophysiol 2001; 18:128–147.
5. Merlino G, Piani A, Dolso P, et al. Sleep disorders in patients with end-stage renal disease undergoing dialysis therapy. Nephrol Dial Transplant 2006; 21:184–190.
6. Siddiqui S, Kavanagh D, Traynor J, Mak M, Deighan C, Geddes C. Risk factors for restless legs syndrome in dialysis patients. Nephron Clin Pract 2005; 101:C155–C160.
7. Davis IR, Baron J, O'Riordan MA, Rosen CL. Sleep disturbances in pediatric dialysis patients. Pediatr Nephrol 2005; 20:69–75.
8. Mucsi I, Molnar MZ, Ambrus C, et al. Restless legs syndrome, insomnia and quality of life in patients on maintenance dialysis. Nephrol Dial Transplant 2005; 20:571–577.
9. Unruh ML, Levey AS, D'Ambrosio C, Fink NE, Powe NR, Meyer KB. Choices for Healthy Outcomes in Caring for End-Stage Renal Disease (CHOICE) Study. Restless legs symptoms among incident dialysis patients: association with lower quality of life and shorter survival. Am J Kidney Dis 2004; 43:900–909.
10. Mucsi I, Molnar MZ, Rethelyi J, et al. Sleep disorders and illness intrusiveness in patients on chronic dialysis. Nephrol Dial Transplant 2004; 19:1815–1822.
11. Gigli GL, Adorati M, Oolso P, et al. Restless legs syndrome in end-stage renal disease. Sleep Med 2004; 5(3):309–315.

12. Bhowmik D, Bhatia M, Tiwari S, et al. Low prevalence of restless legs syndrome in patients with advanced chronic renal failure in the Indian population: a case controlled study. Ren Fail 2004; 26(1):69–72.
13. Takaki J, Nishi T, Nangaku M, et al. Clinical and psychological aspects of restless legs syndrome in uremic patients on hemodialysis. Am J Kidney Dis 2003; 41:833–839.
14. Goffredo Filho GS, Gorini C, Puryslco AS, Silva HC, Elias IE. Restless legs syndrome in patients on chronic hemodialysis in a Brazilian city: frequency, biochemical findings and comorbidities. Arquivos de Neuro-Psiquiatria 2003; 61(3B):723–727.
15. Bhowmik D, Bhatia M, Gupta S, Agarwa S, Tiwari D, Dash S. Restless legs syndrome in hemodialysis patients in India: a case controlled study. Sleep Med 2003; 4:143–146.
16. Kutner NG, Bliwise DL. Restless legs complaints in African-American and Caucasian hemodialysis patients. Sleep Med 2002; 3:497–500.
17. Cirignotta F, Mondini S, Santoro A, Ferrari G, Gerardi R, Burzzi G. Reliability of a questionnaire screening restless legs syndrome in patients on chronic dialysis. Am J Kidney Dis 2002; 40:302–306.
18. Sabbatini M, Minale B, Crispo A, et al. Insomnia in maintenance hemodialysis patients. Nephrol Dial Transplant 2002; 17(5):852–856.
19. Miranda M, Araya F, Castillo JL, Duran C, Gonzalez F, Aris L. Restless legs syndrome: a clinical study in adult general population and in uremic patients. Rev Med Chil 2001; 129(2):179–186.
20. Hui DS, Wong TY, Ko FW, et al. Prevalence of sleep disturbances in Chinese patients with end-stage renal failure on continuous ambulatory peritoneal dialysis. Am J Kidney Dis 2000; 36:783–788.
21. Virga G, Mastrosimone S, Amici G, Munaretto G, Gastaldon F, Bonadonna A. Symptoms in hemodialysis patients and their relationship with biochemical and demographic parameters. Int J Artificial Organs 1998; 21(12):788–793.
22. Collado-Seidel V, Kohnen R, Samtleben W, Hillebrand GF, Oertel WH, Trenkwalder C. Clinical and biochemical findings in uremic patients with and without restless legs syndrome. Am J Kidney Dis 1998; 31:324–328.
23. Winkelman JW, Chertow GM, Lazarus JM. Restless legs syndrome in end-stage renal disease. Am J Kidney Dis 1996; 28:372–378.
24. Walker S, Fine A, Kryger MH. Sleep complaints are common in a dialysis unit. Am J Kidney Dis 1995; 26(5):751–756.
25. Stepanski E, Faber M, Zorick F, Basner R, Roth T, Sleep disorders in patients on ontinuous ambulatory peritoneal dialysis. J Am Soc Nephrol 1995; 6(2):192–197.
26. Holley JL, Nespor S, Rault R. Characterizing sleep disorders in chronic hemodialysis patients. ASAIO Transactions 1991; 37(3):M456–M457.
27. Roger SD, Harris DC, Stewart JH. Possible relation between restless legs and anemia in renal dialysis patients. Lancet 1991; 337:1551.
28. Bastani B, Westervelt FB. Effectiveness of clonidine in alleviating the symptoms of "restless legs" [letter]. Am J Kidney Dis 1987; 10(4):326.
29. Nielsen V. The peripheral nerve function in chronic renal failure. Acta Med Scand 1971; 190:105–111.
30. Hui DS, Wong TY, Li TS, et al. Prevalence of sleep disturbances in Chinese patients with end stage renal failure on maintenance hemodialysis. Med Sci Monit 2002; 8: CR331–CR336.
31. Vecchi A, Finazzi S, Padalino R, et al. Sleep disorders in peritoneal and hemodialysis patients as assessed by self-administered questionnaire. Int J Artif Organs 2000; 23:237–242.
32. Walters AS. Toward a better definition of the restless legs syndrome. The International Restless Legs Syndrome Study Group. Mov Disord 1995; 10:634–642.
33. Allen RP, Picchietti D, Hening W, Trenkwalder C, Walters AS, Montplaisi J. Restless legs syndrome: diagnostic criteria, special considerations, and epidemiology. A report from the Restless Legs Syndrome Diagnosis and Epidemiology Workshop at the National Institute of Health. Sleep Med 2003; 4:101–119.
34. Winkelmann J, Wetter TC, Collado-Seidel V, et al. Clinical characteristics and frequency of the hereditary restless legs syndrome in a population of 300 patients. Sleep 2000; 23:597–602.

35. Molnar MZ, Novak M, Ambrus C, et al. Restless Legs Syndrome in patients after renal transplantation. Am J Kidney Dis 2005; 45(2):388–396.
36. Rijsman RM, de Weerd AW, Stam CJ, Kerkhof GA, Rosman JB. Periodic limb movement disorder and restless leg syndrome in dialysis patients. Nephrology (Carlton) 2004; 9:353–361.
37. Sloand JA, Shelly MA, Feigin A, Bernstein P, Monk RD. A double-blind, placebo-controlled trial of intravenous iron dextran therapy in patients with ESRD and restless legs syndrome. Am J Kidney Dis 2004; 43:663–670.
38. Benz RL, Pressman MR, Hovick ET, Peterson DD. A preliminary study of the effects of correction of anemia with recombinant human erythropoietin therapy on sleep, sleep disorders, and daytime sleepiness in hemodialysis patients (The SLEEPO Study). Am J Kidney Dis 1999; 34:1089–1095.
39. Maiese K, Li F, Chong ZZ. New avenues of exploration for erythropoietin. JAMA 2005; 293:90–95.
40. Lesage S, Hening WA. The restless legs syndrome and periodic limb movement disorder: a review of management. Semin Neurol 2004; 24:249–259.
41. Wetter TC, Stiasny K, Kohnen R, Oertel WH, Trenkwalder C. Polysomnographic sleep measures in patients with uremic and idiopathic restless legs syndrome. Mov Disord 1998; 13:820–824.
42. Huiqi Q, Shan L, Mingcai Q. Restless legs syndrome (RLS) in uremic patients is related to the frequency of hemodialysis sessions. Nephron 2000; 86(4):540.
43. Trendwalder C, Stiasny K, Pollmacher T, et al. L-dopa therapy of uremic and idiopathic restless legs syndrome: a double blind, crossover trial. Sleep 1995; 18:681–688.
44. Walker SL, Fine A, Kryger MH. L-DOPA/carbidopa for nocturnal movement disorders in uremia. Sleep 1996; 19:214–218.
45. Pieta J, Millar T, Zacharias J, Fine A, Kryger M. Effect of pergolide on restless legs and leg movements in sleep in uremic patients. Sleep 1998; 21:617–622.
46. Pellecchia MT, Vitale C, Sabatini M, et al. Ropinirole as a treatment of restless legs syndrome in patients on chronic hemodialysis: an open randomized crossover trial versus levodopa sustained release. Clin Neuropharmacol 2004; 27:178–181.
47. Read DJ, Feest TG. Clonazepam: effective treatment for restless legs syndrome in uremia. Br Med J (Clin Res Ed) 1981; 283:885–886.
48. Ausserwinkler M, Schimdt P. Successful clonidine treatment of restless legs syndrome in chronic kidney insufficiency. Schweiz Med Wochenschr 1989; 119:184–186.
49. Thorp ML, Morris CD, Bagby SP. A crossover study of gabapentin in treatment of restless legs syndrome among hemodialysis patients. Am J Kidney Dis 2001; 38:104–108.
50. Micozkadioglu H, Ozdemir FN, Kut A, Sezer S, Saatci U, Haberal M. Gabapentin versus levodopa for the treatment of restless legs syndrome in hemodialysis patients: an open-label study. Ren Fail 2004; 26:393–397.
51. Tan J, Derwa A, Sanu V, Rahman N, Woodrow G. Gabapentin in treatment of restless legs syndrome in peritoneal dialysis patients. Perit Dial Int 2006; 26:276–278.
52. Ondo WG. Methadone for refractory restless legs syndrome. Mov Disord 2005; 20: 345–348.
53. Yasuda T, Nishimura A, Katsuki Y, Tsuji Y. Restless legs syndrome treated successfully by kidney transplantation–a case report. Clin Transpl 1986; 1:138–139.
54. Winkelmann J, Stautner A, Samtleben W, Trenkwalder C. Long-term course of restless legs syndrome in dialysis patients after kidney transplantation. Mov Disord 2002; 17:1072–1076.
55. Tanaka W, Morimoto N, Tashiro N, Hori K, Katafuchi R, Fujimi S. The features of psychological problems and their significance in patients on hemodialysis–with reference to social and somatic factors. Clin Nephrol 1999; 51:161–176.
56. Benz RL, Pressman MR, Hovick ET, Peterson DD. Potential novel predictors of mortality in end-stage renal disease patients with sleep disorders. Am J Kidney Dis 2000; 35:1052–1060.

# 19 Restless Legs Syndrome and Neuropathy/Myelopathy

**Birgit Högl and Werner Poewe**

*Department of Neurology, Innsbruck Medical University, Innsbruck, Austria*

## INTRODUCTION

Although secondary restless legs syndrome (RLS) has been associated with a variety of peripheral neuropathies, the exact causal relationship is not clear in most of these reports. This is also true for reports of associations of RLS with different kinds of lesions on the spinal cord. This chapter will review the pertinent literature on secondary RLS in the context of peripheral neuropathies and myelopathy.

## POLYNEUROPATHY, RADICULOPATHY, AND PERIPHERAL NERVE LESIONS

Varying frequencies of RLS have been reported in peripheral neuropathies of different origin, ranging from 1% (1) to 28.6% (2). Conversely, greatly varying rates of neuropathy in RLS populations have also been observed. The presence of polyneuropathy (PNP) in a minor fraction of RLS patients (2 out of 27) has been noted as early as 1965 (3), but from the descriptions it is often difficult to determine if the relationship is causal or not. Some authors consider RLS associated with neuropathy to be underestimated (4); others express doubts, if there is any association at all (5).

Ondo et al. investigated 68 consecutive patients with RLS and stratified them for positive or negative family history. Abnormal nerve conduction velocity (NCV) was present in 25% of RLS patients with a positive family history, and 76.5% of the patients without a positive family history ($p < 0.01$) (6). In another paper, the authors investigated 54 patients who met standard criteria of RLS. Ninety-two percent of the patients with idiopathic RLS, but only 13% of patients with RLS associated with neuropathy had a positive family history. Patients with neuropathy also had a later onset of RLS and usually had a more acute onset. Some patients also had concurrent RLS and a more typical superficial burning neuropathy, usually in the feet. This is an important clinical differentiation and represents two distinct phenotypes, which patients will not usually segregate. RLS actually seldom directly affects the feet. Dopaminergics very effectively reduce the urge to move, but often do not help a concurrent burning neuropathic pain. Finally, Ondo et al. more recently reported that neuropathic RLS patients are less likely to develop augmentation with chronic dopaminergic treatment (7). Based on these findings, Ondo and Jankovic suggest that neuropathies may initiate secondary central nervous system changes; thus RLS in neuropathy may be a peripherally induced movement disorder, adding to tremor, dystonia, and others (8).

Oboler administered a self-administered questionnaire to outpatient veterans. It contained a single question for RLS and a single question for PNP. Out of

515 respondents, the frequency of RLS was 29%, and peripheral neuropathy was 49%. The combination of both RLS and PNP was extremely frequent. Because many respondents did not answer all questions, but all questionnaires were used for the analysis, a response bias might have occurred (9).

Rutkove failed to find an increased prevalence of RLS in a patient population with neuropathy (10). In that study, 154 patients with PNP were prospectively evaluated for RLS. The diagnosis of PNP was made on the basis of American association of electrodiagnostic medicine criteria, the diagnosis of RLS was made on the basis of the International Classification of Sleep Disorders 1990 (11). Only eight patients with polyneuropathy (PNP) (5.2% of the sample) fulfilled RLS criteria (10). The RLS symptoms in two patients with Lyme disease associated neuropathy improved after antibiotic treatment. Although the authors come to a different conclusion, this figure of 5.2% is well within the prevalence of RLS in the general population.

Gemignani reported the presence of RLS in 37% of 27 patients with Charcot Marie Tooth (CMT) disease type-II patients (with axonal neuropathy), but in none of 17 CMT type-I patients (with demyelinating neuropathy) (12). This suggests that axonal neuropathies are more likely to be associated with RLS. This is somewhat corroborated by the absence of any reports associating Guillain-Barré syndrome with RLS. It has been suggested that late-onset RLS may represent the initial manifestation of familial amyloid neuropathy (13). RLS preceded clinical manifestation of neuropathy by one to four years. Restless legs have also been reported in primary amyloidosis (14). Finsterer performed a retrospective analysis of 108 patients who had mitochondriopathies and PNP. Thirty-eight of them had axonal, mixed, or demyelinating neuropathies due to mitochondrial neuropathy; three of those were reported to have RLS. Noteworthy, in this study, restless legs were considered one of several possible causes of PNP, not a separate entity (15). Gemigniani reported 12 patients with essential mixed cryoglobulinemia. Four women, but no men, in this group demonstrated RLS as a major manifestation. All of them had a symmetrical sensory neuropathy (16). Another study suggested that the association of RLS and rheumatoid arthritis (RA) (25% of RA population) was due to spinal or peripheral nerve impairment. However, the frequency of neuropathy was similar in rheumatoid arthritis patients with and without RLS (17). In an adult type-II diabetic population, the frequency of sensory PNP was similar among subjects with and without RLS (8.8% vs. 7.0%) (18). Interestingly, the percentage of type-II diabetics affected with RLS was significantly more than type-I diabetics ($p = 0.02$). This difference, however, may have resulted from the older age of the type-II population.

In a population of 218 patients diagnosed with RLS and/or periodic limb movements of sleep (PLMS), only four had a concomitant diagnosis of PNP (prevalence 3.5%) as made by clinical criteria. In 872 matched controls without RLS, the prevalence of peripheral neuropathy was 0.2%; the difference was not significant (19).

Recently, a large population-based study has shown that the frequency of PNP was not higher in individuals with RLS compared to those without (20). In that study, RLS was diagnosed in personal interviews according to standard criteria, and PNP according to clinical and electrodiagnostic criteria. PNP was present in 2.7% of the subjects with RLS, and 2.4% of the subjects without RLS (20).

Taken together, available studies of the frequency of RLS in cohorts of patients with PNP or the prevalence of peripheral neuropathy in RLS cohorts are inconsistent. Some of these discrepancies may result from different thresholds and criteria for diagnosis both of RLS, but especially of neuropathy.

### Neuropathy Associated with Uremia

Uremia is one of the prime causes for secondary RLS. Early descriptions have linked uremic RLS to uremic neuropathy (21). Callaghan suggested that RLS may be "an early sign of peripheral nerve damage" and also stated that RLS in most cases seems unrelated to any specific disease entity (21). Thomas reported "restless legs" in 17.3% of the patients on a chronic dialysis program in the United Kingdom, approximately 50% of whom had peripheral neuropathy (22). The occurrence of restless legs was positively correlated with the presence of neuropathy in this dialysis population (22). In a population of hemodialysis patients in India, 6.9% had RLS (compared to 0% of controls). Electromyography (EMG) was performed in six patients of this sample, five of whom had neuropathy (23). In a study focusing specifically on RLS, RLS disappeared in all 11 dialysis patients who received successful kidney transplantation (24). Whether or not uremic neuropathy is responsible for RLS in patients with uremia remains unsettled, although the transplant data suggests it does not. Particularly in hemodialysis patients, iron deficiency may be the causative factor in a proportion of the cases.

### Peripheral Neuropathy in Idiopathic RLS

While it remains to be established that classical RLS meeting essential diagnostic criteria can actually be caused by PNP, a number of studies have investigated the peripheral nervous system in clinically defined idiopathic RLS without clinical neuropathy.

Harriman performed a detailed study of biopsies from the peroneus brevis muscle in 10 patients with "Ekbom's syndrome" without clinical signs of PNP. He investigated the specimen with vital staining and electron microscopy, with specific attention to motor end plates. In a subgroup of patients, cutaneous nerve biopsies were also examined. He did not find evidence for systematic changes in the examined muscles (25). In a study of 24 male aged volunteers with PLM alone (the presence of RLS was not indicated), the authors did not find a clear correlation with tibial or peroneal nerve conduction velocities and the presence of periodic limb movements (PLM) (26).

While neuropathy of the large nerves is readily detected by conventional NCV studies, small fiber neuropathy requires skin biopsy (or less well-validated additional studies). Iannacone performed detailed studies of peripheral nerve function in eight patients with idiopathic RLS, all of who had a normal clinical neurological examination. The studies included EMG/NCV, quantitative thermal testing, and sural nerve biopsy. In sural nerve biopsy, seven patients had varying combinations of endoneural fibrosis, acute axonal degeneration, or axonal regeneration and remyelinization. Only one showed the complete absence of pathologic abnormality. When electron microscopy was performed, all eight patients showed axonal atrophy and myelin alterations. Clinical pathological criteria for the diagnosis of motor-sensitive peripheral neuropathy were fulfilled in six out of the eight patients. In addition, warmth perception thresholds were abnormal in seven patients and severely affected in four, cold perception was abnormal in five and severely affected in two. EMG polyphasic potentials were increased in five out of the eight patients (27). In a letter to the editor, Iannacone et al. state that, "the occurrence of RLS and peripheral neuropathy is common. However, it is unclear why it is sometimes present and sometimes not in patients affected by peripheral neuropathy of the same etiology." The authors also refer to unpublished data

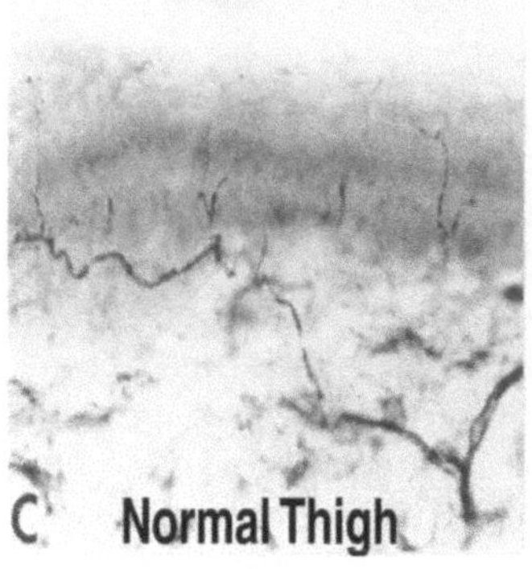

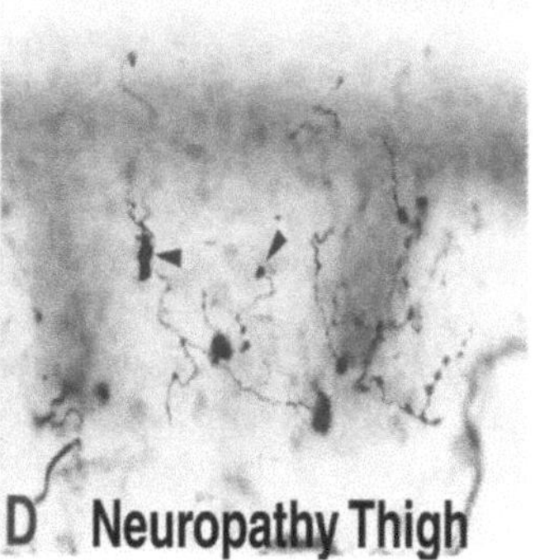


**FIGURE 1** Silver staining showing small fiber neuropathy and control.

indicating that RLS tended to disappear when neuropathy worsened. They suggest that RLS with neuropathy must be differentiated from RLS of "central origin," and that chronic axonal neuropathy is a predisposing factor for RLS (28).

Polydefkis performed EMG for large fiber neuropathy and skin biopsies to investigate small fiber densities in 22 patients with RLS. Some neuropathy was found in eight patients (36%). Out of those, three had pure large fiber neuropathy, three, mixed, and three, isolated small fiber neuropathy, as determined by biopsy (Fig. 1). RLS with small sensory fiber loss was associated with painful dysesthesia, later age of onset and no family history of RLS (29).

## Radiculopathies

It has frequently been stated that RLS may occur in association with radiculopathies, but only few data are available to support this. Walters et al. reported in the nightwalkers survey about a subgroup of 33 patients with RLS who underwent a thorough neurologic evaluation. Among "precipitating factors" lumbosacral radiculopathy was found in four, and diabetic peripheral neuropathy in one. In those patients, RLS was considered to be initially triggered by neuropathy or radiculopathy based on the temporal course of onset of symptoms, examinations, and EMG/NCV findings. Walters also reported a patient with spinal stenosis and a L4/L5 disk herniation, who underwent laminectomy for the L5 radiculopathy, but later had a relapse (30). The patient's wife noted PLM-like movements during sleep, but RLS only occurred again after a second surgical intervention following the relapse.

## Secondary RLS in Myelopathies

A number of case reports and case-series have noted an association of RLS with a variety of insults to the spinal cord suggesting the possibility of a spinal mechanism triggering PLMS, sensory symptoms, and motor restlessness in RLS.

In a polysomnographic study performed by Nogúes et al. in 26 patients with syringomyelia, PLMS during non rapid eye movement sleep were observed in 16, and PLM while awake (PLMA) in three. None of the patients had leg discomfort. In two out of three patients with progressive neurological deterioration, PLM had newly emerged at follow-up polysomnography one to two years after the initial examination. The authors suggest that damage to descending motor pathways, or to inhibitory interneurons by the syrinx may have caused the PLM (31). In a correspondence to this manuscript, Winkelmann reported a 58-year-old woman with a large syrinx extending from C1 to T11 in spinal magnetic resonance imaging. This patient exhibited PLMS, but also had a 15-year history of RLS. Both RLS and PLM responded well to levodopa (32).

Restlessness and lower limb dysesthesia associated with hyperalgesia were observed in a patient with foramen magnum meningioma, which dislocated the brain stem and compressed the spinal cord. This patient had a positive family history of RLS. Prior to surgery, response to levodopa was insufficient, but 2 years after surgery "minimal symptoms" remained, while the patient was on low dose pergolide and clonazepam (33). Lee et al. described three patients with thoracic spinal cord lesions (one schwannoma and two intramedullary lesions) who developed progressive paresis and sleep-related PLM. In one patient, PLM remitted after surgery, in another, marked improvement was experienced with levodopa treatment (34).

Yokota et al. reported 10 patients with PLMS and spinal cord lesions between C4 and T6 due to different etiologies (multiple sclerosis, injury, vascular, and cervical spondylosis). None of them fulfilled the criteria for RLS. Polysomnography was performed, and PLM observed in all. Two had a functionally complete transsection of the spinal cord. Interestingly, in those two patients, PLM also continued throughout REM sleep (35). The authors suggest that transection of the spinal cord may induce or disinhibit an underlying periodic process in the spinal cord, in analogy to periodic rhythmic movements or reflexes in decerebrate cats or animals transected at the lumbar spinal level (35). In a letter to the editor referring to Yokotas report, Hartmann et al. describe three patients with spinal cord lesions, who did fulfil the criteria for RLS, emerging in close temporal association with spinal cord injury (36). The etiology of the spinal cord lesions in this report was (i) multiple sclerosis (in this patient, improvement was achieved with levodopa), (ii) medullary injury due to traumatic atlanto-occipital dislocation (in this patient "satisfactory" relief of symptoms was obtained with levodopa and tramadol, and (iii) spondylotic myelopathy C3 to C6, which responded well to pergolide (36).

Hemmer et al. describe a patient in whom RLS emerged 1 year after treatment of borrelia-induced myelitis (37). Before treatment, the patient had a spastic paraparesis with inability to walk unassisted. When RLS emerged, the pareses had significantly improved and the patient was able to walk again. Polysomnography showed increased PLM. Levodopa treatment significantly improved RLS and reduced PLMS.

Brown et al. reported transverse myelitis associated infectious mononucleosis with RLS and PLMS (38). In this patient, RLS developed immediately after presentation with transverse myelitis, and there was no family history of RLS. RLS and PLM were unresponsive to intrathecal baclopen, but resolved after dopaminergic treatment with pergolide (38). The authors posited that RLS and PLM in spinal lesions resulted from removal of a descending inhibitory drive tonically suppressing a spinal cord reflex (38).

RLS has been reported to occur after spinal anesthesia (39,40). A prospective study reported the occurrence of new-onset RLS in 8.7% of the patients undergoing surgery during their spinal anesthesia. RLS was transient in all cases. The authors felt that the temporal interruption of sensory input or sensorimotor integration may have led to the development of RLS symptoms in susceptible individuals. The association of new-onset RLS in the population, with low mean corpuscular volume and low mean corpuscular hemoglobin points to additional involvement of iron in the pathophysiology of RLS after spinal anesthesia (39).

Maculano and coworkers produced rats with spinal cord lesions at the T9 level (41). Compared to the control group of sham surgery rats, 10 out of 11 rats in the spinal lesion group began to exhibit leg movements during sleep "similar to those observed in PLM patients." The authors suggest that this might be a model for PLM observed in paraplegic patients.

A questionnaire study concerning sleep complaints in postpolio syndrome contained a screening question for RLS. RLS was reported in 9/36 (25%) patients compared to 2/78 (3%) controls taken from the patients' neighborhood. Bruno and coworkers performed polysomnography in seven polio survivors (42). Four had PLM during sleep; two of them also had RLS. Two patients with only PLM responded to lorazepam, two with RLS and PLM responded to levodopa/carbidopa. The author suggested that poliovirus-induced spinal cord damage contributed to the findings (43).

A different report discusses RLS in patients with lumbar spinal stenosis and diminished cardiopulmonary compliance (Vesper's curse). The pathophysiology of RLS in this condition was attributed to increased right atrial filling pressure causing elevated paraspinal filling volumes, lumbar venous plexus engorgement, and a subsequent neurogenic claudication. Symptoms were reported to improve readily after the administration of diuretic medications (44).

The clinical similarity of the Babinski sign or flexion response and periodic movements in sleep was described in 1985 (45). Bara-Jimenez et al. showed state-dependent increased excitability of the spinal flexor reflex in patients with RLS and PLM (46) and secondary RLS due to chronic renal failure (47). Flexor reflex responses showed an increased spatial spread, which was even more marked during sleep compared to controls, and additionally multiple late responses during sleep. The authors concluded that PLMS, which they found to resemble the flexion response, resulted from enhanced spinal cord excitability in RLS patients (46).

## POSSIBLE INTERPRETATIONS OF THE EVIDENCE

The relationship between peripheral neuropathies and RLS seems to be complex. RLS and PNP may co-occur as unrelated comorbidity, but they may also be causally associated. Various degrees and directions of causality have been postulated in the literature reviewed above, e.g., RLS as a heralding sign of PNP (13,21), or a general consequence of PNP; specifically PNP triggering RLS or increasing the propensity to develop RLS (4). Moreover, PNP is also an important differential diagnosis to RLS and may create some diagnostic confusion.

In some of the reviewed literature, RLS was not seen as a separate entity and differential diagnosis, but considered to be one of the symptoms of PNP (15,48). Moreover, the fact that RLS and peripheral neuropathies are not only associated, but may also be confounded, is evidenced by results from a study of patients in primary care practice: Among patients who fulfilled all diagnostic criteria for RLS and had discussed their symptoms with their primary chronic polyarthritis physician, only 25% had been given the diagnosis of RLS. However, a diagnosis of neuropathy had been given to a significant fraction (7.7%) of those patients, and a diagnosis of "back/spinal injury or pain" given to 11% (49). It must also be kept in mind that many studies are based on case observations or lack the power to translate their results to general populations. Moreover, some reports stem from the time before criteria for RLS have been established (or simply ignore established criteria). Other studies report only PLM and it is not always clear if RLS has been ruled out rigorously. In addition, the temporal relationship between the onset of RLS and peripheral neuropathy or spinal diagnosis is not always clear. Many do not specify the time of RLS onset in relation to the lesion.

Therefore, all the literature presented here in aggregate does not convincingly make evident that PNP alone can cause RLS, but more likely is a risk factor for RLS, requiring additional pathology to manifest symptoms.

Regarding the involvement of the spinal cord, several studies have suggested that RLS and PLM are generated or at least modulated at the level of the spinal cord. Whether spinal mechanisms are true RLS/PLM generators or just modulating pathways remains to be established. An enhanced excitability at the spinal cord level has been demonstrated in patients with RLS (45) and multiple mechanisms are conceivable to modulate PLM on a spinal basis (50). Only few dopaminergic neurons exist in the spinal cord of humans (50), but per most reports, spinal lesions that seem to precipitate PLMS and RLS respond to dopaminergic medications (51).

Can a sensorimotor integration deficit be assumed as a common pathogenic mechanism for spinal- or peripheral-induced RLS? Several authors suggest that a disorder of sensory input may be involved in the pathogenesis of RLS (12). It has been suggested that small fiber injury may trigger rewiring in the dorsal horn, contributing to the pathophysiology of RLS in neuropathy (4), or a pain-modulated increase in spinal excitability (52). The presence of abnormal findings in functional studies of the sensory symptoms in RLS (52–54) does not necessarily reflect a primary feature of RLS, but might well be a consequence of long-term disorder.

From a clinical point of view, the occurrence of RLS and PLM during and at the end of spinal anesthesia (39,40) point toward a disorder of sensorimotor integration or sensory input to the brain more than a deficit at the peripheral level itself.

Those findings support the theory that spinal lesions may lead to an altered spinal neuronal excitability. It remains to be determined if these lesions are sufficient to induce denovo RLS in any individual or if they can only aggravate or bring to awareness otherwise "subclinical" RLS in susceptible or at-risk individuals.

Therefore, although many textbook contributions and review articles list spinal and peripheral nerve lesions as causes for secondary RLS, the precise relationship is still insufficiently understood.

## REFERENCES

1. Rotta FT, Sussman AT, Bradley WG, et al. The spectrum of chronic inflammatory demyelinating polyneuropathy. J Neurol Sci 2000; 173(2):129–139.
2. Melli G, Marbini A, Gross R, et al. Restless legs syndrome in peripheral neuropathy (abstract). J Peripher Nerv Syst 2001; 6:52.
3. Gorman CA, Dyck PJ, Pearson JS. Symptom of restless legs. Arch Intern Med 1965; 115:155–160.
4. Gemignani F, Marbini A. Restless legs syndrome and peripheral neuropathy. J Neurol Neurosurg Psychiatry 2002; 72:555.
5. Allen RP, Earley CJ. Restless legs syndrome: a review of clinical and pathophysiologic features. J Clin Neurophysiol 2001; 18(2):128–147.
6. Ondo W, Tan EK, Mansoor J. Rheumatologic serologies in secondary restless legs syndrome. Mov Disord 2000; 15(2):321–323.
7. Ondo WG, Romanyshyn J, Vuong K, Lai D. Long-term treatment of restless legs syndrome with dopamine agonists. Arch Neurol 2004; 61:1393–1397.

8. Ondo W, Jankovic J. Restless legs syndrome: clinicoetiologic correlates. Neurology 1996; 47(6):1435–1441.
9. Oboler Sk, Prochazka AV, Meyer TJ. Leg symptoms in outpatient veterans. West J Med 1991; 155(3):256–259.
10. Rutkove SB, Matheson JK, Logigian EL. Restless legs syndrome in patients with polyneuropathy. Muscle Nerve 1996; 19(5):670–672.
11. Thorpy MJ. Classification of sleep disorders. J Clin Neurophysiol 1990; 7(1):67–81.
12. Gemignani F, Marbini A, Di Giovanni G, et al. Charcot-Marie-Tooth disease type 2 with restless legs syndrome. Neurology 1999; 52(3):1064–1066.
13. Salvi F, Montagna P, Plasmati R, et al. Restless legs syndrome and nocturnal myoclonus: initial clinical manifestation of familial amyloid polyneuropathy. J Neurol Neurosurg Psychiatry 1990; 53(6):522–525.
14. Heinze EG Jr, Frame B, Fine G. Restless legs and orthostatic hypotension in primary amyloidosis. Arch Neurol 1967; 16(5):497–500.
15. Finsterer J. Mitochondrial neuropathy. Clin Neurol Neurosurg 2005; 107(3):181–186.
16. Gemignani F, Marbini A, Di Giovanni G, et al. Cryoglobulinaemic neuropathy manifesting with restless legs syndrome. J Neurol Sci 1997; 152(2):218–223.
17. Salih AM, Gray RE, Mills KR, Webley M. A clinical, serological and neurophysiological study of restless legs syndrome in rheumatoid arthritis. Br J Rheumatol 1994; 33(1):60–63.
18. Skomro R, Ludwig S, Salamon E, Kryger MHl. Sleep complaints and restless legs syndrome in adult type 2 diabetics. Sleep Med 2001; 2:417–422.
19. Banno K, Delaive K, Walld R, Kryger MH. Restless legs syndrome in 218 patients: associated disorder. Sleep Med 2000; 1(3):221–229.
20. Högl B, Kiechl S, Willeit J, et al. Restless legs syndrome: a community-based study of prevalence, severity, and risk factors. Neurology 2005; 64(11):1920–1924.
21. Callaghan N. Restless legs syndrome in uremic neuropathy. Neurology 1966; 16(4): 359–361.
22. Thomas PK. Screening for peripheral neuropathy in patients treated by chronic hemodialysis. Muscle Nerve 1978; 1(5):396–399.
23. Bhowmik D, Bhatia M, Tiwari S, et al. Low prevalence of restless legs syndrome in patients with advanced chronic renal failure in the Indian population: a case controlled study. Ren Fail 2004; 26(1):69–72.
24. Winkelmann J, Stautner A, Samtleben W, Trenkwalder C. Long-term course of restless legs syndrome in dialysis patients after kidney transplantation. Mov Disord 2002; 17(5):1072–1076.
25. Harriman DG, Taverner D, Woolf AL. Ekbom's syndrome and burning paraesthesia. A biopsy study by vital staining and electron microscopy of the intramuscular innervation with a note on age changes in motor nerve endings in distal muscles. Brain 1970; 93(2):393–406.
26. Bliwise DL, Ingham RH, Date ES, Dement W. Nerve conduction and creatinine clearance in age subjects with periodic movements in sleep. J Gerontol 1989; 44(5):M164–M167.
27. Iannaccone S, Zucconi M, Marchettini P, et al. Evidence of peripheral axonal neuropathy in primary restless legs syndrome. Mov Disord 1995; 10(1):2–9.
28. Iannaccone S, Quattrini A, Sferrazza B, Ferini-Strambi L. Charcot-Marie-Tooth disease type 2 with restless legs syndrome. Neurology 2000; 54(4):1013–1014.
29. Polydefkis M, Allen RP, Hauer P, et al. Subclinical sensory neuropathy in late-onset restless legs syndrome. Neurology 2000; 55(8):1115–1121.
30. Walters AS, Hickey K, Maltzman J, et al. A questionnaire study of 138 patients with restless legs syndrome: the "Night-Walkers" survey. Neurology 1996; 46(1):92–95.
31. Nogúes M, Cammarota A, Leiguarda R, et al. Periodic limb movements in syringomyelia and syringobulbia. Mov Disord 2000; 15(1):113–119.
32. Winkelmann J, Wetter TC, Trenkwalder C, Auer DP. Periodic limb movements in syringomyelia and syringobulbia. Mov Disord 2000; 15(4):752–753.
33. Glasauer FE, Egnatchick JE. Restless legs syndrome: an unusual cause for a perplexing syndrome. Spinal Cord 1999; 37:862–865.
34. Lee MS, Choi YC, Lee SH, Lee SB. Sleep-related periodic leg movements associated with spinal cord lesions. Mov Disord 1996; 11(6):719–722.

35. Yokota T, Hirose K, Tanabe H, Tsukagoshi H. Sleep-related periodic leg movements (nocturnal myoclonus) due to spinal cord lesion. J Neurol Sci 1991; 104:13–18.
36. Hartmann M, Pfister R, Pfadenhauer K. Restless legs syndrome associated with spinal cord lesions. J Neurol Neurosurg Psychiatry 1999; 66(5):688–689.
37. Hemmer B, Riemann D, Glocker FX, et al. Restless legs syndrome after a borrelia-induced myelitis. Mov Disord 1995; 10(4):521–522.
38. Brown LK, Heffner JE, Obbens EA. Transverse myelitis associated with restless legs syndrome and periodic movements of sleep responsive to an oral dopaminergic agent but not to intrathecal baclofen. Sleep 2000; 23(5):591–594.
39. Högl B, Frauscher B, Seppi K, et al. Transient restless legs syndrome after spinal anesthesia: a prospective study. Neurology 2002; 59(11):1705–1707.
40. Moorthy SS, Dierdorf SF. Restless legs during recovery from spinal anesthesia. Anesth Analg 1990; 70:334–337.
41. Esteves AM, de Mello MT, Lancellotti CL, et al. Occurrence of limb movement during sleep in rats with spinal cord injury. Brain Res 2004; 1017:32–38.
42. Van Kralingen KW, Ivanyi B, van Keimpema AR, et al. Sleep complaints in postpolio syndrome. Arch Phys Med Rehabil 1996; 77(6):609–611.
43. Bruno RL. Abnormal movements in sleep as a post-polio sequelae. Am J Phys Med Rehabil 1998; 77(4):339–343.
44. LaBan MM, Viola SL, Femminineo AF, Taylor RS. Restless legs syndrome associated with diminished cardiopulmonary compliance and lumbar spinal stenosis – a motor concomitant of "Vesper's curse." Arch Phys Med Rehabil 1990; 71(6):384–388.
45. Smith RC. Relationship of periodic movements in sleep (nocturnal myoclonus) and the Babinski sign. Sleep 1985; 8(3):239–243.
46. Bara-Jimenez W, Aksu M, Graham B, et al. Periodic limb movements in sleep: state-dependent excitability of the spinal flexor reflex. Neurology 2000; 54(8):1609–1616.
47. Aksu M, Bara-Jimenez W. State dependent excitability changes of spinal flexor reflex in patients with restless legs syndrome secondary to chronic renal failure. Sleep Med 2002; 3(5):427–430.
48. Muller-Felber W, Landgraf R, Wagner S, et al. Follow-up study of sensory-motor polyneuropathy in type 1 (insulin-dependent) diabetic subjects after simultaneous pancreas and kidney transplantation and after graft rejection. Diabetologia 1991; 34(suppl 1): S113–S117.
49. Hening W, Walters AS, Allen RP, et al. Impact, diagnosis and treatment of restless legs syndrome (RLS) in a primary care population: the REST (RLS epidemiology, symptoms, and treatment) primary care study. Sleep Med 2004; 5(3):237–246.
50. Trenkwalder C, Paulus W. Why do restless legs occur at rest? – pathophysiology of neuronal structures in RLS. Neurophysiology of RLS (part 2). Clin Neurophysiol 2004; 115:1975–1988.
51. de Mello MT, Lauro FA, Silva AC, Tufik S. Incidence of periodic leg movements and of the restless legs syndrome during sleep following acute physical activity in spinal cord injury subjects. Spinal Cord 1996; 34(5):294–296.
52. Stiasny-Kolster K, Magerl W, Oertel WH, et al. Static mechanical hyperalgesia without dynamic tactile allodynia in patients with restless legs syndrome. Brain 2004; 127: 773–782.
53. Happe S, Zeitlhofer J. Abnormal cutaneous thermal threshold in patients with restless legs syndrome. J Neurol 2003; 250(3):362–365.
54. Schattschneider J, Bode A, Wasner G, et al. Idiopathic restless legs syndrome: abnormalities in central somatosensory processing. J. Neurol 2004; 251(8):977–982.

# 20 Restless Legs Syndrome in Pregnancy

**Luigi Ferini-Strambi and Mauro Manconi**

*Department of Neurology, Sleep Disorders Center, University Vita-Salute, IRCCS H San Raffaele, Milan, Italy*

## INTRODUCTION

During pregnancy, changes in sleep pattern and sleep duration are commonly reported, as are sleep complaints associated with the physical changes of the pregnant condition. The physiologic and biochemical changes of pregnancy may place women at risk of developing specific sleep disorders, including obstructive sleep apnea and restless legs syndrome (RLS). Hedman et al. (1) studied sleep habits in women during pregnancy and reported a mean increase in sleep duration of 0.7 hours during the first trimester, compared to the prepregnancy period. Other authors (2) found a mean increase of more than 30 minutes of total nocturnal sleep time at 11 to 12 weeks of gestation in a group of women who underwent in-home polysomnography prior to conception and during each trimester of pregnancy. However, sleep efficiency and the percentage of slow-wave sleep decreased significantly compared to the prepregnancy period (2). In the second trimester (13–24 weeks of gestation), total nocturnal sleep time falls (2). A significant increase in the percentage of slow-wave sleep compared to the first trimester is observed (3); however, sleep complaints increase (4).

During the third trimester, the majority of the women report altered sleep (1,4,5). Decreases in the percentages of the slow-wave sleep (2) and rapid eye movement (REM) sleep (2,3) have been reported. Despite increased waking time after sleep onset and decreased nocturnal sleep time compared to the first two trimesters (2,6), total nocturnal sleep time approximates prepregnancy sleep duration (2). Moreover, the majority of the pregnant women report taking daytime naps (5), which may add more than an hour to the total 24-hour sleep time. Thus, in the third trimester, total sleep time may exceed prepregnancy sleep time (7). Nevertheless, gravid women maintain a clear diurnal rhythm in serum melatonin levels during pregnancy, without evidence of a shift in circadian phase (8). In the last trimester, common etiologies of sleep disturbance include general discomfort (including backache), urinary frequency, and spontaneous awakenings or restless sleep (7). Fetal movement, leg discomfort, fatigue, and difficulty falling asleep or maintaining sleep are also frequently reported (9,10). Interestingly, sedating and hypnotic effects of reproductive hormones have been observed in animal studies and the levels of estrogen and progesterone markedly increase in the third trimester of pregnancy (7). This suggests that the dramatic changes in reproductive hormone levels in the last part of pregnancy could directly cause altered sleep patterns.

Following delivery, the greatest degree of maternal sleep disturbance occurs during the first month (2), with a mean 24-hour total sleep time at 2 weeks postpartum of less than 6 hours, including more than 1 hour of nap-time (11). Total maternal sleep time and sleep efficiency increase gradually as the infant's circadian rhythm matures, with a transition from interrupted to uninterrupted sleep usually occurring approximately at the 12th postpartum week (12).

Concerning specific sleep disorders, RLS related to pregnancy was probably the first of the secondary RLS forms to be described. Mussio-Fournier and Rawak (13) first reported this new and strange association because of the presence of "pruritus, urticaria, and paresthesias" of the lower limbs appearing during rest in three subjects of the same family: a member of that family referred to a characteristic aggravation of RLS symptoms during pregnancy. Since then, higher rates of RLS during pregnancy have been well-documented.

## EPIDEMIOLOGY

In 1945, Ekbom performed the first structured epidemiological study on this topic, finding a prevalence of RLS of 11.3% among 486 pregnant women (14). Several years later, Jolivet, as documented on his degree thesis in medicine, reviewing a population of 100 pregnant women, observed 27 cases of RLS (15). The same topic was further investigated by several other epidemiological studies (Table 1), which found RLS prevalence during pregnancy ranging from 11% to 27% (14–19). The high variability of these rates could be explained by several factors: standard diagnostic criteria for the RLS were used in only one study; the diagnosis was assessed either by self-administered questionnaire or by face-to-face medical interview; often the authors neglected to specify the minimal threshold of frequency of occurrence of symptoms; studies have been performed in different geographic areas and on different racial populations; and the prevalence may be influenced by the time of pregnancy in which the survey has been assessed.

In a large cross-sectional study of approximately 16,000 pregnant women in Japan, Suzuki et al. (18) observed a significant relationship between RLS and the duration of pregnancy, with 15% of the patients reporting RLS symptoms at 3 to 4 months of gestation, which increased to 23% at term. Furthermore, women with RLS reported significantly lower average sleep time, more difficulty in initiating and maintaining sleep, more early morning awakenings, and more excessive daytime somnolence than did women without RLS. In multiple regression analysis, risk factors for RLS included primiparity, duration of pregnancy, less than 7 hours of sleep, absence of daytime napping, current employment, smoking, and the use of medication or alcohol.

Suzuki et al. estimated the prevalence using a self-administered questionnaire in which the RLS was explored only by this question: "Is your sleep interrupted by a sensation of insects running across the skin or hot flashes inside your legs after you go to bed at night?" This question alone, however, does not adequately diagnose RLS (20).

**TABLE 1** Frequency of Restless Legs Syndrome During Pregnancy

| Authors | No. of cases | Prevalence (%) |
|---|---|---|
| Ekbom | 486 | 11.3 |
| Jolivet | 100 | 27.0 |
| Ekbom | 202 | 12.4 |
| Goodman et al. | 500 | 19 |
| Suzuki et al. | 16.528 | 19.9 |
| Manconi et al. | 606 | 26.6 |

When the prevalence rate is ascertained by applying the standard diagnostic criteria through a structured medical interview on a wide and homogenous population of women throughout the entire pregnancy course, Manconi et al. found a 26% prevalence (19). This percentage included either subjects who were already affected by RLS before the pregnancy, or subjects who experienced RLS for the first time during pregnancy. These pregnancy onset cases, in the study of Manconi et al. (19), represent the majority, while the percentage of women affected by a preexisting RLS ranges between 5% and 10%. The higher prevalence of RLS during pregnancy compared to the general female population and, overall, the close temporal relationship between the symptoms' occurrence and the pregnancy time, are the two fundamental findings that argue to include this particular RLS among the secondary/symptomatic forms. However, the term "symptomatic" seems not completely appropriate because pregnancy is a physiological and not a pathological condition. Pregnancy induces RLS only in a minority of women. Therefore, it would be more correct to consider pregnancy as a strong risk factor for RLS, able to increase the probability of disease by approximately two to four times, similar to the way that obesity is a risk factor for arterial hypertension.

## CLINICAL COURSE

The prevalence of RLS is not uniform during pregnancy. It increases progressively starting from the third to fourth month of gestation and reaches a peak during the third trimester, especially at the eighth month, in which the highest rate is observed. After that it rapidly declines during the ninth month and resolves shortly after delivery. No exacerbations generally occur during the puerperium, when the prevalence returns to prepregnancy values. Figure 1 shows the results of a study in a large sample of subjects throughout the pregnancy course (19). In women not previously affected by RLS, the mean duration of RLS symptoms during pregnancy usually is about 3 to 5 months. No data are actually available about long-term followup, and it is unknown if the appearance of the symptoms during the period of pregnancy may be a risk factor for RLS in the future. One epidemiologic study in Germany reported that multiparity was a risk factor for later life RLS, but prospective trials have not been done (20).

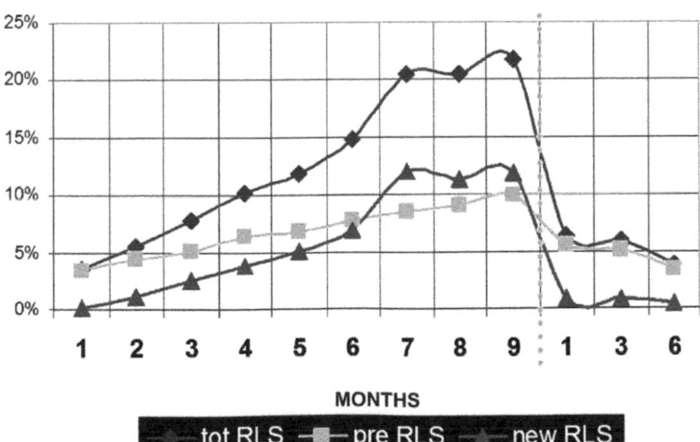


**FIGURE 1** Restless legs syndrome (RLS) course. Percentage of women affected by RLS from preconception to six months after delivery.

The intensity and the frequency of occurrence of the symptoms seem to follow the same trend of the prevalence, characterized by a significant worsening at the third trimester, both in the women already affected by the disease before pregnancy, and in women with symptoms for the first time.

Multipara women often complain of the same symptomatology during all of their pregnancies (17,19). The main features of the RLS during pregnancy such as the quality of symptoms, the anatomic distribution, the circadianity and the motor activity for relieving the disturbance, are similar to those of the idiopathic form (19). Familiar RLS history is a common finding, especially for women affected by a preexisting form of RLS.

The consequences of the symptoms on the sleep of pregnant women are usually not dramatic. Compared to unaffected pregnant subjects, women who experience RLS in pregnancy may refer higher sleep latency, excessive daytime sleepiness, lower total sleep time, and more frequently insomnia (19). In a minority of the cases, the symptoms became very disagreeable, making evening relaxation and sleep onset very difficult (21).

It is also difficult to evaluate the real impact of the RLS "per se" on sleep because the pregnancy itself is a condition that induces insomnia, particularly during the third trimester when nocturia, fetal movements, gastroesophageal reflux, snoring, sleep apneas, forced alteration in bed body position, and anxiety for the delivery, may all impair the sleep quality (22).

The polysomnographic pattern of RLS in pregnant women has never been systematically studied; however, periodic leg movements during pregnancy have been described (23). Although periodic limb movement of sleep (PLMS) are common in individuals with RLS (24), whether PLMS contribute significantly to sleep disruption during pregnancy were assessed is just beginning to be studied. When a series of 10 multiparus women in the third trimester of pregnancy, were assessed PLMS was present in all subjects, with a frequency of 21.7 events per hour (23). In this study, only four subjects reported symptoms of RLS associated with the pregnancy, suggesting that PLMS may be present even in the absence of RLS; however, the authors did not report the frequency of arousals due to PLMS (23).

## ETIOPATHOGENETIC HYPOTHESES

The temporal relationship between the RLS symptoms and the third trimester of pregnancy suggests that during this period some pregnancy-related factors could cause or exacerbate the RLS. How and which pregnancy-related factors could induce the RLS is still not entirely clear. Culpable factors could be present only in the women who develop RLS during pregnancy (~25%) but absent in the rest of the women, or they could involve all women, being correlated in general to the pregnant condition itself, but inducing RLS only in the women predisposed to the syndrome. The first hypothesis is less sustainable because if this possible pathogenetic process involved only approximately one-quarter of the women, we would expect that it involved similarly about one-quarter of the women already affected by RLS before the pregnancy, causing a worsening of the symptoms in them. In truth, a great majority of women with preexisting RLS, not just 25%, report a worsening of symptoms during late pregnancy. Therefore, a more plausible pathogenetic model posits that one or more unknown factors linked generally to the pregnant condition reduce the RLS symptomatic threshold during late pregnancy in all women, provoking the RLS only in subjects with preexisting low symptomatic threshold. In other words, the presence and the duration of RLS would depend mainly on the individual predisposition to the symptomatic threshold. A woman without a predisposition to RLS moves closer to the symptomatic threshold during pregnancy, but without reaching it she never will experience RLS during the pregnancy.

The nature of these hypothetical risk factors has not yet been identified. Some studies support the hypothesis that RLS in pregnant women may be caused by an iron or folate deficiency (25,26). Iron and folate deficiency are well-known conditions correlated with RLS (27). Plasma iron and folate levels could easily decrease in pregnant women, particularly during the second half of pregnancy (28). In a recent study (19), the dose and duration of supplemental iron and folate therapy have been evaluated: no difference was found between women with and without RLS. The same study, however, reported a significant difference in plasma iron storage indicators during pregnancy found between normal and affected women, supporting the hypothesis that a relative iron deficit could have an etiopathogenetic burden in RLS. It should be noted that the accuracy of serum ferritin in assessing iron stores during pregnancy is unclear. Because iron supplementation failed to prevent RLS symptoms, it could be hypothesized that (i) women who became symptomatic during pregnancy could have a lower iron storage already before pregnancy, and the supplementation therapy is not sufficient to prevent the symptoms (26); (ii) a possible defective oral iron absorption in RLS patients could explain past failed attempts to improve RLS by supplemental iron therapy (29); and (iii) there is evidence that RLS patients could have normal serum iron storage indicators, but low cerebrospinal fluid concentrations of ferritin and transferrin (30,31). Contrary to the iron theory is the fact that the majority of RLS women have a remission of symptoms around the delivery, with the largest loss of blood and iron (at least 3 months are needed to recover this loss) (28).

The trend of RLS prevalence and of the symptom severity throughout the pregnancy is quite similar to that of the main sexual hormones. In fact estrogen, progesterone, and prolactin rise throughout pregnancy and peak in the third trimester of pregnancy, falling rapidly after delivery, except for the prolactin that continues to assume a pulsatile secretion. This likeness suggested a possible hormonal influence in RLS appearance. Because dopamine strongly inhibits hypothalamic secretion of the prolactin releasing factor, it could be possible that increased prolactin during pregnancy is associated with reduced dopamine levels, thus lowering the RLS symptomatic threshold (19,32). On the other hand, it has been demonstrated that the estrogens exert an antidopaminergic effect at the basal ganglia, and they increase animal behavior motor activity (32–35). One study observed elevated estradiol in pregnant women with RLS, compared to those without RLS, which resolved shortly after delivery (36). Furthermore, the excitability of several nervous centers may be raised by progesterone: increased respiratory center sensitivity to $CO_2$ and common hyperreflexia are observed during late pregnancy (37).

Several other postulated but less likely mechanisms include the possibilities that the growing fetus size creates a mechanical strain on the mother's nerve roots that recover upon delivery, the reduction in the mother's normal motor activity (more sedentary), and the general increased stress of the late pregnancy. The etiology of RLS in pregnancy may also be multifactorial.

## TREATMENT

The majority of pregnant women who present with RLS to their physician are worried about the unusualness and strangeness of the symptoms, and about the possible consequences on the outcome of the pregnancy and, in general, on the fetus' well-being. The first medical therapeutic approach should be the reassurance of the women on the benign nature of the symptoms and on their probable disappearance at the end of the pregnancy, with no effects on the development and health state of the fetus (19).

Although folate supplementation specifically for pregnancy-associated RLS has been reported in only one small preventative trial (25), oral folate is widely recommended during the periconception and early pregnancy period for the prevention of fetal neural tube defects. Iron supplementation of 30 to 60 mg per day throughout the second and third trimesters of pregnancy is also recommended (38). As symptoms of RLS become more common over the course of pregnancy, a trial of folate supplementation and evaluation for iron deficiency with a serum ferritin level is a reasonable approach in pregnant women who develop RLS.

Conservative treatments such as walking, stretching, massaging the affected limbs, applying heat, and performing relaxation techniques, may also be helpful. Abstinence from tobacco and alcohol should be reinforced, and adequate time should be set aside for sleep because these may be risk factors for RLS in pregnant women (18). For women with severe symptoms who continue to experience clinically significant sleep disruption, consideration may be given to standard pharmacologic therapies for idiopathic RLS, such as dopaminergic, opiate, and benzodiazepine medications. However, there are no controlled clinical trials upon which to base treatment recommendations.

McParland and Pearce reported two severe cases of RLS in pregnancies, which were successfully treated by carbamazepine after there was no improvement by benzodiazepines (temazepam and diazepam) and phenobarbitol (21). Low evening doses (0.5 mg) of clonazepam could improve RLS symptoms (39). However, current consensus discourages use of benzodiazepines during pregnancy (40).

For short-term use, oxycodone and pergolide are currently classified as Class B in pregnancy according to the Food and Drug Administration (Class B = animal studies have failed to demonstrate fetal risk, and no adequate studies in pregnant women exist or animal studies have shown adverse fetal effects, but studies in pregnant women have failed to demonstrate risks for the fetus. Possibility of fetal harm is remote). Gabapentin, pramipexole, and ropinirole have been classified as Class C (Class C = animal studies have shown adverse fetal effects, and no adequate studies in humans exist. Benefits from the use of the drug may be acceptable despite potential risk).

Some days after delivery, the majority of patients with pregnancy-associated RLS report symptom resolution (17,18). In a few women, symptoms may persist beyond the month following delivery (17). These cases can be managed using standard therapies, although consideration should be given to the excretion of opioids, benzodiazepines, and anticonvulsant medications in breast milk and to the possibility that lactation may be diminished by the use of dopaminergic medications, because of their inhibition of prolactin secretion via D2 receptor agonism.

Because there is currently inadequate information on the management of RLS in pregnant subjects (41), the pharmacological treatment would be used only during the third trimester, and at the lowest efficacious dosage. Interestingly, a recent prospective study in a group of women in their ninth month of pregnancy tested the hypothesis that sleep disturbance in late pregnancy is associated with labor duration and delivery type (42). Objective (48-hour wrist actigraphy) and subjective (sleep logs and questionnaires) measures were used to predict labor outcomes. Controlling for infant birth weight, women who slept less than 6 hours at night had longer labors and were 4.5 times more likely to have cesarean deliveries. Women with severely disrupted sleep had longer labors and were 5.2 times more likely to have cesarean deliveries. The authors suggested that health care providers should prescribe 8 hours of bed time during pregnancy to assure adequate sleep (42). Thus, RLS should be recognized by physicians taking care of pregnant patients as a frequent condition of sleep disruption.

## REFERENCES

1. Hedman C, Pohjasvara T, Tolonen U, et al. Effects of pregnancy on mother's sleep. Sleep Med 2002; 3:37–42.
2. Lee KA, Zaffke ME, McEnany G. Parity and sleep patterns during and after pregnancy. Obstet Gynecol 2000; 95:14–18.
3. Driver HS, Shapiro CM. A longitudinal study of sleep stages in young women during pregnancy and postpartum. Sleep 1992; 15:449–453.
4. Schweiger MS. Sleep disturbance in pregnancy. A subjective survey. Am J Obstet Gynecol 1972; 114:879–882.
5. Mindell JA, Jacobson BJ. Sleep disturbances during pregnancy. J Obstet Gynecol Neonat Nurs 2000; 29:590–597.
6. Brunner DP, Munch M, Briedermann K, et al. Changes in sleep and sleep electroencephalogram during pregnancy. Sleep 1994; 17:576–582.
7. Pien GW, Schwab RJ. Sleep disorders during pregnancy. Sleep 2004; 27(7):1405–1417.
8. Kivela A. Serum melatonin during human pregnancy. Acta Endocrinol 1991; 124:233–237.
9. Lee KA, De Joseph JF. Sleep disturbances, vitality and fatigue among a select group of employed childbearing women. Birth 1992; 19:208–213.
10. Baratte-Beebe KR, Lee K. Sources of midsleep awakenings in childbearing women. Clin Nurs Res 1999; 8:386–397.
11. Shinkoda H, Matsumoto K, Park YM. Changes in sleep-wake cycle during the period from late pregnancy to puerperium identified through the wrist actigraph and sleep logs. Psychiatry Clin Neurosci 1999; 53:133–135.
12. Horiuchi S, Nishihara K. Analyses of mothers' sleep logs in post-partum periods. Psychiatry Clin Neurosci 1999; 8:386–397.
13. Mussio-Fournier JD, Rawak F. Familiäres auftreten von pruritus, urtikaria und parästhetischer hyperkinese der unteren extremitäten. Confin Neurol 1940; 3:110–114.
14. Ekbom KA. Restless legs syndrome. Acta Med Scand 1945; 158(suppl):4–22.
15. Jolivet B. Paresthésies agitantes nocturnes des membres inférieurs, impatiences. Thése de Paris, 1953.
16. Ekbom K. Akroparestesier och restless legs under graviditet. Lakartidningen 1960; 57:2597–2603.
17. Goodman JDS, Brodie C, Ayida GA. Restless leg syndrome in pregnancy. BMJ 1988; 297:1101–1112.
18. Suzuki K, Ohida T, Sone T, et al. The prevalence of restless legs syndrome among pregnant women in Japan and relationship between restless legs syndrome and sleep problems. Sleep 2003; 26(6):673–677.
19. Manconi M, Govoni V, De Vito A, et al. Restless legs syndrome and pregnancy. Neurology 2004; 63:1065–1069.
20. Berger K, Luedemann J, Trenkwalder C, John U, Kessler C. Sex and the risk of restless legs syndrome in the general population. Arch Intern Med 2004; 164:196–202.
21. McPharland P, Pearce JM. Restless legs syndrome in pregnancy. Case reports. Clin Exp Obstet Gynecol 1990; 17(1):5–6.

22. Santiago JR, Nolledo MS, Kinzler W, Santiago TV. Sleep and sleep disorders in pregnancy. Ann Intern Med 2001; 134:396–408.
23. Nikkola E, Ekblad U, Ekholm E, Mikola H, Polo O. Sleep in multiple pregnancy: breathing patterns, oxygenation, and periodic leg movements. Am J Obstet Gynecol 1996; 174:1622–1625.
24. Allen RP, Earlui CJ. Restless legs syndrome: A review of clinical and pathophysiologic futures. J Clin Neurophysiol 2001; 18:128–147.
25. Boetz MI, Lambert B. Folate deficiency and restless legs syndrome in pregnancy. N Engl J Med 1977; 297:670.
26. Lee KA, Zaffke ME, Baratte-Beebe K. Restless legs syndrome and sleep disturbance during pregnancy: the role of folate and iron. J Women's Health Gen Med 2001; 10:335–341.
27. O'Keeffe ST, Gavin K, Lavan JN. Iron status and restless legs syndrome in the elderly. Age Ageing 1994; 23:200.
28. Puolakka J, Jänne O, Pakarinen A, et al. Serum ferritin as a measure of iron stores during and after normal pregnancy with and without iron supplements. Acta Obstet Gynecol Scand 1980; 95(suppl):43–51.
29. Davis BJ, Rajput A, Rajput ML, Aul EA, Eichhorn GR. A randomized, double-blind placebo-controlled trial of iron in restless legs syndrome. Eur Neurol 2000; 43:70–75.
30. Earley CJ, Connor JR, Beard JL, Malecki EA, Epstein DK, Allen RP. Abnormalities in CSF concentrations of ferritin and transferrin in restless legs syndrome. Neurology 2000; 54:1698–1700.
31. Sun ER, Chen CA, Ho G, Earley CJ, Allen RP. Iron and restless legs syndrome. Sleep 1998; 21:371.
32. Wetter TC, Collado-Seidel V, Oertel H, et al. Endocrine rhythms in patients with restless legs syndrome. J Neurol 2002; 249:146–151.
33. Euvrard C, Oberlander C, Boissier JR. Antidopaminergic effect of estrogens at the striatal level. J Pharmacol Exp Ther 1980; 214(1):179–185.
34. Ogawa S, Chan J, Gustafsson JA, Korach KS, Pfaff DW. Estrogen increases locomotor activity in mice through estrogen receptor alpha: specificity for the type of activity. Endocrinology 2003; 144(1):230–239.
35. Morgan MA, Pfaff DW. Estrogen's effects on activity, anxiety and fear in two mouse strains. Behav Brain Res 2002; 132(1):85–93.
36. Fulda S, Dzaja A, Lancel M, et al. Sleep and periodic leg movements in late term pregnancy and postpartum in women with and without RLS. J Sleep Res 2004; 13:(suppl 1):252.
37. Roberts JM. Pregnancy related hypertension. In: Creasy RK, Resnik R, eds. Maternal-Fetal Medicine: Principle and Practice. 2nd ed. Philadelphia: Saunders, 1989:783–808.
38. Haram K, Nilsen ST, Ulvik RJ. Iron supplementation in pregnancy–evidence and controversies. Acta Obstet Gynecol Scand 2001; 80:683–688.
39. Manconi M, Govoni V, De Vito A, et al. Pregnancy as a risk factor for restless legs syndrome. Sleep Med 2004; 5:305–308.
40. Briggs GG, Freeman RK, Yaffe SJ. Drugs in pregnancy and lactation. 5th ed. Baltimore: Williams and Wilkings, 1998.
41. Early CJ. Clinical practice. Restless legs syndrome. N Engl J Med 2003; 348:2103–2109.
42. Lee KA, Gay CL. Sleep in late pregnancy predicts length of labor and type of delivery. Am J Obstet Gynecol 2004; 191(6):2041–2046.

# 21 Restless Legs Syndrome and Parkinson's Disease

**Vandana Dhawan**

*Regional Movement Disorders Unit, King's College Hospital, University Hospital Lewisham, London, U.K.*

**K. Ray Chaudhuri**

*Regional Movement Disorders Unit, National Parkinson Foundation Centre of Excellence, Department of Neurology, King's College Hospital, Denmark Hill, and University Hospital Lewisham, and Guy's, King's, and St. Thomas' School of Biomedical Medicine, London, U.K.*

## BACKGROUND

Parkinson's disease (PD) is a common neurodegenerative disorder characterized by an underlying dopaminergic deficiency principally affecting the nigrostriatal system that is responsive to dopaminergic treatment. Restless legs syndrome (RLS) also consistently and reproducibly responds to dopaminergic treatment albeit at much lower doses of the dopaminergic drugs compared to doses administered in PD (1–5). This observation and also the fact that symptoms resembling RLS can occur as a nonmotor manifestation of PD, have strengthened the hypothesis that there is likely to be a link between PD and RLS (6–8). In more recent reports, RLS has also been cited as a possible marker for the preclinical stage of PD based on cases where RLS has preceded development of PD (9). Few studies have systematically addressed the issue of RLS occurring in PD in a prospective case-control manner. This issue is compounded by the fact that RLS is often treated by dopaminergic drugs, and some symptoms of RLS may resemble some symptoms seen in PD, especially akathisia and wearing-off dystonia (9).

## PATHOPHYSIOLOGY

The precise underlying pathology of RLS or periodic limb movements of sleep (PLMS) is unknown, although recent evidence suggests a complex interplay between the dopaminergic, opioid, and iron regulatory systems within the brain (10–12). In RLS, dysfunction of the central dopaminergic system due to cellular loss in the mesocorticolimbic dopamine systems could be indirectly implicated by the beneficial effects of various dopaminergic agents in the treatment of RLS (13). However, striatal deafferentation due to nigral dopaminergic cell loss that characterizes PD has not been noted in RLS, at least in some very preliminary neuropathological reports (14–16). In fact, RLS brains tend to demonstrate modestly more nigral dopaminergic cells than normal controls (Conner, personal communication). In PD, cell loss, both dopaminergic and nondopaminergic, has been linked to sleep disruption, which is also a key symptom of RLS. Evidence favors the hypothesis that the mesocorticolimbic dopamine pathways are involved in some aspects of the sleep–wake cycles in PD, while dysfunction within the diencephalospinal dopaminergic system may result in the sensorimotor syndrome that characterizes RLS (13).

Functional imaging can be used to investigate central dopamine and other receptor status in an effort to understand the link between RLS and PD, but reports on RLS have been conflicting and generally inconclusive. Eisenhsehr et al. (17) showed no differences in presynaptic (dopamine transporter) or postsynaptic ($^{123}$I-IBZM) $D_2$ receptor binding in patients with RLS. However, an intermittent decreased dopamine turnover with relatively normal intrasynaptic dopamine levels or dysfunction of alternative dopamine-dependent pathways such as the diencephalospinal pathways or orexin (hypocretin) neuropeptide-related neuronal dysfunction causing symptoms of RLS cannot be excluded (13). Orexin pathways project to the substantia nigra and also to the pedunculopontine nucleus (18). In another study, Linke et al. studied the striatal dopamine transporter with (123) I IPT (a tropane ligand) using single photon emission tomography (SPECT) in 28 RLS, 29 early PD patients, and 23 age-matched controls. They reported no difference in IPT binding between RLS and controls (19). This study, therefore, further disputes the link between RLS and PD based on nigrostriatal presynaptic dopaminergic dysfunction. A recent study by Mrowka et al. investigated RLS patients and controls using a three-dimensional ultrasound-based movement analysis before and after a levodopa test dose and [2 beta-carbomethoxy-3 beta-(4-iodophenyl) tropaine (beta-CIT)]-SPECT scans (20). No significant change in movement analysis in response to levodopa or signals in caudate or putamen were observed. However, a slight but significant change in the relative $^{123}$I-beta-CIT SPECT in putamen versus the caudate nucleus was observed with lower quotient of ratios in RLS. The clinical significance of this is unclear. Schmidaeur and colleagues showed reduced midbrain echogenecity suggesting reduced iron (20a) using transcranial Doppler ultrasound sonography in RLS patients compared to controls and PD. Therefore, overall there is no good evidence to suggest that PD and RLS have similar pathology.

PLMS and periodic limb movements of wakefulness also accompany RLS and are likely to have a dopaminergic basis. It has been suggested that PLMS arise from a loss of supraspinal inhibitory impulses resulting in enhanced spinal flexor reflex facilitation. Spinal flexor reflexes appear to be under partial dopaminergic control (21). Arnulf et al. have suggested that routine polysomnography evaluation in PD would unmask PLM in 15% of cases, and increased PLM index has also been reported in untreated PD patients (22). In Parkinsonian animal models of both rats and nonhuman primates with bilateral striatal dopamine depletion, excessive nocturnal movements resembling PLM are seen (23,24). PLM and rapid eye movement (REM) sleep-related atonia may be mediated via the indirect circuits that link the basal ganglia outflow with the pedunculopontine nucleus and the pontomedullary reticulospinal pathways, so this may be modulated by dopamine (18,23,24). Spinal dopamine receptors also may be involved as has been suggested from animal studies (25,26).

An association of PD and RLS has also been noted in a large family underlining the possible role of Parkin gene (27). This family (family LA) with RLS, when tested for Parkin gene mutation, showed Parkin mutation in 8 out of 17 patients, some of whom developed signs of PD. Spinocerebellar ataxia (SCA), caused by unstable mutations in the form of expanding trinucleotide repeat sequences, leads to Parkinsonism in some cases. Schols et al. reported that RLS was present in 45% of SCA3 patients but was rare in other types of autosomal dominant cerebellar ataxias; RLS is a frequent and treatable cause of disabling sleep disturbance in SCA3 (28,29). This study provides evidence that the expanded cytosine-adenine-guanine (CAG) repeat in the SCA3 gene is a molecular factor causing both RLS and PD. The prevalence of RLS occurring in other mediated forms of Parkinsonism needs to be investigated further. Poewe and Hogl (2004) recently opined that the similarities in treatment response between PD and RLS would suggest a common dopaminergic basis underlying both conditions. However, the ascertainment of RLS in PD is complicated by the methodological problem of clinical assessments of true RLS in PD as "wearing off"-related lower limb discomfort and restlessness, and akathisia may overlap (30).

## CLINICAL SURVEYS

In 1987, Lang and Johnson examined 100 consecutive PD patients for RLS although the international restless legs syndrome study group (IRLSSG) criteria were not used (31). They reported no patients who had RLS, although two patients reported an inability to remain quiet in the evening or at night, which was suggestive of akathisia (Table 1).

Ondo et al. were the first to formally report the association of RLS and PD based on an observational study (32). In this study, they interviewed and examined 303 consecutive PD patients specifically for symptoms of RLS and additionally used measures of daytime sleepiness [the Epworth Sleepiness Scale (ESS)]. Sixty-three (20.8%) had symptoms of RLS, a substantially higher rate than that seen in the general population. The authors specifically differentiated RLS from general akathisia and nocturnal dystonia, but the diagnosis of RLS was still difficult to make at times and was often ephemeral. Patients seldom considered it apart from their other PD symptoms. The presence of RLS was not related to the demographics of the PD patients and treatment was not received. Lower serum ferritin levels, however, were significantly associated with RLS symptoms in PD patients. In 68% of PD-RLS patients, the PD symptoms preceded the RLS symptoms, and the PD-RLS patients were older than a control group of idiopathic RLS patients and were much less likely to have a family history of RLS. In those PD-RLS patients, where the RLS clearly preceded PD, most had a family history of RLS. The authors did not feel that this population of patients with early onset RLS, who later developed PD, was different than what would be seen by chance occurrence alone.

Simuni et al. reported similar results in their evaluation of 200 patients presenting to a movement disorders clinic with PD (33). Overall, 42 patients (21%) met diagnostic criteria for RLS. Only three of these reported RLS symptoms prior to the onset of their PD, so the authors concluded that RLS does not evolve into PD.

In a case controlled study based on PD patients attending a movement disorders clinic in a regional centre in Delhi, India, Krishnan et al. explored the prevalence of RLS in PD using a structured questionnaire (34). About 126 consecutive PD patients and 128 age- and sex-matched controls were studied, and RLS was present in 10 (7.9%) of cases. This lower rate of RLS in PD, compared to that reported by Ondo et al., needs to be considered in light of the fact that the rate of RLS in the control population studied by Krishnan et al. was extremely low (0.8%, 1 out of 128) (32,34).

Recently, Nomura et al. addressed the clinical significance of RLS occurring in PD in 165 PD cases and 131 age and sex matched controls in a Japanese population (34a). Prevalence of RLS was significantly higher in PD compared to controls (12% vs. 2.3% respectively) with a high Pittsburgh sleep of 0.1 index being registered in PD patients.

**TABLE 1** Reports Examining the Occurrence of Restless Legs Syndrome (RLS) in PD Patients and Extrapyramidal Symptoms in RLS Patients

| Authors | Year | Type of study | Conclusions |
|---|---|---|---|
| Lang and Johnson | 1987 | 100 PD pts, observational | No RLS, 2 reported akathisia |
| Ondo et al. | 2002 | 303 PD pts, observational | 63 (20.8%) had RLS (satisfied IRLSSG criteria) |
| Krishnan et al. | 2003 | 126 PD pts and 128 controls, observational | 10 (7.9%) of PD pts had RLS; 1 (0.8%) of controls had RLS |
| Tan et al. | 2001 | 125 PD pts, observational | 19 (15.2%) had motor restlessness; 1 (0.8%) had RLS |
| Banno et al. | 2000 | 218 RLS pts, observational | 40 (40%) of pts had extrapyramidal dysfunction; 0.2% of controls had extrapyramidal function |
| Chaudhuri et al. | 2004 | 406 PD pts, observational | 18% of PD (>75 yrs) pts had RLS |
| Rye and Delong | 1999 | 1 PD pt underwent posteromedial pallidotomy for control of PD symptoms | Improvement in RLS symptoms |
| Kedia et al. | 2004 | 195 PD pts underwent STN DBS | 11 pts reported RLS postoperatively |
| Linke et al. | 2004 | 28 RLS pts; 29 early PD pts; 23 controls; all had $^{123}$I IPT SPECT study for striatal dopamine transporter | No significant difference reported in IPT binding between RLS and controls |
| Mrowka M et al. | 2005 | 10 RLS pts had 3-D computerized ultrasound-based movement analysis; 6 pts of these also had (123)I]beta-CIT-SPECT scan | No difference between patients and controls regarding beta-CIT-signals in putamen or caudate nucleus |
| Ratnagopal and Tan | 2005 | 200 PD pts, observational | 1 (0.05%) pt. had RLS; 23 (11.5%) had motor restlessness |
| Lüssi et al. | 2005 | 113 PD pts, observational | 28 (24%) pts had RLS |
| Nomura et al. | 2006 | 165 PD pts, 131 controls | 12% PD had RLS vs. 2.3% controls |

*Abbreviations*: PD, Parkinson's disease; STN, subthalamic nucleus; IRLSSG, International Restless Legs Syndrome Study Group; DBS,; CIT-SPECT, carbomethoxy-3 beta-(4-iodophenyl) tropaine–single photon emission tomography.

Few studies have explored the prevalence of RLS in non-White populations. In a door-to-door response survey–based study, Tan et al. reported a very low rate of RLS in residents of Singapore (0.6 for general population and 0.1% for clinic population) (35). In a further study, they evaluated 125 consecutive PD patients using the IRLSSG diagnostic criteria for RLS (36). None of the patients satisfied the IRLSSG criteria for diagnosis of RLS in keeping the extremely low figures for prevalence of RLS in this population (0.6% and 0.1%). One patient (0.8%) had wearing off–related RLS-like symptoms. In a more recent study, Ratnagopal and Tan found a very low rate of occurrence of RLS by administering IRLSSG questionnaire and ESS on 200 consecutive PD patients (37). One patient (0.5%) had RLS, and 23 (11.5%) patients had motor restlessness. These patients with motor restlessness had a higher propensity for hypersomnolence (37).

Both Mrowka et al. and Banno et al. have examined RLS patients for extrapyramidal signs (20,38). Banno et al. found extrapyramidal dysfunction in 17% of men and 23% of women, out of a total of 218 RLS patients, while a corresponding prevalence in the control (nonRLS) population was 0.2%.

In a nationwide audit-based multicenter study addressing quality of life changes in PD, the IRLSSG questionnaire was also administered to a subset of PD patients by Chaudhuri et al. (39). In older PD patients (above 75 years age), the rate of RLS was 18%, comparing favorably with the figure quoted by Ondo et al. A syndrome resembling RLS but not necessarily satisfying the IRLSSG criteria for RLS, the syndrome of "nocturnal restlessness" has also been reported in PD in a survey using the newly developed PD Sleep Scale (7). This may also represent nocturnal akathisia. In another study, using a novel nonmotor symptom questionnaire, symptoms resembling RLS were quoted in a significantly higher number of unselected PD patients across all stages of disease severity compared to an age-matched control group (9).

Lüssi et al. reported a twofold increase on the reported local prevalence of RLS in their prospective survey on 113 PD patients (40). Twenty-eight (24%) of the patients satisfied the IRLSSG criteria [classified as PD/RLS (+)]. Members of the PD/RLS (+) group were younger than PD/RLS (−) group (63 vs. 69 years, $p=0.004$) and had a similar duration of PD (8.8 vs. 9.5 years, $p=0.57$). RLS preceded the onset of PD in only 5 of 27 cases. About 61% of PD/RLS (−) patients reported an urgency to move legs or unpleasant sensations related to wearing-off periods, raising the possibility of RLS phenocopies in fluctuating PD patients. This study supports the observation made by Ondo and colleagues, although the occurrence of RLS was more prevalent in younger people and even a lower number of patients had RLS preceding symptoms of PD.

A complex and debated relationship exists between essential tremor and PD. In a recent study conducted on 100 consecutive patients presenting with essential tremor, Ondo ascertained a high rate of undiagnosed RLS, 33% (Chapter 23). Unlike most other "secondary" forms of RLS, this was associated with a high familial presence of RLS (58%), suggesting that they share some genetic similarities (41).

Further evidence of association of RLS and PD comes from a few case report–based observations. Rye and Delong reported the amelioration of symptoms of RLS in a limb of a patient with dyskinetic PD, who underwent posteromedial pallidotomy for control of PD symptoms (42). In some PD patients, PLM, closely associated with RLS, may be virtually eliminated by pallidotomy (43,44). However, others have noted contradictory effects. Kedia et al. have reported the appearance of RLS following subthalamic nucleus (STN) stimulation in PD (45). In 11 out of 195 patients undergoing STN stimulation, symptoms of RLS became evident when the antiparkinsonian medication was reduced. In contrast, others have reported improvement of RLS following STN stimulation (45a).

## CONCLUSIONS

The issue of the association of PD and RLS remains unclear and somewhat perplexing in spite of considerable efforts to identify a link between the two. The beneficial effect of dopaminergic treatment for both RLS and PD and the fluctuation of responses to treatment is the strongest link that provides evidence of a link between RLS and PD, while imaging studies provide controversial evidence. The central nervous system (CNS) pathology of the two diseases is quite distinct and, in some measures, opposite. RLS has reduced CNS iron and possibly greater dopamine cell counts, whereas PD has increased CNS iron and markedly reduced dopamine cell counts. There is clearly more than a single pathology associated with PD, and likely will be multiple etiologies and pathologies of RLS, which is only currently diagnosed by clinical criteria. At present there appears to be little or no real risk of RLS being a predictive marker for the subsequent development of PD, a fear that affects many patients with RLS. However, clinical observations in a few studies do suggest that RLS, as currently defined, does occur in PD at a rate considerably higher than that quoted for the healthy Caucasian population. Further large-scale, population-based studies addressing the issue of RLS in PD and longitudinal natural history studies in patients with RLS are required to address this issue.

## REFERENCES


1. Akpinar S. Restless legs syndrome treatment with dopaminergic drugs. Clin Neuropharmacol 1987; 10:69–79.
2. Chaudhuri KR, Appiah-Kubi L, Trenkwalder C. Restless legs syndrome. J Neurol Neurosurg Psychiatry 2001; 71:143–146.
3. Montplaisir J, Lorrain D, Godbout R. Restless legs syndrome and periodic movements in sleep: the primary role of dopaminergic mechanism. Eur Neurol 1991; 31(1):41–43.
4. Chaudhuri KR. The restless legs syndrome. Time to recognize a very common movement disorder. Pract Neurol 2003; 3:204–213.
5. Tse W, Koller W, Olanow CW. Restless legs syndrome: differential diagnosis and treatment. In: Chaudhuri KR, Odin P, Olanow CW, eds. Restless Legs Syndrome. London and New York: Taylor-Francis and Thomson Publishing Services, 2004; 85–108.
6. Chaudhuri KR, Schapira AHV, Martinez-Martin P, et al. The holisitic management of Parkinsons' using a novel nonmotor symptom scale and questionnaire. Adv Clin Neurosci Rehab 2004; 4:20–24.
7. Chaudhuri KR, Martinez-Martin P, Schapira AHV, Ondo W, Sethi K. Members of the PD NMS Scale Development Group. An international multicentre study validation the first screening questionnaire (NMS–quest) for competitive assessment of nonmotor symptoms of Parkinson's disease. Mov Disord 2005; 20(10):50.
8. Thorpy MJ. Sleep disorders in Parkinson's disease. Clin Cornerstone 2004; 6(1AS):7–15.
9. Chaudhuri KR, Healy D, Schapira AHV. The non motor symptoms of Parkinson's disease. Diagnosis and management. Lauret Neurol 2006; 5:235–245.
10. Appiah-Kubi L, Pal S, Chaudhuri KR. Restless legs syndrome, Parkinson's disease and sustained dopaminergic therapy for RLS. Sleep Medicine 2002; 3(suppl 1):S51–S55.
11. Mrowka M, Chaudhuri KR, Odin P. Pathophysiology of restless legs syndrome. In: Chaudhuri KR, Odin P, Olanow CW, eds. Restless Legs Syndrome. London and New York: Taylor-Francis and Thomson Publishing Services, 2004:37–48.
12. Allen R. Dopamine and iron in the pathophysiology of restless legs syndrome (RLS). Sleep Med 2004; 5(4):385–391.
13. Rye DB. Parkinson's disease and RLS: the dopaminergic bridge. Sleep Med 2004; 5(3):317–328.
14. Garcia-Borreguero D, Odin P, Serrano C. Restless legs syndrome and PD: a review of the evidence for a possible association. Neurology 2003; 61(3):S49–S55.
15. Pittock SJ, Parrett T, Adler CH, et al. Neuropathology of primary restless leg syndrome: absence of specific tau- and alpha-synuclein pathology. Mov Disord 2004; 19:695–699.
16. Connor JR, Boyer PJ, Menzies SL, et al. Neuropathological examination suggests impaired brain iron acquisition in restless legs syndrome. Neurology 2003; 61: 304–309.
17. Eisenhsehr I, Wetter TC, Linke R, et al. Normal IPT and IBZM SPECT in drug naïve and levodopa treated idiopathic restless legs syndrome. Neurology 2001; 57:1307–1309.
18. Silber M, Rye D. Solving the mysteries of narcolepsy. The hypocretin story. Neurology 2001; 56:1616–1618.

19. Linke R, Eisensehr I, Wetter TC, et al. Presynaptic dopaminergic function in patients with restless legs syndrome: are there common features with early Parkinson's disease? Mov Disord 2004; 19(10):1158–1162.
20. Mrowka M, Jobges M, Berding G, Schimke N, Shing M, Odin P. Computerized movement analysis and beta-CIT-SPECT in patients with restless legs syndrome. J Neural Transm 2005; 112(5):693–701.
20a. Schmidaver C, Sajer M, Sippi K, et al. Transcranial ultrasound shows nigral hypoechogenecity in restless legs syndrome. Ann Neurol 2005; 58(4):630–634.
21. Ruottinen HM, Partinen M, Hublin C, et al. An FDOPA PET study in patients with periodic limb movement disorder and restless legs syndrome. Neurology 2000; 502–504.
22. Arnulf I, Konofal E, Merino-Andreu M, et al. Parkinson's disease and sleepiness: an integral part of PD. Neurology 2002; 58:1019–1024.
23. Decker M, Keating G, Freeman A, Rye D. Parkinsonian-like sleep wake architecture in rats with bilateral striatal 6-OHDA lesions. Soc Neurosci Abstr 2000; 26:1514.
24. Daley J, Turner R, Bliwise D, Rye D. Nocturnal sleep and daytime alertness in the MPTP-TREATD PRIMATE. Sleep 1999; 22(suppl):S218–S219.
25. Van Dyck H, Dijk J, Voom P, Holstege JC. Localisation of dopamine D2 receptor in rat spinal cord identified with immunocytochemistry and in situ hybridisation. Eur J Neurosci 1996; 8:621–628.
26. Gladwell SJ, Pyner S, Barnes NM, Coote JH. D (1)-like dopamine receptors on retrogradely labelled sympathoadrenal neurones in the thoracic spinal cord of the rat. Exp Brain Res 1999; 128:377–382.
27. Maniak S, Kabakei K, Pichler I, Kramer PL, Pramstaller C. Restless legs syndrome (RLS) in a large family (Family LA) with Parkin-associated Parkinson's disease (PD). Mov Disord 2004; 19(9):S354.
28. Schols L, Haan J, Riess O, Amoiridis G, Przuntek H. Sleep disturbance in spinocerebellar ataxias: is the SCA3 mutation a cause of restless legs syndrome? Neurology 1998; 51(6):1603–1607.
29. Abele M, Burk K, Laccone F, Dichgans J, Klockgether T. Restless legs syndrome in spinocerebellar ataxia types 1, 2, and 3. J Neurol 2001; 248(4):311–314.
30. Poewe W, Hogl B. Akathisia, restless legs and periodic limb movements in sleep in Parkinson's disease. Neurology 2004; 63(8):S12–S16.
31. Lang AE, Johnson K. Akathisia in idiopathic Parkinson's disease. Neurology 1987; 37:477–481.
32. Ondo WG, Vuong KD, Jankovic J. Exploring the relationship between Parkinson disease and restless legs syndrome. Arch Neurol 2002; 59(3):421–424.
33. Simuni T, Wilson R, Stern MB. Prevalence of restless legs syndrome in Parkinson's disease. Platform presentation. 14th Annual symposia on etiology, pathogenesis and treatment of PD and other movement disorders. Chicago 2001. Abstract P1043: Mov Disord 2000; 15(5):1043.
34. Krishnan PR, Bhatia M, Behari M. Restless legs syndrome in Parkinson's disease: a case controlled study. Mov Disord 2003; 18:181–185.
34a. Nomura T, Inove Y, Miyake M, Yasvi K, Nakashima K. Prevalence and clinical characteristics of restless legs syndrome in with Parkinson's disease. Mov Disord 2006; 21: 380–384.
35. Tan EK, Seah A, See SJ, Lim E, Wong MC, Koh KK. Restless legs syndrome in an Asian population: a study in Singapore. Mov Disord 2001; 16:577–579.
36. Tan EK, Lum SY, Wong MC. Restless legs syndrome in Parkinson's disease. J Neurol Sci 2002; 196:33–36.
37. Ratnagopal P, Tan EK. Restless legs syndrome in Parkinson's disease. Parkinsonism Relat Disord 2005; 11(S2):209.
38. Banno K, Delaive K, Walld R, Kryger MH. Restless legs syndrome in 218 patients: associated disorders. Sleep Med 2000; 1:221–229.
39. Chaudhuri KR, Taurah LS, MacMahon DG, et al. PD LIFE—A prospective multicentre longitudinal audit of quality of life in Parkinson's disease across the UK. J Neurol Neurosurg Psychiat 2004; 75:516–522 (P 005).

40. Lüssi F, Peralta C, Wolf E, et al. Restless legs in idiopathic Parkinson's disease. Parkinsonism Relat Disord 2005; (11)S2:207–208.
41. Ondo WG. The association of restless legs syndrome and essential tremor. Move Disord 2005; 20(suppl 10):S171, p579.
42. Rye D, DeLong M. Amelioration of sensory limb discomfort of restless legs syndrome by pallidotomy. Ann Neurol 1999; 46:800–801.
43. Rye D. Contributions of the pedunculopontine region to normal and altered REM sleep. Sleep 1997; 20:757–788.
44. Rye DB. Modulation of normal and pathologic motor neuron activity during sleep: insights from the neurology clinic, Parkinson's disease, and comments on parkinsonian related sleepiness. Sleep Med 2002; 3(suppl 1):S43–S49.
45. Kedia S, Moro E, Tagliati M, Lang AE, Kumar R. Emergence of restless legs syndrome during subthalamic stimulation for Parkinson disease. Neurology 2004; 63(12): 2410–2412.
45a. Driver-Dunckley E, Evidente VG, Adler CH, et al. Restless legs syndrome in Parkinson's disease patients may improve with subthalamic stimulation. Mov Disord 2006.

# 22 Iatrogenic Restless Legs Syndrome

**Changkook Yang**
*Sleep Disorders Clinic, Department of Psychiatry, Dong-A University College of Medicine, Busan, Korea*

**John W. Winkelman**
*Division of Sleep Medicine, Brigham and Women's Hospital, Harvard Medical School, Boston, Massachusetts, U.S.A.*

## INTRODUCTION

Restless legs syndrome (RLS) is a debilitating neurologic disorder characterized by unpleasant, deep-seated paresthesias in the legs and sometimes in the arms. Symptoms predominately occur at rest and worsen at night, resulting in sleep disturbance. They are temporarily alleviated by movement.

RLS is most commonly idiopathic but can be often secondary to several medical or neurological disorders. There is also evidence from published case reports that RLS symptoms may be caused or worsened by medications, including commonly prescribed psychotropic agents such as antidepressants and antipsychotics. It is not known why some persons taking a precipitating medication develop RLS symptoms whereas most others do not.

The pathophysiology of RLS is still poorly understood. Current pathophysiologic models for RLS focus on the central dopaminergic system, central iron pathways, and endogenous opioid system dysfunction (1). On the other hand, serotonergic, noradrenergic, and GABAergic systems may also be implicated, at least in part, in RLS (2,3). Thus, drugs that affect the above neurotransmitter systems may influence the expression of RLS.

Medication-induced movement disorders include extrapyramidal symptoms (EPS) related to antipsychotic use (i.e., Parkinsonism, tardive dyskinesia, akathisia, and neuroleptic malignant syndrome). They are now included in the DSM-IV (4), demonstrating the potential untoward influences of prescribed medications, their contribution to treatment noncompliance, and the importance of measures to prevent and/or treat such iatrogenic disorders.

However, medication-induced RLS has not been included in this category or in any other separate diagnostic criteria. In fact, little attention has been paid to iatrogenic RLS, possibly due to a lack of understanding of RLS symptoms, and the means of distinguishing RLS from other movement disorders. One of the major difficulties in understanding the literature on iatrogenic RLS is that such cases may have been misdiagnosed as akathisia.

Drugs that have been reported to induce movement disorders and RLS share some common pharmacologic characteristics: antidopaminergic, antiserotonergic, antiadrenergic, anticholinergic, and antihistaminergic effects. Although drug-induced RLS has been infrequently reported compared with other iatrogenic movement disorders, clinicians should be aware of the potential for its occurrence when initiating a precipitating medication, because RLS symptoms, as well as being debilitating, may result in noncompliance, and may contribute to significant psychosocial and occupational impairment. This chapter addresses an analysis of case reports and related studies indicating the association of RLS and medications. Possible underlying mechanisms for the development of iatrogenic RLS are also briefly described.

## ANTIDEPRESSANTS

Evidence that antidepressants may provoke or exacerbate RLS is accumulating. For instance, Leutgeb and Martus (5) reported that 27.0% of a highly selected population treated with tricyclic antidepressants (TCAs) and selective serotonin reuptake inhibitors (SSRIs) had RLS. Antidepressants have been associated with various movement disorders such as EPS (i.e., akathisia, dystonia, and Parkinsonism) and tardive dyskinesia (6,7), although certainly to a much lesser degree than antipsychotics. It has also been demonstrated that a higher incidence of periodic leg movement of sleep (PLMS) is found among patients treated with serotonergic antidepressants such as SSRIs and venlafaxine (8). PLMS has been closely associated with RLS, and it has been suggested that RLS and drug-induced akathisia may share some aspects of pathophysiology, while being distinct in other respects (9).

Although the data are not sufficient to make definite conclusions, the case reports available suggest that SSRIs and other newer antidepressants may be more common offenders than TCAs in inducing RLS.

### Tricyclic Antidepressants

TCAs inhibit the reuptake pumps for both serotonin and norepinephrine, and to a lesser extent, dopamine (10). While TCA-induced movement disorders, including akathisia, have frequently been reported in the literature, case reports or studies of TCA-induced RLS have been very limited. However, given the pharmacological profiles of TCAs, the potential for them to induce RLS is feasible. Morgan (11) described his experience with drug-induced RLS and cited nortriptyline and amitriptyline as causes. On the other hand, Ginsberg (12) reported the case of a 47-year-old female patient who developed RLS on cessation of long-term treatment of imipramine 75 mg/day and showed prompt suppression of the symptoms after a rechallenge of imipramine at 50 mg/day. The author concluded that the abrupt withdrawal of imipramine resulted in RLS.

### Selective Serotonin Reuptake Inhibitors

SSRIs demonstrate not only a high degree of selectivity in blocking the neuronal uptake of serotonin, but also lesser degrees of actions at other neurotransmitter receptors, including those for norepinephrine and dopamine (10). Several epidemiologic studies and case reports have reported an association between SSRIs and RLS. A general population survey in five European countries found that users of SSRI were more likely to have RLS [odds ratio (OR) 3.11] (13). In recent years, there have been several case reports of RLS as a result of treatment with SSRIs. For example, fluoxetine treatment has been implicated in causing RLS; Bakshi (14) reported a 22-year-old female patient, who developed a dose-dependent exacerbation of preexisting mild RLS. RLS symptoms occurred two weeks after she began taking fluoxetine 20 mg/day for depression and became considerably worse after the dose was increased to 40 and then 60 mg/day, requiring discontinuation of the drug. Sertraline also exacerbated preexisting mild RLS in a 71-year-old male patient with depression (15). In this case, RLS symptoms, which were successfully controlled with lorazepam 1 mg/day were intensified one week after beginning sertraline 25 mg/day and then resolved within three to four days after discontinuation of the sertraline. A case of RLS worsened by paroxetine has also been reported in a 33-year-old male patient (16). From the second week of treatment with paroxetine 20 mg/day, the patient described the reappearance of RLS symptoms, which he had experienced before. His RLS symptoms disappeared within days after he stopped the drug, but, when the paroxetine was restarted, the RLS symptoms reappeared with even greater intensity. On the other hand, Dimmitt and Riley (17) observed that most of their patients treated with SSRIs experienced improvement of preexisting RLS, although some patients reported development or worsening of RLS symptoms. However, the authors did not describe which SSRIs were prescribed.

Knowing how SSRIs induce RLS in some patients but may improve symptoms in others might provide helpful information for understanding the pathophysiology of RLS. However, all such potential mechanisms remain speculative at this time. There are diffuse interconnections between serotonergic and dopaminergic nuclei in the central nervous system (CNS). Serotonin inhibits dopamine release from dopaminergic axon terminals in dopamine pathways, which causes dopamine depletion (10). SSRIs, therefore, may cause or exacerbate RLS through enhanced serotonergic availability and secondarily decreased dopaminergic effects. Serotonin projections from the dorsal raphe also descend into the spinal cord, where they stimulate the intermediolateral nucleus (10a). This same spinal nucleus is inhibited by diencephalic-spinal dopaminergic (A11) projections that are postulated to prevent RLS when fully functional (10b). Therefore increased serotonin availability from SSRI medication may also cause PLMS or RLS directly. However, most serotonergic antidepressants have at least some noradrenergic activity, either primarily or through active metabolites. Thus, it is difficult to exclude the possibility of the involvement of the noradrenergic system in SSRI-induced RLS.

### Venlafaxine

Venlafaxine is not only a serotonin–norepinephrine reuptake inhibitor, but it also modestly inhibits dopamine reuptake, especially at high doses (10). In one prospective study, two (25.0%) of eight healthy volunteers, who first received 75 mg for two nights and then 150 mg for the following two nights, developed RLS, and six (75%) developed PLMS (18).

### Mirtazapine

Several cases of mirtazapine-induced RLS have been reported (19–21,21a). Agargun et al. (19) described a 45-year-old male patient who, having started on mirtazapine 15 mg/day for depression, developed RLS after the dosage was increased to 30 mg/day one week later. After clonazepam 1 mg/day was added to the mirtazapine, his RLS improved. Bahk et al. (20) reported a 56-year-old female patient with major depression who was on mirtazapine of 15 mg/day and alprazolam of 0.5 mg/day. On the fifth day of mirtazapine intake, she developed RLS. After switching the mirtazapine to paroxetine, her RLS symptoms completely disappeared. Bonin et al. (21) also reported that a 33-year-old male with depression developed RLS symptoms after seven days of mirtazapine 15 mg/day in combination with valpromide 300 mg/day. On the other hand, Pae et al. (22) have reported two cases that did not show reappearance of RLS with mirtazapine after it was readministered, following an initial episode of RLS provocation upon the first exposure to the drug.

Mirtazapine is a noradrenergic and specific serotonergic antidepressant. Mirtazapine has potent antagonist properties of presynaptic alpha-2 heteroreceptors and alpha-2 autoreceptors, which lead to increased release of both serotonin and norepinephrine. In addition, it is a potent 5-$HT_{2A}$, 5-$HT_{2C}$, and 5-$HT_3$ receptor antagonist, and also exhibits relatively potent antihistaminic activity (10). The main mechanism involved in mirtazapine-induced RLS is presumed to be the stimulation of 5-$HT_2$ receptors that induce an inhibitory action on dopamine release. Antihistaminergic properties may also be culpable. It should, however, be remembered that mirtazapine also has intrinsic 5-$HT_2$ receptor–blocking properties.

### Mianserin

Mianserin, which enhances adrenergic activity but does not significantly affect dopaminergic function, has been reported to cause RLS (23,24). Paik et al. (24) first reported three cases of mianserin-induced RLS. All three patients were female and were in their late 40s. They developed RLS symptoms one to two weeks after initiating mianserin, but none of them developed RLS until the dose was 60–90 mg daily, suggesting RLS development is dose-dependent. The RLS symptoms remitted after mianserin was either discontinued or reduced. The authors hypothesized that noradrenergic mechanisms were involved in their cases, because mianserin is a norepinephrine potentiator.

Markkula and Lauerma (23) also presented six cases (two males and four females, ages between 29 and 78) of mianserin-induced RLS. Half of them had a family history of RLS, and it is uncertain whether they had preexisting RLS. They had been prescribed mianserin 30–90 mg/day as monotherapy or in combination, and discontinuing or decreasing the dose of mianserin, or changing to another antidepressant, or both, invariably relieved the symptoms. The authors suggested that mianserin might cause RLS by potentiating noradrenergic and serotonergic transmission.

### Bupropion

To our knowledge, there are no published cases of bupropion-induced RLS. Given the role of dopamine in RLS and the agonistic effects of bupropion on central dopaminergic function (10), it is conceivable that bupropion might not be linked to iatrogenic RLS. Some studies support this possibility indirectly. In a retrospective case series, Nofzinger et al. (25) found that bupropion was not associated with drug-induced periodic limb movement disorder (PLMD), rather its use reduced objective measures of PLMD in five depressed patients with the disorder. Yang et al. (8) have also reported that bupropion does not produce PLMS. Although RLS symptoms were not documented in these two studies, given the evidence that PLMS is often associated with RLS, and that both disorders may share the same pathophysiology, it is likely that bupropion is not associated with drug-induced RLS, although it is too premature to conclude.

## ANTIPSYCHOTICS

Evidence from case reports suggests that typical antipsychotics, which are dopamine antagonists, can worsen RLS (Table 1). Given the robust efficacy of dopamine agonists in the treatment of RLS, this is not surprising. Blom and Ekbom (26) reported three

**TABLE 1** List of Medications (Mostly Dopamine Antagonists) Thought to Worsen Restless Legs Syndrome

| Generic name | Brand/trade name® |
|---|---|
| Acetophenazine | Tindal |
| Aripiprazole[a] | Abilify |
| Chlorpromazine | Largactil, Megaphen, Thorazine |
| Clorprothixene | Taractan |
| Clozapine[a] | Clozeril |
| Droperidol | Inapsine |
| Fluphenazine | Permitil, Prolixin |
| Haloperidol | Haldol |
| Loxapine | Loxitane |
| Mesoridazine | Serentil |
| Metoclopramide | Reglan |
| Molindone | Moban |
| Olanzapine | Zyprexa |
| Perphenazine | Etrafon, Trilafon, Triavil |
| Pimozide | Orap |
| Piperacetazine | Quide |
| Prochlorperazine | Combid, Compazine |
| Promazine | Sparine |
| Promethazine | Phenergan, Stopayne, Synalgos, |
| Risperidone | Risperdal |
| Quetiapine[a] | Seroquel |
| Thiethylperazine | Torecan |
| Thioridazine | Mellaril |
| Thiothixene | Navane |
| Trifluoperazine | Stelazine |
| Triflupromazine | Versprin |
| Trifluoperazine | Stelazine |
| Trimeprazine | Temaril |
| Triflupromazine | Versprin |
| Trimethobenzamide[a] | Tigan |
| Trimeprazine | Temaril |

[a]Dopaminergic antagonism mild and/or restless legs syndrome worsening not established.

patients who developed mixed symptoms of RLS and akathisia while they were being treated with different phenothiazine derivatives (perphenazine, prochlorperazine, and thiopropazate). Morgan (11) described his experience with RLS and concluded that antipsychotics, such as trifluoperazine, promethazine, prochlorperazine, and perphenazine, may provoke RLS. Ekbom (27) also proposed promethazine and prochlorperazine as causes of RLS. Pimozide was reported to worsen RLS symptoms (28), and pretreatment with pimozide prevented the improvement of RLS with codeine (29). Levomepromazine also appears to induce RLS in a dose-dependent manner (30). All of the above reports suggest that RLS symptoms can be caused or worsened in vulnerable individuals by dopamine-blocking agents, including typical antipsychotics such as haloperidol, loxapine, thioridazine, molindone, thiothixene, fluphenazine, trifluoperazine, triflupromazine, chlorpromazine, and perphenazine.

Some novel antipyschotics, such as olanzapine (31), risperidone (32), and quetiapine (33), have been implicated in the development of PLMS. Of the atypical antipsychotics, olanzapine (31) and risperidone (32) have been reported to induce RLS.

Kraus et al. (31) reported the case of a 41-year-old male patient who developed RLS and PLMS with olanzapine. The RLS symptoms developed 36 hours after an increase in dose from 10 to 20 mg, but a reduction back to 10 mg resulted in a slight amelioration, and the symptoms immediately disappeared after withdrawal of the drug. The periodic leg movement index was also significantly higher when the patient was on olanzapine compared to when he was off it.

Wetter et al. (32) reported the case of a 31-year-old female patient with schizoaffective disorder who did not show RLS symptoms on clozapine 200 mg/day but developed RLS and PLMS on risperidone 6 mg/day. Because RLS symptoms continued even after decreasing the dose to 4 mg/day, the authors decided to change risperidone 4 mg/day to haloperidol 10 mg/day, but the RLS symptoms continued. However, after changing to quetiapine 400 mg/day, RLS completely disappeared, with PLMS measurements returning to normal. The authors speculated that dopamine-blocking effects of risperidone and haloperidol might induce RLS, while the low affinity of clozapine and quetiapine for dopamine $D_2$ receptor may protect the patient from RLS.

Most people associate dopamine antagonists with antipsychotic medications; however, they are often marketed and used for nausea and to increase gastric motility. Prochlorperazine (Compazine®), metoclopramide (Reglan®), promazine (Sparine®), droperidol (Inapsine®), promethazine (Phenergan®), and trimethobenzamide (Tigan®) are all dopamine antagonists, listed in descending order of $D_2$ antagonist potency. Domperidone (Motilium) is also a $D_2$ antagonist but does not readily cross the blood–brain barrier and has been used successfully to treat nausea associated with medications used to treat RLS.

Finally, in controlled settings, dopamine antagonists have been shown to negate the clinical improvement from both dopamine agonists and opioid medications (29,34).

## HISTAMINE-RECEPTOR ANTAGONISTS

Drugs that belong to this category have not only antagonistic properties on histamine receptors but also dopamine-blocking activity. For these reasons, $H_1$ receptor antagonists have been prescribed as antihistamines, antiemetics, and antipruritics.

Antihistamines may be the most common agents associated with iatrogenic RLS (35). The most frequent offender seems to be diphenhydramine (Benadryl®). A wide variety of over-the-counter medications for cold, hay fever, sinus infections, and sleep disturbance presently contain it. People may take these medications as sleeping aids only to find they provoke their RLS symptoms. Some may simply report that these sleeping aids do not work or make them restless, because they are not familiar with RLS (35). Some people report "allergies" to the medications, and it is not common for antihistamines to provoke latent RLS in patients whom have never otherwise experience it. Many antidepressants, such as amitriptyline and doxepin, also have strong antihistaminergic properties and can worsen RLS "Non sedating" anti-histamines do not easily cross the blood–brain barrier and have been less associated with RLS exacerbation.

Many antiemetics, such as metoclopramide (Reglan®) and prochlorperazine (Compazine), and antipruritics, such as hydroxyzine (Vistaril®, Atarax®) also induce RLS symptoms partially through antihistaminergic. However, in one controlled study, metoclopramide administration did not provoke RLS symptoms in individuals with preexisting RLS (36).

## LITHIUM

Lithium can worsen RLS. Heiman and Christie (37) reported the case of a 48-year-old female patient with bipolar disorder, whose preexisting mild RLS was aggravated by treatment with lithium 1800 mg/day. This case showed a relatively clear association between serum lithium concentration and severity of RLS symptoms. Terao et al. (30) also reported the case of an 18-year-old male with obsessive-compulsive disorder, who developed RLS symptoms two weeks after he started lithium 1000 mg/day. RLS symptoms were relieved after the lithium dose was decreased to 400 mg/day, in accordance with increases and then decreases of serum-3-methoxy-4-hydroxyphenylglycol (MHPG), respectively. The development and resolution of his RLS symptoms were closely related to lithium dose and serum-free MHPG, suggesting that RLS development is dose dependent. Lithium is known to inhibit the release of norepinephrine and dopamine but not serotonin (38).

## ANTIEPILEPTICS

Antiepileptic drugs such as carbamazepine and gabapentin have been found to effectively treat RLS patients. However, there are some case reports of RLS being induced by antiepileptic drugs. Drake (39) reported two patients, a 30-year-old female and a 56-year-old male, who developed RLS on initiation of therapy with methsuximide and phenytoin, respectively, that subsided when these drugs were changed to other antiepileptics, valproate sodium, and carbamazepine, respectively.

Chen et al. (40) reported a case of zonisamide-induced RLS in a 27-year-old female with a seizure disorder. During titration of zonisamide, she began to experience typical RLS symptoms. The intensity of her RLS symptoms was clearly correlated with a subsequent increase in the dosage of zonisamide. Zonisamide is a broad-spectrum antiepileptic agent, and it is reported to have enhancing effects on dopaminergic activity, while, at supratherapeutic doses, it may inhibit dopamine function (40). The authors speculated that the dopamine-modulating activity of zonisamide was associated with the development of RLS in their patient.

## SMOKING

Three recent epidemiologic studies found a significant correlation between smoking and RLS (13,41,42). The Kentucky Behavioral Risk Factors Surveillance Survey smokers (41) found a significant association of cigarette smoking with RLS for those individuals smoking at least one pack per day (OR 2.06), but not for lighter smokers. A population-based interview study in a Turkish population found that individuals who smoke more than 10 cigarettes a day had a higher risk of developing RLS than nonsmokers (42). Another study, using telephone interviews in five European countries, also found that smoking more than 20 cigarettes a day increased the risk of having RLS (OR 1.72) (13). On the other hand, a Canadian population-based study failed to find a significant association of smoking with RLS (43). A major limitation of this latter study is that it did not take into account the number of cigarettes smoked or the degree of dependence. For reference, Menza et al. (44) reported significantly more akathisia in smokers than in nonsmokers. Of course, all such associations are cross-sectional and are thus unable to determine if there is a causal relationship between smoking and RLS (or akathisia), and if so, the direction of causation.

Nicotine directly stimulates nicotinic cholinergic receptors, which in turn cause release of dopamine. Nicotine also promotes the release of dopamine acutely. However, the data on the effect of chronic nicotine intake are mixed, with studies indicating either a continued increase or a decrease in dopamine function because of excessive dopamine stimulation (10).

## CAFFEINE

Caffeine has long been implicated in the worsening of RLS symptoms (45,46). However, this observation has never been demonstrated in a well-designed study. On the basis of therapeutic experience with 62 patients over an 11-year period, Lutz (47) observed that the occurrence of RLS in some patients coincided with their initial consumption of caffeine-containing beverages, while in others it followed their increased consumption. Lutz (47) concluded that caffeine is a major factor in the development of RLS. However, one of the epidemiologic studies found that coffee drinking was a protective factor for RLS, while it was a risk factor for PLMD (13). Caffeine has dopamine agonist-like effects and also shows various effects on serotonergic, adrenergic, GABA, adenosin, and cholinergic receptors (48). A PET study showed caffeine-related blood flow decreases in the striatum and the thalamus, together with changes in dopamine $D_2$ receptor–binding characteristics (i.e., increase in the striatum and decrease in the thalamus) (49).

## ALCOHOL

The general population telephone survey in five European countries found that individuals drinking at least three alcoholic beverages a day were more likely to have RLS (OR 1.47) (13). Among a sample from a general sleep disorders clinic, women who consumed two or more drinks a day were more likely to report RLS symptoms and to be diagnosed with RLS, while the risk of PLMS, a disorder that frequently accompanies RLS, was increased threefold; a similar relation was found among men (50). Sanz-Fuentenebro et al. (16) reported that symptoms of paroxetine-induced RLS were intensified by alcohol ingestion. On the other hand, one epidemiologic study revealed that RLS was associated with alcohol abstinence (41).

Alcohol's action mechanism is nonspecific, because alcohol can have effects in a wide variety of neurotransmitter systems including $\gamma$-amino butyric acid (GABA), *N*-methyl-d-aspartate (NMDA), dopamine, and opioid (10).

## MISCELLANEOUS

Tramadol is a central analgesic, and it has been found to be effective in the treatment of RLS (51). Its abrupt withdrawal has been implicated in the development of RLS. Freye and Levy (52) reported a case of RLS, which developed as a symptom of acute abstinence-like syndrome in a 45-year-old female patient, who had taken tramadol for over one year followed by a sudden abstinence from the drug. They speculated that long-term use of tramadol might result in a monoaminergic withdrawal of 5-HT at the spinal level, with ensuing peripheral sensory symptoms such as RLS, because tramadol inhibits the neuronal reuptake of noradrenaline and serotonin.

In a study using a multivariate logistic regression model, Leutgeb and Martus (5) found RLS to be associated with the intake of analgesics among patients on TCAs or SSRIs. They concluded that regular intake of analgesics, rather than the pain comorbidity itself, is a risk factor of RLS.

In a population-based survey of the elderly (53), RLS patients were found to take more estrogen compared with non-RLS cases. The authors suggested the possibility that the postmenopausal intake of estrogen may play a role in the clinical manifestation of RLS in elderly women.

One case report to date described interferon-α (IFNα) -induced RLS (54). A 60-year-old male patient with chronic hepatitis developed RLS two months after beginning IFNα, his RLS symptoms resolved with its discontinuation, and then they recurred on resumption. IFNα has been linked to several movement disorders including parkinsonism, akathisia, and chorea (55). The authors speculated that IFNα may cause RLS via direct or indirect effects on the dopaminergic and opiate receptor systems, because IFNα can directly inhibit dopaminergic activity, and it can also exert effects on opiate systems in the brain.

## AUGMENTATION

Augmentation has been defined as a worsening of underlying RLS, manifested either by a temporal extension (symptoms beginning earlier in the day), anatomical extension (involvement of body parts, usually upper extremities, which were not originally involved), or worsening of symptom intensity, as a result of pharmacologic intervention, discussed in detail in Chapter 26. Allen and Early (56) reported that 82% of their patients treated with a nighttime dose of levodopa/carbidopa over a period of two months complained that RLS symptoms had increased in the afternoon and the evening prior to taking the next nightly dose. Clinically, augmentation may begin about three to four weeks after the start of treatment. Increasing the dose of the drug transiently improves symptoms but causes further augmentation and may result in the patient suffering from RLS symptoms day and night. Augmentation may be greater for subjects with more severe RLS symptoms and for patients on higher doses (≥50/200 mg carbidopa/levodopa) (56). Severe augmentation requires discontinuation of levodopa, whereas mild symptoms may be treated by dose changes.

In general, it is now recognized that augmentation complicates about 50–80% of patients with RLS on chronic levodopa treatment. However, augmentation appears not to be exclusive to levodopa; it is observed in 27% of cases of RLS treated with the dopamine agonist pergolide (57), and in 10–30% of cases of RLS treated with the pramipexole (58–60). Currently, there are no reports of augmentation with the use of cabergoline (59).

## CONCLUSION

Many case reports and epidemiologic studies indicate that various medications, either through intake or withdrawal, may contribute to developing or worsening RLS symptoms. However, because the majority of associations are based on case reports, and the prevalence of RLS in the general population is relatively high (5–10% of Caucasian), any causal interpretations should be made with extreme caution. Well-designed prospective studies may help with clarification regarding the prevalence and pathophysiology of drug-induced RLS.

The main mechanism underlying drug-induced RLS is likely to be associated with serotonergic, dopaminergic, and histaminergic systems in the CNS. However, other neurotransmitter systems or other mechanisms could certainly contribute to the pathogenesis of drug-induced RLS. For example, SSRIs may also induce RLS via the thyroid axis, because the SSRI paroxetine has been implicated in reducing thyroid hormone (61), and hypothyroidism has been associated with RLS (62).

It is possible that some patients are more vulnerable than others to drug-induced RLS. Information from available case reports, however, does not support any consistent risk factor for drug-induced RLS, although some risk factors worth considering may include total daily dose of the drug, rapidity of dose escalation, and endogenous iron stores. Several patient-dependent and pharmacokinetic variables may also determine the likelihood that RLS will develop. For example, SSRIs have been reported to increase serum levels of antipsychotics. Such drug combinations may increase the likelihood of RLS. In addition, medications that normally do not cause RLS could, when combined with a drug, such as an SSRI that may worsen RLS, predispose a patient to RLS via reduced hepatic clearance due to competitive metabolism of the P450 cytochrome enzymes.

In summary, because drug-induced RLS has potentially occurred in different situations with different possible contributing factors, and because the other drugs that have not so far been reported to cause or worsen RLS may yet be found to do so, we may conclude only that a greater awareness of the possibility of drug-induced RLS will increase its recognition and prevent drug-induced morbidity. Clinicians should also list drug-induced RLS as a possible candidate for the cause of treatment-emergent insomnia or hypersomnia, even though a patient may not spontaneously report the typical symptoms of RLS. At present, it would appear that the most judicious means of treating drug-induced RLS is to decrease or discontinue the offending agent.

## REFERENCES

1. Allen R. Dopamine and iron in the pathophysiology of restless legs syndrome (RLS). Sleep Med 2004; 5:385–391.
2. Trenkwalder C, Paulus W. Why do restless legs occur at rest?—Pathophysiology of neuronal structures in RLS. Neurophysiology of RLS (part 2). Clin Neurophysiol 2004; 115:1975–1988.
3. Wetter TC, Pollmacher T. Restless legs and periodic leg movements in sleep syndromes. J Neurol 1997; 244(suppl 4):S37–S45.
4. American Psychiatric Association. Diagnostic and Statistical Manual of Mental Disorders. 4th ed. Washington, D.C.: American Psychiatric Association, 1994:678–680.
5. Leutgeb U, Martus P. Regular intake of nonopioid analgesics is associated with an increased risk of restless leg syndrome in patients maintained on antidepressants. Eur J Med Res 2002; 7:368–378.
6. Gill HS, DeVane CL, Risch SC. Extrapyramidal symptoms associated with cyclic antidepressant treatment: a review of the literature and consolidating hypotheses. J Clin Psychopharmacol 1997; 17:377–389.
7. Leo RJ. Movement disorders associated with the serotonin selective reuptake inhibitors. J Clin Psychiat 1996; 57:449–454.
8. Yang CK, Winkelman JW, White DP. The effects of antidepressants on leg movements [abstr]. Sleep 2004; 27(suppl):697–698.
9. Walters AS, Hening W, Rubinstein M, Chokroverty S. A clinical and polysomnographic comparison of neuroleptic-induced akathisia and the idiopathic restless legs syndrome. Sleep 1991; 14:339–345.

10. Stahl SM. Essential Psychopharmacology: Neuroscientific Basis and Practical Applications. Cambridge: Cambridge University Press, 2000:199–295, 499–537.
10a. Clemens S, Rye D, Hochman S. Restless legs syndrome: revisiting the dopamine hypothesis from the spinal cord perspective. Neurology 2006; 67:125–130.
10b. Ondo WG, He Y, Rajasekaran S, Le WD. Clinical correlates of 6-hydroxydopamine injections into A11 dopaminergic neurons in rats: a possible model for restless legs syndrome. Movement Disorders 2000; 15:154–158.
11. Morgan LK. Restless limbs: a commonly overlooked symptom controlled by "Valium". Med J Aust 1967; 23:589–594.
12. Ginsberg HN. Propranolol in the treatment of restless legs syndrome induced imipramine withdrawal. Am J Psychiat 1986; 143:938.
13. Ohayon MM, Roth T. Prevalence of restless legs syndrome and periodic limb movement disorder in the general population. J Psychosom Res 2002; 53:547–554.
14. Bakshi R. Fluoxetine and restless legs syndrome. J Neurol Sci 1996; 142:151–152.
15. Hargrave R, Beckley DJ. Restless leg syndrome exacerbated by sertraline. Psychosomatics 1998; 39:177–178.
16. Sanz-Fuentenebro FJ, Huidobro A, Tejadas-Rivas A. Restless legs syndrome and paroxetine. Acta Psychiatr Scand 1996; 94:482–484.
17. Dimmitt SB, Riley GJ. Selective serotonin receptor uptake inhibitors can reduce restless legs symptoms. Arch Intern Med 2000; 160:712.
18. Salin-Pascual RJ, Galicia-Polo L, Drucker-Colin R. Sleep changes after 4 consecutive days of venlafaxine administration in normal volunteers. J Clin Psychiat 1997; 58:348–350.
19. Agargun MY, Kara H, Ozbek H, Tombul T, Ozer OA. Restless legs syndrome induced by mirtazapine. J Clin Psychiat 2002; 63:1179.
20. Bahk WM, Pae CU, Chae JH, Yun TY, Kim KS. Mirtazapine may have the propensity for developing a restless legs syndrome? A case report. Psychiat Clin Neurosci 2002; 56:209–210.
21. Bonin B, Vandel P, Kantelip JP. Mirtazapine and restless leg syndrome: a case report. Therapie 2000; 55:655–656.
21a. Chang CC, Shiah IS, Chang HA, Mao WC. Does domperidone potentiate mirtazapine-associated restless legs syndrome? Prog Neuropsychopharmacol Biol Psychiatry 2006; 30:316–318.
22. Pae CU, Kim TS, Kim JJ, et al. Readministration of mirtazapine could overcome previous mirtazapine-associated restless legs syndrome? Psychiatr Clin Neurosci 2004; 58:669–670.
23. Markkula J, Lauerma H. Mianserin and restless legs. Int Clin Psychopharmacol 1997; 12:53–58.
24. Paik IH, Lee C, Choi BM, Chae YL, Kim CE. Mianserin-induced restless legs syndrome. Br J Psychiat 1989; 155:415–417.
25. Nofzinger EA, Fasiczka A, Berman S, Thase ME. Bupropion SR reduces periodic limb movements associated with arousals from sleep in depressed patients with periodic limb movement disorder. J Clin Psychiat 2000; 61:858–862.
26. Blom S, Ekbom KA. Comparison between akathisia developing on treatment with phenothiazine derivatives and the restless legs syndrome. Acta Med Scand 1961; 170:689–694.
27. Ekbom KA. Restless legs syndrome. Neurology 1960; 10:868–873.
28. Akpinar S. Treatment of restless legs syndrome with levodopa plus benserazide. Arch Neurol 1982; 39:739.
29. Montplaisir J, Lorrain D, Godbout R. Restless legs syndrome and periodic leg movements in sleep: the primary role of dopaminergic mechanism. Eur Neurol 1991; 31:41–43.
30. Terao T, Terao M, Yohimura R, Abe K. Restless legs syndrome induced by lithium. Biol Psychiat 1991; 30:1167–1170.
31. Kraus T, Schuld A, Pollmacher T. Periodic leg movements in sleep and restless legs syndrome probably caused olanzapine. J Clin Psychopharmacol 1999; 19:478–479.
32. Wetter TC, Brunner J, Bronisch T. Restless legs syndrome probably induced by risperidone treatment. Pharmacopsychiatry 2002; 35:109–111.
33. Cohrs S, Rodenbeck A, Guan Z, et al. Sleep promoting properties of quetiapine in healthy subjects. Psychopharmacology (Berl) 2004; 174:421–429.

34. Akpinar S. Restless legs syndrome: treatment with dopaminergic drugs. Clin Neuropharmacol 1987; 10:69–79.
35. Ondo W. Secondary restless legs syndrome. In: Chaudhuri KR, Odin P, Olanow CW, eds. Restless Legs Syndrome. London and New York: Taylor & Francis, 2004:57–84.
36. Winkelmann J, Schadrack J, Wetter TC, Zieglgansberger W, Trenkwalder C. Opioid and dopamine antagonist drug challenges in untreated restless legs syndrome patients. Sleep Med 2001; 2:57–61.
37. Heiman EM, Christie M. Lithium-aggravated nocturnal myoclonus and restless legs syndrome. Am J Psychiat 1986; 143:1191–1192.
38. Baldessarini RJ, Tarazi FI. Drugs and the treatment of psychiatric disorders: psychosis and mania. In: Hardman JG, Limbird LL, Gilman AG, eds. Goodman and Gilman's The Pharmacological Basis of Therapeutics. 10th ed. McGraw-Hill, Medical Publishing Division, 2001:485–520.
39. Drake ME. Restless legs with antiepileptic drug therapy. Clin Neruol Neurosurg 1988; 90:151–154.
40. Chen JT, Garcia PA, Alldredge BK. Zonisamide-induced restless legs syndrome. Neurology 2003; 60:147.
41. Phillips B, Young T, Finn L, Asher K, Hening W, Purvis C. Epidemiology of restless legs symptoms in adults. Arch Intern Med 2000; 160:2137–2141.
42. Sevim S, Dogu O, Camdeviren H, et al. Unexpectedly low prevalence and unusual characteristics of RLS in Mersin, Turkey. Neurology 2003; 61:1562–1569.
43. Lavigne GJ, Lobbezoo F, Rompre PH, Nielsen TA, Montplaisir J. Cigarette smoking as a risk factor or an exacerbating factor for restless legs syndrome and sleep bruxism. Sleep 1997; 20:290–293.
44. Menza MA, Grossman N, Van Horn M, Cody R, Forman N. Smoking and movement disorders in psychiatric patients. Biol Psychiatry 1991; 30:109–115.
45. Missak SS. Does the human body produce a substance similar to caffeine? Med Hypotheses 1987; 24:161–165.
46. Jeddy TA, Berridge DC. Restless leg syndrome. Br J Surg 1994; 81:49–50.
47. Lutz E. Restless legs, anxiety and caffeinism. J Clin Psychiat 1978; 39:693–698.
48. Shi D, Nikodijevic O, Jacobson KA, Daly JVV. Chronic caffeine alters the density of adenosine, adrenergic, cholinergic, GABA, and serotonin receptors and calcium channels in mouse brain. Cell Mol Neurobiol 1993; 13:247–261.
49. Kaasinen V, Aalto S, Nagren K, Rinne JO. Dopaminergic effects of caffeine in the human striatum and thalamus. Neuroreport 2004; 15:281–285.
50. Aldrich MS, Shipley JE. Alcohol use and periodic limb movements of sleep. Alcohol Clin Exp Res 1993; 17:192–196.
51. Lauerma H, Markkula J. Treatment of restless legs syndrome with tramadol: an open study. J Clin Psychiatry 1999; 60:241–244.
52. Freye E, Levy J. Acute abstinence syndrome following abrupt cessation of long-term use of tramadol (Ultram®): a case study. Eur J Pain 2000; 4:307–311.
53. Rothdach AJ, Trenkwalder C, Haberstock J, Keil U, Berger K. Prevalence and risk factors of RLS in an elderly population: the MEMO study. Neurology 2000; 54:1064–1068.
54. LaRochelle JS, Karp BI. Restless legs syndrome due to Interferon-α. Mov Disord 2004; 19:730–731.
55. Sunami M, Nishikawa T, Yrogi A, Shimoda M. Intravenous administration of levodopa ameliorated a refractory akathisia case induced by interferon-alpha. Clin Neuropharmacol 2000; 23:59–61.
56. Allen RP, Early CJ. Augmentation of the restless legs syndrome with carbidopa/levodopa. Sleep 1996; 19:205–213.
57. Silber MH, Shepard JW Jr., Wisbey JA. Pergolide in the management of restless legs syndrome: an extended study. Sleep 1997; 20:878–882.
58. Ondo W, Romanyshyn J, Vuong KD, Lai D. Long-term treatment of restless legs syndrome with dopamine agonists. Arch Neurol 2004; 61:1393–1397.
59. Tse W, Koller W, Olanow CW. Restless legs syndrome: differential diagnosis and treatment. In: Chaudhuri KR, Odin P, Olanow CW, eds. Restless Legs Syndrome. London and New York: Taylor & Francis, 2004:85–107.

60. Winkelman JW, Johnston L. Augmentation and tolerance with long-term pramipexole treatment of restless legs syndrome (RLS). Sleep Med 2004; 5:9–14.
61. Konig F, Hauger B, von Hippel C, Wolfersdorf M, Kaschka WP. Effect of paroxetine on thyroid hormone levels in severely depressed patients. Neuropsychobiology 2000; 42:135–138.
62. Banno K, Delaive K, Walld R, Kryger MH. Restless legs syndrome in 218 patients: associated disorders. Sleep Med 2000; 1:221–229.

# 23 Other Restless Legs Syndrome Associations

**Irfan Lalani**

*Section of Pain Management, Department of Anesthesiology, M.D. Anderson Cancer Center, Houston, Texas, U.S.A.*

**William G. Ondo**

*Department of Neurology, Baylor College of Medicine, Houston, Texas, U.S.A.*

## INTRODUCTION

Restless legs syndrome (RLS) has been described in conjunction with a variety of clinical conditions. Well-known associations with RLS include iron deficiency, uremia, pregnancy, neuropathy, and Parkinson's disease. These associations have been addressed earlier in this text.

Other causes of secondary RLS are less well established. These include fibromyalgia, rheumatoid arthritis (RA), ataxia, tremor, Tourette's syndrome (TS), stroke, sleep apnea, and hyperparathyroidism. Some of these associations have only been described as case reports and, thus, may represent coincidental cooccurrence. Whereas others may be true associations. We will discuss these less well-established associations.

## RHEUMATOLOGICAL DISORDERS

The literature suggests a possible association between RLS and Sjogren's syndrome (SS), RA, and fibromyalgia.

Two studies report a high prevalence of RLS in patients presenting with RA. Both used their own definitions of RLS. Reynolds et al. found that 30% of 70 patients with RA had RLS symptoms, compared to 6% of 70 age-matched controls (1). Salih et al. reported that 25% of 46 patients with RA met their RLS criteria versus 4% of 30 osteoarthritis (OA) controls (2). Patients with RA and RLS had worse RA and were more likely to be female. However, in this study, RA patients were also more likely than OA patients to have neuropathy, evidence of subtle myelinopathy based on slightly abnormal evoked potentials, and low ferritin levels. The low ferritin level was not commented upon but is particularly important, given the now accepted risk that low iron stores impart. Overall, potential confounding variables were not controlled in the study.

Using a written questionnaire, Gudbjornsson et al. looked at sleep disturbances in patients with RA and SS. Of 40 SS patients, 24% had RLS symptoms. In contrast to the other reports, only 2% of 42 RA patients had RLS (3). SS patients also reported more sleep disturbance, nocturnal pain, and fatigue. Again, this study predated the adaptation of standardized criteria for RLS.

Using a different approach, we screened 68 patients who presented with RLS at our movement disorders clinic for the presence of rheumatoid factor (RF) and SSA (Ro) and SSB (La) antibodies (4). A positive RF was seen in 3.6% of RLS patients and a positive SSA/SSB was seen in 3.1%, which is similar to the rate of positive antibody titers seen in the general population. None of the study patients exhibited overt signs of rheumatological disease. However, they were not examined by a rheumatologist as part of the study.

These seemingly disparate results may stem in part from different assessment tools used to make the diagnosis of RLS. Moreover, the diagnosis itself may be more difficult to make in these inherently painful conditions, where joint pain may be worse at night and may mimic RLS symptoms.

Yunus et al. examined the relationship between RLS and fibromyalgia (5). They reported that 31% of 135 female patients with fibromyalgia had RLS symptoms, whereas RLS symptoms occurred in only 2% of 88 women controls. In addition, leg cramps were also found to occur more commonly in fibromyalgia patients than in controls.

Interestingly, in a case reported by San Pedro et al., pain-dependent decreased regional blood flow in the caudate nucleus was demonstrated in two related RLS patients (5a). A similar pattern of decreased blood flow has also been reported in fibromyalgia. The pathogenesis of fibromyalgia remains obscure, and treatment options are limited. Dopamine agonists, which have proven efficacy in treating RLS are also being evaluated for use in patients with fibromyalgia.

## ATAXIA

In 2001, Abele et al. reported the presence of RLS in 28% of 58 subjects with genetic ataxias [spinocerebellar ataxia (SCA) 1, SCA2, SCA3] (6). This was significantly higher than the 10% incidence of RLS that they found in their control population. The average age at onset of RLS was 49 years. SCA patients with RLS had a similar incidence of neuropathy as did SCA patients without RLS. The risk of developing of RLS in SCA patients increased with increasing age but was unrelated to age of onset of ataxia and to CAG-repeat length. Thus, the period of time patients live with the triplet-repeat expansion appeared to influence the development of RLS.

Schols et al. evaluated 89 patients with genetically defined subtypes of autosomal dominant cerebellar ataxias for sleep abnormalities by history, polysomnogram, and nerve conduction studies. RLS was present in 45% of the 51 SCA3 patients in the study. However, none of 6 SCA1 patients, 2 of 11 SCA2 patients, and 1 of 21 SCA6 patients had RLS. RLS was more common in SCA patients with clinically overt polyneuropathy (7).

In a separate report, Van Elfen et al. described RLS symptoms in a family with intermediate CAG-repeat lengths for SCA3 (8). While all four affected members of the family had RLS, only three of the four had sensorimotor polyneuropathy, and two of the four had signs of central nervous system dysfunction (i.e., tremor, parkinsonism, and pyramidal signs). Thus, the molecular lesion in SCA3 caused central and peripheral nervous system dysfunction, and RLS may be the result of a combination of these effects.

Desautels et al. explored a possible association between CAG-repeat lengths in the SCA3 gene in patients with primary RLS (9). Similar repeat lengths were found in 125 RLS patients and 188 healthy controls. This finding suggests that the SCA3 locus is unlikely to be linked to the development of primary RLS.

Konieczny et al. went on to test 215 RLS patients with confirmed PLMS for SCA1, SCA2, SCA6, SCA7, and SCA17 (10). Only one subject possessed an "intermediate" length CAG expansion for SCA 17. Therefore, it does not appear that these conditions can present with RLS symptoms.

## TREMOR

In 2005, our center reported a large family with essential tremor (ET) linked to chromosome 2, in which RLS largely cosegregated with ET (11). Another case report also demonstrated the cooccurrence of these two conditions (12).

We recently prospectively evaluated for ET in patients presenting with National Institutes of Health criteria–defined RLS, as well as looked for RLS in patients presenting to us with established criteria for ET (13–15).

Of 100 consecutive patients presenting with ET (60 female, and 75 with a family history of ET) seen over 19 weeks, the age was $65.2 \pm 16.3$ years, and the age at tremor onset was $37.8 \pm 19.9$ years. Arm postural tremor severity (0–4) was rated as 1 (19 subjects), 2 (37 subjects), 3 (25 subjects), and 4 (19 subjects). Concurrent dystonia was seen in 19: neck (6), arm/hand (5), voice (5), and cranial (3). DBS of the ventral intermediate (VIM) nucleus had been performed in 24 patients. Thirty-three met all criteria for RLS, of which 25 had never been previously diagnosed. A family history of RLS was reported in 57.6% of these 33 patients and was the only significant predictor of RLS in the ET population. Family history of tremor, tremor severity, tremor duration, concurrent dystonia, sex, and patient status did not predict RLS. The onset of ET preceded the onset of RLS in 19, RLS preceded ET in 10, and 4 reported a simultaneous onset. Their international RLS rating scale score was $16.6 \pm 8.1$ (range: 0–40), which is generally less severe than those presenting to us for RLS.

We also examined 68 consecutively seen RLS patients (63.2% female and 54.4% with a family history of RLS) for the presence of tremor. Their age was $55.8 \pm 14.4$ years, and the age at RLS onset was $33.7 \pm 19.5$ years. No RLS patient demonstrated any rest tremor. No patient demonstrated a postural tremor of greater than 1, and only a single patient demonstrated a kinetic tremor of 2. Mild tremor, however, was very common. With posture, 10 patients (14.7%) were rated as 0.5, and 11 (16.2%) were rated as 1.0 in their worst hand. During finger to nose, 22 patients (32.4%) were rated as 0.5, and 18 (26.5%) were rated as 1.0 in their worst hand. Only four patients had any tremor anatomy aside from their hands. Clinically, we felt these very low amplitude tremors represented an "enhanced physiological tremor" rather than ET. The tremor did not cause any subjective disability in any case. Only a family history of ET was significantly associated with tremor in this RLS population, odds ratio = 6.6 [95% CI: (1.8, 24.5)], ($p = 0.005$). Worse RLS ($p = 0.09$) and higher ferritin ($p = 0.10$) tended to correlate.

The findings are consistent with the report of Walters et al., who only diagnosed ET in 3 of 56 patients presenting with RLS, based on criteria that required subjective disability and a minimum amplitude on examination (16). They did not include very low amplitude tremor (Walter, personal communication).

Overall, we found a very high rate of undiagnosed RLS in patients presenting for tremor, but unlike most other "secondary" forms of RLS, this was also associated with a high familial history of RLS, suggesting that they share some genetic similarities. Conversely, meaningful tremor is not often observed in people presenting with RLS. We have also noted that successful treatment of ET with deep brain stimulation to VIM nucleus does not improve RLS (17).

## TOURETTE'S SYNDROME

TS and RLS share certain clinical characteristics. Both manifest a partially suppressible urge to move, strong genetic components, presumed involvement of dopaminergic systems, and sleep disturbances. Lesperance et al. studied the prevalence of RLS in 144 patients with TS and chronic tics and in the parents of the affected probands (18). They found that 10% of affected probands and 23% of parents had RLS. Interestingly, the risk of RLS in probands was related to the presence of RLS in the mothers but not fathers, suggesting the role of a genetic modifier such as imprinting in differential phenotypic expression.

Clinical evidence indicates that the pathophysiology of RLS is likely different from other symptoms of TS. For example, RLS symptoms usually worsen with increasing age, whereas tics improve with time. TS-associated obsessive-compulsive symptoms respond to serotonin specific re-uptake inhibitors, whereas RLS may often be aggravated by them.

Dopaminergic antagonists (antipsychotics) are commonly used to treat patients with TS but usually exacerbate idiopathic RLS. The effects of antipsychotics on RLS symptoms in TS patients have not been systematically studied. However, Lipinski et al. reported treating 32 TS patients with the dopaminergic agonist pergolide and found significant improvement in tic severity (19). Interestingly, 59% of the patients were diagnosed with concomitant RLS, and this group of patients responded particularly well to pergolide, both for the RLS symptoms and for tics. This counter intuitive result might be explained by nondopaminergic affinities of pergolide, including its affinity for the alpha-2 receptors, similar to that of clonodine, another medicine used to treat tics. An open-label report, however, also suggests efficacy of the more specific dopamine agonist, ropinirole (20).

In the author's experience, differentiating tics from RLS in a pediatric population can be difficult. Tics may involve an urge to move the legs and often improve with intense mental activity. If these happen to occur more at night, this would overlap with the diagnostic criteria for RLS.

## MULTIPLE SCLEROSIS

RLS has been observed in multiple sclerosis (MS) (21,22). Manconi et al. recently found that 30 of 83 (36%) patients presenting with MS also met criteria for RLS based on interview (20). They found that the presence of RLS was associated with greater overall MS impairment and radiographic involvement of the cervical cord. Specifically, RLS correlated with diffusion tensor magnetic resonance imaging (MRI) and fractional anisotropy abnormalities independent of T2 lesions. Based on anatomical correlations with this MRI pattern in MS, they posited that RLS resulted for "a loss of alignment of axons" rather than direct cord demyelination. Systemic therapeutic trials in MS populations have not been reported.

## SLEEP APNEA

Ohayon et al. found that 5.5% of a European cohort of 18,980 individuals had RLS based on International Classification of Sleep Disorders criteria (23). The odds of having RLS were significantly associated with a history of loud snoring and the presence of obstructive sleep apnea (OSA) as determined by a questionnaire. RLS, however, was also associated with older age, female sex, the presence of musculoskeletal disease, heart disease, cataplexy, doing physical activities close to bedtime, and the presence of a mental disorder. Polysomnographic testing to confirm the presence of OSA was not done. Recently, Lakshminarayanan et al. reported that 8.3% of 60 patients with polysomnography-proven sleep apnea had RLS (24). The rate of RLS in age-matched spousal controls was 2.5%, and the difference was not statistically significant. Therefore, a clear and reproducible association between these disorders has not been established at this time. There is little doubt that OSA can produce periodic limb movements of sleep (PLMS); however, the pathogenic mechanisms of this may or may not be similar to PLMS associated with RLS.

## MISCELLANEOUS ASSOCIATIONS

Several other conditions have been reported with RLS. Huntington's disease was reported with RLS in a single family (25). We have also seen undiagnosed chorea patients who meet all criteria for RLS. RLS was reported to occur in acute intermittent porphyria (26), hypothyroidism treated with Colchimax (27), chronic respiratory insufficiency (28), venous insufficiency and varicose veins (29), peripheral microembolism (30), hyperparathyroidism (31), Isaac's syndrome (32), stroke (33), and telangiectasia (34). However, data from large cohorts or well-designed association studies are lacking for these conditions. Given the high prevalence of RLS in the general population, it is far from clear that any of these associations represent more than chance occurrence.

## CONCLUSION

In addition to the better-known associates such as uremia, iron deficiency, pregnancy, neuropathy, and Parkinson's disease, there are reasonable data to support a true association of RLS with SCA3 and ET. Rheumatological conditions, such as SS, RA, and fibromyalgia, may be associated with RLS; however, phenotypic overlap between nocturnal pain symptoms and pure RLS symptoms may cloud this association. TS and MS are possibly associated, but this requires verification. Other reported associations are less well established and may result from chance occurrences.

## REFERENCES


1. Reynolds G, Blake DR, Pall HS, et al. Restless leg syndrome and rheumatoid arthritis. Br Med J (Clin Res Ed) 1986; 292(6521):659–660.
2. Salih AM, Gray RE, Mills KR, et al. A clinical, serological, and neurophysiological study of restless legs syndrome in rheumatoid arthritis. Br J Rheumatol 1994; 33(1):60–63.
3. Gudbjornsson B, Broman JE, Hetta J, et al. Sleep disturbances in patients with primary Sjogren's syndrome. Br J Rheumatol 1993; 32(12):1072–1076.
4. Ondo W, Tan EK, Mansoor J. Rheumatologic serologies in secondary restless legs syndrome. Mov Disord 2000; 15(2):321–323.
5. Yunus MB, Aldag JC. Restless legs syndrome and leg cramps in fibromyalgia syndrome: a controlled study. BMJ 1996; 312(7042):1339.

5a. San Pedro EC, Mountz JM, Mountz JD, et al. Familial painful restless legs syndrome correlates with pain dependent variation of blood flow to the caudate, thalamus, and anterior cingulate gyrus. J Rheumatol 1998; 25:2270–2275.

6. Abele M, Burk K, Laccone F, et al. Restless legs syndrome in spinocerebellar ataxia types 1, 2, and 3. J Neurol 2001; 248(4):311–314.
7. Schols L, Haan J, Riess O, Amoiridis G, Przuntek H. Sleep disturbance in spinocerebellar ataxias: is the SCA3 mutation a cause of restless legs syndrome? Neurology 1998; 51:1603–1607.
8. van Alfen N, Sinke RJ, Zwarts MJ, et al. Intermediate CAG repeat lengths (53,54) for MJD/SCA3 are associated with an abnormal phenotype. Ann Neurol 2001; 49(6):805–807.

9. Desautels A, Turecki G, Montplaisir J, et al. Analysis of CAG repeat expansions in restless legs syndrome. Sleep 2003; 26(8):1055–1057.
10. Konieczny M, Bauer P. Tomiuk J, et al. CAG repeats in Restless Legs syndrome. Am J Med Genet B Neuropsychiatr Genet 2006; 141:173–176.
11. Higgins JJ, Lombardi RQ, Pucilowska J, Jankovic J, Tan EK, Rooney JP. A variant in the *HS1–BP3* gene is associated with familial essential tremor. Neurology 2005; 64:417–421.
12. Larner AJ, Allen CM. Hereditary essential tremor and restless legs syndrome. Postgrad Med J 1997; 73(858):254.
13. Allen RP, Picchietti D, Hening WA, Trenkwalder C, Walters AS, Montplaisi J. Restless legs syndrome: diagnostic criteria, special considerations, and epidemiology. A report from the restless legs syndrome diagnosis and epidemiology workshop at the National Institutes of Health. Sleep Med 2003; 4(2):101–119.
14. Bain P, Brin M, Deuschl G, et al. Criteria for the diagnosis of essential tremor. Neurology 2000; 54(11 suppl 4):S7.
15. Ondo WG. The association of restless legs syndrome and essential tremor. Mov Disord 2006; 21(4):515–518.
16. Walters AS, LeBrocq C, Passi V, et al. A preliminary look at the percentage of patients with restless legs syndrome who also have Parkinson disease, essential tremor or Tourette Syndrome in a single practice. J Sleep Res 2003; 12(4):343–345.
17. Ondo WG. VIM deep brain stimulation does not improve preexisting restless legs syndrome in patients with essential tremor. Park Dis Rel Disord 2006; 12(2):113–114.
18. Lesperance P, Djerroud N, Diaz Anzaldua A, et al. Restless legs in Tourette syndrome. Mov Disord 2004; 19(9):1084–1087.
19. Lipinski JF, Sallee FR, Jackson C, et al. Dopamine agonist treatment of Tourette disorder in children: results of an open-label trial of pergolide. Mov Disord 1997; 12(3):402–407.
20. Anca M, Giladi N, Korczyn A. Ropinirole in Gilles de la Tourette syndrome. Neurology 2004; 62:1626–1627.
21. Rae-Grant AD, Eckert N, Bartz S, et al. Sensory symptoms in multiple sclerosis: a hidden reservoir of morbidity. Mult Scler 1999; 5:179–183.
22. Auger C, Montplaisir J, Duquette P. increased frequency of restless legs syndrome in a French-Canadian population with multiple sclerosis. Neurology 2005; 65:1652–1653
23. Ohayon MM, Roth T. Prevalence of restless legs syndrome and periodic limb movement disorder in the general population. J Psychosom Res 2002; 53(1):547–554.
24. Lakshminarayanan S, Paramasivan KD, Walters AS, et al. Clinically significant but unsuspected restless legs syndrome in patients with sleep apnea. Mov Disord 2005; 20:501–503.
25. Evers S, Stogbauer F. Genetic association of Huntington's disease and restless legs syndrome? A family report. Mov Disord 2003; 18(2):225–227.
26. Stein JA, Tschudy DP. Acute intermittent porphyria. A clinical and biochemical study of 46 patients. Medicine 1970; 49(1):1–16.
27. Bon E, Rolland Y, Laroche M, et al. Hypothyroidism on Colchimax revealed by restless legs syndrome. Rev Rhum Engl Ed 1996; 63(4):304.
28. Spillane JD. Restless legs syndrome in chronic pulmonary disease. BMJ 1970; 4(738):796–798.
29. McEwan AJ, McArdle CS. Effect of hydroxyethylrutosides on blood oxygen levels and venous insufficiency symptoms in varicose veins. BMJ 1971; 2(754):138–141.
30. Harvey JC. Cholesterol crystal microembolization: a cause of the restless leg syndrome. South Med J 1976; 69(3):269–272.
31. Lim LL, Dinner D, Tham KW, et al. Restless legs syndrome associated with primary hyperparathyroidism. Sleep Med 2005; 6(3):283–285.
32. Lugaresi E, Cirignotta F, Coccagna G, et al. Nocturnal myoclonus and restless legs syndrome. Adv Neurol 1986; 43:295–307.
33. Anderson KN, Bhatia KP, Losseff NA. A case of restless legs syndrome in association with stroke. Sleep 2005; 28(1):147–148.
34. Metcalfe RA, MacDermott N, Chalmers RJ. Restless red legs: an association of the restless legs syndrome with arborizing telangiectasia of the lower limbs. J Neurol Neurosurg Psychiatr 1986; 49(7):820–823.

# 24 Treatment Overview

**William G. Ondo**

*Department of Neurology, Baylor College of Medicine, Houston, Texas, U.S.A.*

## SCALES FOR RESTLESS LEGS SYNDROME

Many medications have been shown to improve restless legs syndrome (RLS) in clinical trials. One must remember, however, that what these medicines really improve is the scales we use to assess RLS. Any detailed understanding of the treatment data subsequently presented in the following chapters requires a critical review of the assessment scales that support that data. Because this disease has only recently been carefully studied, most of our scales are relatively new. Most trials conducted prior to 2000 employed their own unvalidated scales, making comparison among studies, which is always difficult, even more problematic. Several assessments are now widely used in most large RLS trials. They can be broken down into questionnaire data regarding subjective symptoms and physiological data assessing sleep, periodic limb movements (PLM), or other motor activity (Table 1).

The 10-question International Restless Legs Syndrome Rating Scale (IRLS) has been used in most multicenter trials over the past five years (1,1a). Development of this scale began in the late 1990s and it underwent several modifications prior to final extensive metric evaluations. It should be noted, however, that version 2.0 underwent these validation studies, whereas version 2.1, which is currently used, differs semantically. It is not generally felt that these minor changes should mitigate against the validity assessments. The scale is meant to be administered by an RLS expert who can clarify the questions if needed. Another self-administered version was also developed but it has not undergone the same validation trials and has not been used in treatment trials (2).

The IRLS contains 10 equally weighted questions taken from a pool of germane clinical RLS features offered by a group of RLS researches (Appendix A). Each is scored 0 to 4 (total score 0–40) and they possess identical polarity. Five questions directly query the intensity and frequency of RLS symptoms and five query consequences of RLS, including nocturnal sleep and daytime fatigue and mood. The scale was validated at 20 centers from six countries. It was separately administered twice to each patient by two different researchers. The first test was given to 196 RLS patients and two to four weeks later was repeated in 187 of those subjects. These were compared to 110 normal controls and 99 controls with other sleep disorders. Criteria validity was compared to a clinician-assessed eight-item clinical global impression (CGI) scale.

Overall metric assessments of the scale were excellent. The interexaminer intraclass coefficient (ICC) was 0.93. The intraexaminer test-retest reliability yielded an ICC of 0.87. Criteria validity compared to the CGI was good, $r = 0.73$, $p < 0.001$. Discriminant validity was excellent. Only 17 of 176 controls scored greater than zero on the scale, but this is not surprising given that all of the

**TABLE 1** Subjective Questionnaires

| |
|---|
| International RLS rating scale |
| Johns Hopkins restless legs rating scale |
| RLS scale-6 |
| Clinical global impressions |
| Visual analogue scales |
| Pittsburgh sleep scale |
| Medical outcomes survey |
| Physiological assessments |
| Polysomnogram with limb electromyogram for PLMs |
| Actigraphy (accelerometers) |
| Suggested immobilization test |

*Abbreviation*: PLMs, periodic limb movements.

questions end with "from your RLS." Correlation among the 10 individual items (item convergent validity) was very high. Item 3, concerning relief while walking, was the least correlated with other questions. A factor analysis of the scale revealed that a single factor accounted for 74% of variance. A separate factor analysis from the self-administered Internet scale defined two primary factors (3). Six items (questions 1, 2, 4, and 6–8) resulted in 42% of variance. Three questions (3, 9, and 10) loaded together to account for 23% of variance.

Overall, the scale is short, simple to administer, and has excellent metrics. However, there are some potential shortcomings. First, studies using this scale have demonstrated a fairly robust placebo effect, although this is also seen in global clinical evaluations (4,5). Second, there may be a ceiling effect. Based on the exact semantics, even a single minute of mild RLS could easily result in a score of 6 to 8. Combined with the placebo response, this could minimize a real treatment effect. The uniform nature and polarity of questions has also been criticized.

The scale, in English and other languages, can be obtained from MAPI Research Institute (6). It is free to academic researchers, and there is a minor fee for profit organizations.

The Johns Hopkins restless legs rating scale (JHRLS) is a single question based on RLS time of onset (7). It segregates severity into 0 = no symptoms, 1 = symptoms only at bedtime, 2 = symptom onset at or after 6 pm, and 4 = symptom onset before 6 pm. This showed correlation to PSG sleep efficiency and PLMS. The scale is a very good mechanism to grossly stratify patients, similar to the Hoen and Yahr scale in Parkinson's disease. Because it only measures one aspect of RLS, it is only rarely used in treatment trials.

A six-question RLS rating scale (RLS-6) has been used in several European trials (8,9). Although this scale is easy to use and appears to possess a smaller placebo response, it has not undergone extensive published validation assessments (Appendix B). Preliminary data demonstrate acceptable metrics. Recent European trials have often used the IRLS as their primary efficacy point and the RLS-6 as a secondary point.

A RLS Quality of Life has recently undergone psychometric evaluations (10,11). The final version contains 18 questions regarding how RLS affects a variety of life functions (Appendix C). The questionnaire was validated in 85 RLS patients. Sixty-two returned an identical survey two weeks later. Internal consistency (Cronbach's alpha = 0.92) and test–retest reliability (ICC = 0.79) were good. This is also available through the MAPI Research Institute. See Chapter 15 for more detail on quality of life in RLS.

Several other scales that do not directly measure RLS have been used in clinical trials. The Epworth sleepiness scale is an eight-question survey that asks how likely one would "doze" in various daytime activities (12). Because RLS symptoms prevent people from falling asleep, this tends not to be very abnormal in RLS. The Medical Outcomes Study (MOS) sleep scale (13) and the Pittsburgh sleepiness scale (14) query both nocturnal and daytime sleepiness issues. Subscales within the MOS in particular have shown marked improvement from RLS treatments (15). The short-form 36 questionnaire is a widely used scale for overall health status (16,17). Patients with severe RLS have markedly abnormal scores, worse than most other chronic diseases such as heart failure. The effects of therapeutic intervention on this scale are not clear.

### Physiological Assessment

Overnight polysomnogram with electromyographic assessment for periodic limb movements (PLM) is the gold standard for sleep measures, including in RLS (18). PLM generally correlate with RLS severity (7,19) and consistently improve with most treatments of RLS. In fact, dopaminergics can completely eliminate PLM in many patients in a dose-dependent manner. Other sleep measures, including total sleep time, have variably improved with dopaminergics and other medications (15,20,21).

Actigraphy employs accelerometers to assess a variety of movements. Actigraphy can be used with reasonable accuracy to determine total sleep time, although this often requires subjective diary input (22–24). Actigraphy that employs a higher sampling rate can also be used to specifically assess PLM. These have generally correlated very well with PLM scores done with EMG during PSG (25,26). There are several brands currently available: Actiwatch® by Mini-Mitter Co., Inc., Bend, Oregon, U.S.A.; PAM-RL by IM Systems, Baltimore, Maryland, U.S.A., and Actiwatch Plus by Cambridge Neurotechnology, Cambridge, U.K. These are less costly and more convenient than polysomnogram (PSG) and are beginning to be used in clinical trials.

The suggested immobilization test (SIT) has been developed as a specific measure for RLS (27–29). It assesses both the motor component and sensory component of RLS. The SIT is administered about 9 pm, often before a PSG. During this test, subjects remain in bed, reclined at a 45° angle with their legs outstretched. Subjects are instructed to avoid moving voluntarily.

To assess movement, surface EMG from right and left anterior tibialis muscles are attached to quantify leg movements. Scoring criteria recommend scoring all movements lasting 0.5 to 10 seconds, separated by an interval of between 4 and 90 seconds, and occurring in a series of four consecutive movements. The SIT PLM index represents the number of periodic leg movements per hour of immobility.

Leg discomfort is measured during the SIT by a visual analog scale (VAS) connected to an electronic device. This apparatus gives an auditory signal every five minutes, at which time the patient is required to estimate his or her leg discomfort on a 100 mm horizontal bar. The descriptors "no discomfort" and "extreme discomfort" are used at the left and right endpoints of the VAS. The scoring of leg discomfort is automatically converted to a 0 to 100 scale. A total of 12 values are obtained (one every 5 minutes for 60 minutes) (Fig. 1).

Overall, the SIT has proven sensitive and specific for the diagnosis of RLS and sensitive to treatment effects. It is a labor- and cost-intensive test. So, it will likely remain a research tool.

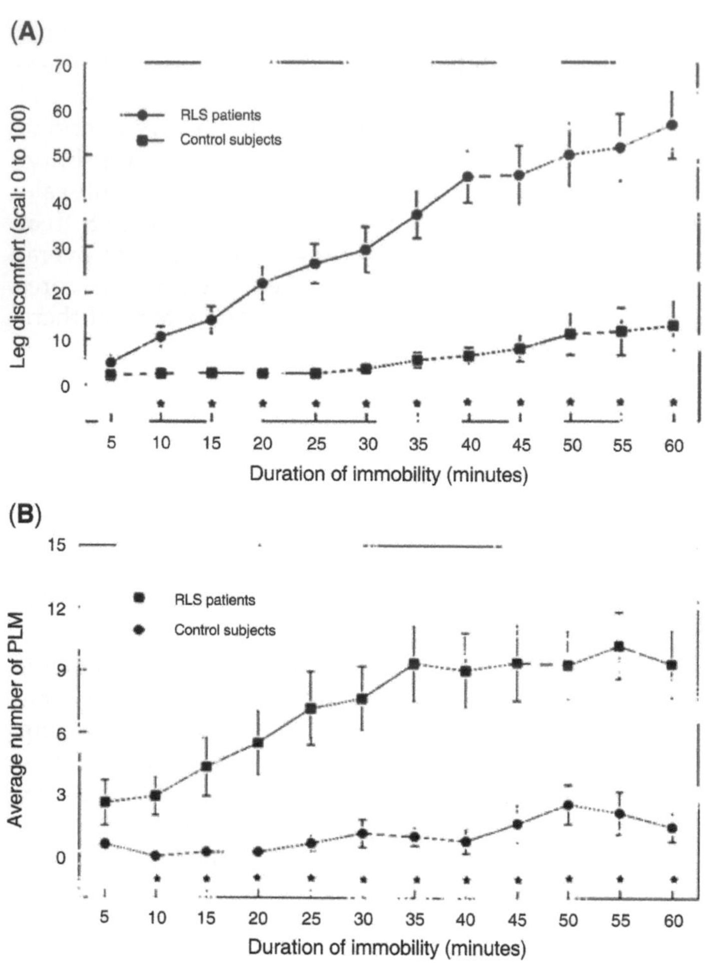


**FIGURE 1** Results from SIT comparing RLS to controls.

## TREATMENT OVERVIEW

Numerous medications improve RLS symptoms. All are felt to provide only symptomatic relief rather than "cure" the condition. Therefore, treatment should only be initiated when the benefits are felt to justify any potential adverse effects and costs. This varies individually and relates to both frequency and intensity of symptoms, and how those symptoms affect quality of life.

There is no minimum frequency that justifies chronic treatment, but most drug efficacy data come from trials that require at least 15 nights of symptoms per month. However, if severe RLS results in sleep deprivation one or two nights per week, most clinicians would recommend treatment. This scenario might warrant *pro re nata* dosing, but no data on *prn* use of any medication have yet been published. Furthermore, most oral medications require 30 to 90 minutes to improve RLS symptoms. Often, mild-to-moderate RLS will last only an hour per night, thus limiting the utility of taking a medicine only after symptom onset. Anecdotally, medicines may not work as well if taken after symptom onset, but this is not clearly established. Certainly some people take medications in situations where planned immobility, such as on an airplane, will likely result in RLS symptoms. Again this strategy has never been formally assessed but is anecdotally successful.

RLS is usually a chronic condition; therefore, selection of medicines should take into account potential long-term complications and be individualized to the particular needs of the patient. Both dosing and medication changes are often required to maximize benefit and minimize the risk of tolerance and adverse effects. Most physicians will titrate up to the minimally effective dose. Because RLS is circadian, timing of the dose may also greatly impact efficacy. Many advocate initial dosing shortly before the onset of symptoms. Multiple doses may be required if the drug's pharmacokinetics demand additional dosing to suppress symptoms until the early morning. As a general rule, morning doses are only required in the most severe cases. The amount and timing of dose will likely change over time, but data concerning this and all aspects of optimized dosing strategies are very limited. Finally, patients with severe RLS often take more than a single medication, usually from different classes of drugs. Polypharmacy has never been formally evaluated but anecdotally may have a role. The individual drug classes will be discussed briefly below and in much more detail in the subsequent chapters.

### Dopamine Agonists

Dopamine agonists (DA) are clearly the best-investigated and probably the most effective treatments for RLS. The improvement is immediate and often very dramatic. Adverse events are fewer and milder than when the medications are used for parkinson's disease (PD). RLS patients almost never experience hallucinations or orthostatic hypotension. This may result from the lower doses but probably also concerns differences in the disease states. There have been no comparative trials among the DA, but all are felt to provide roughly similar efficacy. Several DA are now approved for RLS or petitioning for registration in North America and Europe.

### Levodopa

Levodopa has been used for more than 20 years to treat RLS. It is clearly effective and possesses a relatively rapid onset of action. It may be less effective than DA, but this is based upon only small amounts of trial data and anecdotal evidence. Levodopa may also confer a higher rate of augmentation than DA. These differences may result from its shorter half-life or the fact that levodopa incurs presynaptic uptake by dopamine transporter protein and subsequent physiological release into the synapse. DA directly stimulate the postsynaptic receptors and therefore obviates both the presynaptic neurons and the synapse itself.

### Opioids

Opioid medications, also known as narcotics, have long been known to successfully treat RLS and in fact were first reported for RLS in the 17th century (30). Open label trials consistently demonstrate good initial and long-term results without difficulty with tolerance, dependence, or addiction. There exist, however, only minimal controlled data. We tend to prefer methadone (a $\mu$-specific opioid agonist) in RLS patients who have failed DA, but there are no data that compare different opioids. One apparent advantage of opioids is the apparent absence of augmentation, often seen in dopaminergics. We have seen little dependency or addiction, but these remain legitimate concerns.

## Benzodiazepines

Despite their past widespread use, there is very little data to support the use of benzodiazepines for RLS. In the opinion of most experts, benzodiazepines do help facilitate sleep but seldom improve RLS cardinal features if they are severe. Benzodiazepines can be used successfully in mild cases of RLS and as adjunct therapy for residual insomnia. Because antihistamines often exacerbate RLS, benzodiazepines are the preferred sleep aid for patients with RLS. Nonbenzodiazepine sedatives such as zolpidem (Ambien®), zaleplon (Sonata®), and eszopiclone (Lunesta®) have not been formally tested in RLS but seem to behave similar to benzodiazepines.

## Other Agents

Numerous other agents, including other antiepileptic medications, clonidine, baclofen, tramadol, and magnesium, have been reported to help RLS but because of limited data, and with the possible exception of gabapentin, cannot be recommended as either first- or second-line therapy. Oral iron is poorly absorbed and has improved RLS only in open label trials. Intravenous iron has shown dramatic benefits in some patients but has some potentially serious risks. Controlled trials are ongoing.

## REFERENCES


1. Waslters AS, LeBrocq C, Dhar A, et al. Validation of the International Restless Legs Syndrome Study Group rating scale for restless legs syndrome. Sleep Med 2003; 4(2): 121–132.

1a. Abetz L, Arbuckle R, Allen RP, et al. The reliability, validity and responsiveness of the International Restless Legs Syndrome Study Group rating scale and subscales in a clinical-trial testing. Sleep Med 2006; 7:340–349.

2. Allen R, Abetz L, Kirsch J. Development and validation of the Restless Legs Syndrome Rating Scale-Patient Version (RLSRS-PV). Eur J Neurol 2002; 9(suppl 2):P3159.
3. Allen RP, Kushida CA, Atkinson MJ. Factor analysis of the International Restless Legs Syndrome Study Group's scale for restless legs severity. Sleep Med 2003; 4(2):133–135.
4. Walters AS, Ondo WG, Dreykluft T, Grunstein R, Lee D, Sethi K. Ropinirole is effective in the treatment of restless legs syndrome. TREAT RLS 2: a 12-week, double-blind, randomized, parallel-group, placebo-controlled study. Mov Disord 2004; 19(12):1414–1423.
5. Trenkwalder C, Garcia-Borreguero D, Montagna P, et al. Ropinirole in the treatment of restless legs syndrome: results from the TREAT RLS 1 study, a 12 week, randomised, placebo controlled study in 10 European countries. J Neurol Neurosurg Psychiatr 2004; 75(1):92–97.
6. www.mapi-research.fr/t_03_serv_dist_user.htm.
7. Allen RP, Earley CJ. Validation of the Johns Hopkins restless legs severity scale. Sleep Med 2001; 2(3):239–242.
8. Stiasny-Kolster K, Kohnen R, Schollmayer E, Moller JC, Oertel WH. Patch application of the dopamine agonist rotigotine to patients with moderate to advanced stages of restless legs syndrome: a double-blind, placebo-controlled pilot study. Mov Disord 2004; 19(12):1432–1438.
9. Kohen R, Oertel H, Stiasney-Kolster K, Benes H, Trendwalder C. Severity rating of restless legs syndrome: validation of the RLS-6 scales. Sleep 2004; 27(suppl 1):A304.
10. Abetz L, Allen R, Follet A, et al. Evaluating the quality of life of patients with restless legs syndrome. Clin Ther 2004; 26(6):925–935.
11. Abetz L, Arbuckle R, Allen R, Mavraki E, Kirsch J. The reliability, validity and responsiveness of the Restless Legs Syndrome Quality of Life questionnaire (RLSQoL) in a trial population. Health Qual Life Outcomes 2005; 3(1):79.
12. Johns MW. A new method for measuring daytime sleepiness: the Epworth sleepiness scale. Sleep 1991; 14(6):540–545.

13. Hayes RD, Stewart AL. Sleep measures. In: Stewart AL, Ware JC, eds. Measuring Functioning and Well-Being: The Medical Outcomes Study Approach. Durham and London: Duke University Press, 1992.
14. Nofzinger EA, Reynolds CF III. Sleep impairment and daytime sleepiness in later life. Am J Psychiatr 1996; 153(7):941–943.
15. Allen R, Becker PM, Bogan R, et al. Ropinirole decreases periodic leg movements and improves sleep parameters in patients with restless legs syndrome [see comment]. Sleep 2004; 27(5):907–914.
16. Ware JE. SF-36 Health Survey—Manuel and Interpretation Guide. Boston: The Health Institute, New England Medical Center, 1993.
17. Lyons RA. Evidence for the validity of the Short-form 36 Questionnaire (SF-36) in an elderly population. Age Ageing 1994; 23(3):182–184.
18. Atlas Task Force of the American Sleep Disorders Association. Recording and scoring leg movements. Sleep 1993; 16:748–759.
19. Garcia-Borreguero D, Larrosa O, de la Llave Y, Granizo JJ, Allen R. Correlation between rating scales and sleep laboratory measurements in restless legs syndrome. Sleep Med 2004; 5(6):561–565.
20. Montplaisir J, Nicolas A, Denesle R, Gomez-Mancilla B. Restless legs syndrome improved by pramipexole: a double-blind randomized trial. Neurology 1999; 52(5): 938–943.
21. Garcia-Borreguero D, Larrosa O, de la Llave Y, Verger K, Masramon X, Hernandez G. Treatment of restless legs syndrome with gabapentin: a double-blind, cross-over study. Neurology 2002; 59(10):1573–1579.
22. Morrish E, King MA, Pilsworth SN, Shneerson JM, Smith IE. Periodic limb movement in a community population detected by a new actigraphy technique. Sleep Med 2002; 3(6):489–495.
23. Ancoli-Israel S, Cole R, Alessi C, Chambers M, Moorcroft W, Pollak CP. The role of actigraphy in the study of sleep and circadian rhythms. Sleep 2003; 26(3):342–392.
24. Kushida CA, Chang A, Gadkary C, Guilleminault C, Carrillo O, Dement WC. Comparison of actigraphic, polysomnographic, and subjective assessment of sleep parameters in sleep-disordered patients. Sleep Med 2001; 2(5):389–396.
25. Sforza E, Johannes M, Claudio B. The PAM-RL ambulatory device for detection of periodic leg movements: a validation study. Sleep Med 2005; 6(5):407–413.
26. King MA, Jaffre MO, Morrish E, Shneerson JM, Smith IE. The validation of a new actigraphy system for the measurement of periodic leg movements in sleep. Sleep Med 2005; 6(6):507–513.
27. Michaud M, Poirier G, Lavigne G, Montplaisir J. Restless legs syndrome: scoring criteria for leg movements recorded during the suggested immobilization test. Sleep Med 2001; 2(4):317–321.
28. Michaud M, Lavigne G, Desautels A, Poirier G, Montplaisir J. Effects of immobility on sensory and motor symptoms of restless legs syndrome. Mov Disord 2002; 17(1): 112–115.
29. Montplaisir J, Boucher S, Nicolas A, et al. Immobilization tests and periodic leg movements in sleep for the diagnosis of restless leg syndrome. Mov Disord 1998; 13(2): 324–329.
30. Willis T. Two Discourses Concerning the Soul of Brutes. London: Dring, Haeper and Leigh, 1683.

## APPENDIX A

### International Restless Legs Syndrome Study Group Rating Scale (IRLS)
(Investigator Version 2.2)

Have the patient rate his/her symptoms for the following ten questions. The patient and not the examiner should make the ratings, but the examiner should be available to clarify any misunderstandings the patient may have about the questions. The examiner should mark the patient's answers on the form.

In the past week ...

(1) Overall, how would you rate the RLS discomfort in your legs or arms?

☐ Very severe
☐ Severe
☐ Moderate
☐ Mild
☐ None

In the past week ...

(2) Overall, how would you rate the need to move around because of your RLS symptoms?

☐ Very severe
☐ Severe
☐ Moderate
☐ Mild
☐ None

In the past week ...

(3) Overall, how much relief of your RLS arm or leg discomfort did you get from moving around?

☐ No relief
☐ Mild relief
☐ Moderate relief
☐ Either complete or almost complete relief
☐ No RLS symptoms to be relieved

In the past week ...

(4) How severe was your sleep disturbance due to your RLS symptoms?

☐ Very severe
☐ Severe
☐ Moderate
☐ Mild
☐ None

In the past week ...

(5) How severe was your tiredness or sleepiness during the day due to your RLS symptoms?

☐ Very severe
☐ Severe
☐ Moderate
☐ Mild
☐ None

In the past week ...

(6) How severe was your RLS as a whole?

☐ Very severe
☐ Severe
☐ Moderate
☐ Mild
☐ None

In the past week ...

(7) How often did you get RLS symptoms?

☐ Very often (This means 6 to 7 days a week)
☐ Often (This means 4 to 5 days a week)
☐ Sometimes (This means 2 to 3 days a week)
☐ Occasionally (This means 1 day a week)
☐ Never

In the past week ...

(8) When you had RLS symptoms, how severe were they on average?

☐ Very severe (This means 8 hours or more per 24 hour day)
☐ Severe (This means 3 to 8 hours per 24 hour day)
☐ Moderate (This means 1 to 3 hours per 24 hour day)
☐ Mild (This means less than 1 hour per 24 hour day)
☐ None

In the past week ...

(9) Overall, how severe was the impact of your RLS symptoms on your ability to carry out your daily affairs, for example, carrying out a satisfactory family, home, social, school, or work life?

☐ Very severe
☐ Severe
☐ Moderate
☐ Mild
☐ None

In the past week ...

(10) How severe was your mood disturbance due to your RLS symptoms, for example, angry, depressed, sad, anxious, or irritable?

☐ Very severe
☐ Severe
☐ Moderate
☐ Mild
☐ None

## APPENDIX B

### RLS-6 Rating Scales

To be completed by the subject. The subject and not the examiner should make the ratings, but the examiner should be available to clarify any misunderstandings the subject may have about the questions.

Please evaluate the following questions for the last 7 days or nights:

How satisfied are you with your sleep during the last 7 nights?

completely satisfied ☐ ☐ ☐ ☐ ☐ ☐ ☐ ☐ ☐ ☐ ☐ completely dissatisfied

How severe were your RLS symptoms during the last 7 nights or days in the following situations?

At falling asleep

none ☐ very mild ☐ ☐ ☐ ☐ ☐ ☐ ☐ ☐ ☐ ☐ very severe

During the night

none ☐ very mild ☐ ☐ ☐ ☐ ☐ ☐ ☐ ☐ ☐ ☐ very severe

During the day when you were at rest (sitting, lying)

none ☐ very mild ☐ ☐ ☐ ☐ ☐ ☐ ☐ ☐ ☐ ☐ very severe

During the day when you were not at rest but engaged in activities (walking, activities in your job, homework, leisure activities)

none ☐ very mild ☐ ☐ ☐ ☐ ☐ ☐ ☐ ☐ ☐ ☐ very severe

How tired or sleepy were you during the day (between getting up in the morning and bedtime in the evening) within the last 7 days ?

not at all ☐ very mild ☐ ☐ ☐ ☐ ☐ ☐ ☐ ☐ ☐ ☐ very severe

Subject's signature: ______________________________

## APPENDIX C

### Johns Hopkins Restless Legs Syndrome Quality of Life Questionnaire (RLS-QOL)

The following are some questions on how your restless legs syndrome might affect your quality of life. Answer each of the items below in relation to your life experience in the past 4 weeks. Please mark only one answer for each question.

1. In the past 4 weeks how distressing to you were your restless legs?
☐ Not at all ☐ A little ☐ Some ☐ Quite a bit ☐ A lot

2. How often in the past 4 weeks did your restless legs disrupt your routine evening activities?
☐ Never ☐ A few times ☐ Sometimes ☐ Most of the time ☐ All the time

3. How often in the past 4 weeks did restless legs keep you from attending your evening social activities?
☐ Never ☐A few times ☐ Sometimes ☐ Most of the time ☐ All the time

4. In the past 4 weeks how much trouble did you have getting up in the morning due to restless legs?
☐ None ☐ A little ☐ Some ☐ Quite a bit ☐ A lot

5. In the past 4 weeks how often were you late for work or your first appointments of the day due to restless legs?
☐ Never ☐ A few times ☐ Sometimes ☐ Most of the time ☐ All the time

6. How many days in the past 4 weeks were you late for work or your first appointments of the day due to restless legs?

Write in number of days:

7. How often in the past 4 weeks did you have trouble concentrating in the afternoon?
☐ Never ☐ A few times ☐ Sometimes ☐ Most of the time ☐ All the time

8. How often in the past 4 weeks did you have trouble concentrating in the evening?
☐ Never ☐ A few times ☐ Sometimes ☐ Most of the time ☐ All the time

9. In the past 4 weeks how much was your ability to make decisions affected by sleep problems?
☐ Not at all ☐ A little ☐ Some ☐ Quite a bit ☐ A lot

10. How often in the past 4 weeks would you have avoided traveling when the trip would have lasted more than two hours?
☐ Never ☐ A few times ☐ Sometimes ☐ Most of the time ☐ All the time

11. In the past 4 weeks how much interest did you have in sexual activity?
☐ None ☐ A little ☐ Some ☐ Quite a bit ☐ A lot

☐Prefer not to answer

12. In the past 4 weeks how much did restless legs disturb or reduce your sexual activities?

☐ Not at all ☐ A little ☐ Some ☐ Quite a bit ☐ A lot

☐ Prefer not to answer

13. In the past 4 weeks how much did your restless legs disturb your ability to carry out your daily activities, for example, carrying out a satisfactory family, home, social, school, or work life?

☐ Not at all ☐ A little ☐ Some ☐ Quite a bit ☐ A lot

14. Do you currently work (full or part time, paid work, unpaid or volunteer)? (mark one box)

☐ YES If Yes please answer questions #15 through #18

☐ NO, because of my RLS — Thank you, you have now completed the questionnaire.

☐ NO, due to other reasons — Thank you, you have now completed the questionnaire.

15. How often did restless legs make it difficult for you to work a full day in the past 4 weeks?

☐ Never ☐ A few times ☐ Sometimes ☐ Most of the time ☐ All the time

16. How many days in the past 4 weeks did you work less than you would like due to restless legs?

Write in number of days:

17. On the average, how many hours did you work per day in the past 4 weeks?

Write in number of hours per day:

18. On days you worked less than you would like, on average about how many hours less did you work per day due to your restless legs?

Write in number of hours per day:

Thank you, you have now completed the questionnaire.

# 25 Dopaminergic Therapy for Restless Legs Syndrome

**Philip M. Becker**

*Department of Psychiatry, University of Texas Southwestern Medical Center at Dallas, Dallas, Texas, U.S.A.*

## INTRODUCTION

Dopaminergic agents are considered as first-line therapy for restless legs syndrome (RLS) according to practice guidelines of the American Academy of Sleep Medicine (1) as well as the medical advisory board of the RLS foundation (2). Double-blind, placebo-controlled trials in patients with moderate to severe RLS have demonstrated the efficacy of levodopa (3–6), pergolide (7–10), pramipexole (11,12), ropinirole (13–18), and cabergoline (19). Other dopamine agonists are also under investigation. Dopaminergic therapy is well tolerated by most patients with RLS, particularly because the dosages that are prescribed are significantly lower than those typically used with Parkinson's disease (PD) patients. The primary limitation for the long-term usage of dopaminergic therapy in the chronic illness of RLS is augmentation. This chapter reviews the efficacy, adverse events (AE), and long-term experience with various dopaminergic agents in patients with RLS.

## PROPOSED THERAPEUTIC ACTION

Dopamine receptors are categorized into two classes, D1-like receptors and D2-like receptors, based upon activity. In 1979, Kebabian and Calne discussed the effect of dopamine on the binding to these two receptors and their subtypes (20). D1-like receptors include subtype D1 receptors, which are primarily found in the nigrostriatum and cortex, and subtype D5 receptors that are principally found in the hippocampus and enterorhinal cortex. The D1 and D5 receptors activate adenylate cyclase through the $G_s$-coupled mechanism. The D2-like receptor includes the subtypes D2, D3, and D4 that were identified by cloning and homologic techniques. These inhibit cyclic adenosine monophosphate (cAMP) production through the $G_i$-coupled mechanism. D2 and D3 subtypes are found in the highest concentrations in the mesolimbic tract, while the D2 subtype receptors also show high activity in the nigrostriatum. The D4 subtype is rather broadly distributed with slightly higher concentrations in the cortex. Table 1 summarizes the distribution of the receptor subtypes in the central nervous system (CNS).

The etiologic mechanism of RLS and its relationship to specific dopamine receptor activity remain unknown. However, the consistent therapeutic response to selective dopaminergic therapy suggests dysregulation of dopamine as the most likely etiologic mechanism. D2 subtype receptors are the most actively investigated (21). The probable site of action is within the central nervous system rather than within the peripheral nervous system. Brain involvement best explains the four core symptoms of primary RLS, although spinal mechanisms appear to generate periodic limb movements (PLM) (22). Current investigations of iron and RLS speculate that

**TABLE 1** Dopamine Receptor Subtypes and Their Distribution in the Brain

| Class | Subtype | Mesolimbic | Nigrostriatum | Hippocampus | Cortex | Enterorhinal cortex |
|---|---|---|---|---|---|---|
| D2-like | D-2 | +++ | +++ | | | |
| | D-3 | +++ | + | + | + | + |
| | D-4 | ++ | + | ++ | +++ | ++ |
| D1-like | D-1 | +/– | +++ | + | +++ | + |
| | D-5 | + | +/– | +++ | + | +++ |

iron interacts with dopamine to precipitate RLS symptoms (23). The therapeutic response to opiates has also been suggested to arise from their ability to upregulate central dopaminergic activity. Naloxone, an opioid antagonist, does not block the therapeutic effect of dopaminergic medications (4). In contrast, a dopamine antagonist will block the therapeutic effects of opioids, suggesting that opioids require dopaminergic systems to improve RLS symptoms (24). However, neither dopamine antagonists nor opioid antagonists markedly worsen untreated RLS (25). Therefore, this relationship remains unclear.

Agonists of dopamine receptor subtypes D2 and D3 are consistently associated with therapeutic improvement in RLS (26). D2–D3 agonists represent the principal agents in use to improve the four core symptoms of RLS, whereas isolated D1 agonist drugs are much less abundant and have not been tested in patients with RLS. It is not known whether the D2 subtype or the D3 subtype is more important.

## PHARMACOLOGY OF COMMON DOPAMINERGIC AGENTS

Levodopa is the immediate precursor of dopamine. It is usually given with either carbidopa or benserazide. These compounds inhibit the peripheral metabolism of levodopa to dopamine by inhibiting l-aromatic acid decarboxylase. Dopamine in the periphery cannot easily cross the blood–brain barrier to the brain, and increased nausea results. More recently the carbonic-O-methyl transferase inhibitors entacapone and tolcapone have also been used to inhibit peripheral levodopa metabolism and thus funnel more levodopa into the brain.

Dopamine agonists can be segregated by whether or not they are ergotamine based. The ergotamine derivative dopamine agonists, bromocriptine, pergolide, and cabergoline have received active investigation for RLS. Bromocriptine is a weaker, primarily D2 receptor agonist, while cabergoline and pergolide prove to be potent agonists of the D1, D2, and D3 receptor subtypes. The therapeutic activity of nonergotamine agonists, pramipexole and ropinirole, both show high affinity for D2 and D3 receptors and very low affinities for D1 receptors.

Table 2 lists the pharmacological properties of common dopaminergic agonists that have been studied as RLS treatments. Levodopa has a more rapid onset of action in the immediate release formulation but has the shortest half-life of any dopaminergic agents. The controlled release form of levodopa extends this somewhat. Ropinirole has approximately a one-hour onset to action and a six-hour half-life. Propensity to augmentation, however, is much less with ropinirole. Pramipexole takes approximately two hours to reach a therapeutic serum level but sustains benefit for 8 to 10 hours. The longer-acting dopamine agonists such as pergolide and cabergoline offer some therapeutic advantages for the patient

**TABLE 2** Pharmacological Properties of Common Dopaminergic Agents for Restless Legs Syndrome

| Agent | Dosing range in RLS | Time to peak plasma level (minutes) | Half-life (hours) | Mode of elimination |
|---|---|---|---|---|
| Levodopa | 100–400 mg/day | 30 | 1.5–3 | Hepatic |
| C/L dopa ER | 150–500 mg/day | 120 | 6–8 | Hepatic |
| Bromocriptine | 2.5–10 mg/day | 45–60 | 3–4 (up to 40) | Hepatic |
| Pergolide | 0.1–0.75 mg/day | 60 (est.) | 27 | Renal |
| Cabergoline | 0.25–3.0 mg | 120 | 63–68 | Hepatic |
| Pramipexole | 0.25–1.5 mg/day | 120 | 8–12 | Renal |
| Ropinirole | 0.5–4.0 mg/day | 60–120 | ~6 | Hepatic |

*Abbreviation*: ER, extended release.

with severe RLS with all-day symptoms, but they are initially associated with a higher degree of side effects, necessitating a more gradual upward titration of therapy. Pretreatment to prevent nausea with peripheral acting dopamine antagonists such as domperidone (Motilium®) may mitigate some AE. Table 3 describes the proposed prescribing recommendations for the most commonly used dopaminergic agents.

AE are a class effect, appearing consistently across dopaminergic agents. All dopaminergic medications commonly produce gastrointestinal (GI) side effects of dyspepsia, nausea, and vomiting during initial exposure. The GI side effects are transient, often resolving over a few days. Discontinuation of dopaminergic therapy may be required in 5% to 10% of patients experiencing GI upset. GI side effects are best managed with antinausea therapy such as domperidone taking the medicines with food and a more gradual titration of the dopaminergic agent. Occasional side effects include headache, joint or muscular aches, insomnia,

**TABLE 3** Proposed Dosing Regimen for Bedtime Restless Legs Syndrome

| Agent | Initial dose (p.o.) (mg) | | Dosage timing | Each dose adjustment | Recommended maximum dose (mg) |
|---|---|---|---|---|---|
| Levodopa (+ inhibitor) | 100 mg | 1/2–1 | 0.5 hour | 1 q 3d | 300 (total) |
| Levodopa ER (+ inhibitor) | 100 mg | 1 | 2 hr before h.s. | 1 q 3d earlier pm | 300 (total) |
| Bromocriptine | 2.5 mg | 1/2–1 | 1 hour | 1/2 supper and h.s. q 3d | 20 |
| Pergolide | 0.05 mg | 1 | Supper and/ or h.s. | 1 q 2–3d | 1–2 |
| Cabergoline | 0.5 mg | 1/2; | Supper | 1/2; to 1 q wk | 1–3 |
| Pramipexole | 0.125 | 1 | 2 hr before h.s. | 1 q 2–3 d | 1.5–3 |
| Ropinirole | 0.25 | 1 | 1–2 hr before h.s. | 1 q 2–3 d | 3–6 |

*Note*: If restless legs syndrome (RLS) symptoms present earlier in the evening or in the late afternoon, medication should be dosed at the indicated dosage timing, but substitute the typical time of day that the RLS symptoms present rather than use just h.s. dosing. (For example, symptoms presenting at 6:00 P.M. in a patient who is to receive ropinirole would result in a recommended initial 0.25 mg tablet at 5:00 P.M. and another 0.25 mg tablet one hour before bedtime with the maximum daily dose not to exceed 3 to 6 mg.)

somnolence, edema, etc. Edema is quite underrecognized, because it usually occurs months or even years after initiation of therapy. The etiology of dopaminergic edema is unknown, and no clear risk factors have been established (27).

In general, the lower doses of dopaminergics required to treat RLS, and the different disease pathology, produce less serious side effects than when dopaminergics are used to manage PD. In particular, the serious side effect of sudden onset of sleep is associated with dopaminergic therapy for PD patients (28). It appears that PD is the primary reason for daytime sleepiness on dopaminergic agents, because the combined presence of RLS in patients with PD does not alter daytime sleepiness according to the Epworth sleepiness scale (29). Daytime sleepiness does not worsen when dopaminergics are used to treat RLS, instead, it usually tends to improve (29a). Organic psychosis that manifests primarily as visual hallucinations is very common in PD patients treated with dopamine agonists but is almost completely absent in RLS. Likewise, orthostatic hypotension is a much less common adverse event in RLS. Finally, increased impulsivity such as gambling and spending more money, has been seen with dopamine agonists. This also appears to be less common with RLS than PD (29b). The long-term consequences of augmentation and fibrotic injury are discussed later in the chapter.

## Levodopa

Akpinar in 1982 (30) and then Montplaisir (31) offered the initial reports that levodopa improved leg restlessness, movements, and sleep in patients with RLS. The excellent results encouraged further research.

Von Scheele compared levodopa plus benserazide to a lactose pill and reported that 17 of 20 RLS patients chose levodopa over placebo for its benefits (3). Akpinar went on to complete a double-blind, placebo-controlled trial of levodopa in 13 patients (4) that established a statistically significant improvement in subjective sleep parameters. Brodeur et al. showed a similar subjective improvement in six RLS patients in a double-blind, placebo-controlled study of levodopa while offering the first description of the suggested immobilization test (SIT) to objectively evaluate PLM when awake (5).

Long-term therapy with levodopa in 30 Swedish RLS patients (32) and 47 American patients (33) indicated sustained benefit of therapy for six months or longer in 70% to 80% of the patients. Only two patients in the Swedish group ended therapy because of significant side effects, primarily nausea. In the American study, eight of 49 patients experienced nausea or other side effects, and a total of five did not continue because of side effects. Although the term "augmentation" had not yet been coined, both long-term studies reported that approximately one-third of the sample received progressive increases in their dosing of levodopa, with the American study indicating that eight of 47 patients developed rebound morning restlessness while taking the short-acting formulation of levodopa/carbidopa. Becker and colleagues described a mean nightly dose of levodopa of 160 mg in 33 of 47 patients who continued on therapy for nine months.

In 1993, Guilleminault et al. published the first paper that described in detail the rebound phenomena of dopaminergic therapy, principally the use of levodopa, in 20 RLS patients (34). Both short- and long-term formulations of carbidopa/levodopa demonstrated a propensity to worsen symptoms in the early morning because the serum level of medication fell over the night, and the intensity of the restlessness complaint in the hours before bedtime increased. The "rebound" phenomena could be managed by initiating a dosage of levodopa just prior to or at the time of symptom onset. Later, this phenomenon was subsumed under the term "augmentation." Rebound now refers to the early morning wearing-off associated with serum levels.

Studies support the high initial therapeutic response to levodopa in secondary cases of RLS. Sandyk demonstrated that levodopa could lessen the complaints of leg restlessness in uremic patients who are undergoing hemodialysis (35). Trenkwalder et al. subsequently completed a comparative study of levodopa and placebo in 11 uremic patients with secondary RLS and 17 idiopathic RLS patients, reporting clinical and statistical significant improvement in RLS and sleep parameters for both patient groups as well as reductions in the frequency of PLM during sleep at doses of 100 to 200 mg of levodopa (36).

Numerous subsequent studies have evaluated different preparations of levodopa and compared this to other RLS treatments. The largest double-blind, placebo-controlled, multicenter crossover trial included 32 German patients with moderate to severe RLS, and demonstrated immediate response to therapy from levodopa (6). In a small double-blind, placebo-controlled trial, levodopa proved superior to propoxyphene in suppressing symptomatic complaints and PLM (37). Additional studies have further confirmed a 70% to 90% initial therapeutic response of the standard formulation of levodopa, longer duration of the therapeutic benefit of the slow-release formulation of levodopa (38), the efficacy of levodopa for RLS associated with hemodialysis (39), and the complications of augmentation and rebound of RLS with levodopa (40). Response to levodopa has even been proposed as a method to confirm the diagnosis of RLS (41). Stiasny-Kolster et al. recently reported that a single dose of 100 mg L-dopa improved RLS by at least 50% in 80–88% of subjects, but that no subjects without RLS improved (41a). Therefore the specificity of the L-dopa test was 100%. Overall 83–90% of subjects could be diagnosed based exclusively on the L-dopa challenge test. Levodopa is labeled for the treatment of RLS in Germany and Switzerland.

### Bromocriptine

Bromocriptine, an ergot derivative, was tested at the same time that levodopa became a common therapy for RLS. Akpinar described its use in 1987 against placebo in three RLS patients (4). The first double-blind, placebo-controlled crossover study of bromocriptine 7.5 mg at bedtime in RLS was reported in 1988 by Walters et al., and showed that five of six patients received a mild-to-moderate reduction in symptomatology, and a 40% to 50% reduction in the frequency of PLM during sleep (42). Case reports show that bromocriptine has also improved RLS symptoms (43). As is true for other ergot derivatives, bromocriptine has been associated with the infrequent but serious complication of fibrosis of soft tissues that results in pleuropulmonary complications, pericarditis, and valvular heart disease (44–46). Because bromocriptine has a relatively low affinity for the dopamine receptors, its reduced potency results in less usage as a therapy for RLS compared to the newer, higher potency dopamine receptor agonists.

### Pergolide

Pergolide is an ergotamine derivative that is active at the D2 and D3 receptor subtypes. It is a potent dopamine receptor agonist that shows a fairly rapid onset of action and an extended half-life of up to 20 hours. The first report of the therapeutic benefit of pergolide was an open-label study completed by Earley and Allen in patients with fairly severe RLS who had been taking levodopa (47). Because approximately 70% of the 51 patients experienced augmentation on levodopa, the alternative therapy of pergolide was offered. By the study end, 39% of levodopa patients remained on therapy, while 50% had been changed to pergolide that was given at supper time and bedtime at doses ranging from 0.05 to 0.25 mg. This initial study reported a reduced incidence of side effects of pergolide with only 15% of the patients reporting symptoms consistent with augmentation. It should be noted that patients received prior treatment with domperidone 10 mg po tid (unavailable in the United States) at the first sign of nausea, the most common side effect with pergolide.

In a German study by Staedt et al., initial efficacy of pergolide 0.125 mg and short-acting levodopa 250 mg in combination with carbidopa was evaluated in 11 patients who received 16 days of alternating night randomized therapy with either agent with a washout period between treatment arms (8). The final doses averaged 0.16 mg pergolide and 363 mg of levodopa. Pergolide demonstrated superiority in therapeutic response (9 of 11 patients reported relief or near relief of symptoms) when compared to levodopa (1 of 11 received complete relief). Pergolide also showed a more significant reduction of PLM during sleep (79% vs. 45%, $p < 0.001$) and increased total sleep time (421 minutes vs. 325 minutes, $p < 0.05$) when compared to levodopa. Pergolide was associated with significant nausea in nine patients, which was relieved with domperidone. In a randomized, double-blind, placebo-controlled study of eight subjects, Earley and Allen reported significant improvements of RLS with pergolide offered in early evening and one hour before bedtime, compared to placebo. Side effects were considered mild to moderate by the authors and did not necessitate the discontinuance of pergolide (7). In a larger placebo-controlled trial of pergolide in 30 medication-free patients with idiopathic RLS, a single evening dose that reached a mean of 0.5 mg two hours before bedtime proved superior to placebo by reducing symptomatic complaints, increasing total sleep time, and reducing PLM during sleep (9). Again, domperidone was used to reduce peripheral dopaminergic side effects, resulting in good tolerance. As an extension of the polysomnographic study, the same group was followed in a one-year, open-label, continuation study (48). Pergolide was continued at a mean dose of 0.37 mg daily by 79% of 28 patients who reported satisfaction with the therapy. Six patients discontinued medication, with the most common reason being augmentation.

A large multicenter double-blind, placebo-controlled trial in 100 patients documented the therapeutic response of pergolide over six weeks of therapy, followed by an open-label extension for one year (10). Pergolide at 0.25 to 0.75 mg two hours before bedtime proved superior to placebo in reductions of the international restless less syndrome rating scale (IRLS) and the frequency of arousals related to PLM during sleep. Sleep efficiency as measured by polysomnography was unchanged, although at the one-year follow-up, sleep onset and sleep efficiency remained improved according to patient reports, and sleep testing continued to show reductions in PLM during sleep and associated arousals. The principal side effects were headaches and nausea.

Successful use of pergolide requires initiation at the lowest dose of 0.05 mg and will be facilitated by pretreatment with a peripheral-acting dopamine antagonist such as domperidone. Because domperidone is not available in the United States, some experts have advocated the usage of Zofran® to manage the nausea that occurs with pergolide. There remains concern that significant fibrotic consequences can arise with the use of ergotamine derivatives such as pergolide in a small but significant number of patients (49). Most recently, heart valve fibrosis has been reported; however, it is debated whether this is an ergotamine effect or is related to serotoninergic effects (50–52). Large clinical trials of pergolide as an RLS treatment in the United States are not expected.

### Cabergoline

Cabergoline is a potent D2 dopamine agonist with a half-life of around 60 hours that is used to suppress prolactin-secreting hypothalamic tumors. In 2000, Stiasny et al. evaluated the open-label benefits of cabergoline in nine idiopathic RLS patients who remained symptomatic while being treated with levodopa (53). Five patients continued on levodopa during the early phase of therapy. All patients were pretreated with domperidone 20 mg po tid that was later tapered and discontinued without recurrence of nausea. Over the 12 weeks, patients showed an excellent therapeutic response from cabergoline at a mean dose of 2.1 mg, with a significant improvement in polysomnographic measures of total sleep time, PLM during sleep, associated arousals, and sleep efficiency. Augmentation from previous use of levodopa resolved.

Zucconi et al. reported on 12 moderate-to-severe RLS patients treated in an open-label study over two months (54). Actigraphy was used to assess sleep and movements. Ten patients completed the trial at a mean dose of cabergoline of 1.1 mg with clinically significant reductions in subjective parameters of RLS as measured by the IRLS, as well as on actigraphic movements at the end of two months of therapy. Nine of the patients continued for 12 months on cabergoline without significant side effects, including no reports of augmentation. A small open label Japanese study also showed good improvement on the IRLS at 1 mg. (54a).

Stiasny-Kolster et al. reported the efficacy of cabergoline compared to placebo in a large multicenter, double-blind trial that was completed on 85 patients with moderate-to-severe RLS who were assessed with the RLS-6, IRLS, and a questionnaire about sleep (19). On the primary measure, RLS-6, the three test dosages of cabergoline 0.5, 1, and 2 mg produced significant reductions of RLS symptoms at bedtime and during the day. All measures of efficacy showed positive change. An open-label extension allowed for observation over a mean of 47 weeks. About 78% of the patients continued on cabergoline at a mean dose of 2.2 mg. From the study beginning to the end of open-label extension, 11 of the 85 patients discontinued therapy because of AE, two of whom had obvious augmentation and four had probable mild augmentation.

A long-term study of cabergoline was completed at 37 centers in Germany on 302 RLS patients with moderate-to-severe symptoms (55). At the mean follow-up of six months, 82% of the patients continued on cabergoline at a mean dose of 1.5 mg daily. As a group, the patients showed significant improvement in their IRLS and RLS-6, as well as subjective sleep parameters. Initial side effects of nausea, dizziness, headache, and others were experienced by 48% of the sample, but therapy continued in over 94% of the patients, because the AE were mild and transient. In 5% of the 302 patients, RLS symptoms worsened, another 6% had a poor response, and 3% were reported to experience augmentation.

Recently a large multicenter European study compared 2 to 3 mg of cabergoline (Cabaseril®, Pfizer) versus 200 to 300 mg of levodopa (56). Patients were initially titrated to the lower dose but could increase to the higher dose if needed. The study evaluated short-term efficacy after four weeks of a stable dose (six or eight weeks) with IRLS and other measures. Long-term efficacy concentrated on time of discontinuation due to either augmentation or lack of efficacy. In the cabergoline group, 148/178 (83.1%) remained on the lower dose, whereas only 102/183 (55.7%) of the levodopa group remained on the lower dose ($p < 0.001$). Initial IRLS improvement strongly favored cabergoline ($15.6 \pm 10.8$ vs. $8.8 \pm 10.7$, $p < 0.001$). Long-term discontinuation rates also favored cabergoline: lack of efficacy discontinued (3.9% cabergoline vs. 9.8% levodopa, $p < 0.05$) and augmentation discontinued (7.9% cabergoline vs. 14.2% levodopa, $p < 0.05$). AE were somewhat higher in the cabergoline group (total related AE 68.0% vs. 50.3%) but were consistent with other dopaminergic medications.

Long-term studies indicate that cabergoline is well tolerated by the majority of patients after an adjustment phase, principally with complaints of nausea, during the first weeks of therapy. It is of note that daytime sleepiness has not been a significant complaint in these long-term trials. Pulmonary and cardiac fibrosis with cabergoline may be a serious adverse event in a small number of patients as is the case for any of the ergotamine derivatives.

### Pramipexole

Over the last five years, the nonergot derivatives have become the more commonly used agents for the treatment of RLS. Pramipexole, a nonergotamine D2–D3 subtype receptor agonist, has seen increasing use since open-label reports of efficacy for RLS in 1998. Lin et al. treated 16 patients who had insufficient therapeutic response to prior therapies for RLS (57). At a mean dose of 0.3 mg over two to three months of therapy, 60% to 75% of the patients showed improvements in the typical symptoms of RLS. In the same year, Becker et al. reported on their experience of 23 previously treated patients with moderate to severe RLS with an early version of IRLS (58). Nineteen patients showed significant reductions in their ratings of restless legs symptoms, and 17 of the 19 indicated a preference for pramipexole over any prior therapy. Over the three months of treatment, one patient developed augmentation. The side effects of sleepiness and dyspepsia were considered quite mild, resulting in no discontinuation of therapy.

Montplaisir et al. first reported a double-blind, placebo-controlled trial of pramipexole in 1999 (11). Their own RLS scale improved by 87% compared to 29% on placebo. A suggested immobilization test (SIT) also significantly improved. Polysomnographic testing was included in 10 RLS patients who were treated for one month. Although total sleep time did not improve, PLM during sleep dramatically improved from a mean of 60 to 1 per hour on drug at the nightly dosage of 0.75 to 1.5 mg. Subsequently, seven of the 10 patients were followed for a mean of 7.8 months and continued to show an excellent response without significant AE (59). Saletu et al. provided further evidence of pramipexole efficacy in 11 RLS patients who received standard subjective measures and polysomnography to compare the effects of pramipexole to placebo over one month of therapy (12). At a mean dosage of 0.27 mg, pramipexole was superior to placebo in improvements of objective and subjective sleep quality, PLM during sleep, and reports of RLS symptoms. Daytime function, including assessment of subjective sleepiness with the Epworth Sleepiness Scale, demonstrated modest improvement.

Partinen et al. reported a three-week, double-blind, placebo-controlled, single-center, comprehensive polysomnographic study of 109 RLS patients (60).

The primary endpoint was reduction in periodic limb movements during time in bed index (PLMI), and secondary endpoints included RLS severity score (IRLS), and the Clinical Global Impression Improvement Scale (CGI-I). They found a significant dose-dependent improvement in both PLMI and IRLS between 0.125 and 0.5 mg. Overall, the 0.75 mg dose was not superior to the 0.5 mg dose.

Oertel et al. presented data from a 345-patient, six-week, placebo-controlled trial, followed by a 46-week open-label phase (61). Patients were randomized 2:1 to pramipexole at a dose titrated from 0.125 to 0.75 mg per night. At the end of six weeks, the IRLS improved by a mean of 12.4 points on drug compared to 5.8 points on placebo, $p < 0.0001$. AE during the controlled and open-label portions were mild and predictable.

Winkelman et al. presented another large trial evaluating three doses of pramipexole (0.25, 0.5, and 0.75 mg) compared to placebo in a double-blind, fixed dose, parallel group design (62). The study evaluated mean change from baseline to end of study in the IRLS and CGI-I scale score at week 12, assessed by different raters. Weeks one to four were used to up-titrate patients to their randomized dose group. Patients were then on maintenance treatment from week five at the latest dose to the end of the study. Three hundred and forty-five patients (129 male, 38%) were randomized to treatment, and 339 patients could be analyzed. Pramipexole produced significantly greater improvements than placebo in IRLS total score at week 12 in all dose groups (adjusted mean change from baseline, placebo −9.3, pramipexole 0.25 mg −12.8; $p = 0.0086$, pramipexole 0.5 mg −13.8; $p = 0.0011$, pramipexole 0.75 mg −14; $p = 0.0005$). Similarly, pramipexole treatment was associated with significantly greater improvement than placebo in CGI-I scores as measured by the percentage of patients meeting the criterion for a responder (much/very much improved): placebo 51.2%; pramipexole 0.25 mg 74.7%; $p = 0.0005$, pramipexole 0.5 mg 67.9%; $p = 0.0484$, pramipexole 0.75 mg 72.9%; $p = 0.0038$. Pramipexole was generally well tolerated. The most frequent AEs were nausea (19%), headache 17.8%, RLS 12.8%, insomnia 10.5%, somnolence 10.1%, dizziness 9.7%, nasopharyngitis 6.6%, and fatigue 5%. Two patients reported an episode of sudden onset of sleep with pramipexole, one patient with placebo.

Two open-label studies have been completed to look at the long-term effectiveness of pramipexole over one or two years of use (63,64). Both studies supported the continuing efficacy of pramipexole with limited side effects. Mild-to-moderate augmentation was noted in up to 35% of the pramipexole-treated patients. Augmentation could often be well managed by adding a second dosage of medication in the late afternoon or early evening. The authors of both studies were of the opinion that the degree of augmentation was less than is typical for patients treated with levodopa. Other side effects of interest included dyspepsia, headache, fluid retention, and insomnia. Although the nonergotamine derivatives appear to present little risk for the development of fibrosis as had been noted for ergotamines, a recent paper by Chaudhuri raises questions that will need to be considered about the long-term fibrotic consequences of nonergotamine agents (46).

### Ropinirole

Ropinirole is labeled for the treatment of RLS in the United States and is the most studied agent for the treatment of RLSs, with over 3000 subjects having participated in various trials around the world (14,16,64a,64b,64c). Ondo first reported an open-label study showing the efficacy and favorable side effect profile in 16

RLS patients who received ropinirole at a mean dose of 2.8 mg per day (65). Small-scale sleep laboratory studies of ropinirole and placebo groups further documented the efficacy of ropinirole therapy (13,15,18,66,67).

The first of three similarly designed large-scale, multicenter trials to be published included 284 moderate-to-severe patients from 10 countries who met National Institutes of Health (NIH) consensus criteria for RLS and were not receiving any other RLS or sleep therapy (14). The study consisted of a double-blind, placebo-controlled, protocol-defined flexible dosing comparison of ropinirole 0.5 to 4.0 mg and placebo. Dosage increased from 0.25 to 0.5 mg over the first week, then increased by 0.5 mg increments on a weekly basis, until it was felt that dosage was optimized. Over the 12-week trial, ropinirole showed superiority over placebo as early as the first week of therapy, although both groups showed clinically significant reductions of symptoms throughout the 12-week trial. Utilizing last-observation-carried-forward methodology, this large sample of patients showed that ropinirole produced a 33% greater reduction of baseline ratings on the IRLS over placebo.

A subsequent multicenter study that was conducted in North America on 267 patients utilizing a similar protocol demonstrated essentially the same results with improvements in patient ratings, clinician impression of change, and the patient's self-ratings of quality of life (16). The mean dosage of ropinirole in both studies was 1.9 mg. AE were typically mild and temporary when compared to placebo, showing a higher incidence of nausea, lightheadedness, and body aches. Less than 3% of the patients ended participation in the research trials because of AE.

A third almost identical trial of 372 patients conducted in the United States showed a similar treatment effect (64b). Interestingly, both the placebo response and the drug response were somewhat greater in this study.

A recent ropinirole trial employed twice-daily dosage, up to a maximum of 3 mg in the late afternoon and 3 mg at night (68). The entry IRLS scores were somewhat more severe (mean 26.0) than the previous trials. The mean daily dose for the 178 ropinirole patients was $3.1 \pm 1.9$ mg versus $4.4 \pm 1.9$ mg for the 189 placebo patients. The IRLS improved by 15.6 versus 11.4 on placebo. AE were generally mild with only 3% of ropinirole patients dropping out because of AE. The somewhat greater treatment response supports the role of individualized dosing.

Another placebo-controlled withdrawal study of ropinirole demonstrated the expected worsening of RLS in those who were relegated to placebo, but there were no unexpected AE or rebound exacerbation, and in fact, the mean IRLS were still better than prior to their baseline before ever receiving ropinirole (64c).

Recently, Leibowitz and Black systematically evaluated ropinirole in patients with mild-to-moderate RLS who require only intermittent dosing (Black, personal communication). Twenty-one patients completed the 12-week open-label testing period. The IRLS-scale score decreased from $17.9 \pm 5.1$ (range 6–27) at baseline to $14.9 \pm 3.2$ (range 9–20; $p < 0.01$) at 12 weeks, and mean RLS visual analogus score decreased from a baseline of $44.3 \pm 20.6$ (range 14–89) to $29.3 \pm 13.4$ (range 6–55, $p < 0.01$). Several secondary endpoints also improved. The dose of ropinirole was $0.50 \pm 0.4$ (range 0.125–2.0), and dosing frequency was $3.3 \pm 1.5$ (range 1–9) doses per week. Somnolence (11.1%), nausea (7.4%), disturbed sleep (25.9%), and headache (18.5%) were the most commonly reported AE, and no other serious AE, occurred. They felt that ropinirole was effective when used as pro re nata (prn) basis for the treatment of mild and/or intermittent RLS symptoms.

In a ropinirole trial that included polysomnographic testing, 65 patients underwent comprehensive diagnostic polysomnography to assess the sleep changes related to ropinirole versus placebo (17). In the 59 patients who had valid data after 12 weeks of therapy, PLM during sleep showed a reduction in the ropinirole group (mean dose of 1.8 mg) from 48 per hour to 12 per hour, while the placebo group showed a minor change from 36 to 34 per hour ($p < 0.0001$). A similar significant change in PLM when awake was also noted, and arousals associated with sleep-related leg movements were robustly and statistically reduced by ropinirole. Sleep onset latency was improved as was the amount of stage-II sleep, but there was only a trend toward improvement of total sleep time and sleep efficiency.

Overall, these studies demonstrated superior efficacy with modest AE. In fact, the total dropout rates were identical for drug and placebo. Nausea was by far the most common AE, but in most cases resolved within four days of any dose (69). It could return upon dose increase. As has been true for other clinical trials that have been reported for RLS, the high placebo response requires that controls be utilized to assess efficacy. In the four large placebo-controlled parallel trials, this placebo response may have been further augmented by the large number of scheduled dose increases, each resulting in additional placebo improvement. Overall, the percentage of placebo patients that increased eight times up to the maximum dose was much higher in those taking placebo (48% vs. 22%) than those taking drug. Trials with a controlled extended release preparation of ropinirole are ongoing. Both 12 hour and 24 hour formulation are in preparation.

## INVESTIGATIONAL DOPAMINE AGONISTS

Other dopamine agonists have shown efficacy in generally small-scale or preliminary studies. Rotigotine, a nonergotamine patch preparation, was studied in 63 RLS patients during a one-week proof-of-principle study to test the initial response and tolerability of therapy (70). Rotigotine was administered daily at 1.125, 2.25, 4.5 mg and placebo patch in treatment groups of approximately 15 subjects each. In a dose-dependent manner, the ratings on the IRLS showed improvement of two points, four points, and eight points at the respective rotigotine doses over placebo response. Only the 4.5 mg dosage was statistically significant over placebo at $p < 0.01$.

A double-blind, six-arm, parallel group, randomized, placebo-controlled dose-finding study with the rotigotine patch enrolled 371 subjects at 34 centers in Austria, Germany, and Spain (71). Patients were treated with 1.125, 2.25, 4.5, 6.75, or 9 mg rotigotine/day or placebo in a seven-week trial. The primary efficacy measure was the IRLS, and secondary measures included CGI, RLS-6, and a RLS quality of life scale. The baseline IRLS total score of the 340 randomized patients (age $58 \pm 10$ years, 70% females) was $27.9 \pm 6.0$. The adjusted mean changes from baseline to week 6 in the IRLS total score were: placebo −9.2 points, 1.125 mg −10.6 points; 2.25 mg −15.1 points; 4.5 mg −15.7 points; 6.75 mg, −17.5 points; 9 mg, −14.8 points. The treatment difference was significant for all rotigotine doses except the 1.125 mg dose. Comparable results were found with CGI and RLS-6 scales. The most common AE (incidence greater than or equal to 5% in a treatment group) were application site reaction, nausea, fatigue, influenza-like symptoms, and headache. Three placebo-treated patients and 12 rotigotine-treated patients discontinued prematurely due to an AE. The most frequent reasons were GI symptoms (nausea, vomiting) in six patients and skin reactions in four patients.

Aside from skin reactions, the AE profile of rotigotine was generally consistent with oral dopamine agonists.

There is interest in rotigotine in view of its ability to sustain therapeutic blood levels throughout 24 hours, potentially of significant value for the most severe patients, and in those having shown augmentation to shorter-acting agents. Additional multicenter-controlled trials are ongoing.

Apomorphine, a potent, short-acting parentally administered dopamine agonist used for rescue therapy in PD, has been tested as a therapy for RLS. Reuter et al. first reported improvement in two patients with RLS (72). Tribl et al. tested intravenous apomorphine in nine patients with moderate-to-severe disease after pretreatment with domperidone to lessen nausea and vomiting (73). Challenge to the therapeutic response was then tested with the opioid antagonist naloxone or D2 antagonist metoclopramide. Visual analogue ratings by patients and measurement of periodic limb movement of wake (PLMW) on a modified daytime suggested immobilization test (SIT) showed significant reductions in both parameters with apomorphine and maintenance of benefit upon challenge with a trend to increased periodic limb movements with metoclopramide administration. Apomorphine may not prove to be a practical solution for RLS due to its very short half-life but may have a role as a rescue therapy.

Research in the management of RLS is ongoing with other agents that enhance dopaminergic action. Entacapone has extended the benefit of levodopa (74). D2 agonists or partial agonists such as terguride (75), talipexole (76), alpha-dihydroergocriptine (77), and piribedil (78), have shown reductions in RLS symptoms in open-label trials of short duration. Both oral and a transdermal patch of lisuride have also shown efficacy (78a, 78b). More investigation, however, is required before any of these agents could be recommended for therapeutic consideration for RLS.

## AUGMENTATION DUE TO DOPAMINERGIC THERAPY

Augmentation (discussed in detail in Chapter 26) represents the primary impediment to successful long-term therapy with dopaminergic agents. Rebound restlessness and increased daytime symptoms were first recognized with the use of levodopa (34). The term "augmentation" in patients treated with levodopa was first reported in the literature in 1996 (40). The consensus definition of "augmentation" is listed in Table 4 and was derived at an NIH conference in 2003 (41).

Augmentation is most problematic with levodopa. Treatment with levodopa results in augmentation in up to 80% of RLS patients (40). Long-term studies with dopamine agonists suggest a rate of augmentation between 15% and 40% of RLS

**TABLE 4** Definition of Augmentation

| |
|---|
| Key feature: two hours or greater shift in RLS symptoms compared to baseline and/or |
| Increased intensity with increased dose |
| Decreased intensity with decreased dose |
| Shorter latency to the onset of symptoms as compared to baseline |
| Urge to move expands to other limbs or body parts |
| Duration of benefit is shorter than at baseline |
| Periodic limb movements when awake appear or worsen |

*Abbreviation*: RLS, restless legs syndrome.
*Source*: From Ref. 39.

patients (7,63,64,79). Garcia-Borreguerra has opined that dopamine agonists produce a lower propensity and milder presentation of augmentation than levodopa (80). Studies with pergolide (7) and cabergoline (8) suggest that the longer-acting agents lessen the risk for augmentation. As the onset to augmentation appears to take many months with dopamine agonists, it is necessary to monitor the risks of augmentation for up to 18 months before having confidence that the problem will not impact continued dopaminergic therapy.

Management of augmentation depends upon the agent (2). The goal of any RLS therapeutic intervention is to initiate effective treatment prior to symptom onset. Applying this strategy to levodopa often results in a cycle of escalation of dosage and further augmentation that becomes very distressing for the patient. Augmentation that is related to levodopa therapy is best managed by changing to a dopamine agonist such as pramipexole or ropinirole. When dopamine agonists result in augmentation, earlier dosing is often sufficient to help manage the symptom. Some would advocate consideration of pergolide or cabergoline because of their long half-lives (7,8), but the concern for side effects, particularly for ergotamine-derived fibrosis, might raise some concern about the long-term use of these therapies. If continued earlier shift of RLS symptoms occurs with the earlier dosage of the dopamine agonist, a change in therapeutic class would be recommended. Options include gabapentin or opiates. In particularly severe RLS patients, the use of high-potency, long-acting opiates such as methadone have been demonstrated to be of benefit (81).

## CONCLUSION

The etiology of RLS remains unknown. Although medical research continues on pathophysiologic mechanisms, clinical research has established the benefit of dopaminergic therapy for RLS, and practice guidelines consider dopaminergic agents to be the first-line therapy for patients with moderate-to-severe symptoms. Levodopa as an RLS treatment has been used for over 20 years in controlled clinical trials and long-term follow-up studies. The primary limitation to the ongoing use of levodopa is its high rate of augmentation that requires escalating doses that eventually worsen overall symptoms. Dopamine agonists have proven efficacious in both short and longer trials that have included the largest number of patients under controlled conditions. Ropinirole is the first Food and Drug Administration (FDA)-approved medication in the United States for the treatment of RLS with the expectation that other dopamine agonists such as pramipexole and rotigotine will also receive approval over the next few years. Cabergoline, pergolide, and rotigotine may offer particular advantage in severe patients who need therapy earlier in the day, as they offer medication coverage for 20 or more hours. AE, particularly nausea, are usual transient and manageable to the patient. Daytime sleepiness is an infrequent side effect of therapy, and sudden onsets of sleep have not been systematically demonstrated at the dosages of dopamine agonists that are currently recommended for RLS patients. Long-term issues with agonists include augmentation that appears of lesser severity than levodopa. There remains concern that the ergotamine derivatives (and still a question for nonergotamine derivatives) produce abnormal fibrosis of pleura, pericardium, cardiac valves, or perineum in some patients. There is no current data for clinicians to judge whether one agent is superior to another as to efficacy in the management of a specific or different groups of patients, leaving the choice of therapeutic agent to the experience of the clinician.

## REFERENCES


1. Littner MR, Kushida C, Anderson WM, et al. Standards of Practice Committee of the American Academy of Sleep Medicine. Practice parameters for the dopaminergic treatment of restless legs syndrome and periodic limb movement disorder. Sleep 2004; 27(3):557–559.
2. Silber MH, Ehrenberg BL, Allen RP, et al. Medical Advisory Board of the Restless Legs Syndrome Foundation. An algorithm for the management of restless legs syndrome. Mayo Clin Proc 2004; 79(7):916–922.
3. von Scheele C. Levodopa in restless legs. Lancet 1986; 2(8504):426–427.
4. Akpinar S. Restless legs syndrome treatment with dopaminergic drugs. Clin Neuropharmacol 1987; 10(1):69–79.
5. Brodeur C, Montplaisir J, Godbout R, Marinier R. Treatment of restless legs syndrome and periodic movements during sleep with L-dopa: a double-blind, controlled study. Neurology 1988; 38(12):1845–1848.
6. Benes H, Kurella B, Kummer J, Kazenwadel J, Selzer R, Kohnen R. Rapid onset of action of levodopa in restless legs syndrome: a double-blind, randomized, multicenter, crossover trial. Sleep 1999; 22(8):1073–1081.
7. Earley CJ, Yaffee JB, Allen RP. Randomized, double-blind, placebo-controlled trial of pergolide in restless legs syndrome. Neurology 1998; 51(6):1599–1602.
8. Staedt J, Wassmuth F, Ziemann U, Hajak G, Ruther E, Stoppe G. Pergolide: treatment of choice in restless legs syndrome (RLS) and nocturnal myoclonus syndrome (NMS). A double-blind randomized crossover trial of pergolide versus L-Dopa. J Neural Transm 1997; 104(4–5):461–468.
9. Wetter TC, Stiasny K, Winkelmann J, Buhlinger A, Brandenburg U, Penzel T, et al. A randomized controlled study of pergolide in patients with restless legs syndrome. Neurology 1999; 52(5):944–950.
10. Trenkwalder C, Hundemer HP, Lledo A, et al. Efficacy of pergolide in treatment of restless legs syndrome: the PEARLS Study. Neurology 2004; 62(8):1391–1397.
11. Montplaisir J, Nicolas A, Denesle R, Gomez M. Restless legs syndrome improved by pramipexole: a double-blind randomized trial. Neurology 1999; 52(5):938–943.
12. Saletu M, Anderer P, Saletu-Zyhlarz G, Hauer C, Saletu B. Acute placebo-controlled sleep laboratory studies and clinical follow-up with pramipexole in restless legs syndrome. Eur Arch Psychiatry Clin Neurosci 2002; 252(4):185–194.
13. Saletu B, Gruber G, Saletu M, et al. Sleep laboratory studies in restless legs syndrome patients as compared with normals and acute effects of ropinirole. 1. Findings on objective and subjective sleep and awakening quality. Neuropsychobiology 2000; 41(4):181–189.
14. Trenkwalder C, Garcia-Borreguero D, Montagna P, et al. Therapy with Ropinirole: Efficacy and Tolerability in RLS 1 Study Group. Ropinirole in the treatment of restless legs syndrome: results from the TREAT RLS 1 study, a 12-week, randomized, placebo controlled study in 10 European countries. J Neurol Neurosurg Psychiatry 2004; 75(1): 92–97.
15. Adler CH, Hauser RA, Sethi K, et al. Ropinirole for restless legs syndrome: a placebo-controlled crossover trial. Neurology 2004; 2762(8):1405–1407.
16. Walters AS, Ondo WG, Dreykluft T, Grunstein R, Lee D, Sethi K. TREAT RLS 2 (Therapy with Ropinirole: Efficacy and Tolerability in RLS 2) Study Group. Ropinirole is effective in the treatment of restless legs syndrome. TREAT RLS 2: a 12-week, double-blind, randomized, parallel-group, placebo-controlled study. Mov Disord 2004; 19(12):1414–1423.
17. Allen R, Becker PM, Bogan R, et al. Ropinirole decreases periodic leg movements and improves sleep parameters in patients with restless legs syndrome. Sleep 2004; 27(5):907–914.
18. Bliwise DL, Freeman A, Ingram CD, Rye DB, Chakravorty S, Watts RL. Randomized, double-blind, placebo-controlled, short-term trial of ropinirole in restless legs syndrome. Sleep Med 2005; 6(2):141–147.
19. Stiasny-Kolster K, Benes H, Peglau I, et al. Effective cabergoline treatment in idiopathic restless legs syndrome. Neurology 2004; 63(12):2272–2279.
20. Kebabian JW, Calne DB. Multiple receptors for dopamine. Nature 1979; 277(5692):93–96.

21. Turjanski N, Lees AJ, Brooks DJ. Striatal dopaminergic function in restless legs syndrome: 18F-dopa and 11C-raclopride PET studies. Neurology 1999; 52(5): 932–937.
22. Bara J, Aksu M, Graham B, Sato S, Hallett M. Periodic limb movements in sleep: state-dependent excitability of the spinal flexor reflex. Neurology 2000; 54(8):1609–1616.
23. Allen RP, Earley CJ. Restless legs syndrome: a review of clinical and pathophysiologic features. J Clin Neurophysiol 2001; 18(2):128–147.
24. Montplaisir J, Lorrain D, Godbout R. Restless legs syndrome and periodic leg movements in sleep: the primary role of dopaminergic mechanism. Eur Neurol 1991; 31:41–43.
25. Winkelmann J, Schadrack J, Wetter TC, Zieglgansberger W, Trenkwalder C. Opioid and dopamine antagonist drug challenges in untreated restless legs syndrome patients. Sleep Med 2001; 2:57–61.
26. Hening WA, Allen RP, Earley CJ, Picchietti DL, Silber MH. Restless Legs Syndrome Task Force of the Standards of Practice Committee of the American Academy of Sleep Medicine. An update on the dopaminergic treatment of restless legs syndrome and periodic limb movement disorder. Sleep 2004; 27(3):560–583.
27. Tan EK, Ondo WG. Clinical Characteristics of Pramipexole Induced Peripheral Edema. Arch Neurol 2000; 57:729–732.
28. Kaynak D, Kiziltan G, Kaynak H, Benbir G, Uysal O. Sleep and sleepiness in patients with Parkinson's disease before and after dopaminergic treatment. Eur J Neurol 2005; 12(3):199–207.
29. Ondo WG, Dat Vuong K, Khan H, Atassi F, Kwak C, Jankovic J. Daytime sleepiness and other sleep disorders in Parkinson's disease. Neurology 2001; 57(8):1392–1396.
29a. Moller JC, Korner Y, Cassel W, et al. Sudden onset of sleep and dopaminergic therapy in patients with restless legs syndrome. Sleep Med 2006; 7:333–339.
29b. Ondo WG. Risk factors for gambling and other impulsive behaviors in patients taking dopamine agonists for Parkinson's disease and restless legs syndrome. World Congress of Movement Disorders, Kyoto 2006.
30. Akpinar S. Treatment of restless legs syndrome with levodopa plus benserazide. Arch Neurol 1982; 39(11):739.
31. Montplaisir J, Godbout R, Poirier G, Bedard MA. Restless legs syndrome and periodic movements in sleep: physiopathology and treatment with L-dopa. Clin Neuropharmacol 1986; 9(5):456–463.
32. von Scheele C, Kempi V. Long-term effect of dopaminergic drugs in restless legs. A 2-year follow-up. Arch Neurol 1990; 47(11):1223–1224.
33. Becker PM, Jamieson AO, Brown WD. Dopaminergic agents in restless legs syndrome and periodic limb movements of sleep: response and complications of extended treatment in 49 cases. Sleep 1993; 16(8):713–716.
34. Guilleminault C, Cetel M, Philip P. Dopaminergic treatment of restless legs and rebound phenomenon. Neurology 1993; 43(2):445.
35. Sandyk R, Bernick C, Lee SM, Stern LZ, Iacono RP, Bamford CR. L-dopa in uremic patients with the restless legs syndrome. Int J Neurosci 1987; 35(3–4):233–235.
36. Trenkwalder C, Stiasny K, Pollmacher T, Wetter T, Schwarz J, Kohnen R, et al. L-dopa therapy of uremic and idiopathic restless legs syndrome: a double-blind, crossover trial. Sleep 1995; 18(8):681–688.
37. Kaplan PW, Allen RP, Buchholz DW, Walters JK. A double-blind, placebo-controlled study of the treatment of periodic limb movements in sleep using carbidopa/levodopa and propoxyphene. Sleep 1993; 16(8):717–723.
38. Collado-Seidel V, Kazenwadel J, Wetter TC, et al. A controlled study of additional sr-L-dopa in L-dopa-responsive restless legs syndrome with late-night symptoms. Neurology 1999; 52(2):285–290.
39. Janzen L, Rich JA, Vercaigne LM. An overview of levodopa in the management of restless legs syndrome in a dialysis population: pharmacokinetics, clinical trials, and complications of therapy. Ann Pharmacother 1999; 33(1):86–92.
40. Allen RP, Earley CJ. Augmentation of the restless legs syndrome with carbidopa/levodopa. Sleep 1996; 19(3):205–213.

41. Allen RP, Hening WA, Montplaisir J, Picchietti D, Trenkwalder C, Walters AS, et al. Restless legs syndrome: diagnostic criteria, special considerations, and epidemiology: a report from The RLS Diagnosis and Epidemiology Workshop at the National Institutes of Health. Sleep Med 2003; 4:101–119.
41a. Stiasny-Kolster K, Kohen R, et al. Validation of the L-DOPA test for diagnosis of restless legs syndrome. Mov Disord 2006.
42. Walters AS, Hening WA, Kavey N, Chokroverty S, Gidro-Frank S. A double-blind randomized crossover trial of bromocriptine and placebo in restless legs syndrome. Ann Neurol 1988; 24(3):455–458.
43. Montplaisir J, Lapierre O, Warnes H, Pelletier G. The treatment of the restless leg syndrome with or without periodic leg movements in sleep. Sleep 1992; 15(5):391–395.
44. Demonet JF, Rostin M, Dueymes JM, Ioualalen A, Montastruc JL, Rascol A. Retroperitoneal fibrosis and treatment of Parkinson's disease with high doses of bromocriptine. Clin Neuropharmacol 1986; 9(2):200–201.
45. Klaassen RJ, Troost RJ, Verhoeven GT, Krepel HP, van der Lely AJ. Suggestive evidence for bromocriptine-induced pleurisy. Neth J Med 1996; 48(6):232–236.
46. Chaudhuri KR, Dhawan V, Basu S, Jackson G, Odin P. Valvular heart disease and fibrotic reactions may be related to ergot dopamine agonists, but non-ergot agonists may also not be spared. Mov Disord 2004; 19(12):1522–1523.
47. Earley CJ, Allen RP. Pergolide and carbidopa/levodopa treatment of the restless legs syndrome and periodic leg movements in sleep in a consecutive series of patients. Sleep 1996; 19(10):801–810.
48. Stiasny K, Wetter TC, Winkelmann J, Brandenburg U, Penzel T, Rubin M, et al. Long-term effects of pergolide in the treatment of restless legs syndrome. Neurology 2001; 56(10):1399–1402.
49. Agarwal P, Fahn S, Frucht SJ. Diagnosis and management of pergolide-induced fibrosis. Mov Disord 2004; 19(6):699–704.
50. Van Camp G, Flamez A, Cosyns B, Weytjens C, Muyldermans L, Van Zandijcke M, et al. Treatment of Parkinson's disease with pergolide and relation to restrictive valvular heart disease. Lancet 2004; 363(9424):1907–1908.
51. Horowski R, Jahnichen S, Pertz HH. Fibrotic valvular heart disease is not related to chemical class but to biological function: 5-HT2B receptor activation plays crucial role. Mov Disord 2004; 19(12):1523–1524.
52. Horvath J, Fross RD, Kleiner-Fisman G, et al. Severe multivalvular heart disease: a new complication of the ergot derivative dopamine agonists. Mov Disord 2004; 19(6): 656–662.
53. Stiasny K, Robbecke J, Schuler P, Oertel WH. Treatment of idiopathic restless legs syndrome (RLS) with the D2-agonist cabergoline–an open clinical trial. Sleep 2000; 23(3):349–354.
54. Zucconi M, Oldani A, Castronovo C, Ferini-Strambi L. Cabergoline is an effective single-drug treatment for restless legs syndrome: clinical and actigraphic evaluation. Sleep 2003; 26(7):815–818.
54a. Aizawa H, Aburakawa Y, et al. Treatment of Japanese restless legs syndrome patients with cabergobine: an open clinical preliminary triedal. Intern Med 2006; 45(7):453–455.
55. Benes H, Heinrich CR, Ueberall MA, Kohnen R. Long-term safety and efficacy of cabergoline for the treatment of idiopathic restless legs syndrome: results from an open-label 6-month clinical trial. Sleep 2004; 27(4):674–682.
56. Pfizer, Data on file.
57. Lin SC, Kaplan J, Burger CD, Fredrickson PA. Effect of pramipexole in treatment of resistant restless legs syndrome. Mayo Clin Proc 1998; 73(6):497–500.
58. Becker PM, Ondo W, Sharon D. Encouraging initial response of restless legs syndrome to pramipexole. Neurology 1998; 51(4):1221–1223.
59. Montplaisir J, Denesle R, Petit D. Pramipexole in the treatment of restless legs syndrome: a follow-up study. Eur J Neurol 2000; 7(suppl 1):27–31.
60. Partinen M, Hirronen K, et al. Efficacy and safety of pramipexole in idiopathic restless legs syndrome:A polysomnographic dose-finding study-The PRECLUDE study. Sleep Med 2006; 7(5):407–417.

61. Oertel W, Stiasny-Kolster K. Pramipexole is effective in the treatment of Restless Legs Syndrome (RLS): results of a 6-week, multi-centre, double-blind and placebo-controlled study. Mov Disord 2005; 20(suppl 10):S58 P191.
62. Winkelman J, Sethi K, Kushida C, Becker P, Mahowald M. Pramipexole is efficacious and safe in treating RLS patients: results of a 12 weeks placebo controlled, fixed dose study. Sleep Med 2005; 6(suppl 2):S74.
63. Silber M, Girish M, Izurieta R. Pramipexole in the management of restless legs syndrome: an extended study. Sleep 2003; 26:819–821.
64. Winkelman JW, Johnston L. Augmentation and tolerance with long-term pramipexole treatment of restless legs syndrome (RLS). Sleep Med 2004; 5(1):9–14.

64a. Morgan JC, Sethi KD. Ropinisole versus placebo in primary restless legs syndrome. Curr Neurol Neurosci Rep 2006; 6(4):278–280.

64b. Bogan RK, Fry JM, et al. Ropinirole in the treatment of patients with restless legs syndrome: a US-based randomized, double-blind, placebo-controlled clinical trial. Mayo clin Proc 2006; 81(1):17–27.

64c. Montplasis J, Karrasch J, et al. Ropinirole is effective in the long-term management of restless legs syndrome: A randomized controlled trial. Mov Disord 2006.

65. Ondo W. Ropinirole for restless legs syndrome. Mov Disord 1999; 14(1):138–140.
66. Estivill E, de la Fuente V. The efficacy of ropinirole in the treatment of chronic insomnia secondary to restless legs syndrome: polysomnography data. Rev Neurol 1999; 29(9):805–807 (Spanish).
67. Pellecchia MT, Vitale C, Sabatini M, Longo K, Amboni M, Bonavita V, Barone P. Ropinirole as a treatment of restless legs syndrome in patients on chronic hemodialysis: an open randomized crossover trial versus levodopa sustained release. Clin Neuropharmacol 2004; 27(4):178–181.
68. GSK. Data on file.
69. GSK. Data on file.
70. Stiasny-Kolster K, Kohnen R, Schollmayer E, Moller JC, Oertel WH, Rotigotine Sp 666 Study Group. Patch application of the dopamine agonist rotigotine to patients with moderate to advanced stages of restless legs syndrome: a double-blind, placebo-controlled pilot study. Mov Disord 2004; 19(12):1432–1438.
71. Oertel W, Benes H, Geisler P, for Rotigotine SP709 Study Group. Rotigotine patch efficacy and safety in the treatment of moderate to severe idiopathic restless legs syndrome–results from a multi-national double-blind placebo-controlled multi-center dose-finding study. World Association of Sleep Medicine, 2005.
72. Reuter I, Ellis CM, Chaudhuri RK. Nocturnal subcutaneous apomorphine infusion in Parkinson's disease and restless legs syndrome. Acta Neurologica Scandinavica 1999; 100(3):163–167.
73. Tribl G, Sycha T, Kotzailias N, Zeitlhofer J, Auff E. Apomorphine in idiopathic restless legs syndrome: an exploratory study. J Neurol Neurosurg Psych 2005; 76(2):181–185.
74. Sharif AA. Entacapone in restless legs syndrome. Mov Disord 2002; 17(2):421.
75. Sonka K, Pretl M, Kranda K. Management of restless legs syndrome by the partial D2-agonist terguride. Sleep Med 2003; 4(5):455–457.
76. Inoue Y, Mi tani H, Nanba K, Kawahara R. Treatment of periodic leg movement disorder and restless leg syndrome with talipexole. Psychiatry Clin Neurosci 1999; 53(2):283–285.
77. Tergau F, Wischer S, Wolf C, Paulus W. Treatment of restless legs syndrome with the dopamine agonist alpha-dihydroergocryptine. Mov Disord 2001; 16(4):731–735.
78. Evidente VG. Piribedil for restless legs syndrome: a pilot study. Mov Disord 2001; 16(3):579–581.
79. Ondo WG, Romanyshyn J, Vuong K, Lai D. The Long-Term Treatment of Restless Legs Syndrome with Dopamine Agonists. Arch Neurol 2004; 1393–1397.
80. Garcia-Borreguero D. Augmentation: understanding a key feature of RLS. Sleep Med 2004; 5(1):5–6.
81. Ondo WG. Methadone for refractory restless legs syndrome. Mov Disord 2005; 20(3):345–348.

# 26 Dopaminergic Augmentation

**Diego García-Borreguero, Oscar Larrosa, Renata Egatz, Belen Cabrero, and Patrick Tröster**
*Sleep Research Institute, Madrid, Spain*

## INTRODUCTION

Dopaminergic drugs have been used for the treatment of restless legs syndrome (RLS) since the first description of their efficacy in 1982 (1). Since then, the overall long-term efficacy of these drugs has been well established by several retrospective studies (2–5). Side effects are generally mild (4), and contrary to their use in Parkinson's disease (PD), no cases of dyskinesias have been reported to date (4,6–8).

Despite the widespread use of dopaminergic drugs for RLS, it was not until 1996 that the first clinical description of augmentation as a complication of dopaminergic treatment was reported (9). Allen and Earley (9) described a group of 30 RLS patients who had been treated with levodopa (L-DOPA) and described a condition characterized by an earlier onset of symptoms in the afternoon, along with a faster onset of symptoms following resumption of rest, an expansion of symptoms to the upper limbs and the trunk, an overall increase in severity, and a shorter effect of the medication. All patients reported an earlier time of onset of symptoms in the evening, and nearly all (96%) reported an increased intensity of symptoms. In addition, 56% of the sample reported a shorter onset time at rest, and 11% reported an expansion of symptoms to the upper limbs. Augmentation of RLS symptoms occurred in 82% of the patients and was severe enough to require change of treatment in 50% (9,10). The most characteristic feature of this new condition was the fact that it occurred during long-term treatment with L-DOPA with an increase in severity beyond the one seen at baseline, a feature that differentiated it from rebound and from tolerance (i.e., seen with benzodiazepines or in opiates).

## CLINICAL DESCRIPTION AND SIGNIFICANCE

So far, clinical descriptions of the symptoms involved in RLS augmentation have been scarce in the literature. In their first and to date most complete description of 30 RLS patients, Allen and Earley (9) reported that 100% of the patients undergoing augmentation showed an earlier onset of symptoms in the evening following long-term treatment with dopaminergic drugs (mainly L-DOPA). Other characteristic features such as an increase in symptom severity were somewhat less common. Furthermore, a shorter latency to RLS symptoms while at rest and an expansion of symptoms to other parts of the body occurred with far less frequency (33% and 10%, respectively). This impression was confirmed by Collado-Seidel et al. (7) showing a time shift of RLS symptoms to the afternoon or evening during long-term treatment with L-DOPA in 8 out of 30 RLS patients (26.7%), while only two of them reported an expansion of symptoms to additional body parts (6.6%). Similar results were obtained in later studies (11,12).

**TABLE 1** NIH Criteria for Diagnosis of Restless Legs Syndrome Augmentation

RLS augmentation can be diagnosed if either of the following two criteria is met:

*Criteria 1*

- RLS symptoms occur at least two hours earlier than was typical during the initial course of beneficial stable treatment

*Criteria 2*

Two more of the following key features of RLS augmentation are present:

- An increased overall intensity of the urge to move or sensation is temporally related to an increase in the daily medication dosage or a decreased overall intensity of the urge to move or sensation is temporally related to a decrease in the daily medication dosage
- The latency to RLS symptoms at rest is shorter than the latency either during initial therapeutic response or before treatment was instituted
- The urge to move or sensation is extended to previously unaffected limbs or body parts
- The duration of treatment effect is shorter than the duration either during initial therapeutic response or before treatment was instituted
- Periodic limb movements while awake occur for the first time or are worse than either during initial therapeutic response or before treatment was instituted

In addition to meeting one of these two criteria, the diagnosis requires both of the following:

- Augmented symptoms meeting these criteria present for at least one week for a minimum of 5 days, and
- No other medical, psychiatric, behavioral, or pharmacological factors explain the exacerbation of the patient's RLS and the augmented symptoms meeting these criteria

*Abbreviation*: RLS, restless legs syndrome.
*Source*: From Ref. 13.

In an effort to standardize and universalize clinical recognition of augmentation, the NIH-sponsored RLS Diagnosis and Epidemiology Workshop defined clinical criteria for augmentation (13). Accordingly, the primary feature of augmentation is represented by a "shift of RLS symptoms to a time period that is two or more hours earlier than was typical of the time of symptom onset during the initial course of beneficial stable treatment or the state before recently starting treatment" (Table 1). Other medical, psychiatric, behavioral, or pharmacological factors should be previously excluded as an explanation for the time shift. Thus, a time shift in the time of symptoms, if present for at least five days of the week previous to evaluation, would be a sufficient criterion to consider augmentation. In the absence of such a time shift in symptoms, augmentation would also be diagnosed if two or more of a list of six features was present. These features can be shortly summarized as (i) an increase of the RLS symptoms occurring with an increase of daily medication for RLS, or conversely (ii) a decrease in symptoms with a decrease in daily medication, (iii) a shorter latency to symptom onset when at rest, (iv) an expansion of RLS symptoms to additional body parts, (v) a shorter duration of treatment effect than during initial treatment response, or (vi) an onset or worsening (if preexisting) of periodic leg movements while awake. The presence of augmentation does not imply that it is severe. In fact, in many cases, augmentation can be mild and not have any clinical or therapeutic consequences (7).

Thus, both the clinical reports on augmentation and the NIH definition of the condition have included an increase in the overall severity of symptoms and a shorter duration of treatment effects among the symptom constellation of augmentation. This feature along with a shift in the time of onset of RLS symptoms, the expansion to other limbs, and the shorter latency to symptoms at rest, reflect an increase in overall symptom severity. In fact, some authors consider the time of onset of RLS symptoms as the most reliable and stable marker of disease severity (14). In other words, augmentation reflects a drug-induced increase in RLS symptom severity beyond that experienced before treatment was initiated, and this remains the most characteristic feature of dopaminergic augmentation as compared to pharmacologic tolerance.

Several studies have been able to correlate the presence of augmentation during treatment with L-DOPA with the severity of RLS symptoms at baseline and with a higher medication dosage, but not with age or gender (9). Clinical experience shows that severe augmentation can result in a loss of essential RLS features, such as the symptoms no longer being improved during activity or the loss of a circadian pattern, such that symptoms are present 24 hours per day. In severe augmentation, RLS can occur continuously during the day, it can involve the entire body, and it cannot be noticeably affected by rest or activity, showing a remarkable similarity with neuroleptic-induced akathisia. The clinical picture obtained during dopaminergic augmentation resembles the one obtained in severe RLS (15,16). None of the clinical features of dopaminergic augmentation is specific to that condition or can be differentiated from RLS itself. In fact, RLS augmentation reflects a worsening of RLS severity during dopaminergic treatment.

## AUGMENTATION UNDER DOPAMINERGIC AGENTS

Although augmentation seems to be particularly common during treatment with L-DOPA, it has also been observed with other dopaminergic agents, notably with dopamine agonists. Thus, augmentation occurs in 15% to 27% of patients being treated with pergolide (3,17,18), 8% to 56% of patients under long-term treatment with pramipexole (5,19–21), and 3% to 9% of patients under treatment with cabergoline (22,23). No long-term data have been published specifically on other dopamine agonists.

However, any comparative conclusions on augmentation rates across drugs must remain preliminary at this point, because these studies have been performed in a retrospective fashion, using different criteria for augmentation, and none used standardized screening instruments. Furthermore, no data exist on augmentation under placebo treatment. Thus, the specificity of these symptoms to the treatment remains questionable.

## AUGMENTATION UNDER NONDOPAMINERGIC AGENTS

So far, less of an emphasis has been laid on performance of systematic long-term treatments with nondopaminergic treatment, such as opiates, anticonvulsants, or benzodiazepines. Nevertheless, no cases of augmentation have been reported under any such agents in the literature. Until such evidence is provided, it must be concluded that augmentation remains a specific phenomenon of dopaminergic treatment in RLS.

## THE PATHOPHYSIOLOGY OF AUGMENTATION

Augmentation has not been reported following long-term treatment with nondopaminergic drugs, suggesting that it might be specific to the dopaminergic mode of action of these drugs. Preliminary data have shown that occurrence of augmentation during L-DOPA treatment does not necessarily predict similar episodes of augmentation during dopamine agonists therapy (5). Accordingly, augmentation might be caused by a down regulation of either presynaptic or postsynaptic mechanisms. A combination of both mechanisms might also be possible, because dopamine agonists can inhibit endogenous dopamine release from nigrostriatal dopaminergic neurons (24). Furthermore, because specific subtypes of postsynaptic receptors might be involved, a differential effect of increasing doses of dopaminergic agents on postsynaptic receptors might lead to a downregulation of the endogenous dopamine production, aggravating RLS symptoms (9,24–27).

Other mechanisms such as pharmacokinetics might also be involved since the probability of augmentation generally correlates with the half-life of the drug (28). Thus, augmentation is more likely during treatment with agents with a shorter half-life such as L-DOPA (9,11,13), than during treatment with drugs with a longer half-life such as cabergoline (22,29) or even pergolide (30).

In the only report to directly compare augmentation rates from different dopamine agonists (pramipexole, ropinirole, pergolide), Ondo et al. queried all subjects initiated on agonists by the Baylor College of Medicine Movement Disorders Center (31). Patients with PD, uremia, or medications that could affect RLS were excluded. Demographics, efficacy, dosing, adverse events, and augmentation were tracked over time. After eliminating all RLS patients with factors that could affect DA dosing or the accuracy of data, 83 subjects were followed with at least six months use of DA, $39.2 \pm 20.9$ months. Efficacy was maintained over time but at the expense of a moderate but significant increase in mean dose ($p < 0.01$). Augmentation, as defined only by a two hour earlier onset of symptoms, was frequent (48%) but usually modest and was predicted by a positive family history for RLS, and especially the lack of any neuropathy on electromyogram and nerve conduction studies (Fig. 1). There was no difference in augmentation rates among those three agonists. It should be noted that the range of half-lives among those three dopaminergics is relatively narrow (6–19 hours).

It is not clear why drugs with a shorter half-life might lead to augmentation in RLS. This may result from some true biological effect of more continuous dopaminergic stimulation that prevents some iatrogenic neurotransmitter or receptor change, or it may result from the simple fact that longer dopaminergics will occupy receptors for a longer time and thus cover up rather than prevent augmentation. In animal models of PD, pulsatile administration of L-DOPA induces molecular abnormalities such as phosphorylation of *N*-methyl-d-asportate (NMDA) subunits and upregulation of α-amino-5-hydroxy-3-methyl-4-isoxazole propionic acid (AMPA) receptors (32–35). Such a glutamatergic hyperactivity might ultimately lead to increased dopaminergic neuronal firing and to dopamine depletion (34–36). With continued degeneration taking place in PD, as the striatal dopamine deficit increases, an impaired storage capacity develops that might compensate for the changes in dopamine availability associated with the oral administration of L-DOPA, leading to complications such as wearing-off or dyskinesias (37). However, unlike in Parkinson's disease, in RLS there is no cell loss in basal ganglia, and the storage capacity for dopamine is not impaired (38–40). That might explain why motor complications of L-DOPA are not seen in RLS. However, glutaminergic stimulation might initially lead to increased dopaminergic neuronal firing and increased dopamine turnover, and, ultimately, to a compensatory inhibition of endogenous dopaminergic mechanisms.

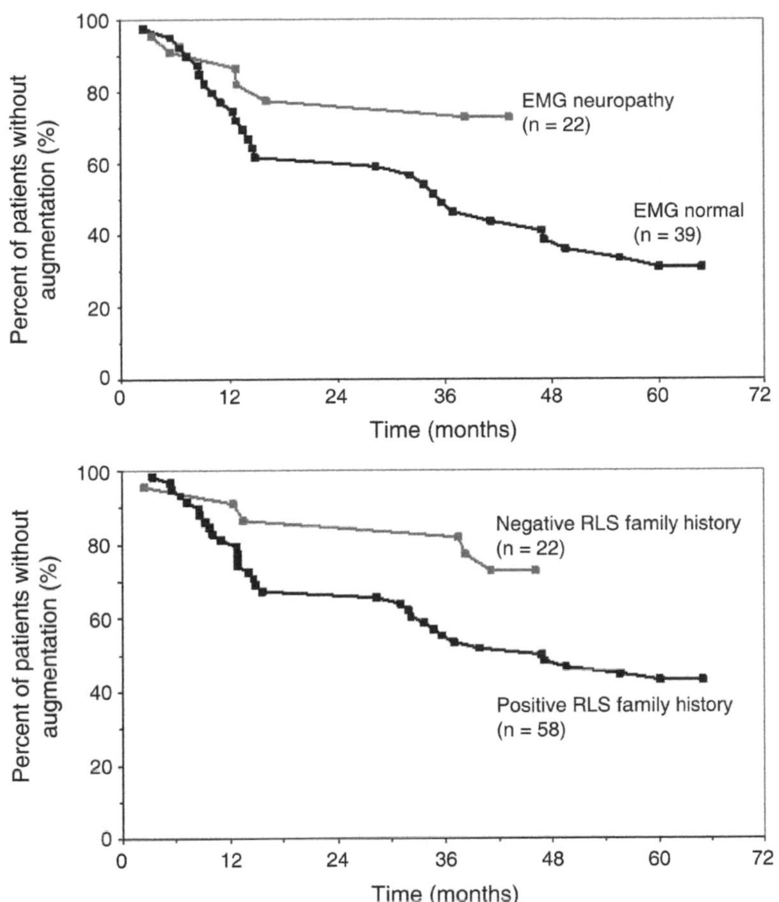


**FIGURE 1** Survival curve for absence of augmentation as defined by at least a 2 hour shift in time of symptom onset. Patients who lack any neuropathy and patients who have a positive family historical of RLS are more likely to experience augmentation. *Source*: W. Ondo.

Hormonal changes in growth hormone (GH) and prolactin (PRL) are seen with dopaminergic therapy in RLS and may contribute to augmentation. This is a difficult field to study, because these hormonal changes could also be mediated by sleep disruption. Sleep deprivation is known to affect hormonal release of both GH and PRL and dopaminergic systems, although no consistent pattern of change has been found (41–45).

Taken together, augmentation seems to be related to a progressive dopaminergic dysfunction during treatment with dopaminergic agents. The precise mechanisms are not clear.

## MEASUREMENT OF AUGMENTATION

Because augmentation reflects an increase in symptom severity of RLS, any measurements of severity can be used to measure augmentation. That is, sleep laboratory measurements of severity (46) such as polysomnography suggested that immobilization test or even actigraphy could be theoretically used to measure augmentation. However, none of these methods has been validated or standardized to date.

Currently, a rating scale that is specifically designed to measure augmentation is being developed by the European Restless Legs Study Group (Table 2) (47), and preliminary results of its multicentric validation were presented recently (12). The scale consists of four items with specific questions on anticipation of symptoms, increased severity, shorter latency to symptoms when at rest, and expansion of symptoms to the arms, which are asked at baseline and during treatment. The scale calculates the difference in scores and measures augmentation as a continuum, rather than as a category. Thus, it assumes that augmentation might be a continuous increase in severity of symptoms and might become clinically relevant after a specific threshold.

## DIFFERENTIAL DIAGNOSIS OF AUGMENTATION

From a clinical point of view, augmentation needs to be differentiated from two main conditions: The first one, early morning rebound, is characterized by the development of RLS in the early morning, rather than earlier onset of symptoms in the evening, as is the case under augmentation. Following rebound in the morning, there is usually a symptom-free period of time until symptoms reappear again in the afternoon or evening. However, in some cases of severe augmentation, particularly when patients suffer symptoms throughout the day, it might be difficult to differentiate from rebound. Rebound is considered to be an end-of-dose effect, related to the half-life of the therapeutic agent. No correlation has been found between the occurrence of augmentation and rebound, supporting the general view that both phenomena reflect separate problems (9).

In contrast to the former, distinguishing augmentation from tolerance might be more difficult from a clinical point of view. In fact, tolerance, defined as a loss of therapeutic effect over time under a given therapeutic dosage, may produce symptom changes that meet two of the criteria (criteria "a" and "e": Table 1) of augmentation. Thus, in the absence of a noticeable anticipation in the time of onset of symptoms (i.e., if only criteria "a" and "e" were met), tolerance and augmentation might take an identical shape. Strictly speaking, even in the worst case of tolerance, severity of symptoms would not be expected to increase over the level of severity occurring without treatment. In contrast, during augmentation, the severity of symptoms during augmentation might well increase beyond that preexisting at baseline. This differentiation might prove to be of more theoretical than practical value in clinical practice, because most patients cannot assess the severity of their symptoms with such precision (14). Furthermore, the absence of specific rating instruments for augmentation as well as the lack of prospective studies to assess the long-term course of the different features of augmentation make the differentiation between both processes particularly difficult.

Augmentation also resembles tolerance in other aspects. Clinical experience shows that following interruption of dopaminergic treatment in patients experiencing augmentation, therapeutic response to the same medication is usually fully restored (48). Thus, augmentation under dopaminergic treatment shares some of the properties of pharmacological tolerance that are frequently seen with opiate medications. Moreover, because the features in augmentation reflect an increase in symptom severity during long-term dopaminergic treatment, possibly as a result in changes in dopamine receptor sensitivity (9), the underlying pathophysiology might not necessarily be different from the one generally accepted for tolerance. Both augmentation and tolerance resolve after discontinuation of treatment.

**TABLE 2** Items of the Augmentation Severity Rating Scale, as Developed by the European Restless Legs Syndrome Study Group

*Item 1.* During the past week, at what time did your RLS symptoms usually start?
Please write down the time when the symptoms usually started (e.g., 22:45)

*Item 2.* During the past week, what was the usual severity of your RLS symptoms?
0—None
1—Mild
2—Moderate
3—Severe
4—Very Severe

*Item 3a.* During the past week, if you were sitting or resting during the daytime (for example, in a car, plane, theater, or watching TV), how soon afterwards did your RLS symptoms usually start?
0—After a very long time or never
1—After a long time (i.e., after about an hour)
2—After a moderate amount of time (i.e., after about half an hour)
3—After a short time (i.e., within a few minutes)
4—Immediately or almost immediately

*Item 3b.* During the past week, at any times you were sitting or resting (for example, in a car, plane, theater, or watching TV), how soon afterwards did your RLS symptoms usually start? *Please indicate the time it takes for symptoms to start at various times during the day (late morning, early afternoon, late afternoon, evening before taking any RLS medication)*
*When sitting in the late morning (i.e., before noon), your symptoms usually started...*
0—After a very long time or never
1—After a long time (i.e., after about an hour)
2—After a moderate amount of time (i.e., after about half an hour)
3—After a short time (i.e., within a few minutes)
4—Immediately or almost immediately
5—Did not sit or rest in the morning over the last week
*When sitting in the early afternoon (i.e., 12:00–15:00), your symptoms usually started...*
0—After a very long time or never
1—After a long time (i.e., after about an hour)
2—After a moderate amount of time (i.e., after about half an hour)
3—After a short time (i.e., within a few minutes)
4—Immediately or almost immediately
5—Did not sit or rest in the early afternoon over the last week
*When sitting in the late afternoon (i.e., 15:00–18:00), your symptoms usually started...*
0—After a very long time or never
1—After a long time (i.e., after about an hour)
2—After a moderate amount of time (i.e., after about half an hour)
3—After a short time (i.e., within a few minutes)
4—Immediately or almost immediately
5—Did not sit or rest in the late afternoon over the last week
*When sitting in the evening (after 18:00, before taking the first dose of RLS medication), your symptoms usually started...*
0—After a very long time or never
1—After a long time (i.e., after about an hour)
2—After a moderate amount of time (i.e., after about half an hour)
3—After a short time (i.e., within a few minutes)
4—Immediately or almost immediately
5—Did not sit or rest in the evening over the last week or took my first dose of RLS medication at or before this time

*Item 4.* During the past week, what parts of your body were usually affected by RLS symptoms? Please let the patient shade in the figure the portions of his/her body affected by RLS symptoms and choose the corresponding score

Please write the corresponding score (0 to 4)
0, none; 1, below the knees; 2, below the hips; 3, arms and legs; 4, most of the body

However, unlike tolerance, augmentation increases the severity of symptoms to levels that exceed any seen without treatment. A "drug holiday" reestablished drug efficacy for both augmentation and tolerance, but for augmentation it also reduces symptoms to the levels experienced before treatment. Anecdotally, this required about a week. Thus, an earlier onset of symptoms to a time that did not occur previously would suggest augmentation and differentiate it from tolerance.

Another situation that needs to be differentiated from augmentation is a progressive worsening of the clinical course of RLS over time. Although data on the long-term spontaneous course in untreated RLS patients are scarce and usually not well controlled, it is believed that any progression is slow unless accentuated by some acute processes, such as hemorrhage or iatrogenic worsening. This could, however, be confounded with a slowly progressive, mild process of augmentation. In this case, however, a drug holiday produces opposite effects, that is, a full expression of the progressive worsening of symptoms, while in augmentation, symptoms would be reduced.

## TREATMENT OF AUGMENTATION

To our knowledge, no studies have been performed on the treatment of augmentation. Various strategies are employed. Moderate augmentation will usually clinically improve by adding additional doses of dopaminergics to coincide with the earlier onset of symptoms. Switching from one dopaminergic to another may help some patients. In general, because augmentation symptoms are known to improve following reduction or interruption of dopaminergic treatment, the most definitive treatment is to either gradually or abruptly stop the dopaminergic treatment. Simultaneous treatment with opiates or other nondopaminergic drugs might also be helpful. It remains a question of controversy whether reinitiating dopaminergic treatment following a period with alternative medication might lead to a repeated episode of augmentation and how quickly this might occur (3,5,21).

## REFERENCES

1. Akpinar S. Treatment of restless legs syndrome with levodopa plus benserazide. Arch Neurol 1982; 39(11):739.
2. von Scheele C, Kempi V. Long-term effect of dopaminergic drugs in restless legs. A 2-year follow-up. Arch Neurol 1990; 47(11):1223–1224.
3. Silber MH, Shepard JW, Wisbey JA. Pergolide in the management of restless legs syndrome: an extended study. Sleep 1997; 20(10):878–882.
4. Happe S, Trenkwalder C. Role of dopamine receptor agonists in the treatment of restless legs syndrome. CNS Drugs 2004; 18(1):27–36.
5. Silber MH, Girish M, Izurieta R. Pramipexole in the management of restless legs syndrome: an extended study. Sleep 2003; 26(7):819–821.
6. Collado-Seidel V, Winkelmann J, Trenkwalder C. Aetiology and treatment of restless legs syndrome. CNS Drugs 1999; 12(1):9–20.
7. Collado-Seidel V, Kazenwadel J, Wetter TC, et al. A controlled study of additional sr-L-dopa in L-dopa-responsive restless legs syndrome with late-night symptoms. Neurology 1999; 52(2):285–290.
8. Winkelmann J, Trenkwalder C. Pathophysiology of restless-legs syndrome. Review of current research. Nervenarzt 2001; (72):100–107.
9. Allen RP, Earley CJ. Augmentation of the restless legs syndrome with carbidopa/levodopa. Sleep 1996; 19(6):205–213.
10. Allen RP. Race, iron status and restless legs syndrome. Sleep Med 2002; 3(6):467–468.

11. Trenkwalder C, Collado-Seidel V, Kazenwadel J, et al. One-Year Treatment with Standard and Sustained-Release Levodopa: Appropriate Long-Term Treatment of Restless Legs Syndrome? Mov Disord 2003; 18(10):1184–1189.
12. Garcia Borreguero D, Högl B, Ferrini-Strambi L, et al. Validation of the Augmentation Severity Rating Scale (ASRS): First results from a study of the European Restless Legs Syndrome Study Group (EU-RLSSG). 1st Congress of the World Association of Sleep Medicine (WASM), Berlin 2005 Sleep Med 2005; 6(suppl 2):S67 (Abstract).
13. Allen RP, Picchietti D, Hening WA, Trenkwalder C, Walters AS, Montplaisir J. Restless legs syndrome: diagnostic criteria, special considerations, and epidemiology. A report from the restless legs syndrome diagnosis and epidemiology workshop at the National Institutes of Health. Sleep Med 2003; 4(2):101–119.
14. Allen RP, Earley CJ. Validation of the Johns Hopkins Restless Legs Severity Scale. Sleep Med 2001; 3:239–242.
15. Allen RP, Walters AS, Montplaisir J, et al. Restless legs syndrome prevalence and impact: REST general population study. Arch Intern Med 2005; 165(11):1286–1292.
16. Walters AS, LeBrocq C, Dhar A, et al. Validation of the International Restless Legs Syndrome Study Group rating scale for restless legs syndrome. Sleep Med 2003; 4(2): 121–132.
17. Earley CJ, Allen RP. Pergolide and carbidopa/levodopa treatment of the restless legs syndrome and periodic leg movements in sleep in a consecutive series of patients. Sleep 1996; 19(10):801–810.
18. Stiasny K, Wetter TC, Winkelmann J, et al. Long-term effects of pergolide in the treatment of restless legs syndrome. Neurology 2001; 56(10):1399–1402.
19. Hening W, Allen R, Earley C, Kushida C, Picchietti D, Silber M. The treatment of restless legs syndrome and periodic limb movement disorder. An American Academy of Sleep Medicine Review. Sleep 1999; 22(7):970–999.
20. Ferini-Strambi L. Restless legs syndrome augmentation and pramipexole treatment. Sleep Med 2002; 3(suppl):S23–S25.
21. Winkelman JW, Johnston L. Augmentation and tolerance with long-term pramipexole treatment of restless legs syndrome (RLS). Sleep Med 2004; 5(1):9–14.
22. Benes H, Heinrich CR, Ueberall MA, Kohnen R. Long-term safety and efficacy of Cabergoline for the treatment of idiopathic restless legs syndrome: results from an open-label 6-month clinical trial. Sleep 2004; 27(4):674–682.
23. Stiasny-Kolster K, Benes H, Peglau I, et al. Effective cabergoline treatment in idiopathic restless legs syndrome. Neurology 2004; 63(12):2272–2279.
24. Scarnati E, Forchetti C, Ciancarelli G, Pacitti C, Agnoli A. Responsiveness of nigral neurons to the stimulation of striatal dopaminergic receptors in the rat. Life Sci 1980; 26(15):1203–1209.
25. Carlson JH, Bergstrom DA, Weick BG, Walters JR. Neurophysiological investigation of effects of the D-1 agonist SKF 38393 on tonic activity of substantia nigra dopamine neurons. Synapse 1987; 1(5):411–416.
26. Heidenreich BA, Mailman RB, Nichols DE, Napier TC. Partial and full dopamine D1 agonists produce comparable increases in ventral pallidal neuronal activity: contribution of endogenous dopamine. J Pharmacol Exp Ther 1995; 273(1):516–525.
27. Mereu G, Collu M, Ongini E, Biggio G, Gessa GL. SCH 23390, a selective dopamine D1 antagonist, activates dopamine neurons but fails to prevent their inhibition by apomorphine. Eur J Pharmacol 1985; 111(3):393–396.
28. Vetrugno R, Contin M, Baruzzi A, Provini F, Plazzi G, Montagna P. Polysomnographic and pharmacokinatic findings in levodopa-induced augmentation of restless legs syndrome. Mov Disord 2006;21:. Eur J Pharmacol 2006; 21:264-258.
29. Zucconi M, Oldani A, Castronovo C, Ferini-Strambi L. Cabergoline is an effective single-drug treatment for restless legs syndrome: clinical and actigraphic evaluation. Sleep 2003; 26(7):815–818.
30. Trenkwalder C, Hundemer HP, Lledo A, et al. Efficacy of pergolide in treatment of restless legs syndrome: the PEARLS Study. Neurology 2004; 62(8):1391–1397.
31. Ondo WG, Romanyshyn J, Vuong K, Lai D. The Long-Term Treatment of Restless Legs Syndrome with Dopamine Agonists. Arch Neurol 2004:1393–1397.

32. Obeso JA, Grandas F, Herrero MT, Horowski R. The role of pulsatile versus continuous dopamine receptor stimulation for functional recovery in Parkinson's disease. Eur J Neurosci 1994; 6(6):889–897.
33. Olanow CW, Obeso JA. Preventing levodopa-induced dyskinesias. Ann Neurol 2000; 47(4 suppl 1):S167–S176.
34. Chase TN, Oh JD. Striatal dopamine- and glutamate-mediated dysregulation in experimental Parkinsonism. Trends Neurosci 2000; 23(suppl):24–33.
35. Chase TN, Bibbiani F, Oh JD. Striatal glutamatergic mechanisms and extrapyramidal movement disorders. Neurotox Res 2003; 5(1–2):139–146.
36. Oh JD, Chase TN. Glutamate-mediated striatal dysregulation and the pathogenesis of motor response complications in Parkinson's disease. Amino Acids 2002; 23(1–3):133–139.
37. Obeso JA, Rodriguez-Oroz M, Marin C, et al. The origin of motor fluctuations in Parkinson's disease: importance of dopaminergic innervation and basal ganglia circuits. Neurology 2004; 62(1 suppl 1):S17–S30.
38. Garcia-Borreguero D, Odin P, Schwarz C. Restless legs syndrome: an overview of the current understanding and management. Acta Neurologica Scand, 2004.
39. Connor JR, Boyer PJ, Menzies SL, et al. Neuropathological examination suggests impaired brain iron acquisition in restless legs syndrome. Neurology 2003; 61:304–309.
40. Pittock SJ, Parrett T, Adler CH, Parisi JE, Dickson DW, Ahlskog JE. Neuropathology of primary restless leg syndrome: Absence of specific tau- and alpha-synuclein pathology. Mov Disord 2004; 19(6):695–699.
41. Baumgartner A, Dietzel M, Saletu B, et al. Influence of partial sleep deprivation on the secretion of thyrotropin, thyroid hormones, growth hormone, prolactin, luteinizing hormone, follicle stimulating hormone, and estradiol in healthy young women. Psychiatry Res 1993; 48(2):153–178.
42. Zhang SQ, Kimura M, Inoue S. Bromocriptine-induced blockade of pregnancy affects sleep patterns in rats. Neuroimmunomodulation 1996; 3(4):219–226.
43. Lal S, Thavundayil J, Nair NP, et al. Effect of sleep deprivation on dopamine receptor function in normal subjects. J Neural Transm 1981; 50(1):39–45.
44. Lal S, Tesfaye Y, Thavundayil JX, Skorzewska A, Schwartz G. Effect of time-of-day on the yawning response to apomorphine in normal subjects. Neuropsychobiology 2000; 41(4):178–180.
45. Ebert D, Kaschka W. Humoral aspects of sleep deprivation. Fortschr Neurol Psychiatr 1995; 63(11):441–450.
46. Garcia-Borreguero D, Serrano C, Egatz R. Diagnosis of the restless legs syndrome: the use of the sleep laboratory. In: Chaudhuri KR, Odin P, Olanow CW, eds. Restless Legs Syndrome. London: Taylor & Francis, 2004:113–134.
47. Garcia-Borreguero D. Augmentation: understanding a key feature of RLS. Sleep Med 2004; 5(1):5–6.
48. Comella CL. Restless legs syndrome: treatment with dopaminergic drugs. Neurology 2002; 58(suppl 1):S87–S92.

# 27 Opioids and the Restless Legs Syndrome: Treatment and Pathogenetic Considerations

**Arthur S. Walters**

*New Jersey Neuroscience Institute, Seton Hall University School of Graduate Medical Education, JFK Medical Center, Edison, New Jersey, U.S.A.*

## INTRODUCTION

Although dopaminergic agents are considered the first line of therapy for restless legs syndrome (RLS), opioids are listed as an appropriate treatment for RLS and periodic limb movement disorder in the practice parameters of the American Academy of Sleep Medicine (1). The National Heart, Lung, and Blood Institute working group on RLS also considers opioids to be an important therapy for RLS, and the medical advisory board of the RLS Foundation in a published algorithm for treatment lists opioids as recommended therapy for intermittent, daily, and refractory RLS (2,3).

The potential for addiction and tolerance with opioid therapy in RLS appears to be low even with long-term therapy, as reported by four groups in two separate publications (4,5). The development or exacerbation of sleep apnea does not appear to be a consequence of short-term therapy of RLS with opioids (6). However, patients should be periodically monitored for the development or exacerbation of sleep apnea by asking appropriate questions about choking or gasping in sleep, because this may be a complication of long-term therapy (5).

## THERAPEUTIC TRIALS OF OPIOIDS IN RESTLESS LEGS SYNDROME/PERIODIC LIMB MOVEMENTS

Willis was the first to document the treatment of RLS by opioids via the description of a case from the 17th century (7–9). Ekbom in 1960 also anecdotally noted that RLS would respond to opioids, but no patient data were provided (10). In 1984, Trzepacz et al. documented improvement in RLS symptoms in three patients (11). Methadone 10 mg at h.s. or oxycodone 2.5 mg h.s., in combination with imipramine 50–100 mg/day provided relief in the three patients. Pretreatment polysomnographic data were reported for two of the three subjects, but posttreatment polysomnographic data were not provided (11). Sandyk et al. published a similar open-label study (12). Six patients were studied on either codeine 60 mg or oxycodone 10–20 mg often administered in combination with benzodiazepines. Patients subjectively reported improvement (12).

More recently an open-label nonpolysomnographic study showed that tramadol (Ultram®) 50–150 mg/day was successful in the treatment of RLS in 10 of 12 patients studied (13). Tramadol has opioid-like properties and for prescribing purposes has the advantage of not being a controlled substance, presumably because of its lower addiction potential. Most recently another open-label nonpolysomnographic study of methadone was performed in RLS patients who had failed dopaminergic agents. These refractory patients were currently taking or previously tried 5.9 ± 1.7 (range: 3–9) different medications for RLS and 2.9 ± 0.8 (range: 2–4) different dopaminergics. Methadone was successful in 17 of the 27 patients who remained on methadone at an average dose of 15.5 mg/day (range 5–40) for an average of 23 months at the time of the report (14). Two dialysis RLS patients died while on methadone, and eight stopped (five for adverse events, two for lack of efficacy, and one for logistical reasons). The authors noted little problem with either addiction or dependency. Tramadol is probably more appropriate for milder cases and methadone for refractory cases.

Intrathecal or epidural morphine infusions have also been used for very severe cases (15,16). Jakobsson et al. reported "complete relief" in two refractory patients who were implanted with a pump device (Isomed) for intrathecal delivery of morphine and bupivacaine. In a case report, Vahedi et al. reported no benefit from epidural bupivacaine, but dramatic relief was obtained by epidural morphine. The maintenance therapy with oral morphine sulfate provided equally good results.

In 1986, two studies of RLS where patients were studied polysomnographically both pre- and posttreatment were published in full paper form (17,18). Both acute treatment and subsequent chronic follow-up studies found similar results (17,18). In those open-label studies, we documented that a variety of opioids including propoxyphene 130–260 mg, codeine 30–120 mg, and methadone 5–20 mg successfully treated the leg discomfort, motor restlessness, periodic limb movements (PLMs) in wakefulness, periodic limb movements in sleep (PLMS), and other sleep parameters in five patients with RLS. Patients were followed for up to six years with no complaints of experiencing any significant side effects or tolerance, and with no need for increased doses (18). A subsequent open-label polysomnographic study suggested that patients with PLMS alone without RLS might also respond to opioids (19). Four patients were studied, and PLMS were dramatically decreased in two patients treated with methadone 5 mg and propoxyphene 195 mg. The other two patients did not show an improvement in PLMS, but one of these patients did show an increase in sleep efficiency from 57% to 74%.

Two double-blind polysomnographic studies employing opioids were subsequently published almost simultaneously (6,20). The first of these was performed on 11 patients with RLS (6), and the second was performed on six patients with PLMS (20). The first study documented that oxycodone at an average dose of 15.9 mg/day improved RLS motor restlessness ($p < 0.009$) and leg paresthesias ($p < 0.006$) as rated by the patients on a 1 to 4 severity scale (6). The following features also significantly improved: PLMS/hour of sleep—baseline 38.8, placebo 52.9, drug 18.4 ($p < 0.004$); sleep efficiency—baseline 52.2, placebo 45.7, drug 70.4 ($p < 0.006$); Arousals/hour of sleep—baseline 39.1, placebo 49.1, drug 26.6 ($p < 0.009$) (6).

The second of these studies documented that propoxyphene at doses of either 100 or 200 mg showed the following significant improvements: shorter rapid eye movement (REM) latency, decreased number of PLMS associated with arousals/hour of sleep, and a decreased percentage of PLMS associated with arousals in the first third of the night (all $p < 0.05$). Leg movements as measured by actigraphy were also significantly improved on high-dose propoxyphene ($p < 0.05$) (20).

In comparing these two double-blind studies at the dosages employed, it was obvious that oxycodone was a far more effective treatment than propoxyphene. This difference in efficacy has been verified recently along with the relative efficacy of other opioids in the treatment of RLS (21). In that open-label study, the order of efficacy as determined by the International RLS Study Group rating scale (22) was levorphanol > hydromorphone > hydrocodone > propoxyphene. All showed significant improvement from baseline. Levorphanol was equivalent to the dopamine agonist pramipexole in efficacy in this study. However, propoxyphene was far less effective than pramipexole (21). This is comparable to the results obtained by Kaplan et al. where propoxyphene was far less effective than L-dihydroxyphenylalanine (L-DOPA) in treating PLMS (20).

A long term study of opioids in RLS has recently been published (5). Twenty-three of the 36 opioid monotherapy patients had failed dopaminergic and other therapeutic agents prior to the initiation of opioid monotherapy. Twenty of the 36 opioid monotherapy patients have continued on monotherapy for an average of 5 years and 11 months (range 1–23 years). Addiction and tolerance were the reasons for discontinuation of opioid monotherapy in only one of 16 cases. Two of the weaknesses of this study were that different opioids were employed and that the patients' self-ratings of sensory symptoms were not done before and after opioid treatment. Polysomnography on seven patients performed after an average of seven years and one month of opioid monotherapy (range 1–15 years) showed a tendency toward improvement in all leg parameters and associated arousals (decrease in PLMS index, PLMS arousal index, and PLM while awake index) as well as all sleep parameters (increase in stages 3 and 4 sleep, REM sleep, total sleep time, sleep efficiency, and decrease in sleep latency). Unfortunately, because only seven patients had repeat long-term polysomnography, a statistical comparison of polysomnographic data could not be done. Although there had been no suppression of breathing during sleep in the short-term studies of opioids in RLS by Walters et al. (6), two of the seven patients studied polysomnographically in the aforementioned long-term study developed sleep apnea, and a third patient had worsening of preexisting apnea (5). We concluded that opioids seem to have long-term effectiveness in the treatment of RLS and PLMS and have low potential for addiction or tolerance; but patients on long-term opioid therapy should be clinically or polysomnographically monitored periodically for the development of sleep apnea (5). The low addiction and tolerance potential of opioids in the long-term treatment of RLS and PLMS have been confirmed by Schenck et al. (4).

## OVERALL THERAPEUTIC RECOMMENDATIONS

Based upon our experience and non-rigorous studies, we would recommend tramadol 50 mg for mild cases of RLS because of its low addiction potential. The fact that it is not a highly controlled substance makes it easy to prescribe. For moderate cases, we would recommend codeine 30 mg or oxycodone 5 mg. For severe refractory cases, methadone 5 mg can be advantageous because of its potency and long half-life. For each medication, we would recommend that the patient be gradually increased from one tablet per day to one tablet every three hours during the symptomatic period. It is our experience that dose increases can be done every four days. Despite longer half-lives of some of these medications, multiple dosage times will ensure adequate peak effects throughout the sleep period and fewer side effects. Dosages given 30 minutes prior to time of usual symptom onset can sometimes prevent symptoms before they begin. However, we usually begin with the first dose 30 minutes prior to h.s. For example, if the patient regularly has symptoms from 6 P.M. to 12 midnight, we start with a single tablet at 11:30 P.M. and after four days add another tablet at 8:30 P.M., and after another four days a third tablet at 5:30 P.M., if necessary. It should be emphasized that these recommendations are based upon personal experience, because there are no controlled head-to-head comparison studies of opioids in RLS.

## ROLE OF THE ENDOGENOUS OPIATE SYSTEM IN THE PATHOGENESIS OF RESTLESS LEGS SYNDROME/PERIODIC LIMB MOVEMENTS

### Naloxone Given to Opiate-Treated RLS Patients

The opiate receptor blocker naloxone was administered under blinded conditions to two RLS patients treated with opioids (17,18). In the first of these patients there were 992 PLMs during wakefulness on a single night recording in the untreated state. There was so little sleep that an adequate number of sleep-related periodic leg movements could not be recorded. When treated with methadone 20 mg, there was almost complete suppression of all of the cardinal features of RLS including sensory discomfort and the need to pace the floor at night as well as associated PLMs, both awake and asleep. In the treated state there were only four PLMs during wakefulness and no sleep-related periodic leg movements on a single night recording. While the patient was awake and on methadone, an intravenous naloxone challenge reactivated the PLMs during wakefulness after she received 0.16 mg. These movements increased in frequency for 15 minutes until they blended into a generalized motor restlessness that lasted for 30 minutes after the naloxone was stopped. During the first 15 minutes she had 96 PLMs during wakefulness. On a separate day, while the patient was on methadone, she received a saline infusion as a placebo, which she believed to be naloxone. This did not reactivate the PLMs during wakefulness (17,18).

The second patient had 458 PLMs in wakefulness and sleep combined on a single night recording in the untreated state. These movements were suppressed and his restlessness alleviated by propoxyphene 195–260 mg at bedtime. In the treated state, there were 97 PLMs in wakefulness and sleep combined on a single night recording. Reactivation of symptoms by naloxone in the opioid-treated state was similar to that seen in the first patient. Lack of reactivation of symptoms by saline in the opioid-treated state was also similar to that seen in the first patient (17,18). Winkelmann et al. anecdotally reported similar results in an undisclosed number of patients: "Patients pre-treated with opioids showed not the typical withdrawal signs but rather a conspicuous provocation of characteristic RLS symptoms almost immediately after naloxone was administered" (23). These results suggest that the opioid effect is specific to the opiate receptor and implicates the endogenous opiate system with its enkephalins and endorphins in the pathogenesis of RLS. Because all of the opioids that are therapeutically successful in the treatment of RLS are μu opiate receptor agonists, it is this receptor subtype that is probably most involved in the pathogenesis of RLS.

### Dopamine Receptor Blocking

Neuroleptic-induced akathisia (NIA) is motor restlessness induced by dopamine receptor-blocking agents. It is characterized by an inner urge to move the entire body, as opposed to RLS where motor restlessness is precipitated by the need to relieve leg discomfort. NIA patients also have PLMS and sleep disturbance, but not to the same degree as in RLS. Because NIA and RLS share motor restlessness and other features, the endogenous dopaminergic system is implicated in the pathogenesis of both (24). In further support of this observation is the fact that three RLS patients successfully treated with dopamine agonists experienced an exacerbation of symptoms when treated with dopamine antagonists (unpublished data).

However, administration of dopamine receptor blocking agents to drug-naive RLS patients does not always exacerbate the motor or sensory symptoms of RLS (23,25). Akpinar administered the dopamine receptor blocker pimozide 10–30 mg to a single drug naive RLS patient for two weeks, which did result in a worsening of the symptoms of RLS (25). Winkelmann et al. administered the dopamine receptor blocker metoclopramide 10 mg to eight drug-naive RLS patients (23). In contrast, there was only a tendency to exacerbate RLS symptoms with metoclopramide, but there were no statistically significant differences from baseline.

### Naloxone Given to Dopamine-Treated RLS Patients and Dopamine Antagonists Given to Opioid-Treated RLS Patients

When dopaminergically treated RLS patients are challenged with naloxone there appears to be no reactivation of symptoms (25). Akpinar reported the results of naloxone challenge to a single RLS patient treated with dopaminergic drugs (25). The patient was treated with bromocriptine 2.5 mg at 9:15 P.M. and 250 mg L-DOPA plus dopa decarboxylase inhibitor at 10:15 P.M. At 11:25 P.M. he was given naloxone intravenously, and there was no subjective reactivation of RLS symptoms. In contrast, when opiate-treated RLS patients are given the dopamine receptor blocker pimozide, there is a reactivation of at least some of the RLS symptoms (26). Montplaisir et al. studied an RLS patient in the untreated state, in the treated state with codeine sulfate 120 mg, and in the treated state with codeine sulfate 120 mg plus the dopamine receptor blocker pimozide 20 mg. After the addition of pimozide, there was a reversal of the therapeutic effect of codeine on the PLMs/hour during wakefulness (baseline 100, codeine 28, codeine + pimozide 78). However, there was no reversal of the effect of codeine sulfate on the spontaneous RLS or PLMS at night (26). These combined results suggest that opiates have their impact on RLS symptoms through their interaction with a dopaminergic system and not vice versa.

### Naloxone Given to Drug-Naive RLS Patients

When RLS patients who have not been treated with opioids are challenged with naloxone, some report no exacerbation of symptoms (17,18,23), whereas others report reactivation (25). In the first of these studies, which were reported in two separate publications, a single untreated RLS patient was challenged with naloxone (17,18). There was no worsening of any of the sensorimotor features of RLS including PLMs awake or asleep. A second more recent and more extensive study, which examined the effect of naloxone 20 mg given under blinded conditions to eight opioid-naive RLS patients, confirmed these results (23). Although there appeared to be a reactivation of PLMs/hour in wakefulness as determined by the suggested immobilization test, there was no significant difference between placebo and naloxone challenges. A third study conducted by Akpinar in a single patient suggests contradictory results. He reported "a week later, one night at 11:25 P.M., 0.8 mg naloxone was given intravenously without giving bromocriptine and L-DOPA plus benserazide during the hours before naloxone. The symptoms appeared more severe compared with the night before he had begun to use L-Dopa. Although he began to get dopaminergic drugs after 1:50 A.M., it was 5:40 A.M. when he finally slept." (25). However, one critique of this last experiment is that the reactivation of RLS symptoms could be due to rebound from dopaminergic drug withdrawal rather than from exacerbation by naloxone.

## IMPLICATIONS OF THE RECEPTOR BLOCKING STUDIES

For naloxone challenge in untreated RLS patients, the bulk of the evidence favors the results obtained by Winkelmann (relatively little effect), because this study was tightly controlled and involved the largest number of patients. The question arises as to how one can explain the contradiction between the results obtained in the opioid-treated versus the untreated RLS patient when challenged with naloxone. The results may have to do with the differential binding of the endogenous opiates (enkephalins and endorphins) to the opiate receptor as opposed to exogenously administered opioids. It may simply be more difficult to remove the endogenous opioids from the opiate receptor with naloxone than it is to remove codeine, propoxyphene, oxycodone, or methadone. Winkelmann and colleagues offer an alternate explanation. They postulate that the opioidergic tone in neural circuits involved in RLS is rather low. The opioidergic circuits involved in RLS may simply not be tonically active (23). They use the same explanation for the lack of effect of the dopamine receptor blocker metoclopramide on the symptoms of RLS in drug-naive patients (23).

Although many of the studies are small and there are some contradictory results, overall, the results favor the following hypothesis:

- Deficiencies of the endogenous opioid and dopamine systems are pathogenetic to the symptoms of RLS. This does not imply, however, that the primary defect in RLS is necessarily in either of these systems.
- Exogenous or endogenous opioids probably indirectly prevent RLS symptoms by means of their impact upon the dopaminergic system. There may or may not be intermediate biochemical steps between the opioids and dopamine.

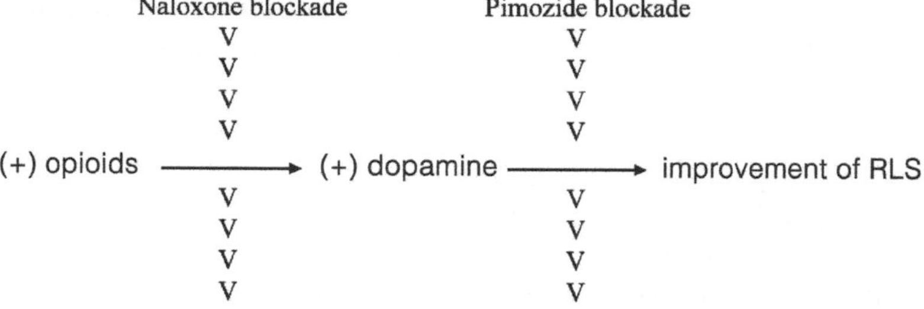


The above diagram illustrates that the opioids may have their impact through the dopaminergic system in RLS. Postsynaptic opiate receptor blocking agents, such as naloxone, block the therapeutic effects of the opioids but not of the dopaminergic agents. Postsynaptic receptor dopaminergic receptor blocking agents, such as pimozide, block the therapeutic effects of opioids as well as those of the dopaminergic agents. Because many of the studies of these blocking agents in RLS are small, they need to be replicated. Other methodologies will also be needed to determine the degree up to which the endogenous system is pathogenetic in RLS.

## OTHER EVIDENCE SUPPORTING A ROLE OF THE ENDOGENOUS OPIATE SYSTEM IN THE PATHOGENESIS OF RESTLESS LEGS SYNDROME

An opiate receptor positron emission tomography (PET) scan study of 15 patients with idiopathic RLS and 12 controls found regional negative correlations between postsynaptic radioligand opiate receptor binding and RLS severity as well as pain severity. It should be noted, however that there was no actual difference in binding between RLS patients and controls. In RLS subjects the binding was correlated to symptom intensity in areas serving the medial pain system including the medial thalamus, amygdala, caudate nucleus, anterior cingulate, gyrus, insular cortex, and orbitofrontal cortex (27). The interpretation of these results by the authors of the study is that the endogenous opiates (e.g., enkephalins and endorphins that are not radioactive) are binding more to their postsynaptic receptors in an attempt to compensate for the discomfort caused by RLS. An alternate explanation is that either the endogenous opiates or their receptors are defective in some way and that the increased binding is an attempt to compensate for this deficiency. This deficiency in the endogenous opiate system could produce the symptoms of RLS. It may be that the use of exogenous opiates as therapy partially overcomes this deficiency.

Regional blood flow was examined using single photon emission computed tomography in patients with RLS. These studies revealed a decrease in regional blood flow in the caudate nucleus with increasing pain. The thalamus and anterior cingulate gyrus showed an increase in regional blood flow with increasing pain (28).

Recent evidence from neurophysiological studies suggests that the pain system may be abnormal in RLS. In a study of 22 secondary and 20 idiopathic RLS patients, there was evidence that temperature perception was abnormal in both groups, even though the secondary RLS patients had evidence of peripheral neuropathy and the idiopathic RLS patients did not have evidence of peripheral neuropathy (29). It was assumed that the problem with temperature perception was due to the peripheral neuropathy in the patients with secondary RLS and that the problem with temperature perception was due to a central processing problem in the patients with idiopathic RLS. The fact that temperature perception is discriminated at the same level of the nervous system as pain lends credence to the idea that the discrimination of pain may be abnormal in RLS.

The concept of abnormal pain discrimination in idiopathic RLS was directly tested in a study of 11 patients with idiopathic RLS and 11 controls. The RLS patients experienced significantly more hyperalgesia to pin prick than controls by a factor of 5.3 to 6.4 (30). This was partially normalized by dopaminergic treatment (30). Based upon this, the authors suggest that the pathophysiology of RLS includes disturbed supraspinal pain modulation involving the basal ganglia and/or descending dopaminergic pathways.

Most recently, Sun et al. created an in vitro animal model of RLS. Because previous research has suggested that low iron levels and low dopamine levels in addition to low levels of the endogenous opiates are pathogenetic to RLS, we showed that decreasing iron by chelating it leads to dopaminergic cell death. This dopaminergic cell death can be prevented by pretreating the cells with opioids (31). This lends further support to the idea that hypofunction of the endogenous opiate system is pathogenetic to RLS. This research suggests that hypofunction of iron, dopamine, and the endogenous opiates may be causally connected in RLS. This further suggests that opioid treatment may be neuroprotective against the symptoms of RLS. This model, of course, will have to be extended to the in vivo situation, and it will have to be determined if animals with low levels of iron, dopamine, and the endogenous opiates are restless.

Further studies looking at the pathophysiology of RLS from the perspective of the endogenous opiate system need to be performed to more accurately determine the primacy of this system in the pathogenesis of RLS. For example cerebrospinal fluid studies of endorphins and enkephalins in patients with RLS versus controls would be helpful in this regard. Additional knowledge regarding opioid abnormalities will clearly facilitate treatment strategies in the future.

## REFERENCES


1. Chesson AL, Wise M, Davila D, et al. Practice parameters for the treatment of restless legs syndrome and periodic limb movement disorder. American academy of sleep medicine report: standards of practice committee of the American academy of sleep medicine. Sleep 1999; 22:961–968.
2. National Heart, Lung, and Blood Institute Working Group on Restless Legs Syndrome. Restless legs syndrome: detection and management in primary care. Am Fam Physician 2000; 62:108–114.
3. Silber MH, Ehrenberg BL, Allen RP, et al. Medical advisory board of the restless legs syndrome foundation. An algorithm for the management of restless legs syndrome. Mayo Clin Proc 2004; 79:916–922.
4. Schenck CH, Halfaker BA, Mahowald MW. Sustained benefit and low risk of major adverse effects during long-term nightly benzodiazepine and/or opiate treatment of injurious parasomnias, restless legs/periodic limb movement disorder and insomnia in 121 adult patients. Sleep Res 1994; 23:81.
5. Walters AS, Winkelmann J, Trenkwalder C, et al. Long-term follow-up on restless legs syndrome patients treated with opioids. Movement Disorders 2001; 16:1105–1109.
6. Walters AS, Wagner ML, Hening WA, et al. Successful treatment of the idiopathic restless legs syndrome in a randomized double-blind trial of oxycodone versus placebo. Sleep 1993; 16:327–332.
7. Willis T. De animae brutorum. London: Wells and Scott, 1672:339.
8. Willis T. Two discourses concerning the soul of brutes. Pordage S, trans. London: Dring, Harper and Leigh, 1683:139.
9. Willis T. The London Practice of Physick. 1st ed. London: Thomas Bassett and William Crooke, 1685:404.
10. Ekbom KA. Restless legs syndrome. Neurology (Minneap) 1960; 10:868–873.
11. Trzepacz PT, Violette EJ, Sateia MJ. Response to opioids in three patients with restless legs syndrome. Am J Psychiatry 1984; 141:993–995.
12. Sandyk R, Bamford CR, Gillman MA. Opiates in the restless legs syndrome. Int J Neurosci 1987; 36:99–104.
13. Lauerma H, Markulla J. Treatment of restless legs syndrome: treatment with tramadol. J Clin Psychiatry 1999; 60:241–244.
14. Ondo WG. Methadone for refractory restless legs syndrome. Movement Disorders 2005; 20:345–348.
15. Jakobsson B, Ruuth K. Successful treatment of restless legs syndrome with an implanted pump for intrathecal drug delivery. Acta Anaesthesiol Scan 2002; 46:114–117.
16. Vahedi H, Kuchle M, Trenkwalder C, Krenz CJ. Peridural morphine administration in Restless Legs status. Anasthesiol Intensivmed Notfallmed Schmerzther 1994; 29:368–370.
17. Walters A, Hening W, Cote L, Fahn S. Dominantly inherited restless legs with myoclonus and periodic movements of sleep: a syndrome related to the endogenous opiates? Adv Neurol 1986; 43:309–319.
18. Hening W, Walters A, Kavey N, Gidro-Frank S, Cote L. Dyskinesias while awake and periodic movements of sleep in restless legs syndrome: treatment with opioids. Neurology 1986; 36:1363–1366.
19. Kavey N, Walters A, Hening W, Gidro-Frank S. Opioid treatment of periodic movements in sleep in patients without restless legs. Neuropeptides 1988; 11:181–184.
20. Kaplan PW, Allen RP, Buchholz DW, Walters JK. A double-blind, placebo-controlled study of the treatment of periodic limb movements in sleep using carbidopa/levodopa and propoxyphene. Sleep 1993; 16:717–723.
21. Becker PM. Efficacy of different opioids in the treatment of restless legs syndrome (RLS): a naturalistic study. Sleep 2001; 24(suppl):A19.

22. Walters AS. Group organizer and correspondent: the international restless legs syndrome study group. Validation of the international restless legs syndrome study group rating scale for restless legs syndrome. Sleep Med 2003; 4:121–132.
23. Winkelmann J, Schadrack J, Wetter TC, Zieglgansberger W, Trenkwalder C. Opioid and dopamine antagonist drug challenges in untreated restless legs syndrome patients. Sleep Med 2001; 2:57–61.
24. Walters AS, Hening W, Rubinstein M, Chokroverty S. A clinical and polysomnographic comparison of neuroleptic-induced akathisia and the idiopathic restless legs syndrome. Sleep 1991b; 14:339–345.
25. Akpinar S. Restless legs syndrome: treatment with dopaminergic drugs. Clin Neuropharmacol 1987; 10:69–79.
26. Montplaisir J, Lorrain D, Godbout R. Restless legs syndrome and periodic leg movements in sleep: the primary role of dopaminergic mechanism. Eur Neurol 1991; 31:41–43.
27. von Spiczak S, Whone AS, Hammers A, et al. The role of opioids in restless legs syndrome: an (11C) diprenorphine PET study. Brain 2005; 128:906–917.
28. San Pedro EC, Mountz JM, Mountz JD, Hong-Gang L, Katholl CR, Deutsch G. Familial painful restless legs syndrome correlates with pain dependent variation of blood flow to the caudate, thalamus, and anterior cingulate gyrus. J Rheumatol 1998; 25:2270–2274.
29. Schattschneider J, Bode A, Wasner G, Binder A, Deuschl G, Baron R. Idiopathic restless legs syndrome: abnormalities in central somatosensory processing. J Neurol 2004; 251:977–982.
30. Stiasny-Kolster K, Magerl W, Oertel WH, Moller JC, Treede R-D. Static mechanical hyperalgesia without dynamic tactile allodynia in patients with restless legs syndrome. Brain 2004; 127:773–782.
31. Sun Y, Hoang-Lee T, Neubauer JA, Walters AS. Opioids protect against substantia nigra cell degeneration under conditions of iron deprivation: a possible model for restless legs syndrome. Sleep 2003; 26:A343.

# 28 Iron Therapy in Restless Legs Syndrome

**Charlene E. Gamaldo and Christopher J. Earley**

*Department of Neurology, Johns Hopkins School of Medicine, Baltimore, Maryland, U.S.A.*

## INTRODUCTION

Once the diagnosis of restless legs syndrome (RLS) has been declared, an appropriate work-up and evaluation should begin prior to or concurrent with therapy. This includes and may be limited to an evaluation of iron status. The appropriate iron status work-up is discussed in Chapters 4 and 17. The treatment options for RLS may include oral or intravenous (IV) iron agents.

## ORAL IRON THERAPY

### Current Studies

In his 1953 case series paper, Nordlander first discussed the efficacy of oral iron therapy for iron deficient RLS patients (1). O'Keeffe observed similar results after giving ferrous sulfate thrice daily for two months in 15 elderly patients (2). In addition, he was able to show complete resolution of symptoms in those with initial ferritin levels below 18 µg/L. Although the above series demonstrated very beneficial results, all were performed under open-label conditions. There has been only one randomized, double-blind, placebo-controlled study with oral iron therapy (3). Twenty-eight RLS patients were evenly divided into the treatment (ferrous sulfate, 325 mg b.i.d.) or placebo groups for 12 weeks. Based on the visual analog scale, no differences could be found in quality of sleep or quality of life between the two groups. However, because of several design flaws, the results are difficult to interpret. Patients with secondary causes of RLS, such as neuropathy, were included, while those with anemia were immediately excluded. The mean serum ferritin for the RLS group was 135 µg/L with a range of 9 to 680, which would predict that the majority of RLS subjects were unlikely to absorb any significant amounts of iron for the duration of the study. It is both interesting and indicative of the study design that the single best measure of effective iron treatment (i.e., post-treatment ferritin) was not given. Finally, subjects were allowed to continue their pretreatment levadopa regimen that may have obscured their response to iron therapy. Unfortunately, this study did not address the efficacy of oral iron treatment in RLS patients with documented iron deficiency.

### Dietary Recommendations

Heme and nonheme are the two dietary forms of iron. The iron found in most plants, cereals, and vegetables is in the nonheme form. This is also the form of iron added to foods that are iron fortified. Heme iron is the type found in meats and fishes. Heme iron is absorbed faster than the nonheme form. Tables 1 and 2 illustrate the amount of iron supplied by a variety of food sources.

**TABLE 1** Selected Food Sources of Heme Iron

| Food | Milligrams per serving | % DV[a] |
|---|---|---|
| Chicken liver, cooked, 3½ ounces | 12.8 | 70 |
| Oysters, breaded and fried, 6 pieces | 4.5 | 25 |
| Beef, chuck, lean only, braised, 3 ounces | 3.2 | 20 |
| Clams, breaded, fried, ¾ cup | 3.0 | 15 |
| Beef, tenderloin, roasted, 3 ounces | 3.0 | 15 |
| Turkey, dark meat, roasted, 3½ ounces | 2.3 | 10 |
| Beef, eye of round, roasted, 3 ounces | 2.2 | 10 |
| Turkey, meat, roasted, 3½ ounces | 1.6 | 8 |
| Chicken leg, meat only, roasted, 3½ ounces | 1.3 | 6 |
| Tuna, fresh bluefin, cooked, dry heat, 3 ounces | 1.1 | 6 |
| Chicken breast, roasted, 3 ounces | 1.1 | 6 |
| Halibut, cooked, dry heat, 3 ounces | 0.9 | 6 |
| Crab, blue crab, cooked, moist heat, 3 ounces | 0.8 | 4 |
| Pork loin, broiled, 3 ounces | 0.8 | 4 |
| Tuna, white, canned in water, 3 ounces | 0.8 | 4 |
| Shrimp, mixed species, cooked, moist heat, 4 large | 0.7 | 4 |

[a]DV represents the percent of daily recommended amount of iron as determined by the Food and Drug Administration. For a more exclusive list of iron food sources, please refer to the U.S. Department of Agriculture's Nutrient Database Web site: (4a).
*Abbreviation*: DV, daily value.
*Source*: From Ref. 4b.

**TABLE 2** Selected Food Sources of Nonheme Iron

| Food | Milligrams per serving | % DV[a] |
|---|---|---|
| Ready-to-eat cereal, 100% iron fortified, ¾ cup | 18.0 | 100 |
| Oatmeal, instant, fortified, prepared with water, 1 cup | 10.0 | 60 |
| Soybeans, mature, boiled, 1 cup | 8.8 | 50 |
| Lentils, boiled, 1 cup | 6.6 | 35 |
| Beans, kidney, mature, boiled, 1 cup | 5.2 | 25 |
| Beans, lima, large, mature, boiled, 1 cup | 4.5 | 25 |
| Beans, navy, mature, boiled, 1 cup | 4.5 | 25 |
| Ready-to-eat cereal, 25% iron fortified, ¾ cup | 4.5 | 25 |
| Beans, black, mature, boiled, 1 cup | 3.6 | 20 |
| Beans, pinto, mature, boiled, 1 cup | 3.6 | 20 |
| Molasses, blackstrap, 1 tablespoon | 3.5 | 20 |
| Tofu, raw, firm, ½ cup | 3.4 | 20 |
| Spinach, boiled, drained, ½ cup | 3.2 | 20 |
| Spinach, canned, drained solids ½ cup | 2.5 | 10 |
| Black-eyed peas (cowpeas), boiled, 1 cup | 1.8 | 10 |
| Spinach, frozen, chopped, boiled ½ cup | 1.9 | 10 |
| Grits, white, enriched, quick, prepared with water, 1 cup | 1.5 | 8 |
| Raisins, seedless, packed, ½ cup | 1.5 | 8 |
| Whole wheat bread, 1 slice | 0.9 | 6 |
| White bread, enriched, 1 slice | 0.9 | 6 |

[a]DV represents the percent of daily dosage recommended amount of iron as determined by the Food and Drug Administration. For a more exclusive list of iron food sources, please refer to the U.S. Department of Agriculture's Nutrient Database Web site: (4a).
*Abbreviation*: DV, daily value.
*Source*: From Ref. 4b.

**TABLE 3** Common Oral Iron Trade Names

| Ferrous fumurate | Ferrous gluconate | Ferrous sulfate |
|---|---|---|
| Femiron | Fergon | Feosol |
| Feostat | Ferralet | Feratab |
| Ferretts | Simron | Mol-Iron |
| Fumasorb | — | Slow Fe |
| Hemocyte | — | Fero-Gadumet |

### Administration of Oral Supplements

Supplemental iron comes in both a ferrous and ferric form. The ferrous salt forms are the best absorbed (5). There are three types of commonly available ferrous salts: ferrous sulfate, ferrous gluconate, and ferrous fumarate. Please see Table 3 for some of the common brand names corresponding to the three salt forms.

Ferrous sulfate is the least expensive as well as the preparation most commonly used in research trials. When the patient purchases their over-the-counter supplement, they should look specifically at the elemental iron content not the total iron content. The elemental amount is the only iron available for absorption. We recommend 50–65 mg of elemental iron with each administration. Depending on the degree of iron deficiency, supplementation can be given one to three times daily. Note that a regular multivitamin tablet with iron usually contains only 18 mg of iron.

Studies have shown an increase in iron absorption when administered along with Vitamin C on an empty stomach (6). Vitamin A can also help with iron repletion by aiding in iron mobilization (7). The following foods can directly inhibit iron absorption and therefore should be avoided one to two hours around administration: cheese, yogurt, eggs, milk, spinach, tea, coffee, soy protein, whole grain breads, cereals, and bran. An adequate amount of stomach acids are necessary for absorption, and therefore, one should avoid taking iron with antacids. The same guidelines apply for calcium, large doses of chromium, zinc, and vitamin E supplements, which can interfere with absorption. Iron is absorbed primarily in the small intestine. A variety of inflammatory conditions and malignancies can affect small bowel function. As a result, these subpopulations may require thrice daily administrations for a longer duration.

### Common Adverse Effects

Gastrointestinal (GI) irritation is the most common adverse effect, which includes constipation, loose stools, dark/tarry stools, and nausea/vomiting. In the case of upper GI irritation such as nausea or vomiting, simply switching to one of the other salt forms may suffice. Ferrous gluconate may cause fewer GI disturbances. Taking the supplements in divided doses tends to be milder on the stomach. Although not conducive to optimal absorption, enteric-coated tablets, extended-release preparations, and/or taking oral iron with food can relieve some of the GI distress.

Staining of tooth enamel may occur, particularly with the liquid elixirs. Mixing the elixir in water or preferably juices high in Vitamin C prevents formation of the iron stains. Using a dropper that places the formulation in the far palate followed by a juice flush may suffice. The stains are usually removed by brushing with baking soda or 3% medicinal hydrogen peroxide.

### Serious Adverse Effects

Less common but serious adverse effects include complications of iron overload. Regardless of the amount of iron intake, iron excretion occurs at a set basal rate. Once iron stores are adequately replete, excess iron is stored in organs such as the liver and heart. Buildup can result in severe organ damage. Hemachromatosis is a genetic disease associated with iron overload. These individuals absorb superfluous amounts of iron. Diagnosis is often made after the excess iron produces irreversible organ damage. Hemachromatosis primarily affects individuals of northern European descent (8). It is worth noting that RLS also occurs with higher prevalence in this demographic group. In fact, cases have even been documented of the two occurring in the same individual (9,10). Iron supplementation can aggravate and accelerate the consequences of hemochromatosis. Therefore, the importance of adequate screening and frequent iron status follow-up cannot be overstated.

Acute iron toxicity can be fatal particularly in children. Incidences of sudden death have occurred at dosages of 200 mg (11). Containers should be kept tightly capped out of the reach of small children. Acute symptoms of iron overdose include diarrhea, abdominal pain/cramping, vomiting, and fever. Acute symptoms may manifest as late as 60 minutes postingestion. Later symptoms include respiratory distress, fatigue, arrhythmias, blue-tinged skin and lips, and seizures. In the case of suspected ingestion, poison control should be contacted immediately.

### Long-Term Complications

Because iron treatment commonly results in a change in stool color, other pathological conditions related to dark stools may be masked. Patients over the age of 50 on long-term iron replacement should follow the current recommendations for endoscopic GI screening.

### Drug Interactions

Iron supplements can affect the metabolism of several different classes of drugs including statins, dopamine agonists, thyroid hormones, fluoroquinolones, and tetracyclines. Therefore, it is imperative that the patient notify his or her other treating physicians and pharmacist in the event of possible interactions.

## INTRAVENOUS IRON THERAPY

### Current Studies

In his two case series reports, Nordlander discusses the dramatic response achieved after one to two injections of Intrafer (iron 2% oxide). Between two and four, 100 to 200 mg IV iron injections were given over a two- to four-day course. All 10 of his iron-deficient anemic patients were "cured" of symptoms for several months. Those who saw a return in symptoms were immediately relieved by follow-up injections. A similar response was noted in patients without anemia and with normal serum iron. However, patients were not included in the study on the basis of any specific RLS clinical criteria. Symptoms such as paresthesia or akathisia in bed qualified as sufficient criteria to include subjects (1,12).

Fifty years later, Earley et al. (13) published a paper attempting to replicate Nordlander's findings. A single 1000 mg IV iron dextran infusion was given to 10 RLS subjects. To qualify, subjects had to report all four cardinal symptoms of RLS and demonstrate a minimum of 20 leg movements per hour during sleep.

Secondary causes of RLS, anemia, ferritin greater than 300 μg/L, percent iron saturation greater than 45%, or other sleep disorders excluded one from the study. A five-day washout period of all other RLS-related medications was required prior to infusion. Subjects were followed about two weeks after infusion to check ferritin and determine response rate. Sixty percent of the patients reported total resolution of their symptoms (Fig. 1A–C). They were able to remain off other RLS treatments from 3 to 36 months postinfusion. Furthermore magnetic resonance imaging especially sequenced to demonstrate brain iron did show increased iron stores in some patients (Fig. 2).

Although the response rate was quite dramatic, it clearly falls below the 95% success rate reported by Nordlander. Compared to Nordlander's study, the Earley group imposed much stricter inclusion criteria and objective outcome measures such as periodic limb movements (PLMs), RLS global rating scales and ferritin. This study, however, was open-label allowing for a strong placebo effect. There was no minimum ferritin cut-off for inclusion into the study. So, some of the patients may have responded just as well to oral treatment. Finally, it is unclear whether the positive response was due to iron therapy or relief from potential augmenting symptoms associated with their previous treatment.

Despite initial response to therapy, subjects in the both studies reported a return in symptoms within approximately six months. To investigate the utility of supplemental iron administrations, Earley developed a spin-off protocol from his original iron single dose study (14). Five subjects who initially responded to the single 1000 mg iron dextran infusion (13) were given 450 mg of iron gluconate upon return of symptoms with repeated treatments of 450 mg if symptoms

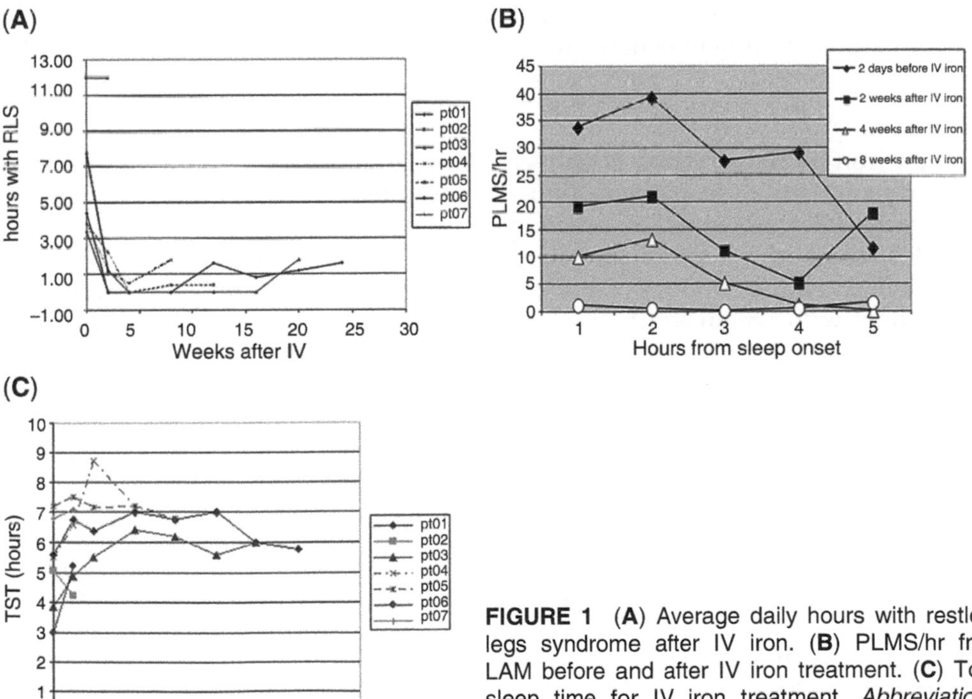


**FIGURE 1** (**A**) Average daily hours with restless legs syndrome after IV iron. (**B**) PLMS/hr from LAM before and after IV iron treatment. (**C**) Total sleep time for IV iron treatment. *Abbreviations*: TST, total sleep time; PLMS, periodic leg movements in sleep.

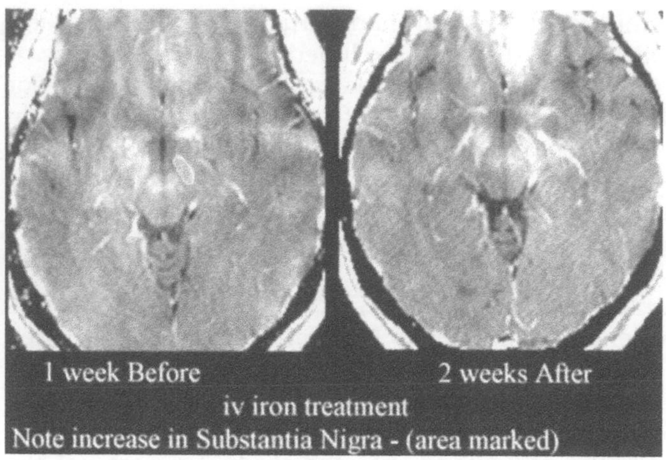


**FIGURE 2** Specially configured MRI shows ions as bright. Improved CNS iron stores after intravenous iron therapy.

returned over a two-year period. Subjects who chose to remain off RLS medications two weeks after the initial infusion were designated "responders." To remain eligible, the subjects had to comply with monthly follow-up visits, stay off all RLS medications, and maintain a monthly ferritin level below 300 μg/L. Over a two-year period, two to four supplemental doses were required to maintain symptomatic improvements. Of more interest was the finding that following IV iron treatments, the serum ferritin levels of the patients declined at rates of 2 to 11 times greater then predicted in the general population despite no indication of blood loss (Fig. 3). This suggested that the infused iron was being rapidly lost by a mechanism as yet unclear. The findings also indicate the reason as to why initial treatment benefits with large IV doses of iron were not sustained.

### Indications

Like oral iron therapy, IV iron is only currently recommended in the case of iron deficiency and in dialysis patients. IV iron is indicated in cases of oral iron therapy failure, side effect intolerance, or severe symptoms with extremely low iron profiles.

Delivering iron intravenously bypasses the GI tract, theoretically allowing one to deliver a larger amount of iron more rapidly. The ability to efficiently absorb iron declines with age. In addition, several inflammatory conditions such as malignancy and the autoimmune arthritides can affect the functioning of the small intestine. A sluggish or absent increase in the iron profile despite an appropriate six-month oral treatment course can be considered in an oral iron nonresponder. IV iron may be a more suitable option in these populations.

### Administration

Available IV formulations include iron dextran, iron sucrose, and sodium ferric gluconate complex (15). Other formulations are under investigation. All three of these agents are colloids. A colloid represents an iron-oxyhydroxide gel core surrounded by a carbohydrate suspension shell. All three IV iron preparations have the same active iron agent at their core but differ in the size of the core and surrounding carbohydrate shell. The molecular weights of the three carbohydrate shells affect the iron core's rate of release as well as the rate of clearance.

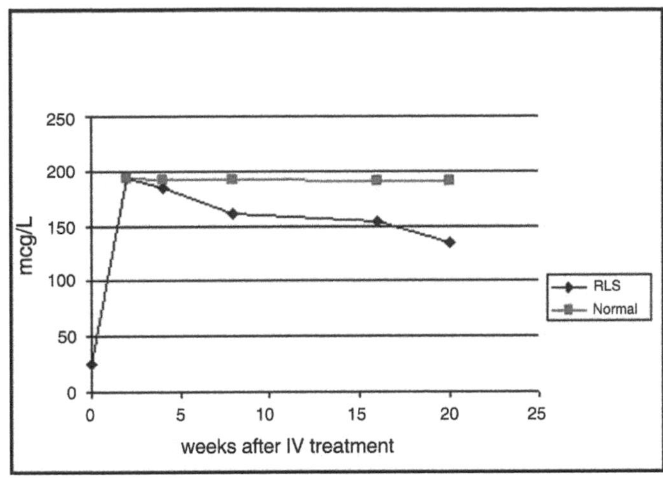


**FIGURE 3** Serum ferritin IV treatment vs. expected normal.

The molecular weight of the shell is directly correlated with the plasma half-life. Oral iron replacement must be discontinued prior to beginning IV therapy.

Iron dextran (Infed) is approved by the Food and Drug Administration (FDA) for iron-deficient individuals for whom oral supplementation is "unsatisfactory or impossible." The total amount of iron dextran required is calculated via a weight-based formula. Prior to administration of the therapeutic infusion, a 0.5 cc test dose should be infused slowly over 30 seconds. The patient should be monitored for signs/symptoms of anaphylaxis for a minimum of one hour. The remaining initial therapeutic infusion can be administered subsequently at a rate not exceeding 1 cc per minute. The majority of anaphylactic responses occur within minutes of the initial infusion. Small incremental administration of 2 cc/day could also be given until the calculated total amount is achieved.

Sodium ferric gluconate (Ferrlecit) is FDA approved as a treatment for iron deficiency anemia for chronic hemodialysis patients receiving erythropoietin treatment. Therefore, the off-label administration for iron-deficient RLS patients is based on clinical trials in this population. Ferrlecit is packaged in 5 cc ampules that contain 62.5 of elemental iron. The FDA recommended initial dosage is 10 cc that may be diluted in 100 cc of 0.9% sodium chloride. The solution should be infused over at least one hour. It can also be infused undiluted slowly at 12.5 mg/minutes. In the dialysis population, an average 1.0 g of total iron given over eight consecutive dialysis sessions were required to obtain the desired hematocrit level. In our experience, most RLS patients are replenished after two to three administrations over the course of one week.

Iron sucrose (Venofer) is FDA approved specifically as an iron replacement treatment for the dialysis population. Each ml of Venofer contains 20 mg of elemental iron. The manufacturers recommend a minimum total dose of 1000 mg administered over the course of 10 consecutive dialysis sessions. The maximum frequency should be three times a week.

Unlike iron dextran, the FDA does not require a preliminary test dose when using Venofer or Ferrlecit. However, a test dose may be prudent in particular subsets such as hemodialysis patients. These preparations should also be used with caution in patients with liver and cardiovascular abnormalities. Those patients manifesting serious anaphylactic responses in the Ferrlecit trials had a similar hypersensitivity response with past administrations of iron dextran. At the doctor's discretion, a 0.5 cc test dose can be infused slowly over one minute. Then, the patient should be monitored for one hour, looking for signs of cardiovascular/respiratory instability before proceeding with the full therapeutic dose.

### Common Adverse Events

Some of the symptoms seen during or immediately following iron administration include hypotension, nausea, headache, cramps, and diarrhea. In the Venofer trials, several patients complained of pruritus, and one manifested a facial rash. Similar reactions were reported in the clinical trial data with Ferrlecit. Side effects occur more commonly with large IV doses infused at faster rates. Most symptoms are self-limited or otherwise relieved with IV fluids, antihistamines, or hydrocortisone.

### Serious Adverse Events

The substantially heavier iron dextran shell results in a plasma half-life that is 60 times longer than its other cohorts. This extended length of release is associated with a more severe toxicity profile. Fatal anaphylactic episodes have been reported with iron dextran (16).

Although less likely with the lighter colloid shells, one must always be aware of the potential for an anaphylactic reaction. In the 231 total patients enrolled in the iron sucrose (Venofer) clinical trials, no fatal or serious anaphylactoid events occurred. Between 1992 and 1999, 8 patients out of the 450,000 treated reported a serious or life-threatening reaction. In Ferrlecit's postmarketing study, there was one reported case of anaphylactoid shock out of the 1097 patients exposed. In the cases of anaphylaxis, dyspnea and/or cardiac instability usually appeared within minutes of initiating infusion. Other common systemic manifestations included fever, abdominal pain, and elevated liver enzymes.

Due to the potential risk of an anaphylactic reaction, administration should always be conducted in a setting equipped to resuscitate and treat anaphylactoid shock.

## FOLLOW-UP

It is important to closely follow the iron status every three months during oral supplementation. Treatment might be discontinued upon acquisition of a therapeutic ferritin level ($\geq$50 µg/mL) or when the saturation level exceeds 40%. There is, however, no data to suggest whether higher serum levels should be sought. In the case of IV administration, individuals may see an immediate improvement in their symptoms. The IV route, however, rapidly floods the system with iron. So, the physician should allow at least two weeks postinfusion before checking an iron panel. Rescreening should be performed should symptoms return or worsen. Finally, anecdotal evidence suggests that patients without overt iron deficiency may also benefit from IV supplementation.

## REFERENCES

1. Norlander. Therapy in restless legs. Act Med Scand 1953; 145(6):453–457.
2. O'Keeffe ST, Gavin K, Lavan JN. Iron status and restless legs syndrome in the elderly. Age Ageing 1994; 23(3):200–203.

3. Davis BJ, Rajput A, Rajput ML, Aul EA, Eichhorn GR. A randomized, double-blind placebo-controlled trial of iron in restless legs syndrome. Eur Neurol 2000; 43(2):70–75.
4a. http://www.nal.usda.gov/fnic/cgi-bin/nut_search.pl.
4b. U.S. Department of Agriculture ARS. USDA Nutrient Database for Standard Reference, Release 16 [online]. Available at: http://www.nal.usda.gov/fnic/foodcamp.
5. Hoffman R, Benz E, Shattil S, et al. Disorders of iron metabolism: iron deficiency and overload. In: Hematology: Basic Principles and Practice. 3rd ed. New York: Churchill Livingstone, Harcourt Brace & Co., 2000.
6. Cook JD. Adaptation in iron metabolism. Am J Clin Nutr 1990; 51:301–308.
7. van Stuijvenberg ME, Kruger M, Badenhorst CJ, Mansvelt EP, Laubscher JA. Response to an iron fortification programme in relation to vitamin A status in 6–12-year old school children. Int J Food Sci Nutr 1197; 48:41–49.
8. Burke W, Cogswell ME, McDonnell SM, Franks A. Genetics and public health in the 21st century: using genetic information to improve health and prevent disease. In: Public Health Strategies to Prevent the Complications of Hemochromatosis. Oxford University Press, 2000.
9. Barton JC, Wooten VD, Acton RT. Hemochromatosis and iron therapy of restless legs syndrome. Sleep Medicine 2001; 2(3):249–251.
10. Earley CJ. Hemochromatosis and iron therapy of restless legs syndrome. Sleep Medicine 2001; 2(3):181–183.
11. Corbett JV. Accidental poisoning with iron supplements. MCN Am J Matern Child Nurs 1995; 20:234.
12. Norlander. Restless legs. Br J Phys Med 1954:160–162.
13. Earley CJ, Heckler D, Allen RP. The treatment of restless legs syndrome with intravenous iron dextran. Sleep Med 2004; 5(3):231–235.
14. Earley CJ, Heckler D, Allen RP. Repeated IV doses of iron provides effective supplemental treatment of restless legs syndrome. Sleep Med 2005; 6(4):301–305.
15. Danielson BG. Structure, chemistry, and pharmacokinetics of intravenous iron agents. J Am Soc Nephrol 2004; 15:S93–S98.
16. Zipf RE. Fatal anaphylaxis after intravenous iron dextran. J Forensic Sci 1975; 20: 326–333.

# 29 Other Therapies in Restless Legs Syndrome

**Joohi Shahed and William G. Ondo**

*Department of Neurology, Baylor College of Medicine, Houston, Texas, U.S.A.*

## INTRODUCTION

Our understanding of the phenomenology and etiopathogenesis of the restless legs syndrome (RLS) has greatly advanced since the first modern description of the disorder by Ekbom (1). There is a strong genetic component to the development of RLS, and many secondary forms are now recognized. In pure idiopathic RLS, there is evidence of dysfunction within dopaminergic pathways and of those controlling iron homeostasis. Initial studies of nondopaminergic medications focused on benzodiazepines, carbamazepine (CBZ), and clonidine. Gabapentin (GBP) later emerged as a viable treatment option for RLS, and by the time the newer dopamine agonists became widely available, physicians had many treatment options available that did not have the potential to cause augmentation. Other nondopaminergic agents (especially antiepileptics) and nonpharmacologic treatments have since been studied in small groups of patients with some efficacy against RLS symptoms, but with insufficient data to advocate routine use.

## ANTIEPILEPTICS

### Gabapentin

The first open-label trials of GBP in RLS (2,3) described subjective improvement in RLS symptoms in a small number of patients. Some patients experienced complete resolution of symptoms for up to six months (2); dosages of GBP ranged up to 2700 mg/day (3).

The first randomized, double-blind, placebo-controlled crossover study of GBP took place in 13 hemodialysis (HD) patients with RLS (4). This study found improvement in 11 patients using dosages of 200 to 300 mg after each HD session for two treatment periods of six weeks, separated by a one-week washout period. The drug was tolerated well, although two additional patients withdrew because of sedation attributed to GBP. It has also been demonstrated objectively by polysomnography that GBP reduces the index of periodic limb movements of sleep (PLMS) while also subjectively reducing RLS symptoms in eight patients (5).

An unpublished report of GBP in RLS patients diagnosed by International RLS Study Group (IRLSSG) criteria (Duntley et al., personal communication) found several more promising results. Ten patients completed (13 total were enrolled) this 14-week, double-blind, placebo-controlled crossover study consisting of two treatment periods separated by a two-week washout. Outcome measures included a sleep diary, a three-question subjective RLS symptom questionnaire, and a polysomnogram. All subjects underwent forced titration to 1800 mg GBP or placebo. GBP resulted in subjective RLS improvement in 9 of 10 subjects ($1.7 \pm 0.51$ vs. $2.8 \pm 0.69$), increased total sleep time ($7.4 \pm 0.26$ vs. $7.0 \pm 0.23$ hours for placebo, $p = 0.03$), and increased sleep efficiency (85.5 ± 0.02 vs. 80.9 ± 0.02% for placebo, $p = 0.02$). Paradoxically, two patients experienced increased PLMS despite an overall trend toward a decrease in such movements. This was attributed to the normal variability of PLMS. The authors also note that the fixed dose protocol may have caused adverse events (mainly drowsiness) in some patients, while it may have been the source of an incomplete response to the drug in others.

A 24 patient randomized, placebo-controlled crossover trial of GBP in RLS (6) evaluated 24 patients (22 with idiopathic RLS, two with iron deficiency) meeting IRLSSG diagnostic criteria. At the end of the six-week arm, at an average dose of 1855 mg/day, GBP was shown to significantly improve several rating scales when compared to placebo, including the IRLSSG Rating Scale (9.5 ± 1.3 vs. 17.9 ± 1.3), Clinical Global Impression ($p < 0.0001$), pain analogue scale ($p < 0.01$), and the Pittsburgh Sleep Quality Index ($p < 0.0001$). A significant benefit was also noticed at four weeks with a mean doses of 1391 mg/day. Patients with a prominent pain component benefited the most. Using polysomnography, this study also demonstrated a greater reduction in the PLMS index for GBP vs. placebo (20.8 ± 3.3 and 11.1 ± 3.3/hour, respectively). Total sleep time (6.0 ± 0.1 vs. 5.5 ± 0.1 hours, $p < 0.01$), sleep efficiency (84.7 ± 1.5% vs. 74.9 ± 1.5%, $p < 0.001$), and slow-wave sleep (104.5 ± 7.2 vs. 82.2 ± 7.2 minutes, $p < 0.05$) all improved on GBP. Other major sleep indices were not changed. Adverse events were modest, with only malaise (six subjects vs. two subjects) occurring more commonly in those taking GBP. Augmentation was not seen.

GBP was later compared to levodopa in an open-label fashion in hemodialysis RLS patients (7) and was found to provide greater reduction in RLS symptoms and sleep quality by multiple questionnaire measurements. When compared to ropinirole in idiopathic RLS, also in an open-label trial (8), GBP was found to be as efficacious for up to 6 to 10 months of follow-up. The main outcome measures were polysomnography and the IRLSSG questionnaire. The GBP mean dosage was 800 ± 397 mg (range 300–1200 mg), while the ropinirole mean dosage was 0.78 ± 0.47 mg (range 0.25–1.50 mg).

In the authors' experience, GBP is relatively more effective when patients report pain in their legs, as opposed to a pure "urge to move." GBP also improves neuropathic pain. Patients with neuropathy associated with RLS may have both conditions, making GBP a parsimonious choice. Finally, GBP is safely used in children for other indications, although no reports of treatment of pediatric RLS have van published. We have generally had good success with GBP in the pediatric population.

The exact mechanism of action of GBP is unknown. In vivo studies in rats have shown that it may antagonize 3,4-diaminopyridine-induced release of dopamine, norepinephrine, and serotonin in the hippocampus, mesolimbic, and striatal regions. This dopaminergic activity may underlie its effectiveness in RLS symptoms (9).

XP13512 (Xenoport, Inc.) is a transported prodrug of GBP designed to facilitate oral absorption. A two-week, 38-patient, multicenter, placebo-controlled, crossover trial reported improved IRLSSG questionnaire scores compared to placebo ($p < 0.0001$) (Xenoport, data on file). Polysomnography demonstrated improved total sleep time, improved slow wave sleep, and reduced awakenings from PLMS. The drug was well tolerated. Phase III trials are ongoing.

### Carbamazepine

CBZ has been used to treat RLS for decades. Three of six patients with RLS treated with CBZ in the first double-blind crossover study experienced benefit in symptoms (10). CBZ was significantly more effective than placebo in a double-blind, between-patient, placebo-controlled study of 174 patients with RLS (11). These studies are limited by the lack of consistent or validated inclusion criteria and outcome measures. No comparison studies have been performed with dopaminergic agents. In the authors' experience, this drug is generally inferior to GBP and dopaminergic agents. However, its low cost and well-established safety factor are advantages.

### Oxcarbazepine

Oxcarbazepine (OXC) (Trileptal®, Novartis) is a derivative of CBZ with fewer potential metabolites. In an open-label study, 17 patients with RLS were treated with an average dose of 900 mg/day of OXC (range 600–1500 mg) (12). In some patients, this was the only RLS treatment, and in others, OXC was added on to stable doses of other RLS medications. Two patients withdrew from the study due to lack of efficacy and two due to side effects. Using an intention to treat/last observation carried forward analysis, IRLSSG rating scales improved from a mean score 28.9 before treatment to 9.1 afterward.

### Lamotrigine

Lamotrigine (Lamictal®, GlaxoSmithKline) is an antiepileptic medication that is also used to treat bipolar disease. Four patients meeting IRLSSG diagnostic criteria for RLS with normal serum ferritin were enrolled in a therapeutic open-label trial of lamotrigine after a three-day drug washout period (13). Three completed the trial, with dosages ranging from 250 to 500 mg/day (average 360 mg/day). A trend toward reduced PLMS was found, and patients reported a subjective improvement in "feelings of restlessness". Lamotrigine has been shown to inhibit monoamine uptake in vitro and to modulate 5-hydroxytryptamine (5HT) uptake in rats, suggesting an affinity for biogenic amine transporters (14), which could account for the efficacy of this drug in RLS.

### Topiramate

Topiramate (Topamax®, Ortho-McNeil) has multiple mechanisms of action including inhibition of voltage gated sodium channels, augmentation of inhibitory chloride ion influx mediated by gamma-aminobutyric acid (GABA), modest inhibition of carbonic anhydrase, and antagonism of the kainate subtype of glutamate receptors. It is used to treat epilepsy, headache, obesity, and tremor. In models of dependence, topiramate has been shown to reduce mesolimbic dopamine levels resulting from nicotine use (15). The extent of this dopaminergic activity throughout the rest of the central nervous system is unknown. A single open-label study showed efficacy at mean doses of $42.1 \pm 18.7$ mg in 19 patients with RLS treated for up to 90 days (16). In some patients, improvement was accompanied by significant weight loss.

### Levetiracetam

Levetiracetam (LEV) (Keppra®, UCB Pharma) is an epilepsy medication with potential applications in treating hyperkinetic movement disorders, including myoclonus and drug-induced dyskinesias. The drug has no affinity for most major neurotransmitter receptors but does seem to oppose the action of GABA(A) antagonists. It has also been demonstrated to antagonize high-voltage N-type calcium channels and affect voltage gated potassium channels. Ten patients were enrolled in an open-label study of LEV in RLS (17). A sleep disorders expert confirmed the diagnosis of RLS and any RLS medications were discontinued for two weeks prior to beginning therapy. LEV dosages were titrated to 1500 mg/day, with assessments at the end of each two-week titration period consisting of the IRLSSG rating scale, Epworth Sleepiness Scale, and Clinical Global Impression scale. Seven patients completed the study; two withdrew due to sedation attributed to LEV. Improvement was seen in all scales and maximally at the end of the 1500 mg dosage titration, but measures of statistical significance were not given. Other case reports also report efficacy with levetiracetam (17a).

## CLONIDINE

Clonidine, an alpha-adrenergic agonist, has been variably reported to improve RLS symptoms in open-label studies and case reports (18–20). A case report and review of the previous literature (21) reported that dosages up to 0.9 mg/day produced benefit in 30 of 41 cases and was generally tolerated well. These studies did not have uniform objective outcome measurements.

A randomized, double-blind, placebo-controlled study (22) was performed in 10 patients with RLS randomized to two weeks of clonidine or placebo. The mean clonidine dose was 0.05 mg/day, and treatment response was measured using a four-point analog RLS severity scale, polysomnography, and actigraphy. In addition to subjective improvement in RLS, the authors found a significant reduction in time to sleep onset (12 vs. 30 minutes for placebo, $p = 0.006$). However, total rapid eye movement (REM) sleep was reduced (4% vs. 16% for placebo, $p = 0.001$), and REM latency was increased in the clonidine group (195 vs. 89 minutes for placebo, $p = 0.028$). No significant change in PLMS was found, but a trend toward decreased motor activity by actigraphic recordings was seen. The authors concluded that clonidine may be an effective treatment for RLS patients who do not have significant PLMS but experience delayed sleep onset due to RLS symptoms.

## BENZODIAZEPINES

Benzodiazepines are commonly used in sleep disorders including insomnia, parasomnias, and REM behavioral disorder. They are generally tolerated well for such uses (23) with relatively low rates of abuse. When used, electroencephalographic recordings show increased amounts of fast frequencies, increased numbers of sleep spindles and reduced slow-wave activity. They induce and maintain sleep by promoting stage 2 sleep while reducing REM, stage 3, and stage 4 sleep (24).

Early case reports suggested that clonazepam was an effective and well-tolerated treatment for RLS in patients with and without uremia (25–28). A randomized, double-blind crossover trial in six patients comparing clonazepam to placebo showed subjective improvement in quality of sleep and sensory symptoms (29). A prospective controlled study in six patients with no other RLS treatment who took clonazepam alternating with placebo for four weeks (30) found that clonazepam was not more effective than placebo in controlling symptoms, using a self-rating score of "feelings of restlessness" as the primary outcome measure.

Clonazepam is known to reduce PLMS and improve sleep quality (31), and these effects are retained in those with RLS and PLMS (32,33). Dosages ranged from 0.5 to 3 mg/day. A more recent study, however, suggests that clonazepam is more effective in improving insomnia and sleep parameters than PLMS in RLS patients (34). In this study, 10 RLS patients and 16 periodic limb movement disorder patients underwent a single-blind, placebo-controlled, unbalanced crossover design study in which they all received 1 mg clonazepam or placebo at bedtime. After one nocturnal polysomnogram for habituation, sleep parameters and subjective sleep scales were measured. In the RLS patients, clonazepam significantly improved sleep efficiency ($88.6 \pm 8.0$ vs. $73.0 \pm 15.3$ for placebo, $p < 0.05$), and improved subjective sleep quality as measured by the Self-Assessment of Sleep and Awakening Quality Scale ($9.6 \pm 4.0$ vs. $15.2 \pm 3/7$, $p < 0.05$). However, no difference was seen in the index PLMS per hour of total sleep time [$31.5 \pm 24.6$ vs. $32.1 \pm 21.0$ for placebo, non-significant (NS)]. No studies using the IRLS questionnaire that specifically addresses change in RLS symptoms have been performed in patients treated with clonazepam.

Alprazolam (35) and triazolam (36) have also been used with some success. Zolpidem is a nonbenzodiazepine hypnotic of the imidazopyridine class that binds to certain benzodiazepine receptors and induces sleep (37). Based on findings that there are high densities of zolpidem binding sites within the output nuclei of the basal ganglia, an open-label study of the drug in eight RLS patients (38) was performed. Without offering objective data, the authors reported that patients treated with 10 mg/day experienced complete relief of symptoms after an average duration of four days, the improvement lasted 12 to 30 months, and symptoms recurred after the drug was discontinued. No adverse events were reported.

## OTHER DRUGS

Two patients with chronic pain, neurogenic claudication, and probable secondary RLS were reported to have experienced improvement in uncomfortable lower extremity sensations within 20 minutes of ingesting oral ketamine (39). One patient was given a 30 mg test dose and the other a 50 mg test dose. Both were maintained on twice daily dosages with sustained improvement up to six months. Ketamine is a noncompetitive *N*-methyl-D-asparatic acid (NMDA) receptor antagonist with analgesic properties. Its mechanism of action in secondary RLS is unknown but may relate to reduced neuroinflammation in patients with known central nervous system injury. Larger studies are needed to confirm this effect.

In one report, 10 cases of secondary RLS were attributed to magnesium deficiency (40). Magnesium was later studied in the treatment of RLS in an open-label pilot study (41). Six patients with mild to moderate RLS and four with PLMS were given 12.4 mmol/day of oral magnesium supplementation administered at night. The findings included reduction in PLMS with arousals ($17 \pm 7$ vs. $7 \pm 7$ for placebo, $p < 0.05$) and without arousals ($33 \pm 16$ vs. $21 \pm 23$ for placebo, $p = 0.07$) and improved sleep efficiency ($75 \pm 12\%$ vs. $85 \pm 8\%$ for placebo, $p < 0.01$). Magnesium also has NMDA antagonistic properties, and its mechanism of action in RLS may be similar to that of ketamine (42).

Tryptophan is an amino acid precursor to the synthesis of serotonin. Acute dietary depletion reduced central 5-HT in humans (43), and a single case report suggests it may improve RLS symptoms (44). The utility of tryptophan supplementation is questionable, however, because the extent to which serotonin and its metabolites are implicated in RLS is not known (45,46), and selective serotonin reuptake inhibitors are known to exacerbate RLS symptoms (47–50).

Folate deficiency has been associated with RLS, especially during pregnancy (51,52). In some pregnant women, low folate levels were more highly correlated with RLS symptoms than low serum ferritin (52). Whether this is due to development of neuropathic changes with subsequent development of secondary RLS or if disorders of folate metabolism are a potential cause of primary RLS is unknown. A systemic study of folate supplementation in the treatment of RLS symptoms has not been performed.

Baclofen is a GABA-ergic drug that mainly has effects at the spinal cord level. Stimulation of GABA receptors promotes endogenous opioid release. This mechanism may underlie reports of successful treatment of RLS with baclofen (53). Similar spinal cord mechanisms have been postulated to account for improvement in RLS symptoms in Parkinson's disease (PD) patients taking amitriptyline (54). Propranolol has been reported to improve secondary RLS symptoms in a patient experiencing withdrawal from imipramine (55).

Three patients with RLS were treated with Botulinum Toxin Type A injections into areas reported by the subjects to be uncomfortable (56). In patient number 1, injections were in the tibialis anterior; patient number 2, the lumbar paraspinals, gastrocnemii, and quadratus femorii; and in patient number 3, in the gastrocnemii. Injections resulted in improved scores on the Epworth Sleepiness Scale in two patients and reduced sleep latency in the third. The two patients on RLS medications were able to stop them after the injections; one patient was reported to experience complete resolution of RLS symptoms, and the other a "great improvement." Effects were seen within two to three days of the injections and wore off within 12 weeks. Reinjection resulted in a similar response. Long-term data are not available.

## NONPHARMACOLOGIC THERAPIES

### Enhanced External Counter Pulsation

Enhanced external counter pulsation (EECP) utilizes sequentially inflated pneumatic devices on the feet to enhance coronary artery diastolic flow and decrease left ventricular afterload (57). Six patients undergoing EECP for this indication who also had RLS completed the IRLSSG rating scale before and 35 days after EECP (58). A significant reduction in scores into the clinically insignificant RLS range was found (average 28.8 before and six after EECP). Long-term follow-up of four patients revealed two with sustained benefit one year after completion of EECP. The authors postulate that impaired vascular flow either centrally or peripherally may contribute to RLS pathogenesis.

### Sclerotherapy

Sclerotherapy is a procedure used to treat varices in different locations. About 1397 patients underwent a screening evaluation for varicose veins and RLS (59). About 113 of 312 patients diagnosed with RLS by the authors' own definition underwent sclerotherapy, with 111 reporting initial unquantified improvement. A recurrence rate of 8% at one year and 28% at two years following treatment was seen.

### Neurosurgical Procedures

One patient undergoing pallidotomy for PD experienced improvement in RLS sensory symptoms after the surgery (60). Another patient with RLS and dystonia experienced remission of RLS symptoms following placement of a deep brain stimulator in the globus pallidus interna (61). Six patients who underwent bilateral deep brain stimulation (DBS) of the subthalamic nucleus for advanced PD and who also had RLS were found to have a 79% improvement in the IRLSSG rating scale (pre-op mean 24.8, post-op mean 5.2) (62). Postoperative rating scales were completed from 2 to 24 months after DBS placement. Improvement occurred despite the reduction in dopaminergic medications that is typical for PD patients treated with this surgery. In contrast, subthalamic nucleus (STN) DBS placement in PD patients has also been reported to precipitate RLS in 11 of 194 patients undergoing the procedure, in association with dopaminergic dose reduction (63). Another report suggested RLS in PD improves after STN DBS (64) in some patients of the ventalis intermedint nucleus used to treat essential tremor did not improve RLS in seven patients with both conditions (65). These conflicting results underscore the need for larger, prospective assessments in patients with neurologic conditions for which there is a high association with RLS. No reports of neurosurgical brain procedures in patients with primary RLS have been published.

### Acupuncture

A single patient with RLS was reported to improve after a series of acupuncture treatments (66). Treatments to the scalp and bilateral foot motor sensory zones were applied, with resolution of symptoms after 15 treatments; improvement was sustained at a single follow-up visit at three months. A larger series of patients has not been studied in a randomized fashion.

## CONCLUSIONS

For patients who are unable to tolerate or who are refractory to dopaminergic agents or opiates for the treatment of RLS, other treatment options exist. Many case reports or series of open-label studies do not employ clear objective measures of RLS symptoms. Of the antiepileptics, GBP is the most rigorously studied and should be tried first. It can be safely used in uremic patients as well with appropriate dosage adjustments. Other antiepileptics have not been sufficiently studied to warrant routine use in RLS patients. These drugs have complicated mechanisms of action, some of which may involve dopaminergic systems. Clonidine, benzodiazepines, and hypnotics are most likely to induce sleep and may also reduce comorbid PLMS, thus enhancing sleep quality. They may also be safe to use in patients with renal failure but may be of most use in RLS patients with prominent sleep complaints. Of the nonpharmacologic therapies, EECP shows the most promise. Neurosurgical therapies used for specific patient populations, especially deep brain stimulation for PD, can improve concomitant RLS symptoms, but larger studies need to be performed.

## REFERENCES

1. Ekbom KA. Restless legs. Acta Med Scand 1945; 158(suppl):1–124.
2. Adler CH. Treatment of restless legs syndrome with gabapentin. Clin Neuropharmacol 1997; 20(2):148–151.
3. Merren MD. Gabapentin for treatment of pain and tremor: a large case series. South Med J 1998; 91(8):739–744.
4. Thorp ML, Morris CD, Bagby SP. A crossover study of gabapentin in treatment of restless legs syndrome among hemodialysis patients. Am J Kidney Dis 2001; 38(1):104–108.

5. Happe S, Klosch G, Saletu B, et al. Treatment of idiopathic restless legs syndrome (RLS) with gabapentin. Neurology 2001; 57(9):1717–1719.
6. Garcia-Borreguero D, Larrosa O, de la Llave Y, et al. Treatment of restless legs syndrome with gabapentin: a double-blind, cross-over study. Neurology 2002; 59(10): 1573–1579.
7. Micozkadioglu H, Ozdemir FN, Kut A, et al. Gabapentin versus levodopa for the treatment of restless legs syndrome in hemodialysis patients: an open-label study. Ren Fail 2004; 26(4):393–397.
8. Happe S, Sauter C, Klosch G, et al. Gabapentin versus ropinirole in the treatment of idiopathic restless legs syndrome. Neuropsychobiology 2003; 48(2):82–86.
9. Pugsley TA, Whetzel SZ, Dooley DJ. Reduction of 3,4-diaminopyridine-induced biogenic amine synthesis and release in rat brain by gabapentin. Psychopharmacology 1998; 137(1):74–80.
10. Lundvall O, Abom PE, Holm R. Carbamazepine in restless legs. A controlled pilot study. Eur J Clin Pharmacol 1983; 25(3):323–324.
11. Telstad W, Sorensen O, Larsen S, et al. Treatment of the restless legs syndrome with carbamazepine: a double blind study. Br Med J 1984; 288(6415):444–446.
12. Youssef IS, Walters AS. An open label study of oxcarbazepine in restless legs syndrome (RLS). Sleep 2004; 27(suppl):A292 (Abstract).
13. Youssef EA, Wagner ML, Martinez JO, et al. Pilot trial of lamotrigine in the restless legs syndrome. Sleep Med 2005; 6(1):89.
14. Southam E, Kirkby D, Higgins GA, et al. Lamotrigine inhibits monoamine uptake in vitro and modulates 5-hydroxytryptamine uptake in rats. Eur J Pharmacol 1998; 358(1):19–24.
15. Schiffer WK, Gerasimov MR, Marsteller DA, et al. Topiramate selectively attenuates nicotine-induced increases in monoamine release. Synapse 2001; 42(3):196–198.
16. Perez Bravo A. Topiramate use as treatment in restless legs syndrome. Actas Esp Psiquiatr 2004; 32(3):132–137.
17. Lacey DM. Efficacy of graduated-dose levetiracetam in treating restless legs syndrome and associated hypersomnia: a pilot study. Sleep 2004; 27(suppl):A302 (Abstract).
17a. Della Marca G, Voliono C, Mariotti P, et al. Levetiracetam can be effective in the treatment of restless legs syndrome with periodic limb movements in sleep: report of two cases. J Neurol Neurosurg Psychiatry 2006; 77:566–567.
18. Handwerker JV, Palmer RF. Clonidine in the treatment of "restless leg" syndrome. N Engl J Med 1985; 313(19):1228–1229.
19. Bamford CR, Sandyk R. Failure of clonidine to ameliorate the symptoms of restless legs syndrome. Sleep 1987; 10(4):398–399.
20. Bastani B, Westervelt FB. Effectiveness of clonidine in alleviating the symptoms of "restless legs." Am J Kidney Dis 1987; 10(4):326.
21. Zoe A, Wagner ML, Walters AS. High-dose clonidine in a case of restless legs syndrome. Ann Pharmacother 1994; 28(7–8):878–881.
22. Wagner ML, Walters AS, Coleman RG, et al. Randomized, double-blind, placebo-controlled study of clonidine in restless legs syndrome. Sleep 1996; 19(1):52–58.
23. Schenck CH, Mahowald MW. Long-term, nightly benzodiazepine treatment of injurious parasomnias and other disorders of disrupted nocturnal sleep in 170 adults. Am J Med 1996; 100(3):333–337.
24. Monti JM. Sleep laboratory and clinical studies of the effects of triazolam, flunitrazepam and flurazepam in insomniac patients. Methods Find Exp Clin Pharmacol 1981; 3(5):303–326.
25. Matthews WB. Treatment of the restless legs syndrome with clonazepam. Br Med J 1979; 1(6165):751.
26. Boghen D. Successful treatment of restless legs with clonazepam. Ann Neurol 1980; 8(3):341.
27. Read DJ, Feest TG, Nassim MA. Clonazepam: effective treatment for restless legs syndrome in uremia. Med J 1981; 283(6296):885–886.
28. Braude W, Barnes T. Clonazepam: effective treatment for restless legs syndrome in uraemia. Br Med J 1982; 284(6314):510.

29. Montagna P, Sassoli de Bianchi L, Zucconi M, et al. Clonazepam and vibration in restless legs syndrome. Acta Neurol Scand 1984; 69(6):428–430.
30. Boghen D, Lamothe L, Elie R, et al. The treatment of the restless legs syndrome with clonazepam: a prospective controlled study. Can J Neurol Sci 1986; 13(3):245–247.
31. Peled R, Lavie P. Double-blind evaluation of clonazepam on periodic leg movements in sleep. J Neurol Neurosurg Psychiatry 1987; 50(12):1679–1681.
32. Horiguchi J, Inami Y, Sasaki A, et al. Periodic leg movements in sleep with restless legs syndrome: effect of clonazepam treatment. Jpn J Psychiatry Neurol 1992; 46(3):727–732.
33. Inami Y, Horiguchi J, Nishimatsu O, et al. A polysomnographic study on periodic limb movements in patients with restless legs syndrome and neuroleptic-induced akathisia. Hiroshima J Med Sci 1997; 46(4):133–141.
34. Saletu M, Anderer P, Saletu-Zyhlarz G, et al. Restless legs syndrome (RLS) and periodic limb movement disorder (PLMD): acute placebo-controlled sleep laboratory studies with clonazepam. Eur Neuropsychopharmacol 2001; 11(2):153–161.
35. Scharf MB, Brown L, Hirschowitz J. Possible efficacy of alprazolam in restless leg syndrome. Hillside J Clin Psychiatry 1986; 8(2):214–223.
36. Tollefson G, Erdman C. Triazolam in the restless legs syndrome. J Clin Psychopharmacol 1985; 5(6):361–362.
37. Swainston-Harrison T, Keating GM. Zolpidem: a review of its use in the management of insomnia. CNS Drugs 2005; 19(1):65–89.
38. Bezerra ML, Martinez JV. Zolpidem in restless legs syndrome. Eur Neurol 2002; 48(3):180–181.
39. Kapur N, Friedman R. Oral ketamine: a promising treatment for restless legs syndrome. Anesth Analg 2002; 94(6):1558–1559.
40. Popoviciu L, Asgian B, Delast-Popoviciu D, et al. Clinical, EEG, electromyographic and polysomnographic studies in restless legs syndrome caused by magnesium deficiency. Rom J Neurol Psychiatry 1993; 31(1):55–61.
41. Hornyak M, Voderholzer U, Hohagen F, et al. Magnesium therapy for periodic leg movements-related insomnia and restless legs syndrome: an open pilot study. Sleep 1998; 21(5):501–505.
42. Fawcett WJ. Ketamine for restless legs syndrome. Anesth Analg 2003; 96(4):1238.
43. Hood SD, Bell CJ, Nutt DJ. Acute tryptophan depletion. Part I: rationale and methodology. Aust N Z J Psychiatry 2005; 39(7):558–564.
44. Sandyk RL. Tryptophan in the treatment of restless legs syndrome. Am J Psychiatry 1986; 143(4):554 555.
45. Earley CJ, Hyland K, Allen RP. CSF dopamine, serotonin, and biopterin metabolites in patients with restless legs syndrome. Mov Disord 2001; 16(1):144–149.
46. Stiasny-Kolster K, Moller JC, Zschocke J, et al. Normal dopaminergic and serotonergic metabolites in cerebrospinal fluid and blood of restless legs syndrome patients. Mov Disord 2004; 19(2):192–196.
47. Bakshi R. Fluoxetine and restless legs syndrome. J Neurol Sci 1996; 142(1–2):151–152.
48. Sanz-Fuentenebro FJ, Huidobro A, Tejadas-Rivas A. Restless legs syndrome and paroxetine. Acta Psychiatr Scand 1996; 94(6):482–484.
49. Hargrave R, Beckley DJ. Restless leg syndrome exacerbated by sertraline. Psychosomatics 1998; 39(2):177–178.
50. Agargun MY, Kara H, Ozbek H, et al. Restless legs syndrome induced by mirtazapine. J Clin Psychiatry 2002; 63(12):1179.
51. Botez MI, Lambert B. Folate deficiency and restless-legs syndrome in pregnancy. N Engl J Med 1977; 297(12):670.
52. Lee KA, Zaffke ME, Baratte-Beebe K. Restless legs syndrome and sleep disturbance during pregnancy: the role of folate and iron. J Womens Health Gend Based Med 2001; 10(4):335–341.
53. Sandyk R, Kwo-on-Yuen PF, Bamford CR. The effects of baclofen in the restless legs syndrome: evidence for endogenous opioid involvement. J Clin Psychopharmacol 1988; 8(6):440–441.
54. Sandyk R, Iacono RP, Bamford CR. Spinal cord mechanisms in amitriptyline responsive restless legs syndrome in Parkinson's disease. Int J Neurosci 1988; 38(1–2):121–124.

55. Ginsberg HN. Propranolol in the treatment of restless legs syndrome induced by imipramine withdrawal. Am J Psychiatry 1986; 143(7):938.
56. Rotenberg J, DiFazio M. Successful use of botulinum toxin A for the treatment of restless legs syndrome: a case series. J Clin Sleep Med 2006; 2(3):275–278.
57. Shea ML, Conti CR, Arora RR. An update on enhanced external counterpulsation. Clin Cardiol 2005; 28(3):115–118.
58. Rajaram SS, Shanahan J, Ash C, et al. Enhanced external counter pulsation (EECP) as a novel treatment for restless legs syndrome (RLS): a preliminary test of the vascular neurologic hypothesis for RLS. Sleep Med 2005; 6(2):101–106.
59. Kanter AH. The effect of sclerotherapy on restless legs syndrome. Dermatol Surg 1995; 21(4):328–332.
60. Rye DB, DeLong MR. Amelioration of sensory limb discomfort of restless legs syndrome by pallidotomy. Ann Neurol 1999; 46(5):800–801.
61. Okun MS, Fernandez HH, Foote KD. Deep brain stimulation of the GPi treats restless legs syndrome associated with dystonia. Mov Disord 2005; 20(4):500–501.
62. Driver-Dunckley ED, Evidente VG, Adler CH, et al. Restless legs syndrome in Parkinson's disease patients improves with subthalamic stimulation. Mov Disord 2006 (in press).
63. Kedia S, Moro E, Tagliati M, et al. Emergence of restless legs syndrome during subthalamic stimulation for Parkinson disease. Neurology 2004; 63(12):2410–2412.
64. Driver-Dunckley E, Evidente VG, Adler CH, et al. Restless legs syndrome in parkinson's disease patients may improve with subthalanic stimulation. Mov Disord 2006 (in press).
65. Ondo WG. VIM Deep brain stimulation does not improve pre-existing restless legs syndrome in patients with essential tremor. Park Dis Rel DisordInk Dispal Disord 2006: 12(2):113–114.
66. Hu J. Acupuncture treatment of restless leg syndrome. Tradit Chin Med 2001; 21(4): 312–316.

# 30 Future Directions

**William G. Ondo**
*Department of Neurology, Baylor College of Medicine, Houston, Texas, U.S.A.*

## INTRODUCTION

Although restless legs syndrome (RLS) was described in the 17th century, most meaningful research concerning RLS phenotype, epidemiology, pathophysiology, and treatment has occurred within the past 10 years. All objective measures of research interest, such as citation index citations numbers and governmental research funding, have increased dramatically over the centuries since then, probably more so than any other neurological disease, and possibly more than any medical disease. A small group of dedicated researchers has grown to a large international community with collaborators in many fields of biosciences. There is much to celebrate.

But like any field of research, an increased volume of knowledge simply expands the surface area of enquiry. As our understanding increases, so does our ability to ask previously unrecognized questions. Let us briefly review our present and future endeavors.

## DIAGNOSIS

We now have widely accepted diagnostic criteria for RLS (1). We have validated written questionnaires, phone questionnaires, and interviews for diagnostic purposes and treatments (2,3). These have undergone extensive psychometric evaluations and are acceptable by any measure.

There are, however, still people who may report all inclusion criteria for RLS, yet in the investigator's view not suffer the syndrome as we envision it. Conversely, there are people who may not meet all of the inclusion criteria yet probably do have the same thing that we define as RLS. Do all four criteria start simultaneously at the same time? This would be unusual in a neurological disease. Should we diagnose people with RLS if it occurs only once or very infrequently? Would people even recognize RLS if it occurred once every six months? What if it occurred in only a very specific unusual situation, such as a midnight flight? Currently, no minimum severity or frequency criteria mitigate the diagnosis. Do people always have RLS if they ever have had it? If not, how long must one be free of symptoms to "not have RLS?" Basic questions regarding the accepted diagnostic criteria remain. Although symptom rarity may mitigate any need for therapeutics, knowing who "really" has RLS is of tremendous importance for RLS research.

Diagnostic criteria in children have been reported but lack any form of validation (1). Attention deficit hyperactivity disorder in children, which is associated with periodic limb movements (PLMS), lower ferritin levels, and parents with RLS is an intriguing finding. Is this a true phenotype of RLS in children, an association, or simply diagnostic overlap between unrelated phenotypes? Likewise, diagnosis in demented patients, or anyone unable to articulate their problem for any reason, is problematic.

An interesting and completely unexplored observation is similarities between RLS and infantile colic. Having had two moderately colicy children myself, I was impressed that the onset coincided with the development of a circadian sleep pattern, and then consistent at 7 P.M. It is then relived by movement, albeit passive, or physical stimulation. Therefore, colic meets $\frac{3}{4}$ RLS criteria, while the "urge to move" is not known. It also can be exacerbated with antihistamines. Improvement of colic also generally correlates with demonstrable accumulation of iron in the brain. At birth, central nervous system (CNS) iron levels are extremely low. We hope to eventually evaluate the associations of pregnancy-induced RLS and colic, and the iron status of the mother and child in this extremely common condition. If it resulted that aggressive iron supplementation improves colic, the researchers would have indeed rendered a tremendous public health service.

One of our main diagnostic shortcomings for RLS is the lack of any biological markers for RLS. This greatly hampers genetic research that relies on a clinical phenotyping, which may be subtle, may not present until later in life, or may not be fully penetrant at all. The absence of any specific RLS gene can be most attributed to phenotyping issues more than any other part of the gene identification process. Can a 35-year-old who does not manifest RLS carry the RLS gene? Of course, but it may not present until they are 40. Obviously, the best biomarker would be identification of RLS genes, but this of course becomes a circuitous argument.

Several potential biological markers do exist, but they lack clear validity and are cumbersome and costly. Imaging of CNS iron via magnetic resonance imaging (MRI) and ultrasound, and measures of CSF iron do separate groups of RLS from controls, but there is some overlap (4–6). Periodic limb movements of sleep are seen in almost 90% of cases with RLS but are not specific for RLS, nor are they part of the diagnostic criteria (7). One functional MRI report demonstrates abnormalities, but this same pattern is seen with other neurological diseases (8). Dopamine imaging shows modest abnormalities but is neither sensitive nor specific for making an RLS diagnosis (9). A variety of other clinical features, such as olfaction testing, neuropsychiatric testing, and neurological examinations are not diagnostically helpful (10). Finally no physiological marker has ever been tested in "presymptomatic" or "at risk" patients for RLS to prospectively evaluate whether this may predict subsequent symptoms.

## EPIDEMIOLOGY

The epidemiology of RLS has been extensively reported, and most reports using currently accepted criteria are fairly homogeneous. Nevertheless, they are only homogeneous in mostly Caucasian populations. Asian population surveys show less RLS but vary. There has never been a rigorous study in Africa, but African Americans anecdotally have less RLS and have been demonstrated to have less RLS in the dialysis population compared to Caucasians (11). Racial and geographical differences need to be clarified. Even the north–south variance within Europe (less RLS in Mediterranean countries) has not been explained. Is this a genetic or environmental etiology?

The severity and course of RLS has never been prospectively followed over decades. There is some suggestion that RLS improves in octogenarians, although different mortality rates could easily explain these findings. Finally, there is also no good epidemiological data on RLS in children.

## DISEASE ASSOCIATIONS

We have discussed multiple other diseases associated with RLS. The relationship between any of these and RLS symptoms is entirely unknown. Do they all have completely different pathologies that result in similar symptoms? Do they all cause some unifying pathology at some point in the genesis of RLS? If so, then where along the presumed rostral–caudal axis do these converge? This of course, is necessarily predicated on understanding the pathology of RLS in general. Why do some people with uremia, neuropathy, pregnancy, and so forth, have RLS symptoms, whereas most do not? Is there some genetic predisposition that would eventually lead to RLS in these patients either way, either possessing a gene that helps cause RLS or lacking a gene that helps prevent it? Is there a genetic predisposition that would specifically cause RLS only with that associated condition? Do some patients only get secondary RLS with two secondary conditions such as neuropathy and iron deficiency (two strikes), or is there just something different in their underlying associated condition (more severe)? Secondary RLS cases are an obvious clue as to the pathogenesis of RLS in general, but with the exception of systemic iron deficiency, little has been learned to date.

## PATHOLOGY

Perhaps the most exciting aspect of RLS research revolves around pathogenesis. There is ample data to support two major lines of inquiry—iron dysregulation and functional dopaminergic deficiency. Both of these, however, are elucidated only at a fundamental level. Iron research suggests altered intracellular homeostatic control, resulting in less iron stores, perhaps associated with iron regulating protein-1 function (12). Currently, however, there is no direct evidence (genetic markers, evidence of toxic intervention, etc.) to support any specific cause of these pathologic observations. It is also not overtly clear that this is the primary pathological process and not an epiphenomenon. Recent animal models show that dopaminergic manipulation can effect iron regulation rather than the other way around, as has been assumed all along. Dopaminergic dysregulation is even less understood. By far, the strongest support for dopaminergic involvement is the dramatic clinical improvement from dopaminergic medications. There is some relatively equivocal dopaminergic imaging data, but one must take into account the fact that the only area large enough to image well is the striatum. Otherwise, there is little physiological or pathological data to support any dopaminergic dysfunction.

The unification of the two areas of enquiry (iron dysregulation and dopaminergic dysfunction) is highly speculative. Three theories exist to explain how iron deficiency might result in dopaminergic dysfunction: (i) iron is required for dopamine synthesis via tyrosine hydroxylase, (ii) iron is required for the dopamine receptor, and (iii) iron is required for Thy-1, which has a role in dopamine synaptic function. None of the three current theories have any direct human evidence to support them. Finally, why does presumed dopaminergic hypofunctioning (again assumed based on treatment response) specifically result in RLS symptoms anyway? What is the anatomy?

In summary, the skeptical view of our current pathological understanding must only concede that we understand (i) clinical symptoms, (ii) reduced iron in the brain in a pattern consistent with homeostatic dysregulation, (iii) dramatic symptom improvement with dopaminergic medication, and (iv) some physiology implicating abnormal energy consumption in nonspecific subcortical structures. Everything else is a "black box."

## TREATMENT

Overall, we have good symptomatic therapy for RLS. In fact, it is the area of research that is most robust and advanced. This fortuitously results from the simple fact that medications designed for other indications, especially Parkinson's disease (PD), improve RLS symptoms. Numerous dopaminergics, opioids, and some epilepsy medications have all demonstrated efficacy in controlled trials and many other medications improve RLS in open-label trials. With the possible exception of intravenous iron, all provide only symptomatic relief that immediately ceases upon discontinuation. In fact, dopaminergics may result in symptom exacerbation upon discontinuation.

Despite the abundance of positive studies, ideal clinical trial assessments have not been established. The questionnaire currently used by almost all treatment trials was never intended as an efficacy measure (13). It appears to suffer from a marked placebo response and probably has a ceiling effect, both of which minimize treatment effect. Older measures such as diaries of RLS symptoms, PLMS and sleep assessments, sleep questionnaires, and analogue scales may better correlate with clinical experience. Therefore, the ideal RLS treatment trial design has yet to be realized.

As with most conditions, individual responses vary. This is further complimented by the heterogeneity of RLS, both the known secondary associations and possible multiple etiologies of primary RLS. No serious effort has been made to identify prognosticators of treatment response. Most associated RLS conditions are excluded from treatment trials, and aside from uremia, these have not been individually studied. Furthermore, comparative trials among different treatments for any RLS are generally lacking.

Perhaps the biggest practical problem in our current treatment armamentarium is dopaminergic augmentation. The mechanism behind this is not known, and it is difficult to study clinically, because most trial designs would necessitate stopping or withholding symptomatically effective medications, which is ethically problematic. Several studies, however, could be performed but lack industry or public agency funding.

Two different aspects of augmentation need to be evaluated. First we should prospectively evaluate treatment strategies after augmentation occurs. Potential options include "cold turkey" drug holidays, dose elevation, switching to other dopaminergic agents, and switching to nondopaminergic agents with or without returning to the original culpable agent. Second and more importantly, we need to initiate prospective trials to evaluate strategies to prevent augmentation. Does the actual dopaminergic drug make a difference, or is it just a feature of pharmacokinetics? Prospective long-term trials with different drugs dosed so they have similar blood levels could help address the first possibility. Different dosing regiments of the same drugs (using the minimum effective nocturnal dose vs. 24 hours, three times per day dosing) could help address the second possibility.

Does continuous dopaminergic stimulation, a popular strategy to prevent dopaminergic dyskinesia in PD, actually prevent augmentation or just cover it up? This would require a staged trial where one group starts with 24-hour continuous therapy then switches to nocturnal therapy, while the other group starts with nocturnal therapy only, clearly a problematic design. Some understanding of augmentation at the cellular level would of course help direct this more costly clinical research.

## SUMMARY

RLS has come a long way in the past 10 years. The abundance of disease and lack of baseline knowledge has fueled tremendous advances in our understanding of clinical features, epidemiology, pathology, and treatment. But as with all good discoveries, this leads to more avenues of research. I am confident that many of the questions I pose in this chapter will be answered within the next decade, and I look forward to new questions to be addressed for the following decade.

## REFERENCES

1. Allen RP, Picchietti D, Hening WA, Trenkwalder C, Walter AS, Montplaisi J. Restless legs syndrome: diagnostic criteria, special considerations, and epidemiology. A report from the restless legs syndrome diagnosis and epidemiology workshop at the National Institutes of Health. Sleep Med 2003; 4:101–119.
2. Abetz L, Vallow SM, Kirsch J, Allen RP, Washburn T, Earley CJ. Validation of the restless legs syndrome quality of life questionnaire. Value Health 2005; 8:157–167.
3. Hening WA, Allen RP, Thanner S, et al. The Johns Hopkins telephone diagnostic interview for the restless legs syndrome: preliminary investigation for validation in a multi-center patient and control population. Sleep Med 2003; 4:137–141.
4. Allen RP, Barker PB, Wehrl F, Song HK, Earley CJ. MRI measurement of brain iron in patients with restless legs syndrome. Neurology 2001; 56:263–265.
5. Earley CJ, Connor JR, Beard JL, Malecki EA, Epstein DK, Allen RP. Abnormalities in CSF concentrations of ferritin and transferrin in restless legs syndrome. Neurology 2000; 54:1698–1700.
6. Mizuno S, Mihara T, Miyaoka T, Inagaki T, Horiguchi J. CSF iron, ferritin and transferrin levels in restless legs syndrome. J Sleep Res 2005; 14:43–47.
7. Montplaisir J, Boucher S, Poirier G, Lavigne G, Lapierre O, Lesperance P. Clinical, polysomnographic, and genetic characteristics of restless legs syndrome: a study of 133 patients diagnosed with new standard criteria. Mov Disord 1997; 12:61–65.
8. Bucher SF, Seelos KC, Oertel WH, Reiser M, Trenkwalder C. Cerebral generators involved in the pathogenesis of the restless legs syndrome. Ann Neurol 1997; 41:639–645.
9. Wetter TC, Eisensehr I, Trenkwalder C. Functional neuroimaging studies in restless legs syndrome. Sleep Med 2004; 5:401–406.
10. Adler CH, Gwinn KA, Newman S. Olfactory function in restless legs syndrome. Mov Disord 1998; 13:563–565.
11. Kutner NG, Bliwise DL. Restless legs complaint in African-American and Caucasian hemodialysis patients. Sleep Med 2002; 3:497–500.
12. Connor JR, Wang XS, Patton SM, et al. Decreased transferrin receptor expression by neuromelanin cells in restless legs syndrome. Neurology 2004; 62(9):1563–1567.
13. Allen RP, Kushida CA, Atkinson MJ. Factor analysis of the International Restless Legs Syndrome Study Group's scale for restless legs severity. Sleep Med 2003; 4:133–135.

# Index


A11 neurons, 93
  identification of, 103
Acroparesthesia, 65
Actigraphy
  reliable diagnosis of PLM, 180
  use of, 277
Active sleep, 3
Acupuncture, 341
Adenosine triphosphate formation, 53
Adenylate cyclase, activation of, 287
ADHD. *See* Attention deficit hyperactivity disorder
Adults
  average sleep requirement of, 3
  RLS prevalence in, 160
African Americans
  RLS prevalence in, 162
  susceptibility to RLS, 221
Age, reversing sleep deprivation and, 130
Age and gender, and adolescent's serum ferritin levels, 175
Akathisia, 256
  drug-induced, 74
  focal, 219
  neuroleptic-induced, 182
  nocturnal, 251
  RLS vs., 152
  smoking and, 261
Alcohol, RLS and, 262
Alpha-amino-5-hydroxy-3-methyl-4-isoxazole propionic acid (AMPA) receptors, 308
Alprazolam, 339
Alzheimer-type changes, 101
American Academy of Sleep Medicine, 315
Amnesia, transient, 1
Amphetamines, 129
Amyloidosis, primary, 230
Analgesics
  nonopioid, role in RLS, 74
  RLS and, 262–263
Anaphylaxis, 331
Anemia, role in RLS, 221
Anesthesia, spinal, 233, 235
Anterior tibialis muscle, 180
Anticonvulsants, 190
Antidepressants, provoking or exacerbating RLS, 256–258
Antiepileptics, RLS and, 261
Antihistamines, 346
Antinociceptive mechanisms, dysfunction of intrinsic, 90
Antipsychotics
  drug-specific action, 260
  worsen RLS, 258–260
Apomorphine, as therapy for PD and RLS, 298
Arm involvement, 148
Arousal, 129
  confusional, 172
Arylalkylamine-*N*-acetyl-transferase (NAT), 34
Asian populations, RLS prevalence in, 162
Asperger syndrome, 172
Ataxia, RLS and, 270
Athens Insomnia Scale (AIS), 225
Atonia, of skeletal muscle, 7
Attention deficit hyperactivity disorder (ADHD), 153
Augmentation, 263
  definition of, 298
  drugs causing, 299
  levodopa on, 291
Autodepolarization, 33

Autosomal dominant transmission, 173
Autosomal recessive model, 118

Babinski sign, 67, 188, 234
Baclofen, 340
Basal ganglia circuitry, schematic of, 20
Basolateral membrane iron export, 52
Benadryl®, 260
Benzodiazepines, 191, 335
  insomnia, 338
  parasomnias, 338
  REM behavioral disorder, 338
  in sleep disorders, 338
  as sleep facilitator, 280
Bereitschafts potential, 71
Blindness postchiasmatic, 32
Blink reflex excitability, 187
Blood–brain barrier, 54, 104, 288
Blood circulation, reduced peripheral, 65
Blood donation, RLS in, 183, 213
Blood flow
  cerebral, 70
  regional, 321
Blood loss, 54, 57
Body pain, diffuse, 74
Body positional discomfort syndrome, 149, 155
Body temperature, decline in, 131
Bone marrow, 53
Botulinum toxin type A injections, 340
Brain
  dopamine subtypes distribution in, 288
  dopamine systems, circadian influences on, 22
  iron homeostasis, 89
  major dopaminergic modulatory systems of, 20
  systematic structural abnormalities of, 68
Brainstem reflexes, 68
Breathing, sleep-disordered, 182, 191
Bromocriptine, RLS treatment by, 291
Burst duration, 181

Cabergoline treatment studies, 293–294
  drug tolerance, 294
  IRLS improvement, 294
[Cabergoline treatment studies]
  long-term discontinuation rates, 294
Caffeine, RLS and, 262
CAG-repeat length, RLS and, 270
Calcineurin activity, stimulation of, 19
Calf muscle, unpleasant sensation in, 147
Carbamazepine (CBZ), 190, 335, 336
  used to treat RLS, 336
Cardiac changes and PLM, 188
Cardiovascular morbidity, chronic sleep restriction and, 131
Carpal tunnel syndrome (CTS), 155
Catastrophes, sleep-related, 5
Cell adhesion molecule, 212
Cell death, opioid use and, 97
  dopaminergic, 187, 247
Cellular iron insufficiency, 105
Central nervous system iron levels, 212, 346
  imaging via magnetic resonance, 346
  excessive, 54
Cerebral blood flow, 70
  PLM and, 188
Childhood RLS
  drug treatment of, 177
  hyperactivity and inattentiveness, association between, 174
  verbalizing discomfort, 171
Circadian rhythm
  disorders, 9
  genes involved in, 22
  phase shift, light stimulus on, 32
  potential environmental factors on, 31
  prime marker of, 75
Circadian sleep pattern, 346
Clinical global impression (CGI) scale, 275
Clock genes, examples of, 33
Clonidine, 338
Cognitive inactivity, 149
Cognitive performance, deficits in, 127
Conners subscale, 176
Cortical or subcortical inhibition, 187
Cortical silent period (CSP), 71
Cryoglubolinemia, 64
Cyclic alternating pattern (CAP), 71
Cytosolic aconitase activity, 105

D2–D3 agonists, principal agents in RLS improvement, 288
D3 receptors, spinal cord excitability and, 94
Dark phase, light exposure during, 37
Data collection strategies, 159
Daytime napping, 130
  during pregnancy, 239
Daytime sleepiness, 126
  self-reported, 127
  for measuring PD/RLS link, 249
  primary reason for, 290
"Dead zone," 32
Deep brain stimulation (DBS), 341
Deep sleep, 181
Delta oscillations, 7
Delta waves, 3
Depression, 112
  incidence of, 28, 160
  RLS and, 74
Dialysis patients
  and RLS, 166, 221–222, 224
  mortality in, 184
3,4-Diaminopyridine, 336
Diencephalospinal pathways, 24, 248
Diurnal modulation, in TH expression, 23
Divalent metal transporter (DMT), 51
Dopamine
  binding, 69
  catabolism, pathways for, 16
  circadian expression of, 41
  dyfunction, behavioral correlates, 20
  enzyme metabolism of, 15
  knockout mice model, 93–95
  metabolic pathway of, 91
  neurons, presence of, 103
  physiological effects of, 19
  production, 15, 17
  receptors
    categories of, 287
    hypersensitivity of postsynaptic, 72
    hypothalamic, 23
    subtypes, 23
  signaling, 22–24
  synthesis, regulation of, 19
  transmission insufficiency, 89
  use of, 8
Dopamine agonists, 279
Dopamine antagonists. *See* Antipsychotics
Dopamine imaging, 346
Dopamine pathways, mesocorticolimbic, 247
Dopamine release, serotonin inhibition of, 257
Dopamine synthesis, 73, 174
Dopamine system integrity, Thy-1 deficiency and, 106
Dopaminergic augmentation, 307
  clinical features of, 307
  differential diagnosis of, 310
  drug efficacy, 312
  hemorrhage worsening, 312
  iatrogenic worsening, 312
  measurement of, 309–310
  molecular abnormalities, 308
  nondopaminergic agents, 307
  pathophysiology of, 307
  pharmacokinetic mechanism, 308
  presynaptic/postsynaptic mechanisms, 308
  standardized screening instruments, 307
  treatment of, 312
Dopaminergic cell death, 321
Dopaminergic drugs, 305
Dopaminergic dysregulation, 347
Dopaminergic neuronal firing, 308
Dopplers, transcranial, 188
Dorsiflexion signal, great toe, 181
Dose–response curve (DRC), 32
Drugs, 339
  class B and C, 244
  dosing strategies, 279
  movement disorders inducing, 255
Dysesthesia, 62
Dyskinesia
  levodopa-induced, 154
  nocturnal, 186
  tardive, 41, 256
Dystonia, 256

Elderly, cognitively impaired, diagnostic criteria for, 151
End-stage renal disease (ESRD) and RLS, 166
Endocytosis, 51

Endogenous opiates
  binding of, 321
  deficiency of, 320
  endorphins, 318, 320
  enkephalins, 318, 320
  hypofunction of, 321
Enhanced external counter pulsation (EECP), 340
Epilepsy variant, 179
Epworth Sleepiness Scale (ESS), 249, 277, 340
Ergot medications, 10
Erythrocytes, mean functional lifetime of, 53
Erythropoiesis, 52
Estrogen replacement therapy, 76
Excessive daytime somnolence (EDS), consequences of, 4
Exercise, benefits of, 129
Extrapyramidal symptoms (EPS), 255

Familial aggregation analysis, 114–117
Family (positive) history and idiopathic RLS, 221
Fatigue, safety problem and, 128
Ferritin, mucosal, 52
Ferroportin, cellular iron export, 104
Ferrous salts, types, 327
Fibromyalgia, 74
  RLS and, 270
Fibrosis
  endoneural, 231
  hepatic, 55
First-degree relative, 221
  correlation coefficient between, 115
  familiar relative risk ratios, 117
Flexion-withdrawal reflex, 67, 179, 234
Fluoro-Gold®, fluorescent tracer, 90
Folate deficiency, 340
  levels, 163
  supplementation, RLS treatment during pregnancy, 244
Foot tapping, 112, 148
Foramen magnum meningioma, 233
F-responses, 64

G-protein–coupled receptors, 18
Gabapentin (GBP), 190, 335
Gamma-aminobutyric acid (GABA), 337
Gastrointestinal irritation, 327
Gastrointestinal side effects, 289
Gene array analysis, 105
Genetic association analysis, 114, 120
Gliosis, 104
Glomerular filtration rate (eGFR), 221
Glutamate receptors, 19
Glutamatergic hyperactivity, 308
Glycine, role in REM sleep, 7
"Growing pains," 171
Guillain–Barre syndrome, 230

Haber–Weiss–Fenton reaction, 49
Hallucinations, 189, 290
Haplotype analysis, 118, 173
Headaches, in RLS, 74
Health risk, associated with sleep level, 4
Heart rate, changes of, 69
Heme iron, 49, 325
  absorption, 50
  food sources of, 326
Hemochromatosis, 214
  familial, 52
  hereditary, 55
Hemodialysis (HD), 335
  patients, levodopa efficacy, for RLS, 291
  renal replacement therapy and RLS prevalence, 219
Hemoglobin levels, lower, 221
Hepcidin gene, plasma regulator of, iron absorption, 51
Heritable trait, 121
H-ferritin, 173
Hindlimb movements (HLM), in rats, 96
Histamine-receptor antagonists, RLS and, 260
Homeostatic control loop, in iron absorption, 51
Homovanillic acid levels, 186
Hopkins RLSQoL summary score, 199
Hormonal theory, RLS during pregnancy, 243
Hormone replacement therapy (HRT), 76
Hormone secretion pattern, 131

H-reflex, 66
impaired excitability curve of, 67
5-$HT_2$ receptors, stimulaton of, 258
Human memory and learning, sleep and REM, 132
Human substantia nigra, immunostaining pattern of, 103
6-Hydroxydopamine (OHDA)–lesioned mice
and iron deprivation studies, results of, 93
TH cells in, 92
Hydroxine replacement, RLS symptoms and, 154
Hydroxyndole-*O*-methyltransferase (HIOM), 34
Hyperalgesia, 74
Hyperlipidemia, 165
Hypersomnolence, 250
Hypnic myoclonus, 1, 182
Hypnotic medications, 37, 188, 190
Hypocretin, 8
Hypotension, orthostatic, 189
Hypothalamus, subparaventricular (SPZ) of, 34
Hypotonia, 3
Hypoxia, and increased iron absorption, 52

Idiopathic RLS and family history, 221
Imaging studies
for PD/RLS link, 248
in PLM, PLMD, and RLS, 188–189
Inheritance models, 113
Inheritance pattern, autosomal recessive, 173
Insomnia, 9, 242
predictor of RLS, 161
Interferon gamma response transcript (IRP), principal iron sensors, 51
International classification of sleep disorders (ICSD), 2
International Restless Legs Syndrome Study Group (IRLSSG), 141–142, 335
rating scale, 282
shortcomings of, 276
Intrafamilial heterogeneity, 118
Intravenous iron therapy
adverse events, 332
in dialysis patients, 330
in RLS patients, 328
indications, 330
serum ferritin, 331
IRLS. *See* International Restless Legs Syndrome Study Group (IRLSSG), rating scale
Iron
absorption regulation of, 50
deficiency, 55–56
dietary forms of, 249
export, basolateral membrane, 52
flux, intraerythrocyte regulation of, 51
heme and nonheme, 325
hepcidin gene as plasma regulator, 51
homeostasis, 54
inherent toxicity, 54
intravenous vs. oral supplementation, 215
management proteins, 103
overload diseases, 55
plasma pool, 52
toxicity, 55
Thy-1 protein expression and, 106
Iron supplementation, 215, 329
Iron deficiency
and other RLS associations, 214
Parkinson's disease, 215
pregnancy, 214
renal failure, 214
RLS and PLM, in children, 213
in RLS children, 173
RLS and, 41, 164–165
Iron deficient anemic patients, 328
Iron deprivation and 6-hydroxydopamine(OHDA)–lesioned mice studies, results of, 90
Iron dextran, 331, 332
for iron-deficient individuals, 331
Iron dysregulation, 347
Iron overload
complications of, 328
symptoms of, 328
systemic, 214
Iron replacement, 174, 215–216
intravenous, 328
oral, 325

Iron stores, low, indicator of, 212
Iron sucrose (Venofer®)
as iron replacement treatment, 331
Iron toxicity | in children, 328

Johns Hopkins Restless Legs Syndrome Quality of Life Questionnaire (RLS-QoL), 285

K complexes, 3
Keppra®, 337
Kidney disease patients, stage 5 chronic, 219
Kleine–Levin syndrome, 9
Kupffer cell lysosomal remnants, 53

Lamotrigine (Lamictal®), 337
Laser capture microdissection (LCM), 104
L-dopa
adverse effect of, 189
in RLS for bipolar disease, 337
Leg discomfort
characterization, difficulty of, 148
measuring, 277
Leg movements and cortical involvement, 71
Levetiracetam (LEV), 337
Levodopa, 143, 279
treatment, 74
effect on RLS and PLMS, 233
treatment studies, 290–291
Lewy bodies and Lewy neurites, 101
Life expectancy, 125
Light sleep, 181
Limb discomfort, 150
Linkage analysis, genetic, 173
Linkage studies, 118–120
Lipid peroxidation reactions, initiating, 49
Lithium, and induction of RLS, 261
Liver. *See* Iron, plasma pool, principal donor to
Logarithm-of-odds (LOD) score, 118, 173
Low-density lipoprotein apheresis (LA), 165
Luminal absorption, of heme iron, 50

Magnesium supplementation, 339
Medication-induced movement disorders, 255
Melatonin, 22
main roles of, 34
sites of action, 35
synthesis
and catabolism, 34–35
rate-limiting enzyme for, 35
Memory deficits, 130
Mesocorticolimbic pathway, 21
Metoclopramide, 72
"Microsleep," 127, 130
Mirtazapine, 257
Mixed linear model approach, 115
Monoamine oxidase (MOA) A and RLS, 120
Monoamines, 93
Monosynaptic "stretch" reflex (MSR) amplitude, 94
Motor-evoked potentials (MEP), 63
Motor activities, 149
Motor limb movements, control over, 187
Motor pathways, damage to, 232
Motor restlessness, 152, 250
Motor thresholds
active vs. resting, 63
of tibialis anterior muscle, 63
Movement disorders
medication-induced, 255
sleep-related, 10
Movements, stereotyped, 67. *See also* PLMS
Multiple sclerosis (MS), RLS and, 272
Multiple sleep latency testing (MSLT), 126
Multivariate logistic regression analysis, 221
Myelopathies, secondary RLS in, 232

Naloxone
in drug-naive RLS patients, 319
as opiate receptor blocker, 318
in opiate-treated RLS patients, 318
Nerve conduction velocity (NCV), abnormal, 229
Nerve entrapment disorder, 155

Neuroleptic-induced akathisia (NIA), 152
by dopamine receptor-blocking agents, 318
Neuromelanin cells, 104, 174
Neuropathy
Charcot–Marie–Tooth, 64
peripheral, 61
peripheral axonal, 63
Neuropathy, and familial RLS, 215
Neurophysiological examination techniques, 63
Neurotransmitter, vesicular release of, 106
Nightwalker survey, 113
Nigrostriatal dysfunction, 186
Nigrostriatal pathway, 19, 23
Nigrostriatal presynaptic dopaminergic dysfunction, 248
*N*-methyl-D-asparatic acid (NMDA)
phosphorylation of, 308
receptor antagonist, 339
1996 Kentucky Behavioral Risk Factor Surveillance, 160
Nociceptor axon reflex, quantitative, 64
Nocturnal habitual sleep period, 126
Nocturnal myoclonus, 179
Nondopaminergic medications studies, 335
gabapentin (GBP), 335
dosages, 335
and levodopa, 336
PLMS index for, 336
in RLS, 335
Nonheme iron, 50
food sources of, 326
Nonrapid eye movement (NREM) sleep, hallmarks of, 7

Obstructive sleep apnea (OSA), 131, 190, 239
Occupations, high-risk, 129
Open-label nonpolysomnographic study
in RLS treatment, 315
Open-label polysomnographic study
in RLS treatment, 316
Opiate-treated RLS patients
naloxone in, 318
Opiate receptor positron emission tomography (PET) scan
Opiates, 190. *See also* Endogenous opiates
Opioids
American Academy of Sleep Medicine, 315
in treatment for
PLM disorder, 315
RLS, 315–317
therapeutic trials in PLM disorder, 315–317
Opioid medications, 279
Opioid monotherapy
addiction and tolerance, 317
PLMS arousal index, decrease in, 317
REM sleep, increase in, 317
and sleep, 317
Opioid receptor binding, RLS severity and, 74
Opioidergic circuits, in RLS, 320
Oppositional Defiant Disorder Scale, 176
Oral contraceptives, to reduce iron loss, 54
Oral iron replacement, 331
Oral iron supplementation, 73, 91
Oral iron therapy, 174
adverse effects, 327–328
complications, 328
drug interactions, 328
efficacy of, 325
placebo-controlled study with, 325
in RLS
patients, 325
Oral iron trade names, 327
Oral supplemental iron, 327
Oral vs. intravenous iron supplementation, 215
Orexin pathways, 248
Oxcarbazepine (OXC), 337
Oxidative deamination, 120
Oxygen
saturation, 1
sensor, 52
Oxytocin release, facilitation of, 21

Pain medications, 74
Painful legs, and moving toes, 155
Pallidotomy, 251

Parasomnias, 10, 172
Parathyroid hormone, low, 221
Paresis, progressive, 233
Parkinson's disease (PD), 348
characteristics of. *See* Cell loss, nigral dopaminergic
daytime sleepiness and, 290
differential diagnosis of, 186
key pathology in. *See* Cell loss, dopaminergic
RLS and, 165, 248, 249
central nervous system pathology, 251
sleep–wake cycles in, 247
and sleep disorder, relationship, 184
*Per* and *Cry* proteins, 33
Pergolide, 189
treatment studies, 291–293
PLM reduction, during sleep, 292
principal side effects | headaches and nausea, 292
therapeutic response, superior, 292
Periodic limb movement disorder (PLMD)
opiods in treatment for, 315
Periodic limb movement index (PLMI), 38, 181
and serum ferritin, association between, 173
Periodic limb movements (PLMs), 329, 345
history and significance of, 179
Periodic limb movements of sleep (PLMS), 335
in RLS patients, 234
low serum ferritin levels with, 213
Peripheral nerve lesions, 155
Peritoneal dialysis and RLS prevalence, 219
PET findings, in sensorimotor processing, 189
Phase-response curve (PRC), 32
Phenoxybenzamine, alpha-receptor blocker, 65
Pimozide, as opiate receptor blocker, 319
Pinealectomy, 22
in rats, 36
Pittsburgh sleepiness scale, 249, 277
Pituitary prolactin (PRL) secretion, hypothalamic dopamine influence on, 41
Plasma pool iron, rate and location of uptake, 53
PLMs. *See* Periodic limb movements
anatomical distribution of, 180
appearance of, 186
cardiac changes, 188
differential diagnosis of, 182
occurrence during sleep, 181
spinal cord level generator for, 188
occurrence of, 233
and ADHD, bidirectional association between, 184
PLMD. *See* Periodic limb movement disorder
anatomical origin of, 187
and depression, 185
drug classes treating, 189–191
epidemiology of, 182–183
first-line treatment for, 189
guidelines for scoring and recording, 180
PLMI. *See* Periodic limb movement index
Polyneuropathy (PNP), 230
axonal, 230
diagnosis criteria, 230
family history and, 229
RLS prevalence in, 230
small fiber, 232
symptoms of, 234
Polysomnography, 309
use in children, 175
profile, in 65-year-old ESRD patient, 223
Pontine, 187
Porphyrin ring structure, 50
Positive airway pressure therapy, 129
Pramipexole, 190
Europe, approved in, 143
studies, 294–295
augmentation, 295
PLM reduction, 294
side effects, 294
SIT improvement, 294
Pregnancy
daytime naps, 239
delivery and RLS symptoms, 243

[Pregnancy]
impaired, 128
plasma iron storage indicators, 243
PLMS occurrence during, 242
risk factor for, RLS and RLS
association between, 162–164, 241
RLS pharmacological treatment, association between, 162–164, 244
RLS prevalence during, 240
RLS symptomatic threshold and, 243
sleep pattern changes in, 239
third trimester total sleep time, 164, 239
treatment for RLS, 244
Psychosis, delusional, 140
Psychosocial dysfunction, 112

Quality of life (QoL)
disease-specific evaluation of, 199
disruption of, 199
chronic disorders vs. RSL sufferers, 200
treatment benefits for, 201
Questionnaires
Johns Hopkins Restless Legs Syndrome Quality of Life (RLS-QoL), 285
nonmotor symptom, 251
subjective, 276

Radiculopathies, 232
lumbosacral, 66
Rapid eye movement (REM) sleep
hallmarks of, 3
phasic, characteristics of, 3
"Rebound" phenomena, 291
Regional blood flow, 321
Renal-failure population, RLS among, 222
Renal transplantation, 231
treatment strategy, 225
Repeat mutation, nucleotide, 114
Rest, 148
Rest-activity cycles, 5
Restless legs syndrome (RLS), 325, 335
acupuncture for, 341

[Restless legs syndrome (RLS)]
age and, 272
age at onset, 89, 114
akathisia, 153
amputation and, 66
analgesics, nonopiod, 74
bedtime, dosing regimen for, 289
biological markers for. *See* Periodic limb movement index (PLMI)
brain iron
content in, 68
homeostasis in, 89
cardinal symptoms of, 328
causes of, 325, 329
cerebrospinal fluid ferritin in, 89, 211
circadian expression of, 77
dopamine and melatonin, 40
circadian pattern in, 38, 89, 149
decreased intracortical inhibition in, 72
development, 335
diagnostic criteria for, 148
diagnosis, 345
disease associations, 347
drug-induced, pathogenesis of, 264
dysesthesias and, 232
environmental factors for, 117
epidemiology, 346–347
etiopathogenesis, 335
extrapyramidal symptoms in, 250
familial, 89
features of, 151, 219
first medical description of, 139
first-line therapy for, 287
folate deficiency, 340
genetic loci for, 121
genetic roles in, 113, 117, 121
headaches in, 74
iatrogenic, common agents associated with, 260
idiopathic, 231, 242
immobility effects on, 148
improvement of, 72
and infantile colic similarity, 346
intravenous iron therapy, 328
iron deficiency and, 41, 73, 164–165
iron regulatory proteins and, 105
iron therapy in, 325
lithium-induced, 261

[Restless legs syndrome (RLS)]
measuring sensory and motor component of, 277. *See* also Suggested immobilization test
mianserin-induced, 258
mimic, 93
mirtazapine-induced, 257
monoamine oxidase A (MOA) and, 120
muscle biopsy studies in, 64
neurodegenerative diseases and, 103
neuropathic, 229
neuropathy and, 336, 64
neurosurgical procedures for, 340–341
nonpharmacologic therapies for, 340
enhanced external counter pulsation (EECP), 340
sclerotherapy, 340
occurrence studies on, 163
origin of, 61
in Parkinson's disease (PD), 340
pathogenesis of, 89
pathophysiology of, 63
phenomenology, 335
phenotype, subtyping, 113
PLM and, 39
positive family history, 149, 232, 233 251, 271
pregnancies, relationship, 161
pregnancy and, 240–241
pregnancy-induced, 346
prevalence of, 89, 114
primary, 211
radiculopathies and, 232
rescue therapy for, 298
rheumatoid arthritis and, 230
risk factor for, 241
scales for, 275–278
secondary, 62, 211, 231, 232, 240
causes of, 214, 215
sensory symptoms of, 147
serum ferritin levels and, 91, 249
severity and PLMI, 39
sleep efficiency in, 89
spinal anesthesia, 233
SSRI and, 256
structural vs. functional abnormality, 62

[Restless legs syndrome (RLS)]
symptoms, 148, 305, 328, 332
characteristic features, 305
clinical recognition of, 306
dopaminergic therapy in, 309
therapeutic consequences, 306
thalmus, role in, 65, 70
transmission of, 114
treatment
baclofen, 340
bromocriptine, 319
bupivacaine, Isomed® for delivery of, 316
carbamazepine (CBZ), 336
clonidine for, 338
dopaminergic agents for, 289, 315, 337
gabapentin (GBP), 335
imipramine, 315
improvements in, 348–349
isomed, 316
lamotrigine for, 337
L-dopa, 319
levetiracetam (LEV) for, 337
levorphanol, 316
magnesium, 339
oxcarbazepine (OXC) for, 337
methadone, 315
for refractory cases, 316
for milder cases, 316
morphine, 316
mu opiate receptor agonist, 318
open-label nonpolysomnographic study, 315
open-label polysomnographic study, 316
opiods, 315, 316
oxycodone, 315
pathogenesis of, 318
pathophysiology of, 321
propoxyphene, 316
topiramate for, 337
tramadol (Ultram®), 315
uremic, 222, 225
vascular pathogenesis of, 65
Retinohypothalamic–pineal tract, 35
Rheumatoid arthritis, 74
Rheumatological disorders, RLS and, 269

Risch's model. *See* First-degree relative, familiar relative risk ratios, estimation for
RLS. *See* Restless legs syndrome
RLS-6 rating scales, 284
Ropinirole, 190, 202
  drug efficacy, 296
  FAO approved drug, 143
  IRLS ratings, 296
  PLM reduction, 297
  side effects, 296
  sleep onset latency improvement, 297
  studies, 295–297
Rotigotine, IRLS improvement and, 297

Sclerotherapy, 65, 340
SCN. *See* Suprachiasmatic nucleus
Segregation analysis, 114, 173
Seizure recurrence, precipitating factor, 130
Selective serotonin reuptake inhibitors (SSRIs), 74, 256
Sensorimotor disorder, 111, 171–172
Sensorimotor integration deficit, 235
Sensory-evoked potentials (SEP), 63
Serum (high) phosphorus, in RLS predicton, 222
Serum ferritin levels
  in adolescents, 175
  age at onset, 214
  familial RLS, 214
  following IV iron treatment, 73
  low, 163, 164, 212. *See also* Iron
  RLS and, 91
  and total body iron stores, 173
Short-Form (SF)-36, 200, 277
Short-form 36 (SF-6), 277
Sibling relationship, correlations for, 115
SIT (suggested immobilization test), 39, 148, 277
Sjogren's syndrome (SS), 269
Skin biopsy, use of, 231
Sleep
  active, 3
  adult requirements, 3
  biochemical determinants of, 8
  circadian and homeostatic control of, 37–38
[Sleep]
  debt, repaying, 132
  deprivation, 4, 37
    animal studies, 132–133
    PET studies, 130
    vs. fragmentation, 126
    immune function and, 131
    neurologic effects of, 130
    reversing, 129
  disorder, classification of, 9
  duration and function of, 126
  homeostasis, 130
  humoral control of, 37
  hypnogram, 2
  needs, 125
  newborn, 3
  ontogeny of, 3
  paralysis, 1
  phylogeny of, 5
  propensity to, 129
  REM, hallmarks of, 3
  unhemispheric, 5
Sleep–wake activity, circadian control of, 34
Sleep–cycle, extension of, 37
Sleep apnea
  development of, 315
  RLS and, 272–273
Sleep complaints
  in postpolio syndrome, 32–34
  and QoL, 200
Sleep deprivation, 23
Sleep fragmentation, 225
Sleep measures, gold standard for, 277
Sleepiness
  countermeasure to, 129
  types of, 5
Sleepwalking, 172
Slow wave sleep (SWS), phenomena associated with, 10
Smoking, RLS and, 261
Snoring, 1
Sodium ferric gluconate (Ferrlecit®)
  for iron deficiency anemia, 331
Spinal cord
  neurodegeneration, 103
  pathological disease states, 188
Spinal cord lesions
  etiology of, 233
  PLMS associated with, 66

Spinal dopamine, sole source of, 24
Spinal dopamine dysfunction, circadian component to, 95
Spinal flexor reflexes, 248
Spinal hyperexcitability, 68
Spinocerebellar ataxia (SCA), 66, 248
Stenosis, lumbar, 155
Striatal deafferentation, 247
Striatal dopamine metabolism, 69
Subthalamic nucleus (STN), 341
Suggested immobilization test (SIT), 39, 148, 277
Suprachiasmatic nucleus (SCN)
  endogenous clock location, 32
  sites of action, 37
Supraspinal inhibitory impulses, 67
  loss of, 67, 248
Supraspinal inhibitory influences, transitory loss of, 67
Sural nerve biopsy, 231
Synapses, stabilizing, 212
Syringomyelia, 66

Tachycardia, transient, 181
Temperature perception, in sensory testing, 63
Tetrahydrobiopterin ($BH_4$), naturally occurring pteridine cofactor, 15
TfR expression, regulation of, 105
Thalamus, activation of, 70
Thy-1 protein expression, iron status and, 106
Thyroid disorders, RLS patients and, 76
Thyroid hormone, rate-limiting enzyme for, dopamine synthesis, 41
Time windows, permissive, 36
Time zone (jet-lag) syndrome, 10
Topiramate (Topamax®), 337
Tourette's syndrome (TS)
  definition of, 153
  RLS and, 271–272
Transcranial magnetic stimulation, 63
Transcriptional–translation loop, circadian autoregulatory, 33
Transferrin (Tf), iron protein complex, example of, 49
Transferrin receptor concentrations, soluble, 161
Transient amnesia, 1
Transient autonomic phenomena, 188
Tremor and PD, 251
Tremor, RLS and, 271
Triazolam, 339
Tricyclic antidepressants (TCA), 256
Trileptal®, 337
Triple flexion, of ankle, knee, and hip, 180
Triple flexion response, 150
Triplet-repeat expansion, RLS and, 270
Tropane ligand, 248
Tryptophan, 339
Tuberoinfundibular and tuberohypophyseal pathways, 21
Twin studies, 117
Tyrosine hydroxylase synthesis, 15, 174

Uremia and RLS, 23, 184

Variance–covariance matrices, 115
Vasopressin (VP), 33
  release, inhibitory modulation of, 21
Venlafaxine, 257
Vertex waves, 2
Vesper's curse, 155, 234
Vigilance tasks, performance on, 129
Visual analog scale (VAS), 39, 277
Visual polysomnogram scoring, 71

Wakefulness
  excess, 125
  stimulating. *See* Dark phase, light exposure during, 37
Wakefulness system, neurotransmitter pathways, 8
Waking alpha rhythm, 130

Zolpidem, 339

Milton Keynes UK
Ingram Content Group UK Ltd.
UKHW050454071024
449327UK00015B/375